ATLAS OF SURGICAL OPERATIONS

ATLAS OF

FOURTH EDITION

SURGICAL OPERATIONS

ROBERT M. ZOLLINGER

M.D., D.Sc. (Hon.), F.A.C.S., F.R.C.S. (Hon.) England and Edinburgh
Emeritus Regents Professor and Chairman of the Department of Surgery, The Ohio State University College of Medicine, and Chief of the Surgical Service, University Hospitals, The Ohio State University; formerly, Assistant Professor of Surgery, Harvard Medical School, and Surgeon at the Peter Bent Brigham Hospital

ROBERT M. ZOLLINGER, Jr.

M.D., F.A.C.S.
Associate Professor of Surgery, Case Western Reserve University School of Medicine and University Hospitals; formerly, Instructor in Surgery, Harvard Medical School and the Peter Bent Brigham Hospital

Illustrations by
CAROL DONNER, MILDRED CODDING,
Paul Fairchild, and William Ollila

Macmillan Publishing Co., Inc.
NEW YORK

Collier Macmillan Canada, Ltd.
TORONTO

Baillière Tindall
LONDON

Copyright © 1975, Macmillan Publishing Co., Inc.

Printed in the United States of America

Earlier editions: *Atlas of Surgical Operations* by Cutler and Zollinger, copyright 1939 and 1949 by Macmillan Publishing Co., Inc.; *Atlas of Surgical Operations,* Vol. I, by Zollinger and Cutler, © 1961 by Macmillan Publishing Co., Inc.; *Atlas of Surgical Operations,* Vol. II, by Zollinger and Zollinger, copyright © 1967 by Macmillan Publishing Co., Inc.

Macmillan Publishing Co., Inc.
866 Third Avenue, New York, New York 10022

Collier Macmillan Canada, Ltd.

Baillière Tindall • London

Library of Congress Cataloging in Publication Data

Zollinger, Robert Milton (date)
    Atlas of surgical operations.

    Previous editions by E. C. Cutler and R. M. Zollinger.
    1. Surgery, Operative—Atlases. I. Zollinger,
Robert Milton (date)   joint author. II. Cutler,
Elliott Carr, 1888–1947. Atlas of surgical operations.
III. Title. [DNLM: 1. Surgery, Operative—Atlases.
WO517 Z84a]
RD41.C8 1975   617'.91   74-23332
ISBN 0-02-431990-2

Printing: 4 5 6 7 8   Year: 8 9 0

TO THE INTERNS AND RESIDENT SURGEONS
OF THE SURGICAL STAFFS OF
THE OHIO STATE UNIVERSITY HOSPITALS, COLUMBUS
THE UNIVERSITY HOSPITALS OF CASE WESTERN RESERVE UNIVERSITY, CLEVELAND
AND THE PETER BENT BRIGHAM HOSPITAL, HARVARD MEDICAL SCHOOL, BOSTON

PREFACE TO THE FOURTH EDITION

The first edition of *Atlas of Surgical Operations* was written with the hope that it would meet the inexperienced young surgeon's need for a concise technical reference on the standard surgical procedures. With subsequent editions, more specialized and less commonly performed procedures were included, as an aid to the established general surgeon who wished to review, often late on the night before surgery, an operation he might have performed only rarely. Although in many cases the procedures that fall into these two categories have changed, the needs of these two readers have continued to serve as guidelines for all decisions on content and presentation in the fourth edition, and in some ways their needs have grown more pressing. Increasingly, the young surgeon finds his period of training being eroded by socioeconomic pressures, and his residency providing not enough direct responsibility for patient care to allow him to develop his surgical expertise. The older general surgeon, perhaps in community practice far from a large medical center, finds himself called upon to perform a procedure under emergency conditions that increased specialization has for some time removed from his repertoire.

The fourth edition of *Atlas of Surgical Operations* combines the two volumes of the third edition, with changes in content to reflect current trends in the field of general surgery. It continues to present in graphic detail the basic surgical procedures that the general surgeon can be expected to perform. Most of these are the "bread and butter" operations that have become largely standardized over the years. However, this body of knowledge must now include new technics not only in gastrointestinal surgery but also in intra-abdominal and sometimes peripheral vascular surgery; consequently the present edition includes new drawings and text on vagotomy, pyloroplasty, enterostomy, tube cecostomy, choledochojejunostomy, splenectomy, resection of abdominal aortic aneurysm, aortofemoral bypass, vena caval interruption, saphenous stripping, and shunting procedures for portal hypertension. Other areas in which the general surgeon must be competent are included in the sections on gynecologic procedures and miscellaneous procedures, covering the various hernia repairs, mastectomies, anorectal procedures, neck surgeries, amputations, minor hand procedures, nerve and tendon repairs, as well as skin grafting. Omitted from this edition are intrathoracic procedures, which have become a well-defined specialty.

Where several procedures exist to achieve the same therapeutic result, we have attempted to include the best established, those that have withstood the test of time. It has not been the intention to champion one procedure over another. The decision to include some and omit others was dictated by the conviction that it is necessary for the young surgeon to be well acquainted with the classic surgical procedures. The inclusion of details that inevitably will be a matter of individual choice has generally been avoided. Suture materials, for instance, are available in such variety that it would be pointless to stipulate specific sutures for each procedure. Throughout the *Atlas*, however, there is constant adherence to the principles of asepsis, careful hemostasis, and a technic that produces the least trauma to organs and tissues.

It is hoped that the return to a single volume will increase the convenience of the *Atlas*. The large-size format has been retained, since it allows reproduction of the illustrations with clarity of detail and provides sufficient space on the opposite page for the accompanying text. As in the past, the text for each procedure includes brief sections on indications for surgery, choice of anesthetic, and pre- and postoperative care, giving the main points of these important aspects of the surgeon's responsibility but not intending to deal with them exhaustively. Again, the three introductory chapters—"Surgical Technic," "Anesthesia," and "Preoperative Preparation and Postoperative Care," revised and updated for this edition, present detailed discussions of these vital topics, while the several plates on surgical anatomy provide further basic reference and review material.

As in the past, the contributions of our colleagues are gratefully acknowledged. Among the many faculty and staff members of The Ohio State University College of Medicine whose opinions and advice were sought, particular thanks are extended to the faculties of the Department of Anesthesiology and the Divisions of Orthopaedics, Plastic Surgery, and Thoracic Surgery. However, our greatest debt is to the members of the Division of General Surgery, whose experience and judgment were indispensable in preparing this new edition of the *Atlas*.

Finally, we must express our gratitude to the artists who have striven for the realistic perspective vital to effective illustrations of surgical procedures. The original drawings for the first edition were made by Miss Mildred Codding, and it is a tribute to her that more than three decades later many of her illustrations have remained unchanged in the present edition. Ms. Carol Donner, having drawn all the illustrations for Volume II of the third edition of the *Atlas*, is responsible for the majority of the plates in the present edition, including all the new drawings. The authors are also grateful to Mr. Paul Fairchild and Mr. William Ollila for their valuable artistic contributions. The editorial assistance of Mrs. Marjorie Barber has enhanced the quality of this edition and is gratefully acknowledged.

ROBERT M. ZOLLINGER, M.D.
ROBERT M. ZOLLINGER, JR., M.D.

CONTENTS

CHAPTER 1 · SURGICAL TECHNIC

Asepsis, hemostasis, and gentleness to tissues are the bases of the surgeon's art. Nevertheless, recent decades have shown a shift in emphasis from the attainment of technical skill to the search for new procedures. Undoubtedly, this attitude resulted from the extraordinary increase in the application of surgical methods to new fields. Such a point of view led to an unremitting search for new procedures when results were unsatisfactory, although faulty technic rather than the procedure itself was the cause of failure. Now that all regions of the body have been explored, it is appropriate to stress the important relationship between the art of surgery and success in surgical therapy. The growing recognition of this relationship should reemphasize the value of precise technic.

The technic described in this book emanates from the school of surgery inspired by William Stewart Halsted. This school, properly characterized as a "school for safety in surgery," arose before surgeons in general recognized the great advantage of anesthesia. Before Halsted's teaching, speed in operating not only was justified as necessary for the patient's safety but also was extolled as a mark of ability. Despite the fact that anesthesia afforded an opportunity for the development of a precise surgical technic that would ensure a minimum of injury to the patient, spectacular surgeons continued to emphasize speedy procedures that disregarded the patient's welfare. Halsted first demonstrated that, with careful hemostasis and gentleness to tissues, an operative procedure lasting as long as four or five hours left the patient in better condition than a similar procedure performed in 30 minutes with the loss of blood and injury to tissues attendant on speed. The protection of each cell with the exquisite care typical of Halsted is a difficult lesson for the young surgeon to learn. The preoperative preparation of the skin, the draping of the patient, the selection of instruments, and even the choice of suture material are not so essential as the manner in which details are executed. Gentleness is essential in the performance of any surgical procedure.

The young surgeon has difficulty in acquiring this point of view, because he is usually taught anatomy, histology, and pathology on tough, dead, chemically fixed tissues by teachers lacking surgical experience. Hence, the student regards tissues as inanimate material that may be handled without concern. He must learn that living cells may be injured by unnecessary handling or dehydration and that they require the surgeon's punctilious care. A review of anatomy, pathology, and associated basic sciences is essential in the young surgeon's daily preparation before he assumes the responsibility of performing a major surgical procedure on his fellow man. The young surgeon is often impressed by the speed of the operator who is interested more in accomplishing a day's work than in teaching the art of surgery. Under such conditions there is little time for consideration of technic, discussion of wound healing, and related basic science aspects of the surgical procedure, or the criticism of results. Wound complications become a distinct problem associated with the operative procedure. If the wound heals, that is enough. A little redness and swelling in and about wounds are taken as a natural course and not as a criticism of what took place in the operating room three to five days previously. Should a wound disrupt, it is a calamity; but how often is the suture material blamed, or the patient's condition, and how seldom does the surgeon inquire into just what did go wrong when the operation took place? Detailed consideration of a common surgical procedure, appendectomy, will serve to illustrate the care necessary to ensure successful results. The patient, an otherwise healthy youth, is anesthetized and wheeled into the operating room. The operating table must be placed where there is maximum illumination and adjusted to present the abdomen and right groin. The patient must be placed so that the site for operation is thrust gently forward. The light must now be focused with due regard for the position of the surgeon and his assistants as well as for the type and depth of the wound. These details must be planned and directed before the skin is disinfected.

Sepsis remains an ever-present threat that requires constant vigilance on the part of the surgeon. The young surgeon must acquire an aseptic conscience and discipline himself to carry out a meticulous hand-scrubbing technic. A knowledge of bacterial flora of the skin and of the proper method of preparing his hands before entering the operating room, and a sustained adherence to a methodical scrub routine are as much a part of the art of surgery as the many other facets that ensure proper wound healing. A cut or burn on the surgeon's hand is as hazardous as the infected scratch on the operative site.

The preoperative preparation of the skin is concerned chiefly with mechanical cleansing. It is important that the patient's skin be shaved immediately before operation, preferably in the operating suite after anesthetization. This eliminates the discomfort to the patient, affords relaxation of the operative site, and is a bacteriologically sound technic. If this is not possible because of the physical arrangement of the operating suite, this preliminary skin preparation should be done with as short a time lapse as possible between shaving and incision, thus preventing contamination of the site by a regrowth of organisms or the possibility of a nick or scratch presenting a source of infection. A stiff lather is developed, and the skin is held taut to present an even, smooth surface as the hair is removed with a sterile, sharp razor. Multiple superficial abrasions and incomplete removal of the hair often result if the skin is not properly shaved with a new blade.

Obviously it is a useless gesture to scrub the skin the night before operation and to send the patient to the operating room with the site of incision covered with a sterile towel. However, some surgeons prefer to carry out a preliminary preparation in elective operations on the joints, hands, feet, and abdominal wall. This involves scrubbing the skin with a cleansing agent several times a day for two or three days before surgery.

In the operating room, after the patient has been properly positioned, the lights adjusted, and the proper plane of anesthesia reached, the final preparation of the operative site is begun. The first assistant scrubs, puts on sterile gloves, and completes the mechanical cleansing of the operative site with sponges saturated in the desired solution. Sterile towels are placed at the upper and lower limits of the operative field to wall off the unsterile drapes. The contemplated site of incision is scrubbed first; the remainder of the field is cleansed with concentric strokes until all of the exposed area has been covered. The skin should appear flushed, indicating that the desquamating epithelium has been thoroughly removed and the germicides are effective. As with all tinctures and alcohols used in skin preparation, caution must be observed to prevent skin blisters caused by puddling of solutions at the patient's side or about skin creases. Some surgeons prefer to paint the skin with an iodine-containing solution or a similar preparation. Some mark the extent of the incision by scratching the skin several times before the anatomic landmarks are covered by drapes or the lines of skin cleavage fixed or distorted by an adherent plastic drape. These hatchmarks aid in the proper reapproximation of the skin at the time of closure. The folded edges of sterile towels are then clipped to the skin, leaving 1 to 2 cm. of skin exposed at either side of the scratch, so that the relatively unsterile surface of the operative field is excluded from the vicinity of the incision. These towels also serve to limit contact of extruding viscera with irritating disinfectants, thereby preventing an insult to delicate tissues.

A transparent sterile plastic drape may be substituted for the skin towels in covering the skin, avoiding the necessity for towel clips through the skin at the corners of the field. The plastic is made directly adherent to the skin by a bacteriostatic adhesive. After application of the drape, the incision is made directly through the material, and the plastic remains in place until the procedure is completed. When, for cosmetic reasons, the incision must accurately follow the lines of skin cleavage, the surgeon gently outlines the incision before the adhesive plastic drape is applied. The addition of the plastic to the drape ensures a wide field that is, surgically, completely sterile, instead of surgically clean as the prepared skin is considered. At the same time the plastic layer prevents contamination should the large drape sheet become soaked or torn.

Superficial malignancies, as in the case of cancer of the breast, lip, or neck, present a problem in that routine mechanical scrub is too traumatic. Malignant cells may be massaged free into the blood stream in this way. Following a gentle lather and shave, a germicidal solution should be applied carefully. Similarly, the burned patient must have special skin preparation. In addition to the extreme tissue sensitivity, many times gross soil, grease, and other contaminants are present. Copious flushing of the burned areas with isotonic solutions is important as mechanical cleansing is carried out with a nonirritating detergent. Germicides of an irritating nature are obviously taboo.

Injuries such as the crushed hand or the open fracture require extreme care, and meticulous attention to skin preparation must be observed. The hasty, inadequate preparation of such emergency surgery can have disastrous consequences. A nylon bristle brush and a detergent are used to scrub the area thoroughly for several minutes. A wide area around the wound edges is then shaved. Copious irrigation is essential after the scrub and shave, followed by a single application of a germicide. An antibacterial sudsing cleanser may be useful for cleansing the contaminated greasy skin of the hands or about traumatic wounds.

Heavy suture materials, regardless of type, are not desirable. Fine silk, cotton, synthetics, or catgut should be used routinely. Every surgeon has his own preference for suture material, and new types are constantly developed. Fine silk is most suitable for sutures and ligatures because it engenders a minimum of tissue reaction, even in potentially infected wounds, and prevents secondary hemorrhage when securely knotted. If a surgeon's knot is laid down and tightened, the ligature will not slip when the tension on the silk is released. A square knot then can be laid down to secure the ligature, which is cut close to the knot. The knots are set by applying tension on the ligature between a finger held beyond the knot in such a plane that the finger, the knot, and the hand are in a straight line. However, it takes long practice to set the first knot and run down the setting, or final knot, without holding the threads taut. This detail of technic is of great importance, for it is impossible to ligate under tension when handling delicate tissue or when working in the depths of a wound. It is important when tying vessels caught in a hemostat that the side of the jaws of the hemostat away from the vessel be presented so that as little tissue as possible be included in the tie. Moreover, the hemostat should be released just as the first knot is tightened, the tie sliding down on tissue not already devitalized by the clamp. One-handed knots and rapidly thrown knots are unreliable. Each knot is of vital importance in the success of an operation that threatens the patient's life.

Some surgeons prefer electrocoagulation to control smaller bleeders rather than ligatures.

As the wound is deepened, exposure is obtained by retraction. If the procedure is to be prolonged, the use of a self-retaining retractor is advantageous, since it ensures constant exposure without fatiguing the assistants. Moreover, the constant shifting of a retractor held by an assistant not only perturbs the surgeon but also stimulates the sensory nerves unless the anesthesia is deep. Whenever a self-retaining retractor is adjusted, the amount of tissue compression must be judged carefully because excessive compression may cause necrosis. Difficulty in obtaining adequate exposure is not always a matter of retraction. Unsatisfactory anesthesia, faulty position of the patient, improper illumination, inadequate and improperly placed incision, and failure to use instruments instead of hands are factors to be considered when visibility is poor.

Handling tissues with fingers cannot be as facile, gentle, or safe as handling with properly designed, delicate instruments. Instruments can be sterilized, while rubber gloves offer the danger that a needle prick may pass unnoticed and contamination may occur. Moreover, the use of instruments keeps hands out of the wound, thus allowing a full view of the field and affording perspective, which is an aid to safety.

After gentle retraction of the skin and subcutaneous tissue to avoid stripping, the fascia is incised in line with its own fibers; jagged edges must be avoided to permit accurate reapproximation. The underlying muscle fibers of the internal oblique and transversalis may be separated longitudinally with the handle of the knife. Blood vessels are divided between hemostats and ligated. Because of the friability of muscle, immediate transfixion and ligation are desirable. After hemostasis is satisfactory, the muscle is protected from trauma and contamination by moist gauze pads. Retractors may now be placed to bring the peritoneum into view.

With toothed forceps the operator seizes and lifts the peritoneum. The assistant grasps the peritoneum near the apex of the tent, while the surgeon releases his hold. This maneuver is repeated until the surgeon is certain that only peritoneum free of intra-abdominal tissue is included in the bite of the forceps. A small incision is made between the forceps with a scalpel. This opening is enlarged with scissors by inserting the lower tip of the scissors beneath the peritoneum for 1 cm. and by tenting the peritoneum over the blade before cutting it. If the omentum does not fall away from the peritoneum, the corner of a moist sponge may be placed over it as a guard for the scissors. The incision should be made only as long as that in the muscle, since peritoneum stretches easily with retraction, and closure is greatly facilitated if the entire peritoneal opening is easily visualized. When the incision of the peritoneum is completed, retractors can then be placed to give the optimum view of the abdominal contents. The subcutaneous fat should be protected from possible contamination by sterile pads or a plastic wound protector. If the appendix or cecum is not apparent immediately, the wound may be shifted about with the retractors until these structures are located.

Although it is customary to wall off the intestines from the cecal region by several moist sponges, we are convinced that the less material introduced into the peritoneal cavity the better. Even moist gauze injures the delicate superficial cells, which thereafter present a point of possible adhesion to another area as well as less of a barrier to bacteria. The appendix is then delivered into the wound, and its blood supply is investigated, the strategic attack in surgery always being directed toward control of the blood supply. The blood vessels lying in the mesentery are more elastic than their supporting tissue and tend to retract; therefore, in ligating such vessels it is best to transfix the mesentery with a curved needle, avoiding injury to the vessels. The vessel may be safely divided between securely tied ligatures, and the danger of its slipping out of a hemostat while being ligated is eliminated. The appendix is removed by the technic depicted in a later chapter, and the cecum is replaced in the abdominal cavity. Closure begins with a search for sponges, needles, and instruments until a correct count is obtained. In reapproximating the peritoneum, a continuous catgut suture or interrupted silk sutures are used to evert the edges of the peritoneum. Successive bites of these sutures should include both the peritoneum and the transversalis fascia, thus ensuring the reapproximation of a

large area of peritoneum reinforced by the strong layer of transversalis fascia.

With the peritoneum closed, the muscles fall together naturally, unless they were widely separated. Several loosely tied sutures may be placed to reapproximate, but not strangle, gaping muscles. The fascia overlying the muscles must, however, be carefully reapproximated with interrupted sutures.

Coaptation of the subcutaneous tissues is essential for a satisfactory cosmetic result. Well-approximated subcutaneous tissues permit the early removal of skin sutures and thus prevent the formation of a wide scar. Subcutaneous sutures are placed with a curved needle, large bites being taken so that the wound is mounded upward and the skin edges are almost reapproximated. The sutures must be located so that both longitudinal and cross-sectional reapproximation is accurate. Overlapping or gaping of the skin at the ends of the wound may be avoided readily by care in suturing the subcutaneous layer.

The skin edges are brought together by interrupted sutures. If the subcutaneous tissues have been sutured properly, the skin sutures may be removed on the fifth to seventh postoperative day, resulting in a fine white line as the ultimate scar. The skin may be approximated by multiple adhesive strips.

Finally, there must be proper dressing and support for the wound. If the wound is closed *per primam* and the procedure has been "clean," the wound should be sealed off, since for at least 48 hours it may be contaminated from without. This may be done with either a dry sponge dressing or a plastic spray dressing.

The time and method of removing skin sutures are important. In the ideal wound closure the approximation of the subcutaneous tissue should be so accurate that the skin sutures can be tied without tension and merely serve to hold the lips of the wound in apposition.

Lack of tension on skin sutures and their early removal, by the fifth to seventh day, eliminate unsightly crosshatching. In other parts of the body, such as the face and neck, the sutures may be removed in 48 hours if the approximation has been satisfactory. When tension sutures are used, the length of time the sutures remain depends entirely on the cause for their use; when the patients are elderly or cachectic or suffer from chronic cough, such sutures may be necessary for as long as 10 to 12 days. A variety of protective devices may be used over which these tension sutures can be tied so as to prevent the sutures from cutting into the skin.

The method of removing sutures is important and is designed to avoid contaminating a clean wound with skin bacteria. At the time of removal the surgeon grasps the loose end of the thread, lifts the knot away from the skin by pulling out a little of the suture from beneath the epidermis, cuts the suture at a point that was beneath the skin, and pulls the suture free. Thus, no part of a suture that was on the outside of the skin will be drawn into the subcutaneous tissues to cause an infection in the wound. The importance of using aseptic technic in removing sutures and subsequent dressing under proper conditions cannot be overemphasized. Adhesive paper strips properly applied can make skin sutures unnecessary in many areas.

The example of the characteristics of a technic that permits the tissues to heal with the greatest rapidity and strength and that conserves all the normal cells demonstrates that the surgeon's craftsmanship is of major importance to the patient's safety. It emphasizes the fact that technical surgery is an art, which is properly expressed only when the surgeon is aware of its inherent dangers. The same principles underlie the simplest as well as the most serious and extensive operative procedure. The young surgeon who learns the basic precepts of asepsis, hemostasis, adequate exposure, and gentleness to tissues has mastered his most difficult lessons. Moreover, once the surgeon has acquired this attitude, his progress will continue, for he will be led to a histologic study of wounds, where the real lessons of wound healing are strikingly visualized. He will also be led to a constant search for better instruments until he emerges finally as an artist, not an artisan.

The surgeon unaccustomed to this form of surgery will be annoyed by the constant emphasis on gentleness and the time-consuming technic of innumerable interrupted sutures. However, if the surgeon is entirely honest, and if he wishes to close all his clean wounds *per primam*, thus contributing to his patient's comfort and safety, he must utilize all the principles that have been outlined. He must use fine suture material—so fine that it breaks when such strain is put on it as will cut through living tissue. He must tie each vessel securely so that the critically important vessel will always be controlled. He must practice asepsis. All this is largely a matter of conscience. To those who risk the lives of others daily, it is a chief concern.

CHAPTER II · ANESTHESIA

Anesthesiology as a special field of endeavor has made clear the many physiologic changes occurring in the patient under anesthesia. The pharmacologic effects of anesthetic agents and technics on the central nervous system and cardiovascular and respiratory systems are better understood. New drugs have been introduced for inhalation, intravenous, spinal, and regional anesthesia. In addition, drugs, such as muscle relaxants and hypotensive drugs, are used for their specific pharmacologic effect. Older anesthetic technics, such as spinal and caudal, have been improved by the refinement of the continuous technic and more accurate methods of controlling the distribution of the administered drug. The areas of marked advances in anesthesia have been in pulmonary, cardiac, pediatric, and geriatric surgery. Improved management of airway and pulmonary ventilation is reflected in the technics and equipment available to prevent the deleterious effects of hypoxia and hypercarbia. An increased understanding of the altered hemodynamics produced by anesthesia in the ill patient has resulted in better fluid, electrolyte, and blood replacement preoperatively in the patient with a decreased blood volume and electrolyte imbalance. This has prevented to a great extent the periods of hypotension previously seen in these patients.

The surgeon, realizing it is impossible to have expert knowledge in all surgical specialties, also realizes that he cannot divorce himself completely from the fundamentals of these other specialities. Although the number of anesthesiologists has increased greatly within recent years, it still is not enough to meet the increased surgical load. The surgeon, therefore, may find that he has to rely upon his untrained colleagues or nurses to administer anesthesia. He must bear in mind that in the absence of a trained anesthesiologist he is legally accountable for the actions of the individual conducting the anesthesia. Under these circumstances the surgeon should limit his choice of anesthetic agents and technics and familiarize himself thoroughly with their indications and complications. Although such caution may occasionally deprive a patient of the benefit of a more physiologic anesthetic agent or technic, this theoretic advantage is outweighed by the surgeon's lack of familiarity with this particular agent or technic. Further, he should familiarize himself with the condition of the patient under anesthesia by observing the color of blood or viscera, the rapidity and strength of the arterial pulsation, and the effort and rhythm of the chest wall or diaphragmatic respirations. Knowing the character of these conditions under a well-conducted anesthesia, he will be able to readily diagnose a patient who is not doing well under anesthesia.

It is this point of view that has caused us to present in this practical volume the following short outline of modern anesthetic principles. This outline makes no pretense of covering fully the physiologic, pharmacologic, and technical details of anesthesiology; but it offers to the surgeon some basic important information.

GENERAL CONSIDERATIONS. The role of the anesthesiologist as a member of the surgical team is threefold: to assure adequate pulmonary ventilation, to maintain a near-normal cardiovascular system, and to conduct the anesthetic procedure itself. One cannot be isolated from the other, and if there is any question as to the anesthesiologist's ability to handle either the patient's pulmonary ventilation or to maintain a near-normal cardiovascular system, then the patient should not receive general anesthesia.

Preventing the subtle effects of hypoxia is the anesthesiologist's most important function. It is well known that severe hypoxia may cause sudden disaster and that hypoxia of a moderate degree may result in slower but equally disastrous consequences. Hypoxia during anesthesia is related directly to some interference with the patient's ability to exchange oxygen. This commonly is caused by allowing the patient's tongue to partially or completely obstruct the upper airway. Foreign bodies, vomitus, profuse secretions, or laryngeal spasm may also cause obstruction of the upper airway. Of these, aspiration of vomitus represents the greatest hazard to the patient. General anesthesia should not be administered in those patients likely to have a full stomach until adequate protection of the airway is assured by the insertion, under topical anesthesia, of a cuffed endotracheal tube. Other conditions known to produce a severe state of hypoxia, but not directly under the anesthesiologist's control, are congestive heart failure, pulmonary edema, asthma, or masses in the neck and mediastinum compressing the trachea. Almost all the aforementioned hazards can be avoided or lessened by having a technically competent individual administering the anesthesia. In addition, one member of the surgical team should be capable of performing endotracheal intubation. This will reduce the possibility of the patient's asphyxiating even though the endotracheal tube is not always a guarantee of a perfect airway.

Before commencing any general anesthetic technic, even open drop ether, facilities must be available to perform positive pressure oxygen breathing, and suction must be available to remove secretions and vomitus from the airway before, during, and after the surgical procedure. Every effort should be expended to perform an adequate tracheobronchial and oropharyngeal cleansing after the surgical procedure, and the airway should be kept free of secretion and vomitus until the protective reflexes return. With the patient properly positioned and observed, all these procedures will help to reduce the incidence of postoperative pulmonary complications.

Fluid therapy during the operative procedure is a joint responsibility of the surgeon and the anesthesiologist. Except in unusual circumstances, anemia, hemorrhage, and shock should be treated by preoperative blood transfusions. During operation transfusions should be used with caution, avoiding whenever possible the use of only one unit of blood for a 500-ml. blood loss. Most patients can withstand this amount of blood loss without difficulty. However, in operative procedures known to require several units of blood, the blood should be replaced as lost and the amount transfused should equal or exceed slightly the amount lost as estimated from the quantity of blood within the operative field, the operative drapes, and the measured sponges and suction bottles. In emergency situations when whole blood is not available, dextran, albumin, or plasma may be administered to maintain an adequate expansion of blood volume. Plasma, unless it is properly processed, is used with caution because of the possibility of transmitting homologous serum hepatitis. Infusions of Ringer's lactate (a balanced electrolyte solution), via a secure and accessible intravenous needle or catheter, should be used during all operative procedures including those in pediatrics. Such an arrangement allows the anesthesiologist to have ready access to the cardiovascular system and thereby a means of treating hypotension promptly.

Anesthesia in the aged patient is associated with an increased morbidity and mortality. Degenerative diseases of the pulmonary and cardiovascular systems are prominent, with the individual less likely to withstand minor insults to either system. Sedatives and narcotics should be used sparingly both in the pre- and postoperative periods. Regional or local anesthesia should be employed in this age group whenever feasible. This form of anesthesia decreases the possibility of serious pulmonary and cardiovascular system complications and at the same time decreases the possibility of serious mental disturbance that can occur following general anesthesia. Induction and maintenance of anesthesia can be made smoother by good preoperative preparation of the respiratory tract by means of positive pressure aerosol therapy and bronchodilators. A detailed cardiac history in preoperative workup will uncover patients with borderline cardiac failure, coronary insufficiency, or valvular disease that require specialized drug treatment and monitoring.

More patients with endocrine disturbances, such as diabetes and adrenal disease, either primary or iatrogenic in origin, are requiring surgery. Local, regional, and spinal anesthesia produce minimal changes in these patients' already disturbed physiology. However, these patients tolerate a well-conducted general anesthesia with any of the commonly used agents if their steroid, insulin, or vasoactive drug therapy is properly managed.

For most adult patients induction of general anesthesia is more pleasant if small doses of thiopental sodium are given intravenously. This provides a rapid induction and eliminates entirely the excitement stage often seen during ether induction. Although thiopental sodium can be used as an anesthetic agent by itself, it is preferable to combine it with nitrous oxide and oxygen in 50 per cent concentration. This reduces the amount of thiopental sodium required and increases the amount of oxygen available to the patients.

Muscle relaxants such as succinyl or curare should be used for those operations requiring muscular looseness if it is not provided by the anesthetic agent. By the use of these drugs adequate muscular relaxation can be obtained in a lighter plane of anesthesia, thereby avoiding the myocardial and peripheral circulatory depression observed in the deeper planes of anesthesia. In addition, the protective reflexes, such as coughing, return more quickly if light planes of anesthesia are maintained. Finally, however, it is important to note that the mycin-derivative antibiotics may interact with curare-like drugs so as to prolong their effect with resultant insufficient spontaneous respiration in the recovery area.

Pediatric surgery in most instances requires the use of general anesthesia. Equipment and technics in recent years have been refined with particular attention directed to assuring adequate pulmonary exchange with minimal resistance and dead space. A sound understanding of the mechanical function of the new equipment and the physiologic principles involved in applying the new technics is essential before clinical experience in their use is undertaken. Therefore, to the anesthesiologist or physician doing occasional pediatric anesthesia, open-drop ether with oxygen insufflation under the mask is still the safest form of anesthesia. Realization of the importance of fluid, electrolyte, and blood replacement has greatly reduced morbidity and mortality. Another problem confronting the anesthesiologist is the lack of integrated control of the central nervous system, which is reflected in the child's poor temperature regulation, irregular respirations, and increased responsiveness of the cardiovascular system to autonomic stimuli. However, means of monitoring and controlling the temperature, the respirations, and the cardiovascular system in pediatric anesthesia mark a great advance in this field. The psychologic disturbances likely to occur following anesthesia and surgery are circumvented by the administration of adequate preoperative sedation consisting of belladonna and a narcotic in doses according to age, weight, and body build.

The patient's position is an important factor both during and after operation. The operating table should be so placed that the benefit of natural lighting is made available to the surgeon whenever possible. The patient should be placed in a position that allows gravity to aid in obtaining optimal exposure. The most effective position for any procedure is the one that causes the viscera to gravitate away from the operative field. Proper position on the table allows adequate anatomic exposure without traumatic retraction and without the use of massive abdominal packs. With good muscular relaxation and an unobstructed airway, the use of exaggerated positions and prolonged elevation of rests becomes unnecessary. The surgeon should bear in mind that extreme positions result in embarrassed respiration, in harmful circulatory responses, and in nerve palsies. When the surgical procedure is concluded, the patient should be returned gradually to the horizontal supine position; sufficient time should be allowed for the circulatory system to become stabilized. When an extreme position is used, elastic extremity wrapping should be applied, and the patient should be returned to the normal position in several stages, with a rest period between each one. Abrupt changes in position or rough handling of the patient may result in unexpected circulatory collapse. After he is returned to bed, the patient should be watched closely until the circulation is stabilized.

In any surgical practice occasions arise in which the anesthesiologist should refuse or postpone the administration of anesthesia. Serious thought should be given before anesthesia is commenced in cases of severe pulmonary insufficiency; elective surgery in the patient with myocardial infarction less than six months prior; severe unexplained anemia; inadequately treated shock; in patients who recently have been or are still on certain drugs such as cortisone, chlorpromazine hydrochloride, and other tranquilizers incompatible with safe anesthesia; and finally, in any case in which the anesthesiologist feels he will be unable to manage the patient's airway, such as Ludwig's angina, or when there are large masses in the neck and mediastinum compressing the trachea.

When the maximum safe dosages of local anesthetic agents are exceeded, the incidence of toxic reactions increases. These reactions, which are related to the concentration of the local anesthetic agent in the blood, may be classified as either central nervous system stimulation, i.e., nervousness, sweating and convulsions, or central nervous system depression, i.e., drowsiness and coma. Either type of reaction may lead to circulatory collapse and respiratory failure. Resuscitative equipment consisting of positive pressure oxygen, intravenous fluids, vasopressors, and an intravenous barbiturate should be readily available during all operative procedures performed under local anesthesia. The quality of intensity of anesthesia produced by the local anesthetic agents depends on the concentration of the agent and on the size of the nerve. As the size of the nerve to be anesthetized increases, a higher concentration of anesthetic agent is utilized. Since the maximum safe dose of procaine is 1 Gm., it is wise, therefore, to use 0.5 per cent procaine when large volumes are needed. A 2 per cent solution of procaine should be reserved for nerve blocks.

The duration of anesthesia can be prolonged by the addition of epinephrine to the local anesthetic solution. Although this prolongs the anesthetic effect and also reduces the incidence of toxic reactions, the use of epinephrine is not without danger. Its concentration should not exceed 1:100,000, i.e., 1 ml. of 1:1,000 solution in 100 ml. of local anesthetic agent. After the operative procedure has been completed and the vasoconstrictive effect of the epinephrine has worn off, bleeding may occur in the wound if meticulous attention to hemostasis has not been observed. If the anesthetic is to be injected into the digits, epinephrine should not be added because of the possibility of producing gangrene by occlusive spasm of these end arteries that have not collaterals. Epinephrine is also contraindicated if the patient has hypertension, arteriosclerosis, or coronary or myocardial disease.

CARDIAC STANDSTILL. Cessation of effective cardiac activity is likely to occur at any time during an anesthetic or operative procedure performed under local or general anesthesia. Many etiologic factors have been cited as producing cardiac standstill; however, acute or prolonged hypoxia is undoubtedly the most common cause. In a few instances undiagnosed cardiovascular disease, such as severe aortic stenosis or myocardial infarction, has been the cause of cardiac standstill. Many sudden cardiac standstills related to anesthetic technic or judgment have been preceded by warning signs long before the castastrophe actually occurred. The anesthetic factors commonly indicated as leading to cardiac standstill are overdosage of anesthetic agents, either in total amount of drug or speed of administration; prolonged and unrecognized partial respiratory obstruction; inadequate blood replacement; delay in treating hypotension; aspiration of stomach contents; and failure to maintain a constant vigilance over the anesthetized patient's cardiovascular system. The last factor is being minimized by the use of the precordial or intraesophageal stethoscope, or continuous ECG on an operating room oscilloscope, or by the various electronic devices for monitoring arterial pressure and cardiac activity.

Mortality and morbidity from cardiac standstill can be minimized further by having all members of the surgical team trained in the immediate treatment of this condition. Successful treatment of cardiac standstill depends upon immediate diagnosis and the institution of therapy without hesitation. Diagnosis is established tentatively by the absence of the pulse and blood pressure as recognized by the anesthesiologist and confirmed by the surgeon's palpating the arteries or observing the absence of bleeding in the operative field. It is imperative that external cardiac compression and the establishment of a clear and unobstructed airway be instituted immediately. Intravenous administration of sodium bicarbonate, glucose, or calcium may be appropriate. If adequate circulation is being produced, a pulse should be palpable in the carotid and brachial artery. Oxygenated blood being circulated through the coronary arteries by external compression will be sufficient many times to start a heart in asystole, and intravenous or intracardiac injection of epinephrine should be utilized. If the heart is fibrillating, it should be defibrillated only after adequate oxygenation of the myocardium. Defibrillation may be accomplished by electrical direct current, which is the preferred method. If all of these resuscitative measures are unsuccessful, then thoracotomy with direct cardiac compression or defibrillation may be considered in an equipped and staffed operating room setting.

The treatment of a patient revived after a cardiopulmonary arrest is directed toward maintaining an adequate cardiopulmonary ventilation and perfusion and toward preventing specific organ injuries such as acute renal tubular necrosis or cerebral edema. This may involve vasoactive drugs, steroids, diuretics, or hypothermia.

CHOICE OF ANESTHESIA. The anesthesiologist's skill is the most important factor in the choice of anesthesia. The anesthesiologist should select the drugs and methods with which he has had the greatest experience. In most instances the effects of drugs used in anesthesia depend to a great degree upon skilled administration. The effects of the drugs are modified by speed of administration, total dose, the interaction of various drugs used, and the technic of the individual anesthesiologist. These factors are far more important than the theoretical effects of the drugs based on responses elicited in animals. With anesthetic agents reported to have produced hepatocellular damage, certain precautions should be observed. This is particularly important in patients who have been administered halogenated anesthetic agents in the recent past or who give a history suggestive of hepatic dysfunction following a previous anesthetic exposure. Further, the halogenated anesthetic agents should be used cautiously in patients whose occupations expose them to hepatocellular toxins or who are having biliary tract surgery.

The proposed operation must be considered: its site, magnitude, and duration, the amount of blood loss to be expected, and the position of the patient on the operating table. The patient should then be studied to ascertain his ability to tolerate the surgical procedure and the anesthetic. Important factors are the patient's age, weight, and general condition as well as the presence of acute infection, toxemia, dehydration, and hypovolemia.

The patient's previous experience and prejudices regarding anesthesia should be considered. Some patients dread losing consciousness, fearing that they will never awaken; others wish for oblivion. Some patients, or their friends, have had unfortunate experiences with spinal anesthesia and are violently opposed to it. An occasional individual may be sensitive to local anesthetics or may have had a prolonged bout of vomiting following ether anesthesia. Whenever possible, the patient's preference regarding the choice of anesthesia should be followed. If his choice is contraindicated, the reason should be explained carefully, and the preferred procedure should be outlined in such a way as to remove his fears. If local or spinal anesthesia is selected, psychic disturbance will be minimized and the anesthetic made more effective if it is preceded by adequate premedication.

Combinations of drugs, formerly considered unwise, now constitute safer anesthesia than a single agent. For example, morphine and scopolamine may be used for premedication. The patient may be rendered unconscious by the intravenous administration of thiopental sodium, light anesthesia then being maintained by cyclopropane and oxygen with a small amount of ether. Muscular relaxation may be obtained by the intravenous administration of muscle relaxants, and after the peritoneum is closed the depth of anesthesia is reduced by changing to nitrous oxide and oxygen.

PRELIMINARY MEDICATION. The patient is visited by the anesthesiologist on the day before operation. The anesthesiologist should acquaint himself with the patient's condition and the proposed operation. He must evaluate personally the patient's physical and psychic state, and he should, at this time, inquire about the patient's previous anesthetic experience and about drug sensitivity. He should question the patient about drugs that he has taken at home and be sure that medicines that require continued administration, such as digitalis or insulin, are continued. Further inquiry should be made concerning drugs (such as corticosteroid drugs, antihypertensive drugs, and tranquilizers) that are potentially incompatible or dangerous if general anesthesia is contemplated. If the patient is taking any of these drugs, proper precautions should be taken to prevent an unsatisfactory anesthetic and surgical procedure.

Preoperative medication is an essential part of the anesthetic procedure. The choice of premedication depends on the anesthetic to be used. Dosage should vary with the patient's age, physical state, and psychic condition. Premedication should remove apprehension, reduce the metabolic rate, and raise the threshold to pain. Upon arriving in the operating suite, the patient should be unconcerned and placid. If a general anesthetic is to be administered, a sedative or narcotic plus atropine or scopolamine should be given subcutaneously one hour before the patient is brought to the operating suite. Although there is some evidence that barbiturates are preferable for premedication, meperidine hydrochloride is our drug of choice. The average healthy patient should receive 100 mg. of merperidine hypodermically. The dose should be reduced for aged and very sick individuals. For very apprehensive individuals 100 mg. of pentobarbital sodium should be administered hypodermically in addition to the merperidine. Atropine and scopolamine prevent increased buccal and bronchial secretions and reduce the vagal effect upon the heart. Scopolamine also produces amnesia and is used in preference to atropine in all individuals except those at the extremes of age. If local or regional anesthesia is used, a barbiturate should be given for premedication, since it tends to reduce the incidence and severity of reactions to local anesthetic drugs.

THE USE OF ANESTHESIA RECORDS. The patient's physical condition should be observed continuously and evaluated during every surgical procedure. Observations of pulse, blood pressure, and respiration should be noted on the record at frequent intervals. The amount of blood loss, the type and quantity of fluids administered, and remarks regarding the patient's condition also should be recorded. The anesthetic drugs, their doses, and the methods used should be noted. The record should be started before the anesthetic is administered, and each observation should be recorded as it is made throughout the procedure. The anesthetic record, in addition to the front sheet shown in **Figure 1**, should contain data on the patient's preoperative condition and his previous operations and responses to anesthetic agents. Space should be available for making postoperative

notes regarding anesthetic or other complications. Study of the anesthetic record contributes greatly to a full understanding of the management of the patient.

ANESTHETICS RECOMMENDED IN SPECIAL FIELDS

I. Neurologic surgery
  A. Intracranial procedures
    1. For cooperative patients, local infiltration with anesthesia monitoring available to monitor vital signs and administer required drugs.
    2. When unconsciousness is desirable, endotracheal anesthesia is preferred for management of ventilation. A nonexplosive anesthetic is required consisting of balanced anesthesia or nitrous oxide and halothane.
  B. Spinal procedures
    1. In the prone position an endotracheal tube assures a patent airway if general anesthesia is required. There is no special indication for any particular agent.
    2. Local infiltration.
  C. Operations on the peripheral nervous system. There are no special indications other than suiting the anesthetic to the disease and the condition of the patient.
II. Thyroid surgery
  A. The maintenance of a patent airway is often difficult during thyroid surgery. The use of an endotracheal tube is recommended.
  B. For toxic or very apprehensive individuals, adequate preoperative sedation should be given. Additional medication can be given intravenously, if needed, after the patient has arrived in the operating room.
  C. Special risk patients. If tracheal compression or deviation exists, endotracheal intubation is mandatory for the prevention of respiratory obstruction during the surgical procedure.
III. Thoracic surgery
  A. Chest wall
    1. Breast. No special indication; deep anesthesia and muscle relaxation are unnecessary.
    2. Empyema
      a. Local infiltration with anesthesia monitoring.
      b. If general anesthesia is desired, a high concentration of oxygen should be provided.
    3. Collapse procedures for tuberculosis
      a. Endotracheal intubation should be performed so that secretions may be easily and promptly removed from the trachea and bronchi by means of a suction catheter passed through the tube.
      b. Intercostal nerve block and local infiltration. These may be supplemented by thiopental sodium and nitrous oxide and oxygen. If the patient loses consciousness, respiratory problems may occur as with general anesthesia.
  B. Pulmonary surgery. The anesthesiologist must maintain adequate pulmonary ventilation. Endotracheal intubation should be used in almost all cases, and special intubations, as with a Carlen's tube, should be possible. The management of the patient during open chest surgery requires the greatest degree of skill and knowledge.
  C. Cardiac surgery. The special considerations of modern cardiac surgery are too complex to be discussed in this work.
IV. Abdominal surgery
  A. Upper abdominal
    1. Profound muscular relaxation must be provided, and muscle relaxants are used for this purpose. Assisted or controlled respiration must be used. Endotracheal intubation ordinarily makes the anesthesiologist's task easier and provides more satisfactory working conditions for the surgeon.
    2. Spinal or continuous spinal anesthesia. Nausea is reduced and the patient's comfort is increased if small amounts of a barbiturate are administered intravenously from time to time. The surgeon must be very gentle in his handling of the viscera, in order to avoid traction reflexes.
  B. Lower abdominal. The requirements in this area are similar to those for upper abdominal work but are less in degree. The doses of drugs used may be reduced.
  C. Poor-risk patients
    1. Local infiltration or intercostal block. The usefulness of these procedures is limited ordinarily to simple palliative operations such as gastrostomy or colostomy. For more extensive work, a splanchnic nerve block should be performed in addition. Utmost gentleness in the handling of the viscera is imperative if the patient is to tolerate the procedure.
    2. If general anesthesia is desired, reduction in the dose of drugs and slow careful administration are necessary for safety. More extensive definitive surgery can be carried out.

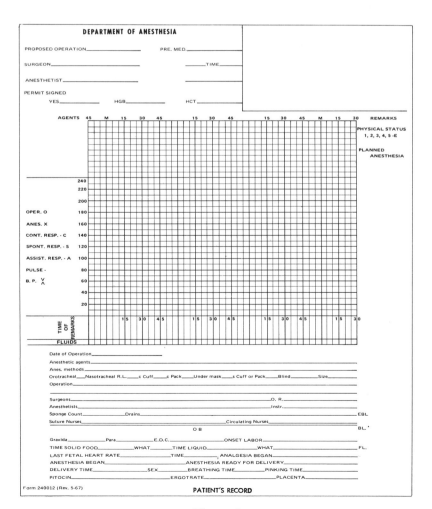

Figure 1

V. Perineal procedures
  A. Urologic surgery is well tolerated by aged individuals when done under low spinal anesthesia.
  B. Gynecologic surgery. No special indication.
VI. Surgery of the extremities
  A. General anesthesia. No special consideration.
  B. Brachial plexus block is often desirable for surgery of the upper extremity.
  C. Spinal anesthesia is often desirable for surgery of the lower extremity.
  D. Local infiltration is often desirable for procedures of lesser magnitude.
  E. Refrigeration is often suitable for amputations in poor-risk patients.

CHAPTER III · PREOPERATIVE PREPARATION AND POSTOPERATIVE CARE

For centuries the surgeon's chief training was in anatomy, almost to the exclusion of other aspects of his art. Only in the twentieth century have the increasing scope of surgery and the unremitting efforts of its leaders to reduce the number of deaths and complications to a minimum led inevitably to the realization that a sound understanding of physiology is of equal importance to thorough grounding in anatomic relationships. This, in turn, has created intense interest in the preoperative and postoperative care of the patient and scientific methods to restore him to a normal physiologic state and maintain him in physiologic equilibrium.

The modern surgeon, therefore, is concerned not only with the proper technical conduct of an operative procedure, but also with all of the problems created by illness in the patient as a whole. He must try to bring the patient to operation in physiologic balance—the food reserves in their normal state, the intestines working normally, the respiratory tract free from infection, the circulation at its optimum efficiency, and the nervous system as undisturbed and peaceful as in daily life. The fact that this often appears to be an unattainable ideal must not deter the surgeon from striving constantly for its realization.

Only 50 years ago it was customary to deny not only the patient awaiting colon surgery but all patients food and water for a day or more before the surgical ordeal, and to purge them routinely. This was based on the assumption that postoperative vomiting and distention were less likely to occur when the intestines were empty. The potential dangers of dehydration and starvation were not understood; nor were tests available to determine the levels of the normal constituents of blood serum. Measures of circulatory efficiency, blood volume, and accurate fluid and electrolyte balance had not been established. The surgeon of today is much better equipped for assaying the patient's physiologic status, and he devotes himself to correcting the abnormalities that he detects.

On the other hand, there is little doubt that sins of commission may be just as unfortunate as sins of omission. It is often noted that a healthy person who suddenly becomes the victim of an accident, and who requires immediate operation without preparation, frequently suffers a minimum of postoperative discomfort. It is likewise well recognized that a long period of hospitalization before surgery, particularly if it involves rest in bed, may be undesirable. The fact that a patient with a simple hernia can tolerate with impunity a preoperative regimen involving a change in diet, enemas, and rest in bed does not justify the unnecessary use of such preparation.

The surgeon should remember that the body spontaneously endeavors to adjust to the physical vicissitudes by which man is beset, and he should attempt to assist the natural physiologic processes rather than arbitrarily impose therapy without reference to the fundamental physiologic reactions of the body.

PREOPERATIVE PREPARATION. Preoperative care properly begins with the family physician. His responsibilities include "oral and respiratory prophylaxis," i.e., the ordering of dental care, treatment of chronic sinusitis, chronic bronchitis, etc., when indicated. Restriction of smoking, combined with expectorants for a few days, will do wonders for the chronic productive cough that is so likely to lead to serious pulmonary complications. He should supervise any special diets that may be required, apprise the family and patient of the routine use of blood transfusions in similar cases, and instill in the patient that peace of mind and confidence which constitute the so-called "psychologic" preparation. He may actually help prevent postoperative complications from catheterizations or distention by encouraging the patient to practice using the urinal and bedpan in the recumbent posture. He should inform the surgeon of any food or drug idiosyncrasies. He will corroborate and supplement the surgeon's own observations concerning the patient as an operative risk.

Before operation, the patient must be carefully appraised from the standpoint of his nutrition and fluid balance, renal function, circulatory efficiency, and pulmonary status. Inquiry should always be made concerning his customary weight and any recent change. A history of significant weight loss suffices to establish the presence of a nutritional deficit. Good kidney function may be assumed usually if the urine is free of albumin and casts and if it concentrates to a specific gravity of about 1.020; an additional check is provided by determining the level of the blood urea nitrogen, nonprotein nitrogen, or creatinine. If kidney function appears impaired, serum and urine tests of urea, creatinine, or osmolarity for urine to plasma ratios (U/P), and urine sodium and potassium concentrations may be of diagnostic value. The vital capacity furnishes a simple check of both cardiac and pulmonary function, since a rather marked decrease will accompany any pronounced loss of efficiency in either. In addition to the complete blood count and urine studies carried out on every patient, a

preoperative X-ray of the chest and electrocardiogram are advisable. Pulmonary pathology may be identified, and the size, configuration, and status of the heart should be noted and compared with the patient's height, weight, and age. Any departure from the norm disclosed by the history, physical examination, or the various procedures enumerated above may call for further investigation and will suggest the type of preoperative preparation required. The surgeon should seek consultation in evaluating the poor-risk patient and in regulating constitutional disorders such as diabetes, chronic nephritis, or congestive heart failure.

The patient should be required to cough to determine if his cough is dry or productive. In the presence of the latter surgery is delayed for the improvement that will follow discontinuance of smoking and the institution of repeated daily pulmonary physiotherapy with expectorants and bronchodilating drugs as indicated. The patient's progress should be documented with formal pulmonary function tests, including arterial blood gases, and patients with other chronic lung problems should be similarly evaluated.

The anesthesiologist should interview each preoperative patient. In those with serious pulmonary or constitutional disease or in need of extensive surgery, the choice of anesthesia is an exacting problem (and an ill-considered decision may have serious consequences).

Chronic malnutrition is to be assumed in every patient who has lost weight, who has long-standing sepsis sufficient to produce even mild fever, or who is a victim of deep-seated malignancy. It is an almost invariable accompaniment of gastrointestinal carcinoma. Dehydration or hemoconcentration can mask a severe anemia or hypoproteinemia; a determination of the blood volume may assist in exposing the true situation. An occasional patient will accumulate edema fluid—especially ascites—at such a rate that there will be no change in total body weight although the patient is actually starving.

Malnutrition results in depletion of liver glycogen, exhaustion of tissue protein, and ultimately in clinical vitamin deficiencies. Its successful correction requires painstaking attention to many details and may tax to the utmost the surgeon's resources. Alimentary feedings are always preferable to parenteral feedings. In some patients who cannot eat but who have an intact gastrointestinal tract, the appropriate high-protein, high-calorie, high-vitamin diet may be given through a fine plastic indwelling nasogastric tube. A gastrostomy or a high jejunostomy may be done for feeding purposes, especially when there is an obstructing lesion in the oropharynx, esophagus, or proximal stomach, or when a neurologic deficit prevents swallowing. Appropriate quantities of meat, eggs, milk, vitamins, and vegetables may be homogenized in a blender for administration by tube, or commercial high-protein, low-residue mixes may be used. Care must be taken not to overload a starving contracted bowel but to resume such feedings gradually. Two dangers must be avoided: diarrhea from too rapid or too concentrated feeding, and uremia from failure to provide enough water for adequate utilization of the protein provided. Accordingly, the patient should have ready access to water by mouth or else diluted solutions should be prepared. The solutions are best tolerated if begun diluted and given at a slow continuous rate using a drip chamber or pump.

Although about 1 Gm. of protein per kilogram of body weight is the average daily requirement of the healthy adult, frequently it is necessary to double this figure to achieve a positive nitrogen balance and to protect the tissues from the strain of a surgical procedure and a long anesthesia. The administered protein may not be assimilated as such unless the total caloric intake is maintained well above basal requirements. If calories are not supplied from sugars and fat, the ingested protein will be consumed by the body like sugar for its energy value. A very rich source of extra oral calories can be provided by the preparation of finely homogenized and flavored fats now available. Alcohol in modest quantities is acceptable to many patients and can provide many extra calories without depressing the appetite. Skim milk powder may be added to fruit juices, milk, and many foods to boost the protein intake. Sometimes tube feedings can be avoided altogether if the patient eats only modestly at meals but takes between-meal supplements rich in proteins and calories. Supplementary parenteral protein by means of any of the standard protein hydrolysates, human albumin, plasma, or whole blood may accelerate the return of a positive nitrogen balance.

Vitamins are not routinely required in patients who have been on a good diet and who enter the hospital for an elective surgical procedure. Vitamin C is the one vitamin usually requiring early replacement, since only a limited supply can be stored in the body at any one time. In some instances (severe burns are one example), massive doses of 1 Gm. daily may be needed. Vitamin B complex is advantageously given daily. Vitamin K is indicated if the prothrombin level is low. This should be suspected whenever the normal formation of vitamin K in the bowel is interfered with by gastric suction, jaundice, the oral administration of broad-spectrum antibiotics, starvation, or prolonged intravenous alimentation.

The success or failure of the whole program may be gauged by weighing the patient at frequent intervals, at least every other day. This exercise has the great value of impressing the patient and the nursing staff with the importance of the nutritional program. In the absence of edema, a modest gain provides a psychologic boost and testifies to a greatly improved tissue reserve for wound healing.

Blood transfusions may be needed to correct anemia or to replace deficits in circulating blood volume. Properly spaced preoperative transfusions can do more to improve the tolerance for major surgery in poor-risk patients than any other measure in preparation. Formerly, blood tended to be given empirically to bolster a patient before a major surgical ordeal. Now the patient's actual volume of circulating blood may be measured with Evans blue dye or isotopes tagging albumin (RISA) or red cells (Radiochromate). Such measurements have shown that the deficit in blood volume parallels the severity of the recent weight loss, regardless of its cause. Such deficits have often been found even when the hemoglobin and hematocrit are normal, as they will be when both plasma volume and red cell volume are contracted together. This situation has been dramatically termed "chronic shock," since all of the normal defences against shock are hard at work to maintain the appearance of physiologic equilibrium in the preoperative period. If the unsuspecting surgeon fails to uncover the recent weight loss and, trusting the hemoglobin, permits the patient to be anesthetized with a depleted blood volume, vasoconstriction is lost and vascular collapse may ensue promptly. In the absence of facilities for the determination of blood volume, the deficit can be estimated as approximately 500 ml. of blood for each 5 kg. of recent weight loss. A common error is to give too little blood, especially in the presence of jaundice or gastrointestinal malignancy of long standing. The hemoglobin level should be brought to approximately 12 Gm. per 100 ml. before elective surgery is undertaken.

Time for the restoration of blood volume and caution are both necessary, especially in older people. If the initial hemoglobin is very low, the plasma volume must be overexpanded. Packed red cells are specifically needed rather than whole blood. Each 500 ml. of blood contains 1 Gm. of salt in its anticoagulant. As a result, cardiac patients may have some difficulty with multiple transfusions from the salt or plasma loading, and diuretics can be very helpful. There also has been some concern about the potassium in blood stored a week or more. This should never prevent a needed transfusion but is a consideration in massive transfusions in emergency situations.

If for any reason the patient cannot be fed via the gastrointestinal tract, parenteral feedings must be utilized. On occasion, a deficient oral intake should be supplemented by parenteral feedings to ensure a daily desirable minimal level of 1,500 calories. Water, glucose, salt, vitamins, blood, plasma, protein hydrolysates, and intravenous fats are the elements of these feedings. Accurate records of intake and output are indispensable. Frequent checks on the blood levels of protein, albumin, blood urea nitrogen, and hemoglobin are essential to gauge the effectiveness of the treatment. One must be careful to avoid giving too much salt. The average adult will require no more than 500 ml. of normal saline each day unless there is an abnormal loss of chlorides by gastrointestinal suction or fistula. Body weight should be determined daily in patients receiving intravenous fluids. Since each liter of water weighs approximately one kilogram, marked fluctuations in weight can give warning of either edema or dehydration. A stable body weight indicates good water and calorie replacement.

In catabolic states of negative nitrogen balance and inadequate calorie intake usually due to inability to eat enough or to a disrupted gastrointestinal tract, parenteral hyperalimentation using a central venous catheter can be life-saving. At present these solutions contain a mixture of protein hydrolysates or amino acids as a protein source and carbohydrates for calories. Fat emulsions provide more calories (9 calories per gram versus 4 for carbohydrates or protein) and to lessen the problems of hyperglycemia. In general, the hyperalimentation solutions contain 20 to 22 per cent carbohydrate as glucose and fructose plus 50 Gm. of protein source per liter. To this are added the usual electrolytes plus calcium, magnesium, phosphates, and multiple vitamins, especially vitamins C and K. Such a solution offers 1,000 calories per liter and the usual adult receives 3 liters per day. This provides 3,000 calories, 150 Gm. of protein, and a mild surplus of water for urine, insensible, and other water losses. Careful monitoring of the patient receiving hyperalimentation is necessary and should include daily weights; intake and output balances; urinalysis for sugar spillage; serum electrolytes, blood sugar and phosphate; hematocrit; and liver function tests with prothrombin levels in specific. Other than catheter-related problems, major complications include hyperglycemia with glucosuria (solute diuresis) and hyperglycemic nonketotic acidosis from too rapid infusion, or reactive hypoglycemia from sudden discontinuance of the infusion (catheter accident). The other major area of complications involves infection, and strict precautions are needed in preparing the solutions and handling the infusion bottles, lines, and catheters. The catheter and its entrance site should be carefully covered with a topical antibiotic and a sterile dressing that is aseptically changed every two to three days. The infusion lines should contain a microporous filter, and all should be changed daily. Fungemia or gram-negative septicemia should be guarded against, and the catheter system should not be violated for drawing blood samples or for infusion of other solutions. Sepsis does not contraindicate the use of intravenous hyperalimentation, but chronic septicemia without obvious etiology is the indication for removal and culturing of these catheters.

Patients requiring treatment for acute disturbances of the blood, plasma, or electrolyte equilibrium present a somewhat different problem. Immediate replacement is in order, preferably with the substances that are being lost, although plasma substitutes such as dextran (500 ml. or 10 per cent of body weight) can provide emergency aid until blood or plasma is available. Thus, in shock from hemorrhage, replacement should be made with electrolyte solutions plus blood. In severe burns, plasma, blood, and normal saline or lactated Ringer's solution are in order. In vomiting, diarrhea, and dehydration, water and electrolytes will often suffice. In many of these patients, however, there is a loss of plasma which is easy to overlook. For instance, in peritonitis, intestinal obstruction, acute pancreatitis, and other states in which large internal surfaces become inflamed, much plasma-rich exudate may be lost, with no external sign to warn the surgeon until the pulse or blood pressure becomes seriously disturbed. Such internal shifts of fluid have been called "third space" losses. These losses always require blood, plasma, or albumin plus electrolyte solutions for proper replacement. It is because of these internal losses that most cases of peritonitis or bowel obstruction will require plasma or some blood during their preoperative preparation.

In all such acute imbalances a minimum of laboratory determinations will include serum or plasma sodium, potassium, chloride, carbon dioxide combining power, and urea nitrogen. Calcium, magnesium, and liver functions may be useful, while arterial blood gases with pH and pCO_2 enable accurate and repeated evaluation of the respiratory and metabolic components involved in an acidosis or alkalosis. If acidosis is present, one-sixth molar sodium lactate or bicarbonate becomes essential; alkalosis usually may be treated with saline alone. In either case, potassium will be needed. It should be given in sufficient quantity to maintain a normal serum level but only after the urine output is adequate to excrete any excess. Although the laboratory data are useful, the key to adequate replacement therapy is found in the patient's clinical course and in his intake-output record. Evidence of restoration is found in a clearing mentality, a stable blood pressure, a falling pulse rate and temperature curve, improved skin turgor, and an increase in urine output.

Chemotherapeutic and antibiotic agents have proved their usefulness in preparing the patient whose condition is complicated by infection or who faces an operation where infection is an unavoidable risk. A day or two of intensive therapy with antibiotics may be desirable before operations upon the lung, and four to five days of treatment with certain oral preparations diminish the bacterial flora of the feces and render resections of the lower bowel more safe. Similar preparation of the bowel helps to reduce the nitrogen and metabolic load on a damaged liver. In jaundiced patients, and in others seriously ill with liver disease, cleansing and sterilizing the bowel may provide the necessary support through a major operative intervention. The beneficial action of these agents must not give the surgeon a false sense of security, however; for in no sense are they substitutes for good surgical technic and the practice of sound surgical principles.

The many patients now receiving endocrine therapy require special consideration. If cortisone or ACTH has been administered within the preceding few months, the same drug must be continued before, during, and after surgery. The dose required to meet the unusual stress on the day of operation is often double or triple the ordinary dose. Hypotension, inadequately explained by obvious causes, may be the only manifestation of a need for more corticosteroids. Some later difficulties in wound healing may be anticipated in patients receiving these drugs.

The diabetic patient may slip easily into shock from either blood loss or insulin excess. His needs for insulin must be thoroughly evaluated preoperatively. In most cases a reduced amount of short-acting regular insulin plus a concurrent and continuous infusion of intravenous glucose will provide an adequate base to which intermittent covering doses of regular insulin may be added every four to six hours, according to urine spillage. This is demonstrated by regular checks of the urine for sugar on the day of surgery and in the immediate postoperative period.

The patient's normal blood pressure should be reliably established by multiple preoperative determinations as a guide to the anesthesiologist. An accurate preoperative weight can be a great help in managing the postoperative electrolyte balance.

The forehanded surgeon will assure himself of a more than adequate supply of properly cross-matched blood. In all upper abdominal procedures, the stomach should be decompressed and kept out of the way. It has a tendency to fill with air during the induction of anesthesia, but this may be prevented by inserting a nasogastric tube just before operation. In cases of pyloric obstruction emptying the stomach will not be easy; nightly lavages with a very large tube may be required. A Foley catheter may be used to keep the bladder out of the way during pelvic procedures. Postoperatively, this can be a great help in obtaining accurate measurements of urine volume at hourly intervals, particularly when there has been excessive blood loss or other reason to expect renal complications. In general, a good hourly urine output of 40 to 50 ml. per hour indicates satisfactory hydration and an adequate effective blood volume for perfusion of vital organs. Finally, the surgeon should forewarn the nursing staff of the expected condition of the patient after operation. This will assist them in having necessary oxygen, aspirating apparatus, syphonage devices, etc., at the patient's bedside upon his return from the recovery room.

POSTOPERATIVE CARE. Postoperative care begins in the operating room with the completion of the operative procedure. The objective, like that of preoperative care, is to maintain in the patient a normal state. Ideally, complications are anticipated and prevented. This requires a thorough understanding of those complications that may follow surgical procedures in general and those most likely to follow specific diseases or procedures.

The unconscious patient or the patient still helpless from a spinal anesthesia requires special consideration. He must be lifted carefully from the table to bed without unnecessary buckling of the spine or dragging of flaccid limbs. The optimum position in bed will vary with the individual case.

Patients who have had operations about the nose and mouth should be on their sides with the face dependent to protect against aspiration of mucus, blood, or vomitus. Major shifts in position after long operations are to be avoided until the patient has regained consciousness; experience has shown that such changes are badly tolerated. In some instances the patient is transferred from the operating table directly to a permanent bed in which he may be returned to his room. After the recovery of consciousness most patients who have had abdominal operations will be more comfortable with the head slightly elevated and the thighs and knees slightly flexed. The usual hospital bed may be raised under the knees to accomplish the desired amount of flexion. If this is done, the heels must also be raised at least as high as the knees, so that statsis of blood in the calves is not encouraged. Patients who have had a spinal anesthesia ordinarily are kept flat in bed for four to six hours to minimize postanesthetic headache and orthostatic hypotension.

Postoperative pain is controlled by the judicious use of narcotics. It is a serious error to administer too much morphine. This will lower both the rate and amplitude of the respiratory excursions, and thus encourage pulmonary atelectasis. Antiemetic drugs minimize postoperative nausea and potentiate the pain relief afforded by narcotics. Some newer antihistamines also sedate effectively without depressing respirations. On the other hand, patients should be instructed to make their pain known to the nurses and to request relief. Otherwise, many stoic individuals, unaccustomed to hospital practice, would prefer to lie rigidly quiet rather than disturb the busy staff. Such voluntary splinting can lead to atelectasis just as readily as does the sleep of morphia.

Although postoperative care is a highly individual matter, certain groups of patients will have characteristics in common. The extremes of life are an example. Infants and children are characterized by the rapidity of their reactions; they are more easily and quickly thrown out of equilibrium with restriction of food or water intake; they are more susceptible to contagious diseases that may be contracted during a long hospitalization. Conversely, the healing processes are swifter, and there is a quicker restoration to normal health. The accuracy of their fluid replacement is a critical matter, since their needs are large and their little bodies contain a very small reserve. Infants require 120 ml. of water for each kilogram of body weight each day; in dehydration, twice this amount may be allowed.

The calculation of fluid needs in infants and children has been related to body surface area. Pocket-sized tables are available for the quick determination of surface area from age, height, and weight. In this system from 1,200 to 1,500 ml. of fluid per square meter are provided for daily maintenance. Parenteral fluids should contain the principal ions from all the body compartments (sodium, chloride, potassium, calcium) but not in high or "normal" concentrations. Solutions containing electrolytes at about half isotonic strength, and balanced for all the ions, are now available. Those containing only dextrose in water are best avoided. Colloids, such as blood, plasma, or albumin, are indicated in severely depleted infants, and whenever acute losses occur, just as in adults. Ten to 20 ml. per kilogram of body weight may be given daily.

The body weight should be followed closely. Very small infants should be weighed each eight hours, and their orders for fluid therapy reevaluated as often. Infants and children have a very low tolerance for overhydration. Since accidents can happen everywhere, the flask for intravenous infusion hanging above an infant should never contain more water than the child could safely receive if it all ran in at once. This is about 20 ml. per kilogram of body weight.

Elderly patients likewise demand special considerations. The aging process leaves its mark on heart, kidneys, liver, lungs, and mind. Response to disease may be slower and less vigorous; the tolerance for drugs is usually diminished; and serious depletions in the body stores may require laboratory tests for detection. Awareness of pain may be much decreased or masked in the aged. A single symptom may be the only clue to a major complication. For this reason it is often wise to listen carefully to the elderly patient's own appraisal of his progress, cater to his idiosyncrasies, and vary the postoperative regimen accordingly. The elderly patient knows better than his physician how to live with the infirmities of age. For him, the routines that have crept into postoperative care can become deadly. Thoracotomy and gastric tubes should be removed as soon as possible. Immobilizing drains, prolonged intravenous infusions, and binders should be held to a minimum. Early ambulation is encouraged. With increasing longevity the geriatric population is swelling, and these people expect the surgeon to be wise in their specific needs.

As long as a postoperative patient requires parenteral fluids, accurate recording of the intake and output is essential for scientific regulation of water and electrolytes. Immediately after surgery the patient's blood volume should be returned to normal by additional transfusions if necessary. Then, the amount and type of fluid to be given each day should be prescribed individually for each patient. His intake should just equal his output for each of the important elements: water, sodium, chloride, and potassium. For each of these a certain loss is expected each day in the physiology of a normal person. In **Table 1** these physiologic losses are listed in Part A. There are two major sources of loss requiring replacement in every patient receiving intravenous fluids: (1) vaporization from skin and lungs, altered modestly by fever, but with a net average of about 800 ml. per day in an adult, and (2) urine flow, which should lie between 1,000 and 1,500 ml. daily. (In the normal stool, the loss of water and electrolytes is insignificant.) About 2,000 ml. of water per day satisfy the normal physiologic requirements. It is a common error to administer too much salt in the form of normal saline in the immediate postoperative period. Normal losses are more than satisfied by the 5.4 Gm. available in 500 ml. of normal saline, and many patients do well on less, unless there is pathologic fluid loss from suction or drainage. The remainder of the normal parenteral intake should be glucose in water, or protein hydrolysates, or fat, as the nutritional requirements of the patient dictate.

To the physiologic output must be added, for replacement purposes, any other loss of body fluids that may result from disease. Some common sources for pathologic external losses are listed in Part B of **Table 1**. In any of these losses appropriate replacement depends upon an accurate intake-output record. If perspiration or fistulae are seeping large quantities of fluid on dressings or sheets, these may be collected and weighed. These fluids should be replaced volume for volume. All of these losses are rich in electrolyte content, and their replacement requires generous quantities of saline, in contrast to the very small amounts needed for

TABLE 1. INTRAVENOUS FLUID REPLACEMENT FOR SOME COMMON EXTERNAL LOSSES

	mEq. per Liter			Replace I.V. with				
	Na+	Cl−	K+	Volume of Water	Saline	Dex/W	Lactate	Add K+
A. Physiologic								
Skin, lungs	0	0	0	800	—	800	—	—
Good urine flow	20	20	20	1,200	500	700	—	—
B. Pathologic				*Volume for Volume*				
Heavy sweating	50	50	4	200 ml./°F fever	½	½	—	—
Gastric suction	60	90	20	ml. for ml.	⅔	⅓	—	Add 30 mEq./L.
Bile	140	100	4	ml. for ml.	⅔	—	⅓	—
Pancreatic juice	140	70	4	ml. for ml.	½	—	½	—
Bowel (long tube)	130	100	20	ml. for ml.	¾	—	¼	Add 30 mEq./L.
Diarrhea	140	100	30		¾	—	¼	Add 30 mEq./L.

normal physiologic replacement. Selection of the appropriate intravenous solutions may be made from a knowledge of the average electrolyte content in the source of the loss. **Table 1** provides some of this data and suggests formulae by which intravenous restitution may be made. Thus, 1,000 ml. of bile may be precisely replaced by 700 ml. of saline and 300 ml. of sodium lactate. Approximations of the formulae to the closest 500 ml. are usually satisfactory in the adult. However, when losses arise from the gastrointestinal system below the pylorus, some alkaline lactate or bicarbonate solutions will eventually be necessary. When large volumes are being replaced, the adequacy of the therapy should be checked by daily weighing and by frequent measurement of serum electrolyte concentrations. When 3 to 6 liters or more of intravenous fluids are required daily, the precise selection of electrolytes in this fluid becomes very important; consideration for calories, proteins, or other substances which slow the rate of administration must be deferred until smaller daily volumes can be given.

The administration of potassium requires special consideration. This is an intracellular ion, and its concentration in the plasma must not be raised above 6 mEq. per liter during any infusion, or serious cardiac arrhythmias may result. Ordinarily, when the kidneys are functioning properly, any excess potassium is quickly excreted and dangerous plasma levels are never reached. Therefore, potassium should be added to the intravenous infusion only after good postoperative urine flow has been established. There are huge intracellular stores of this ion, so that there need be no rush about giving it. On the other hand, pathologic fluid losses from the main intestinal stream—the stomach or bowel—are rich in potassium. After a few days of such losses, sufficient depletion can occur to produce paralytic ileus, uremia, and other disturbances. Therefore, it is best to give potassium generously, once the urine output is clearly adequate, and to monitor its level with plasma electrolyte tests or the height of the T wave in the electrocardiogram in urgent situations.

The surgeon should interest himself in the details of the patient's diet. Prolonged starvation is to be avoided. On the first day the diet may need to be restricted to toast and clear liquids such as tea. Fruit juices may increase abdominal distention and are best omitted until the third postoperative day. In a convalescence proceeding normally, a 2,500-calorie diet with 100 Gm. of protein may often be started on the second or third postoperative day. Weighing should continue at twice-weekly intervals after diet is resumed. This portrays the nutritional trend and may stimulate more efficient feeding, or a search for hidden edema in the case of too rapid a gain.

Ordinarily, constant gastrointestinal suction will be employed after operations upon the esophagus, resections of the gastrointestinal tract, and in the presence of peritonitis, ileus, or intestinal obstruction. If ileus or intestinal obstruction appears postoperatively, a long tube of the Miller-Abbott type is preferred. The tube is kept in place usually for two to five days and removed as normal bowel function returns; this will be evidenced by resumption of peristalsis and the passage of flatus. When gastrointestinal suction is needed for more than a day or two, a gastrostomy placed at operation may provide gratifying comfort to the patient. It has proved efficient in maintaining suction and keeping distention to a minimum, particularly in the elderly patient with chronic lung disease, whose nasopharyngeal space must be kept as clear of contamination as possible. Feeding by way of a jejunostomy or a gastrostomy tube may also be of value, particularly to the patient who is unable to swallow or who has difficulty in maintaining an adequate calorie intake.

No set rule can be laid down for the particular time at which a patient is permitted out of bed. The tendency at present is to have the patient ambulatory at the earliest possible moment, and most patients may be allowed out of bed on the first day after operation. A longer period of rest may be essential to patients who have been in shock recently, who suffer from severe infection, cardiac insufficiency, cachexia, severe anemia, or thrombophlebitis. The principle of early ambulation has unquestionably speeded up the recovery period, accelerated the desire and tolerance for food, and probably decreased the incidence or severity of respiratory complications.

The surgeon should distinguish between ambulation and sitting in a chair; the latter actually may favor deep venous thrombosis. Every surgeon should establish a method of assisting patients out of bed and teach these principles to those responsible for the bedside care. On the evening of operation the patient is encouraged to sit on the edge of the bed, kick his legs, and cough. He is urged to change his position in bed frequently and move his legs and feet. The following day he is turned on his side (wound side down) with the hips and knees flexed. This brings the knees to the edge of the bed, and an assistant then helps him to raise himself sideways to a sitting position as his feet and lower legs fall over the side of the bed. He then swings his legs and moves his feet, stands erect, and breathes deeply and coughs several times. Following this he takes eight or ten steps and sits in a chair for ten minutes. He returns to bed by a reversal of the foregoing steps. Once he has been up, he is encouraged at first to get up twice daily, and later on to be up and walking as much as his condition permits.

It is helpful to determine the vital capacity and to measure the circumference of the calves daily. Sharp changes in the vital capacity may give a clue to impending complications of a pulmonary nature or in proximity to the chest wall or diaphragm. Intermittent positive pressure breathing is a helpful adjunct, particularly for those patients who will not or cannot breathe well for themselves. Frequent deep breathing and coughing in the postoperative period assist in clearing the bronchial tree of fluid collection, whereas ultrasonic or nebulized mists may be needed to loosen dried secretions. Increase in calf circumference may be due to the edema of an otherwise unsuspected deep venous thrombosis. The measurement of the calves should go hand in hand with daily palpation of the calves and adductor canals for tenderness. The onset of phlebitis has been clearly related to slowed venous return from the lower extremities during operation and postoperative immobility. Venous stasis can be reduced by wearing elastic stockings or wrapping to the calves, and this may be a very worthwhile prophylactic measure.

With the occurrence of a deep venous thrombosis, anticoagulant therapy should be instituted at once, so that disabling or fatal pulmonary embolism may be avoided. Thrombosis is to be considered always as a potential complication; it appears to be commoner in elderly and obese individuals, in infective states, and in malignant disease. Early ambulation has not eradicated this dreaded complication.

Disruption of abdominal wounds is fortunately infrequent. It is more common in patients who have extensive surgery for carcinoma or obstructive jaundice. Contributing factors may be vitamin C deficiency, hypoproteinemia, vomiting, abdominal distention, wound infection, or a need to cough excessively if preoperative tracheobronchial toilet was not well accomplished. The disruption is rarely recognized before the seventh day and is exceedingly rare after the seventeenth and eighteenth days. A sudden discharge from the wound of a large amount of orange serum is practically pathognomonic of dehiscence. Investigation may disclose an evisceration with a protruding loop of bowel or merely lack of healing of the walls of the wound. The proper treatment consists of replacing viscera under sterile conditions in the operating room and closing the wound by through-and-through interrupted inert sutures of heavy size (as described in Plate VII).

The surgeon must assume the responsibility for all untoward events occurring in the postoperative period. This attitude is necessary for progress. Too often surgeons are content to explain a complication on the basis of extraneous influences. Although the surgeon may feel blameless in the occurrence of a cerebral thrombosis or a coronary occlusion, it is inescapable that the complication did not arise until the operation was performed. Only as the surgeon recognizes that the sequelae of surgery, good and bad, are the direct results of preoperative preparation, of performance of the operative procedure, or of postoperative care, will he improve his care of the patient and prevent all avoidable complications.

SURGICAL ANATOMY

PLATE I · ARTERIAL BLOOD SUPPLY TO THE UPPER ABDOMINAL VISCERA

The stomach has a very rich anastomotic blood supply. The largest blood supply comes from the celiac axis **(1)** by way of the left gastric artery **(2).** The blood supply to the uppermost portion, including the lower esophagus, is from a branch of the left inferior phrenic artery **(3).** This vessel divides as it reaches the lesser curvature just below the esophagogastric junction. One branch descends anteriorly and the other branch posteriorly along the lesser curvature. There is a bare area of stomach wall, approximately 1 to 2 cm. wide, between these two vessels which is not covered by peritoneum. It is necessary to ligate the left gastric artery near its point of origin above the superior surface of the pancreas in the performance of a total gastrectomy. This also applies when 70 per cent or more of the stomach is to be removed. Ligation of the artery in this area is commonly done in the performance of gastric resection for malignancy so that complete removal of all lymph nodes high on the lesser curvature may be accomplished.

A lesser blood supply to the uppermost portion of the stomach arises from the short gastric vessels **(4)** in the gastrosplenic ligament. Several small arteries arising from branches of the splenic artery course upward toward the posterior wall of the fundus. These vessels are adequate to ensure viability of the gastric pouch following ligation of the left gastric artery as well as of the left inferior phrenic artery. Mobilization of the spleen, following division of the splenorenal and gastrophrenic ligaments, retains the blood supply to the fundus and permits extensive mobilization at the same time. The blood supply of the remaining gastric pouch may be compromised if splenectomy becomes necessary. The blood of the stomach can be mobilized toward the right and its blood supply maintained by dividing the thickened portion of the splenocolic ligament up to the region of the left gastroepiploic artery **(5).** Further mobilization results if the splenic flexure of the colon, as well as the transverse colon, is freed from the greater omentum. The greater curvature is ordinarily divided at a point between branches coming from the gastroepiploic vessels **(5, 6)** directly into the gastric wall.

The blood supply to the region of the pylorus and lesser curvature arises from the right gastric artery **(7)**, which is a branch of the hepatic artery **(8).** The right gastric artery is so small that it can hardly be identified when it is ligated with the surrounding tissues in this area.

One of the larger vessels requiring ligation during gastric resection is the right gastroepiploic artery **(6)** as it courses to the left from beneath the pylorus. It parallels the greater curvature. The blood supply to the greater curvature also arises from the splenic artery **(9)** by way of the left gastroepiploic artery **(5).**

Relatively few key arteries need to be ligated to control the major blood supply to the pancreas. When the duodenum and head of the pancreas are to be resected, it is necessary to ligate the right gastric artery **(7)** and the gastroduodenal artery **(10)** above the superior surface of the duodenum. The possibility of damaging the middle colic vessels **(11)**, which arise from the superior mesenteric artery and course over the head of the pancreas, must always be considered. This vessel may be adherent to the posterior wall of the antrum of the stomach, and it may course over the second part of the duodenum, especially if the hepatic flexure of the colon is anchored high in the right upper quadrant. The anterior and posterior branches of the inferior pancreaticoduodenal artery **(12)** are ligated close to their points of origin from the superior mesenteric artery **(13).** Additional branches directly to the third portion of the duodenum and upper jejunum also require ligation.

The body and tail of the pancreas can be extensively mobilized with the spleen. The splenic artery located beneath the peritoneum over the superior surface of the pancreas should be ligated near its point of origin **(9).** The dorsal pancreatic artery **(14)** arises from the splenic artery near its point of origin and courses directly into the body of the pancreas. Following removal of the spleen, the inferior surface of the body and tail of the pancreas can be easily mobilized without division of major arteries. When the body of the pancreas is divided, several arteries will require ligation. These include the inferior (transverse) pancreatic artery **(15)** arising from the splenic artery and the greater pancreatic artery **(16).**

The blood supply to the spleen is largely from the splenic artery arising from the celiac axis. Following ligation of the splenic artery, there is a rich anastomotic blood supply through the short gastric vessels **(4)**, as well as the left gastroepiploic artery **(5).** The splenic artery is usually serpentine in contour as it courses along the superior surface of the pancreas just beneath the peritoneum. Following division of the gastrosplenic vessels, it is advantageous to ligate the splenic artery some distance from the hilus of the spleen. The gastric wall should not be injured during the division of the short gastric vessels high in the region of the fundus. Small blood vessels entering the tail of the pancreas require individual ligation, especially in the presence of a large spleen and accompanying induration in the region of the tail of the pancreas.

The blood supply to the gallbladder is through the cystic artery **(17)**, which usually arises from the right hepatic artery **(18).** In the triangular zone bounded by the cystic duct joining the common hepatic duct and the cystic artery, Calot's triangle, there are more anatomic variations than are found in any other location. The most common variations in this zone, which is no larger than a 50-cent piece, are related to the origin of the cystic artery. It most commonly arises from the right hepatic artery **(18)** after the latter vessel has passed beneath the common hepatic duct. The cystic artery may arise from the right hepatic artery more proximally and lie anterior to the common hepatic duct. Other common variations include origin of the cystic artery from the left hepatic artery **(19)**, the common hepatic artery **(8),** or the gastroduodenal artery **(10)**, and their relationship to the biliary ductal system. The variations in the hepatoduodenal ligament are so numerous that nothing should be ligated or incised in this area until definite identification has been made.

PLATE I   ARTERIAL BLOOD SUPPLY TO THE UPPER ABDOMINAL VISCERA

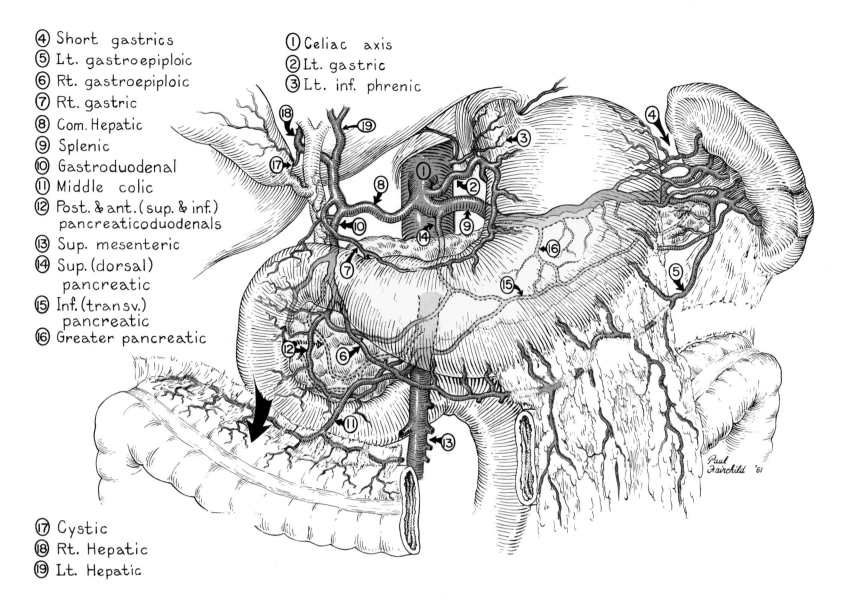

④ Short gastrics
⑤ Lt. gastroepiploic
⑥ Rt. gastroepiploic
⑦ Rt. gastric
⑧ Com. Hepatic
⑨ Splenic
⑩ Gastroduodenal
⑪ Middle colic
⑫ Post. & ant. (sup. & inf.)
   pancreaticoduodenals
⑬ Sup. mesenteric
⑭ Sup. (dorsal)
   pancreatic
⑮ Inf. (transv.)
   pancreatic
⑯ Greater pancreatic

① Celiac axis
② Lt. gastric
③ Lt. inf. phrenic

⑰ Cystic
⑱ Rt. Hepatic
⑲ Lt. Hepatic

Paul
Fairchild '61

PLATE II · VENOUS AND LYMPHATIC SUPPLY TO THE UPPER ABDOMINAL VISCERA

The venous blood supply of the upper abdomen parallels that of the arterial blood supply. The portal vein (1) is the major vessel that has the unique function of receiving venous blood from all intraperitoneal viscera with the exception of the liver. It is formed behind the head of the pancreas by the union of the superior mesenteric (2) and splenic (3) veins. It ascends posterior to the gastrohepatic ligament to enter the liver at the porta hepatis. It lies in a plane posterior to and between the hepatic artery on the left and the common bile duct on the right. This vein has surgical significance in cases of portal hypertension. When portacaval anastomosis is performed, exposure is obtained by means of an extensive Kocher maneuver. Several small veins (4) from the posterior aspect of the pancreas enter the sides of the superior mesenteric vein near the point of origin of the portal vein. Care must be taken to avoid tearing these structures during the mobilization of the vein. Once hemorrhage occurs, it is difficult to control.

The left (coronary) vein (5) returns blood from the lower esophageal segment and the lesser curvature of the stomach. It runs parallel to the left gastric artery and then courses retroperitoneally downward and medially to enter the portal vein behind the pancreas. It anastomoses freely with the right gastric vein (6), and both vessels drain into the portal vein to produce a complete venous circle. It has a significance in portal hypertension in that the branches of the coronary vein, along with the short gastric veins (7), produce the varicosities in the fundus of the stomach and lower esophagus.

The other major venous channel in the area is the splenic vein (3), which lies deep and parallel to the splenic artery along the superior aspect of the pancreas. The splenic vein also receives venous drainage from the greater curvature of the stomach and the pancreas, as well as from the colon, through the inferior mesenteric vein (8). While performing a splenorenal shunt, meticulous dissection of this vein from the pancreas with ligation of the numerous small vessels is necessary. As the dissection proceeds, the splenic vein comes into closer proximity with the left renal vein where anastomosis can be performed. The point of anastomosis is situated proximal to the entrance of the inferior mesenteric vein.

The venous configuration on the gastric wall is relatively constant. In performing a conservative hemigastrectomy, venous landmarks can be used to locate the proximal line of resection. On the lesser curvature of the stomach, the third branch of the coronary vein down from the esophagocardiac junction (5a) is used as a point for transection. On the greater curvature of the stomach the landmark is where the left gastroepiploic vein (9) most closely approximates the gastric wall (9a). Transection is carried out between these two landmarks (5a, 9a).

The anterior and posterior pancreaticoduodenal veins (10) produce an extensive venous network about the head of the pancreas. They empty into the superior mesenteric or hepatic portal vein. The anterior surface of the head of the pancreas is relatively free of vascular structures, and blunt dissection may be carried out here without difficulty. There is, however, a small anastomotic vein (11) between the right gastroepiploic (12) and the middle colic vein (13). This vein, if not recognized, can produce troublesome bleeding in the mobilization of the greater curvature of the stomach, as well as of the hepatic flexure of the colon.

In executing the Kocher maneuver, no vessels are encountered unless the maneuver is carried inferiorly along the third portion of the duodenum. At this point the middle colic vessels (13) cross the superior aspect of the duodenum to enter the transverse mesocolon. Unless care is taken in doing an extensive Kocher maneuver, this vein may be injured.

The lymphatic drainage of the upper abdominal viscera is extensive. Lymph nodes are found along the course of all major venous structures. For convenience of reference, there are four major zones of lymph node aggregations. The superior gastric lymph nodes (A) are located about the celiac axis and receive the lymphatic channels from the lower esophageal segment and the major portion of the lesser curvature of the stomach, as well as from the pancreas. The suprapyloric lymph nodes (B) about the portal vein drain the remaining portion of the lesser curvature and the superior aspect of the pancreas. The inferior gastric subpyloric group (C), which is found anterior to the head of the pancreas, receives the lymph drainage from the greater curvature of the stomach, the head of the pancreas, and the duodenum. The last major group is the pancreaticolienal nodes (D), which are found at the hilus of the spleen and drain the tail of the pancreas, the fundus of the stomach, and the spleen. There are extensive communications among all these groups of lymph nodes. The major lymphatic depot, the cisterna chyli, is found in the retroperitoneal space. This communicates with the systemic venous system by way of the thoracic duct into the left subclavian vein. This gives the anatomic explanation for the involvement of Virchow's node in malignant diseases involving the upper abdominal viscera.

PLATE II   VENOUS AND LYMPHATIC SUPPLY TO THE UPPER ABDOMINAL VISCERA

① Portal
② Sup. mesenteric
③ Splenic

④ Pancreatic
⑤ Coronary
⑥ Rt. gastric

⑩ Pancreaticoduodenal
⑪ Communicating br.
⑫ Rt. gastroepiploic
⑬ Middle colic

⑦ Short gastric
⑧ Inf. mesenteric
⑨ Lt. gastroepiploic

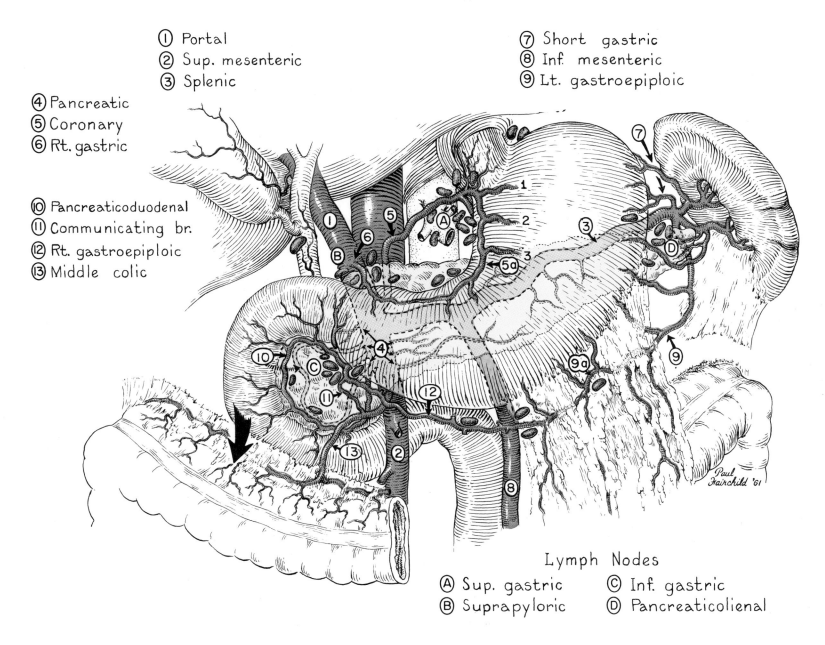

Lymph Nodes

Ⓐ Sup. gastric   Ⓒ Inf. gastric
Ⓑ Suprapyloric   Ⓓ Pancreaticolienal

PLATE III · ANATOMY OF THE LARGE INTESTINE

Because of its embryologic development from both the midgut and hindgut, the colon has two main sources of blood supply: the superior mesenteric (1) and the inferior mesenteric arteries (2). The superior mesenteric artery (1) supplies the right colon, the appendix, and small intestine. The middle colic artery (3) is the most prominent branch of the superior mesenteric artery. The middle colic artery branches into a right and left division. The right division anastomoses with the right colic (4) and the ileocolic (5) arteries. The left branch communicates with the marginal artery of Drummond (6). The middle and right colic and ileocolic arteries are doubly ligated near their origin when a right colectomy is performed for malignancy. The ileocolic artery reaches the mesentery of the appendix from beneath the terminal ileum. Angulation or obstruction of the terminal ileum should be avoided following the ligation of the appendiceal artery (7) in the presence of a short mesentery.

The inferior mesenteric artery arises from the aorta just below the ligament of Treitz. Its major branches include the left colic (8), one or more sigmoid branches (9, 10), and the superior hemorrhoidal artery (11). Following ligation of the inferior mesenteric artery, viability of the colon is maintained through the marginal artery of Drummond (6) by way of the left branch of the middle colic artery.

The third blood supply to the large intestine arises from the middle and inferior hemorrhoidal vessels. The middle hemorrhoidal vessels (12) arise from the internal iliac (hypogastric) (13), either directly or from one of its major branches. They enter the rectum along with the suspensory ligament on either side. These are relatively small vessels, but they should be ligated.

The blood supply to the anus is from the inferior hemorrhoidal (14) vessels, a branch of the internal pudendal artery (15). In low-lying lesions wide excision of the area is necessary with ligation of the individual bleeders as they are encountered.

The venous drainage of the right colon parallels the arterial supply and drains directly into the superior mesenteric vein (1). The inferior mesenteric artery, in the region of the bifurcation of the aorta, deviates to the left and upward as it courses beneath the pancreas to join the splenic vein. High ligation of the inferior mesenteric vein (16) should be carried out before extensive manipulation of a malignant tumor to avoid the vascular spread of tumor cells.

The right colon can be extensively mobilized and derotated to the left side without interference with its blood supply. The mobilization is accomplished by dividing the avascular peritoneal attachments of the mesentery of the appendix, cecum, and ascending colon. Blood vessels of a size requiring ligation are usually present only at the peritoneal attachments of the hepatic and splenic flexures. The transverse colon and splenic flexure can be mobilized by separating the greater omentum from its loose attachment to the transverse colon (see Plate XXIII). Traction on the splenic flexure should be avoided, lest troublesome bleeding result from a tear in the adjacent splenic capsule. The abdominal incision should be extended high enough to allow direct visualization of the splenic flexure when it is necessary to mobilize the entire left colon. The left colon can be mobilized toward the midline by division of the lateral peritoneal attachment. There are few, if any, vessels that will require ligation in this area.

The descending colon and sigmoid can be mobilized medially by division of the avascular peritoneal reflection in the left lumbar gutter. The sigmoid is commonly quite closely adherent to the peritoneum in the left iliac fossa. The peritoneal attachment is avascular, but because of the proximity of the spermatic or ovarian vessels, as well as the left ureter, careful identification of these structures is required. Following the division of the peritoneal attachment and the greater omentum, further mobilization and elongation of the colon can be accomplished by division of the individual branches (8, 9, 10) of the inferior mesenteric artery. This ligation must not encroach on the marginal vessels of Drummond (6).

The posterior wall of the rectum can be bluntly dissected from the hollow of the sacrum without dividing important vessels. The blood supply of the rectum is in the mesentery adjacent to the posterior rectal wall. Following division of the peritoneal attachment to the rectum and division of the suspensory ligaments on either side, the rectum can be straightened with the resultant gain of considerable distance (Plate LXI). The pouch of Douglas, which may initially appear to be quite deep in the pelvis, can be mobilized well up into the wound.

The lymphatic supply follows the vascular channels, especially the venous system. Accordingly, all of the major blood supplies of the colon should be ligated near their points of origin. These vessels should be ligated before a malignant tumor is manipulated. Complete removal of the lymphatic drainage from lesions of the left colon requires ligation of the inferior mesenteric artery (2) near its point of origin from the aorta.

Low-lying malignant rectal lesions may extend laterally along the middle hemorrhoidal vessels (12) as well as along the levator ani muscles. They may also extend cephalad along the superior hemorrhoidal vessels (11). The lymphatic drainage of the anus follows the same pathway but may include spread to the superficial inguinal lymph nodes (17). The lower the lesion, the greater the danger of multiple spread from the several lymphatic systems involved. As a result, the five-year survival is lowest in this group.

PLATE III   ANATOMY OF THE LARGE INTESTINE

① Sup. mesenteric art. & vein
② Inf. mesenteric art.
③ Middle colic art. & vein
④ Rt. colic art. & vein

⑤ Ileocolic art. & vein
⑥ Marginal vessels of Drummond

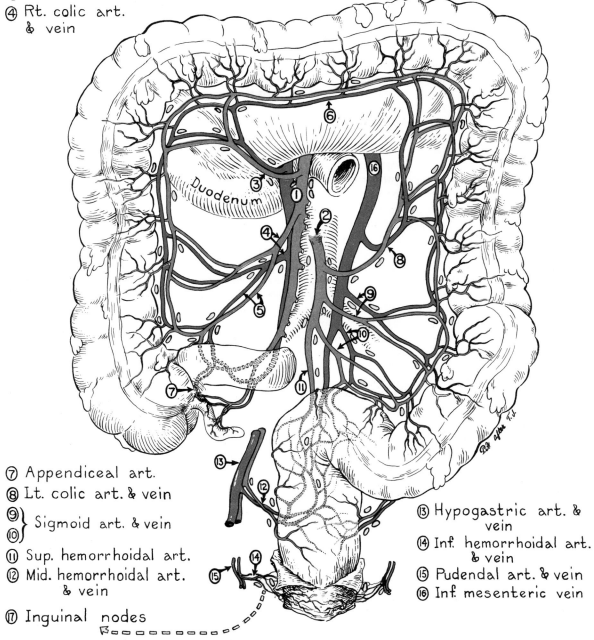

⑦ Appendiceal art.
⑧ Lt. colic art. & vein
⑨ ⎫
⑩ ⎭ Sigmoid art. & vein
⑪ Sup. hemorrhoidal art.
⑫ Mid. hemorrhoidal art. & vein
⑰ Inguinal nodes

⑬ Hypogastric art. & vein
⑭ Inf. hemorrhoidal art. & vein
⑮ Pudendal art. & vein
⑯ Inf. mesenteric vein

PLATE IV · ANATOMY OF THE ABDOMINAL AORTA AND INFERIOR VENA CAVA

The various vascular procedures that are carried out on the major vessels in the retroperitoneal area of the abdominal cavity make familiarity with these structures essential. Likewise, surgery of the adrenal glands and the genitourinary system invariably involves one or more of the branches of the abdominal aorta and inferior vena cava.

The blood supply to the adrenals is complicated and different on the two sides. The superior arterial supply branches from the inferior phrenic artery **(1)** on both sides. The left adrenal receives a branch directly from the adjacent aorta. A similar branch may also pass behind the vena cava to the right side, but a more prominent arterial supply arises from the right renal artery. The major venous return on the left side is directly to the left renal vein **(3)**. On the right side the venous supply may be more obscure, as the adrenal is in close proximity to the vena cava and the venous system **(2)** drains directly into the latter structure.

The celiac axis **(A)** is one of the major arterial divisions of the abdominal aorta. It divides into the left gastric, splenic, and common hepatic arteries. Immediately below this is the superior mesenteric artery **(B)**, which provides the blood supply to that portion of the gastrointestinal tract arising from the foregut and midgut. The renal arteries arise laterally from the aorta on either side. The left renal vein crosses the aorta from the left kidney and usually demarcates the upper limits of arteriosclerotic abdominal aneurysms. The left ovarian (or spermatic) vein **(13)** enters the left renal vein, but this vessel on the right side **(5)** drains directly into the vena cava.

In removing an abdominal aortic aneurysm, it is necessary to ligate the pair of ovarian (or spermatic) arteries **(4)**, as well as the inferior mesenteric artery **(C)**. In addition, there are four pairs of lumbar vessels that arise from the posterior wall of the abdominal aorta **(14)**. The middle sacral vessels will also require ligation **(12)**. Because of the inflammatory reaction associated with the aneurysm, this portion of the aorta may be intimately attached to the adjacent vena cava.

The blood supply to the ureters is variable and difficult to identify. The arterial supply **(6, 7, 8)** arises from the renal vessels, directly from the aorta, and from the gonadal vessels, as well as from the hypogastric arteries **(11)**. While these vessels may be small and their ligation unnecessary, the ureters should not be denuded of their blood supply any further than is absolutely necessary.

The aorta terminates by dividing into the common iliac arteries **(9)**, which in turn divide into the external iliac artery **(10)** and the internal iliac (hypogastric) **(11)** arteries. From the bifurcation of the aorta, the middle sacral vessel **(12)** descends along the anterior surface of the sacrum. There is a concomitant vein that usually empties into the left common iliac vein at this point **(12)**.

The ovarian arteries **(4)** arise from the anterolateral wall of the aorta below the renal vessels. They descend retroperitoneally across the ureters and through the infundibulopelvic ligament to supply the ovary and salpinx **(15)**. They terminate by anastomosing with the uterine artery **(16)** which descends in the broad ligament. The spermatic arteries and veins follow a retroperitoneal course before entering the inguinal canal to supply the testicles in the scrotum.

The uterine vessels **(16)** arise from the anterior division of the internal iliac (hypogastric) arteries **(11)** and proceed medially to the edge of the vaginal vault opposite the cervix. At this point the artery crosses over the ureter ("water under the bridge") **(17)**. The uterine vein, in most instances, does not accompany the artery at this point but passes behind the ureter. In a hysterectomy the occluding vascular clamps must be applied close to the wall of the uterus to avoid damage to the ureter. The uterine vessels then ascend along the lateral wall of the uterus and turn laterally into the broad ligament to anastomose with the ovarian vessels.

The lymphatic networks of the abdominal viscera and retroperitoneal organs frequently end in lymph nodes found along the entire abdominal aorta and inferior vena cava. Lymph nodes about the celiac axis **(A)** are commonly involved with metastatic cancer arising from the stomach and the body and tail of the pancreas. The para-aortic lymph nodes which surround the origin of the renal vessels receive the lymphatic drainage from the adrenals and kidneys.

The lymphatic drainage of the female genital organs forms an extensive network in the pelvis with a diversity of drainage. The lymphatic vessels of the ovary drain laterally through the broad ligament and follow the course of the ovarian vessels **(4, 5)** to the preaortic and lateroaortic lymph nodes on the right and the precaval and laterocaval lymph nodes on the left. The fallopian tubes and the uterus have lymphatic continuity with the ovary, and communication of lymphatics from one ovary to the other has also been demonstrated.

Lymphatics of the body and fundus of the uterus may drain laterally along the ovarian vessels in the broad ligament with wide anastomoses with the lymphatics of the tube and ovary. Lateral drainage to a lesser extent follows a transversal direction and ends in the external iliac lymph nodes **(18)**. Less frequently, tumor spread occurs by lymphatic trunks, which follow the round ligament from its insertion in the fundus of the uterus to the inguinal canal and end in the superficial inguinal lymph nodes **(22)**.

The principal lymphatic drainage of the cervix of the uterus is the preureteral chain of lymphatics, which follow the course of the uterine artery **(16)** in front of the ureters and drain into the external iliac **(18)**, the common iliac **(18)**, and obturator lymph nodes. Lesser drainage is by way of the retroureteral lymphatics, which follow the course of the uterine vein, pass behind the ureter, and end in the internal iliac (hypogastric) lymph nodes **(20)**. The posterior lymphatics of the cervix, less constant than the other two, follow an anteroposterior direction on each side of the rectum to end in the para-aortic lymph nodes found at the aortic bifurcation **(21)**.

The lymphatics of the prostate and bladder, like those of the cervix, are drained particularly by nodes of the external iliac chain **(18)** and occasionally also by the hypogastric **(20)** and common iliac lymph nodes **(19)**.

PLATE IV   ANATOMY OF THE ABDOMINAL AORTA AND INFERIOR VENA CAVA

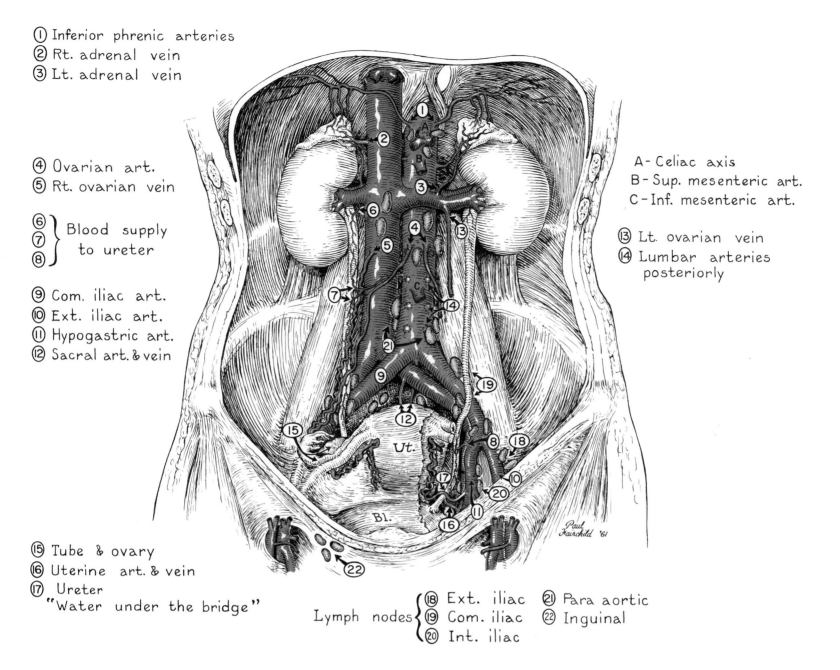

① Inferior phrenic arteries
② Rt. adrenal vein
③ Lt. adrenal vein

④ Ovarian art.
⑤ Rt. ovarian vein

⑥ ⎫
⑦ ⎬ Blood supply
⑧ ⎭   to ureter

⑨ Com. iliac art.
⑩ Ext. iliac art.
⑪ Hypogastric art.
⑫ Sacral art. & vein

A - Celiac axis
B - Sup. mesenteric art.
C - Inf. mesenteric art.

⑬ Lt. ovarian vein
⑭ Lumbar arteries
    posteriorly

⑮ Tube & ovary
⑯ Uterine art. & vein
⑰ Ureter
   "Water under the bridge"

Lymph nodes ⎧ ⑱ Ext. iliac   ㉑ Para aortic
            ⎨ ⑲ Com. iliac   ㉒ Inguinal
            ⎩ ⑳ Int. iliac

GASTROINTESTINAL PROCEDURES

PLATE V · LAPAROTOMY, THE OPENING

OPERATIVE PREPARATION. The principles dealing with the proper preparation of the skin surfaces have been thoroughly covered in Chapter I. However, since the skin can never be rendered absolutely free from bacteria, the less skin exposed, the better the patient is protected. The assistant should ascertain that all hair is completely removed. The incision should not be placed through or near a focus of skin infection. A sterile towel is placed well beyond the upper and lower limits of the operative field to wall off the unsterile drapes. The first assistant scrubs, puts on sterile gloves, and completes the mechanical cleaning of the operative site with sponges saturated with the desired solution (see Chapter I). Some prefer iodinated solutions for skin preparation.

The incision should be carefully planned before the anatomic landmarks are hidden by the sterile drapes. While cosmetic considerations may dictate placing the incision in the lines of skin cleavage in an effort to minimize the subsequent scar, other factors are of greater importance. The incision should be varied to fit the anatomic contour of the patient, provide maximum exposure of the anticipated pathology and probable technical procedures, but involve minimal additional injury to the abdominal wall, especially in the presence of one or more scars from previous surgical procedures. The operative field and adjacent sterile towels are sealed off by a plastic drape.

INCISION AND EXPOSURE. With the edge of a scalpel the operator first scratches superficially the exact position and limits of the incision and may make several superficial crosshatches to aid in proper skin approximation at the time of closure. In making the incision, the operator should hold the scalpel with the thumb on one side and the fingers on the other, with the distal part of the handle resting against the ulnar side of the palm. Some prefer to rest the index finger on top of the knife handle to serve as a sensitive guide to the pressure being applied to the blade. The primary incision may be made in three ways: (1) the surgeon may take gauze in his left hand, pull the skin upward at the upper end of the wound, start to cut in the taut skin immediately below his left hand and, as he progresses, shift the piece of gauze farther down the wound, always keeping the parietes taut so that the knife will separate them more easily; (2) the surgeon may prefer to make the skin taut from side to side by his forefinger and thumb **(Figure 1)**; (3) with the left hand the operator and his first assistant may exert pressure on the skin, over a piece of gauze, and fix the parietes, permitting a scalpel to cut without the soft parts being shifted. The compressing fingers should be separated and flexed to exert pressure downward with a gentle outward pull. This procedure allows the operator full view of the area as he cuts evenly taut skin throughout the entire length of the incision. The incision is then carried down to the underlying fascia. The blade of the knife may be angulated as it is swept downward in order to dissect the fat from the underlying fascia. The fascia should be free of fat for approximately 1 cm. in order that the margins of the fascia may be easily identified at the time of closure. Large vessels are carefully clamped with small curved hemostats and are ligated at this stage, for it is unwise to leave clamps dangling on the delicate superficial tissues. As soon as hemostasis of the superficial fat layer has been accomplished, large gauze pads moistened with normal saline solution are placed in the wound so that the fatty layer is well protected from further desiccation or injury. This also aids in providing a clear view of the underlying parietes.

The fascia is incised whether it is in the midline or overlying the rectus muscle or the oblique muscle. The hands of the surgeon and first assistant give ample exposure without the necessity for retractors **(Figure 2)**. The muscle layer may be split if it is present; however, it is preferable to retract the entire rectus muscle laterally to avoid interfering with its nerve and blood supply. Vessels are encountered most frequently at the tendinous insertions of the rectus muscle. These must be transfixed and ligated with a fine suture. If branches of the epigastric vessels are damaged, they should be carefully ligated. The assistant holds the handle of the hemostat toward the operator to facilitate the placing of the transfixing suture **(Figure 3)**. The ligature is then thrown around the hemostat, and the assistant shifts the handle toward his own side. The point of the hemostat is gently raised, allowing the operator to tighten the first knot without difficulty **(Figure 4)**. It is unwise to include much muscle tissue in any sutures used for this purpose, since muscle is easily strangulated and torn. Moist gauze pads are inserted to the level of the peritoneum. With toothed forceps the operator and first assistant alternately pick up and release the deepest fascial layer and the peritoneum to make certain no viscus is included in their grasp **(Figure 5)**. Both then pull firmly upward, and with the point of the scalpel the operator makes a small opening in the side, not in the vertex, of the tent of elevated peritoneum **(Figure 6)**. The tent formation pulls the peritoneum away from the underlying tissues, and the side opening allows air to rush in and push away any adjacent structure. In the upper abdomen the peritoneum and posterior rectus sheath are separated by a layer of fatty tissue. The operator and assistant may then pick up the preperitoneal fat and peritoneum as previously described, as the abdominal cavity is cautiously opened **(Figure 7)**. A culture is taken at this time if abnormal fluid is encountered. Large collections of fluid in the abdomen should be removed by suction at this time to avoid gross soiling of the field. A moist gauze sponge is placed within this opening to protect the abdominal contents as the peritoneum is incised. Sometimes the flat side of the handle of the forceps may be inserted on top of the gauze as an extra precaution. The edges of the peritoneum, its adjacent fascia, and the edge of a moist gauze pad are grasped in half-length curved clamps, care being taken from this point on to prevent the escape of, or injury to, underlying viscera **(Figure 8)**. Some prefer to insert a plastic wound protector, especially in the presence of sepsis or procedures on the gastrointestinal tract.

By continually elevating the tissues that are to be cut, the surgeon may enlarge the opening with scissors. In cutting the peritoneum with scissors, it is wise to insert only as much of the blade as can be visualized to avoid cutting internal structures that may possibly be adherent to the parietal peritoneum. Tilting the points of the scissors upward affords better visualization of the lower blade **(Figure 9)**. More curved, half-length clamps are placed on the free edges of the peritoneum, including also a bit of the moist gauze pads, so that the edges of the wound may be thoroughly protected against soiling, desiccation, or further trauma from retractors and instruments. The assistant approximates the peritoneum and gauze as the operator applies the curved clamps. Having extended the incision to its uppermost limits, the operator then inserts the index and middle fingers of his left hand downward and divides the peritoneum between the fingers with a scalpel **(Figure 10)**, again attaching the free edge of the peritoneum to the moist gauze. The peritoneal incision should not be as long as the opening in the muscle or fascia **(Figure 11)**. As a general principle, small incisions handicap the surgeon without benefiting the patient.

PLATE V   LAPAROTOMY, THE OPENING

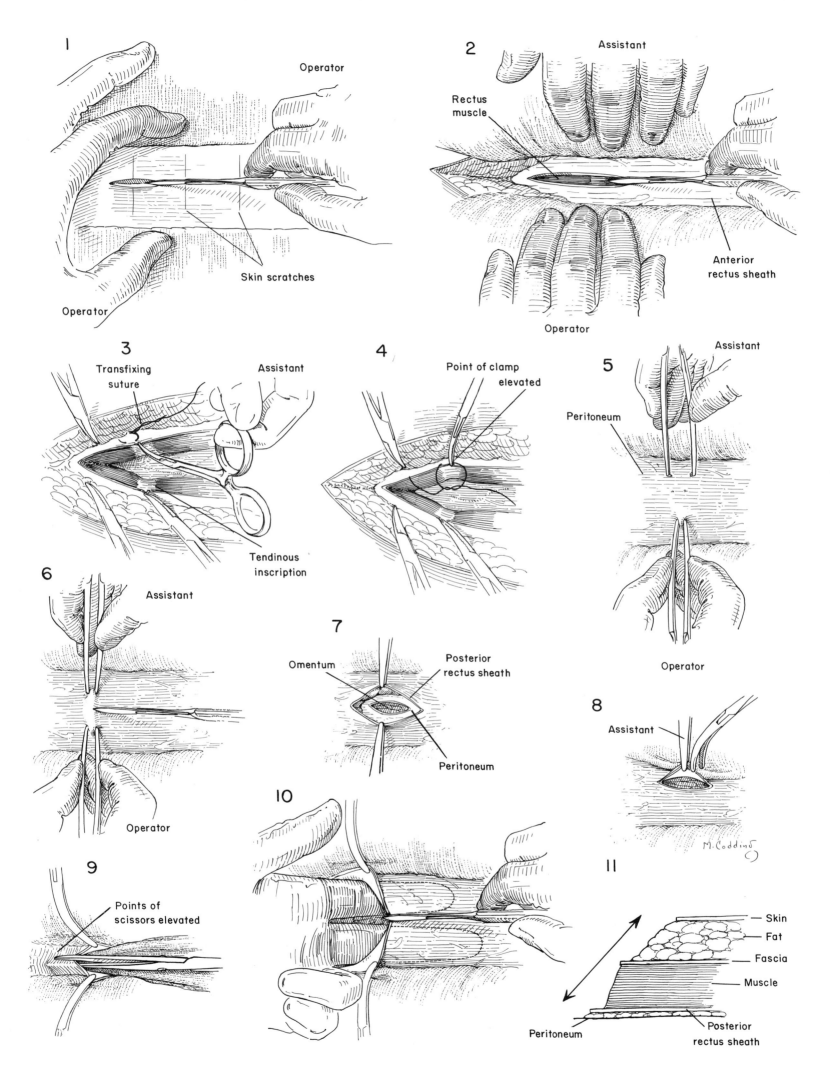

PLATE VI · LAPAROTOMY, THE CLOSURE

CLOSURE. Approximately the same steps are carried out whether the incision is in the midline or over the rectus muscle and whether it is transverse or oblique. If the peritoneum and the posterior rectus sheath are separated, their edges should be approximated by curved, half-length forceps, and the closure of the two layers should be performed as one **(Figure 1).** The peritoneum may be closed with continuous catgut or interrupted mattress sutures of 00 silk. If a continuous suture is used, it is technically simpler to close from the bottom upward, particularly if the surgeon is on the right side of the patient. The suture is started outside the wound at the lowest point of the incision and anchored not in the line of incision but to one side or the other. It is believed that by anchoring the suture to the side and beyond the line of the incision, it will be greatly strengthened **(Figure 2).** The needle is then inserted from the external to the internal surface of the peritoneum **(Figure 3).** As the continuous suture progresses upward, a vertical rather than a horizontal bite of the needle is taken through the internal surface of the peritoneum and posterior rectus sheath to ensure an accurate approximation **(Figure 4).** This is an important factor in avoiding postoperative adhesions and hernia. As the needle enters from the peritoneal surface, it should always include the posterior rectus sheath to give more substance to the bite and greater security to the wound. When the top of the wound is reached, the suture should be brought to the external surface of the peritoneum and anchored beyond and to the side of the incision, similar to the anchoring bite at the beginning of the closure **(Figures 5 and 6).** The finished closure with inner surface to inner surface gives a firm approximation, with slight eversion of the cut edges of peritoneum and posterior rectus sheath **(Figure 16).**

Although more time is consumed in placing interrupted mattress sutures, they give a firmer closure. Fine 00 silk is used. At each end of the wound the peritoneum and posterior rectus sheath are everted by a suture placed through the peritoneal surface immediately beyond the angle of the opening **(Figure 7).** These traction sutures prevent tear and extension of the incision. The assistant pulls upward and outward on these end sutures, approximating the edges of the peritoneum **(Figure 8).** Interrupted mattress sutures are then placed in the peritoneal edges about 1 cm. apart. The far edge of the peritoneum is picked up with mouse-toothed forceps, and the needle is inserted **(Figure 9).** Then the near margin of the peritoneum is grasped with forceps and pulled over toward the point of the needle **(Figure 10).** This allows the first half of the mattress suture to be placed without changing the needle holder on the needle. By a similar procedure the backhand half of the mattress suture is taken, and the suture is tied on the side of the assistant **(Figures 11 and 12).** Mattress sutures placed in this fashion assure the approximation of peritoneal surface to peritoneal surface without fear of inversion of the edges.

As an alternate method of closing by the interrupted technic, mattress sutures may be placed using only the inner surface of the everted peritoneum. This more difficult method ensures approximation of peritoneal surface to peritoneal surface with less chance of injuring any underlying structures **(Figures 13, 14, and 15).** A cross section of the closed, everted peritoneum is shown **(Figure 16).**

The sutures, after being placed, are held under tension by the assistant to define the site of subsequent sutures and to aid in approximation when the sutures are tied. Three throws of the tie should be used for each knot. It seems more convenient to place all the sutures, then tie and cut them all; but each surgeon must standardize his own technic and educate his team to one system or the other in order to reduce the time spent in closing the wound. The wound may be irrigated with warm saline until all obvious particles of fat and blood have been taken up by suction. One or more bleeding points may require ligation following this procedure.

It may not be possible to close the peritoneum in some patients following evisceration and secondary closure. Indeed, the necessity for a peritoneal closure has been questioned, provided the remainder of the incision is securely approximated.

PLATE VI   LAPAROTOMY, THE CLOSURE

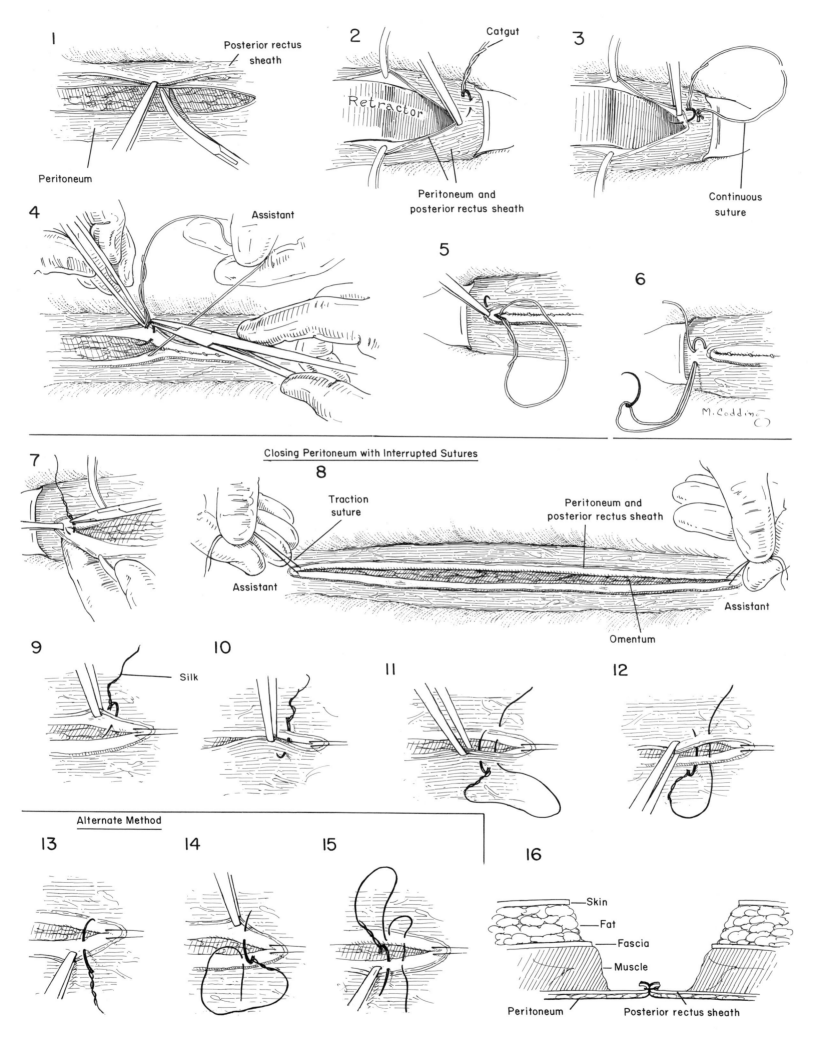

1 Posterior rectus sheath / Peritoneum

2 Catgut / Retractor / Peritoneum and posterior rectus sheath

3 Continuous suture

4 Assistant

5

6 M. Codding

7

Closing Peritoneum with Interrupted Sutures

8 Traction suture / Assistant / Peritoneum and posterior rectus sheath / Assistant / Omentum

9 Silk

10

11

12

Alternate Method

13

14

15

16 Skin / Fat / Fascia / Muscle / Peritoneum / Posterior rectus sheath

PLATE VII · LAPAROTOMY, THE CLOSURE

CLOSURE (*Continued*). The margins of the fascia should be free of fat and well identified. The fascia is usually closed with single interrupted 00 silk sutures taken about 1 cm. apart. The far edge is picked up with the thumb forceps, and a bite is taken with a French or small Ferguson (No. 12) needle near the margin **(Figure 17)**. The opposite margin of the fascia is then picked up with the forceps and pulled over to the point of the needle. By pulling the fascia over to the point of the needle, only one change of grasp with the needle holder is required. The sutures are all placed and held by the assistant. As the operator ties, he may separate one suture from the other with the handle of the thumb forceps **(Figure 18)**. The closure is facilitated if the assistant prepares each suture for the operator by crossing it so that, as the first loop is made, it goes down without being twisted. This crossing of sutures not only speeds the procedure but also relieves any existing tension on the previous suture as the next suture is tied.

After all the knots are placed, the ends of the sutures are held under tension by the assistant and are cut. Silk sutures should be cut within 2 mm. of the knot with the point of straight, blunt scissors. The scissors are steadied by the index finger extended well up along the blade. As the sutures' ends are held directly perpendicular to the wound by the assistant, the scissors are slid down to the knot and rotated one-quarter turn **(Figures 19 and 20)**. Closure of the scissors at this level allows the suture to be cut near the knot without destroying it. When nonabsorbable suture material is used, it is important that all excessive foreign material be eliminated by cutting sutures close to the knot.

To make a particularly firm closure and perhaps avoid using retention sutures, a so-called "eight-pound" stitch using a variety of suture materials may be placed in three steps: (1) a diagonal bite in the far edge of the fascia **(Figure 21)**; (2) a horizontal background bite about 1 cm. from the near edge **(Figure 22)**; and (3) a second diagonal bite crossing the first one on the far edge of the fascia **(Figure 23)**. The suture is then tied, placing the knot about 1.5 cm. back from the opposite margin **(Figure 24)**.

Suturing of the muscle layers together is unwise, since this tissue is easily cut by the suture, and its blood supply is jeopardized. If sutures are ever to be used in the muscle, they must be tied loosely to minimize these dangers.

Occasionally, it is necessary to use a retention or through-and-through suture. This is especially true in debilitated, elderly patients and in cases of malnutrition with malignancy. Retention sutures also should be considered in the very obese or in those patients with a chronic cough. They may be the only type of suture used for the secondary closure of a postoperative evisceration. Through-and-through 000 stainless-steel-wire sutures including all layers of the abdominal wall are especially suitable for grossly contaminated wounds and for the closure of disrupted wounds. A near-and-far type of suture may be used. Curved, half-length forceps are placed on the peritoneum and posterior rectus sheath to make certain that they do not retract beneath the muscle, and a ribbon retractor may be inserted into the wound to protect the underlying viscera. A large, curved needle is inserted through all the layers of the far side of the incision 1 cm. from the edge. From the skin downward, the suture is then carried through to the other side from peritoneum outward and brought out about 2 cm. from the edge **(Figure 25)**. The second turn of the suture is then started on the far edge 2 cm. from the incision **(Figures 26 and 27)** and extended downward through all layers of this side and upward on the near side, to be brought out on the near margin about 1 cm. from the skin border **(Figure 28)**. Except for secondary closure after evisceration, the layers of the abdominal wall are approximated with interrupted 00 silk sutures before the retention sutures are pulled tight and tied. After at least 12 days, the far margins may be cut, and the suture may be pulled out by grasping the near twisted end **(Figure 29)**.

A figure-of-eight suture of 000 stainless steel wire, No. 1 silk, or No. 1 synthetic suture material may be used, including all layers of the abdominal wall except the peritoneum. This suture is introduced after the peritoneum is closed. The wire suture is not tied until the fascia and skin have been carefully approximated.

Many prefer to use No. 4 braided black silk as retention suture material. Interrupted sutures are passed through all layers of the abdominal wall except the peritoneum. The suture is introduced about 2.5 to 3 cm. from the skin margin and brought out about the same distance from the skin margin on the opposite side. These distances may be varied depending on the thickness of the abdominal wall. The sutures are spaced approximately 3 cm. apart. They are tied loosely after the wound, including the skin, has been approximated as usual. Retention sutures are often tied too tightly, leading to tissue necrosis and considerable discomfort to the patient. Good judgment and deliberate planning are required in placing a sufficient number of retention sutures to ensure an effective wound closure without undue tissue necrosis.

PLATE VII   LAPAROTOMY, THE CLOSURE

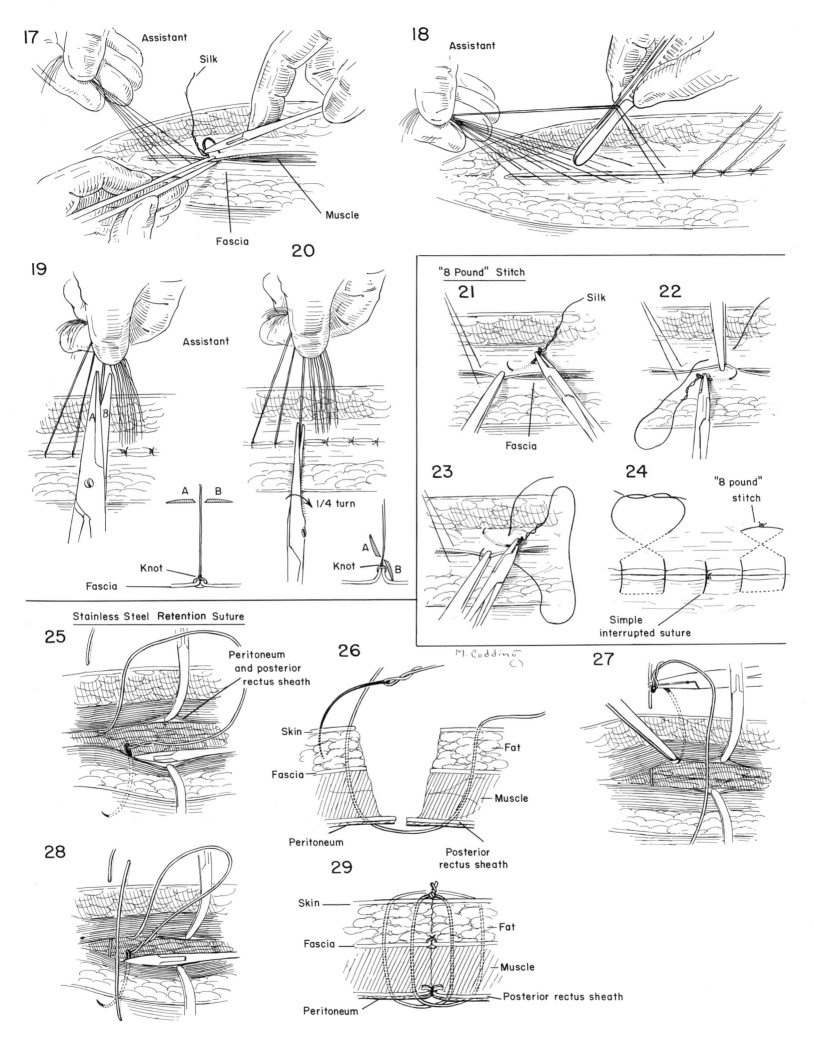

17 Assistant · Silk · Muscle · Fascia

18 Assistant

19 Assistant · A B · A B · Knot · Fascia · Knot

20 Assistant · 1/4 turn · A B · Knot · A B

"8 Pound" Stitch

21 Silk · Fascia

22

23

24 "8 pound" stitch · Simple interrupted suture

M. Coddino

Stainless Steel Retention Suture

25 Peritoneum and posterior rectus sheath

26 Skin · Fascia · Peritoneum · Fat · Muscle · Posterior rectus sheath

27

28

29 Skin · Fascia · Peritoneum · Fat · Muscle · Posterior rectus sheath

PLATE VIII · LAPAROTOMY, THE CLOSURE

CLOSURE (*Continued*). Following the irrigation of the wound the subcutaneous tissue is closed with fine interrupted 0000 silk sutures, small catgut, or synthetic sutures, in one or more layers to eliminate the dead space and to give more accurate approximation. The deeper rows of sutures may be placed with the knot upward, but the superficial row should be placed with the knot downward **(Figure 30)**. It is essential that an adequate number of sutures be placed in the subcutaneous tissue to mound up the wound and thereby reduce the pull on the actual skin sutures **(Figure 31)**. This will decrease considerably the amount of crosshatching in the scar which might occur from pressure of the final layer of superficial skin sutures. Finer suture material is always used for the subcutaneous tissues than for the deeper layers.

Ordinarily, the skin is closed with interrupted 0000 silk sutures placed with straight needles, and the same principles are utilized here that apply to the use of straight needles elsewhere. Thus, when the needle is inserted on one side, it is introduced perpendicularly. If the skin edge is elevated with forceps, a milliner's needle can be directed parallel to the surface of the body yet enter the skin margin at right angles without having to direct the point down and then up **(Figure 32)**. The opposite margin of the wound is similarly held with thumb forceps. The handle of the forceps assists in steadying the opposite skin edge, so that the needle emerges once more parallel to the surface of the body but perpendicular to the skin **(Figure 33)**. Better approximation is achieved and the closure is more rapid if all needles are placed before any sutures are tied. Each needle, when placed, holds the skin in correct position for the next needle. The sutures are pulled through and tied on the near side of the incision. With the thumb forceps the operator pushes downward and forward on the base of the needle, elevating the point, which is grasped by the assistant with a hemostat and pulled through **(Figure 34)**. The ends of the sutures are grasped in one hand and cut evenly about 2 cm. from the knot **(Figure 35)**. The skin may also be closed with interrupted subcuticular sutures of fine catgut or 0000 silk. With this method the suture must lie in the deepest layers of the corium, and the surgeon, when placing it, must see that the needle actually penetrates from the cut edge back into the tissues at least several millimeters **(Figure 36)**. Small bites are then taken on alternate sides of the skin margin in the deepest layers of the corium **(Figures 37 and 38)**. When such a suture is pulled tight, it gives a perfect approximation and a minimal scar **(Figures 39, 40, and 41)**. A continuous suture of fine catgut or absorbable synthetic material may be preferred. The skin margins can be further supported by the application of multiple paper-like adhesive strips.

On the whole, the subcuticular type of sutures takes more time than other methods, but it may be more suitable for short incisions in an exposed area where an inconspicuous scar is desired for cosmetic reasons. In addition, these wounds tend to ensure greater comfort to the patient as well as to avoid the unnecessary concern of some patients in anticipating the possible discomfort during the removal of skin sutures. Regardless of how the skin is closed, the crosshatches made when the initial incision was marked should be accurately approximated in order to give an even symmetrical scar **(Figures 40 and 41)**.

A vertical mattress suture may be used where slight tension on the skin margin is expected or where a fine linear scar is desirable in thick, heavy skin. The first portion of the suture is made by taking deep bites in both margins of the skin, after proper eversion with mouse-toothed forceps **(Figures 42 and 43)**. The final half of the mattress suture is completed by inserting the needle through only the superficial edge of the corium at the skin margins **(Figures 44, 45, and 46)**. Placing the deeper portion of the suture first prevents the needle, contaminated from the superficial skin margins, from carrying infection into the deeper layers of the subcutaneous tissue. This type of suture provides a sealed wound and a well-approximated skin margin regardless of the patient's activity.

PLATE VIII   LAPAROTOMY, THE CLOSURE

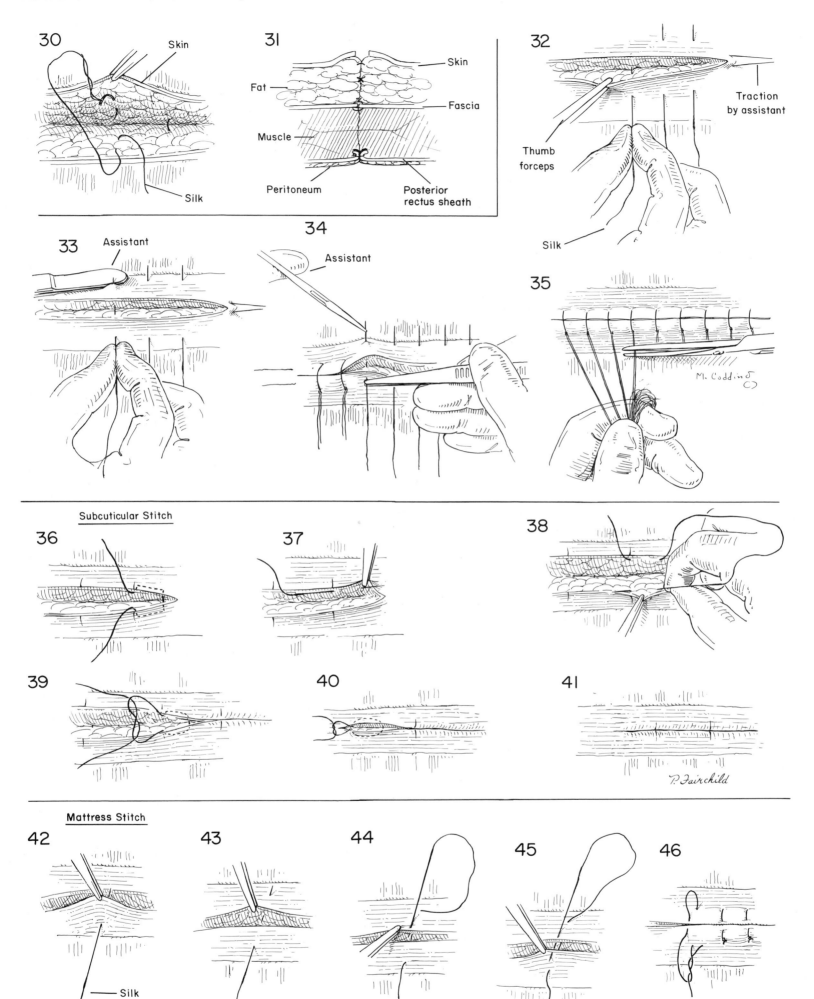

Subcuticular Stitch

Mattress Stitch

PLATE IX · GASTROSTOMY

INDICATIONS. Gastrostomy is commonly utilized as a temporary procedure to avoid the discomfort of prolonged nasogastric suction following such major abdominal procedures as vagotomy and subtotal gastrectomy, colectomy, etc. This procedure should be considered following abdominal operation in those poor-risk or elderly patients prone to pulmonary difficulties or where postoperative nutritional difficulties are anticipated.

Gastrostomy is considered in the presence of obstruction of the esophagus, but it is most frequently employed as a palliative procedure in nonresectable lesions of the esophagus or as the preliminary step in treating the cause of the obstruction. A permanent type of gastrostomy may be considered for feeding purposes in the presence of almost complete obstruction of the esophagus due to nonresectable malignancy. The type of gastrostomy depends upon whether the opening is to be temporary or permanent.

As a temporary gastrostomy the Witzel or the Stamm procedure is used frequently and is easily performed. A permanent type of gastrostomy, such as the Janeway and its variations, is best adapted to patients in whom it is essential to have an opening into the stomach for a prolonged period of time. Under these circumstances the gastric mucosa must be anchored to the skin to ensure long-term patency of the opening. Furthermore, the construction of a mucosa-lined tube with valvelike control at the gastric end tends to prevent the regurgitation of the irritating gastric contents.

PREOPERATIVE PREPARATION. If the patient is dehydrated, his fluid balance is brought to a satisfactory level by the intravenous administration of 5 per cent dextrose in saline. Since these patients may be malnourished, it is frequently desirable to administer proteins and vitamins parenterally. Whole blood transfusion should be given if there is evidence of secondary anemia or a substantial loss of weight. Intravenous hyperalimentation may be indicated.

No special preparation is required for the temporary gastrostomy, since this is usually performed as a minor part of a primary surgical procedure.

ANESTHESIA. Since some patients requiring a permanent gastrostomy are both anemic and cachectic, local infiltration or field block anesthesia is usually advisable. There is no special indication in anesthesia for a temporary gastrostomy, since this is usually a minor technical procedure which precedes the closure of the wound of a major operation.

POSITION. The patient lies in a comfortable supine position with the feet lower than the head, so that the contracted stomach tends to drop below the costal margin.

OPERATIVE PREPARATION. The skin is prepared in the routine manner.

INCISION AND EXPOSURE. A small incision is made high in the left midrectus region, and the muscle is split with as little injury to the nerve supply as possible, if the gastrostomy is the lone surgical procedure planned **(Figure 1)**. The high position is indicated since the stomach may be contracted and high because of the long-term starvation that the patient may have experienced. The usual temporary tube gastrostomy is brought out through a stab wound some distance from the primary incision and away from the costal margin. The site of the stab wound must correspond exactly to the area of the abdominal wall to which the underlying stomach can be attached without tension **(Figure 1)**.

A. Stamm Gastrostomy

This type of gastrostomy is most commonly utilized as a temporary procedure. The midanterior gastric wall is grasped with Babcock forceps, and the ease with which the gastric wall approximates the overlying peritoneum is tested **(Figure 2)**. An incision at right angles to the long axis of the stomach is made in an effort to minimize the number of arterial bleeders. The incision is made with either scissors or a knife. A mushroom catheter of average size, F16 to F18, is introduced into the stomach for a distance of 10 to 15 cm. A Foley-type catheter may also be used. A suture of fine silk is taken through the entire gastric wall on either side of the tube in order to control any bleeding from the divided gastric wall **(Figure 3)**. When all bleeding has been controlled, the gastric wall about the tube is inverted by the usual purse-string suture of 00 silk **(Figure 3)**. The gas-

tric wall should be inverted about the tube to ensure rapid closure of the gastric opening when the catheter is removed **(Figure 6)**.

A point is then selected some distance from the margins of the incision for the placement of the stab wound and subsequent passage of the tube through the anterior abdominal wall **(Figure 4)**. The position of the catheter end should be checked to make certain that a sufficient amount extends into the gastric lumen to ensure efficient gastric drainage. The gastric wall is then anchored to the peritoneum about the tube **(Figure 5)** by four or five 00 silk sutures. Occasionally, additional sutures are necessary. The gastric wall must not be under undue tension at the completion of the procedure. The diagram in **Figure 6** shows the inversion of the gastric wall about the tube and the sealing of the gastric wall to the overlying peritoneum.

B. Janeway Gastrostomy

This procedure is one of the many types of permanent gastrostomies utilized to avoid an inlying tube and prevent the regurgitation of irritant gastric contents. Such a mucosa-lined tube anchored to the skin tends to remain patent with a minimal tendency toward closure of the mucosal opening.

DETAILS OF PROCEDURE. The operator visualizes the relation of the stomach to the anterior abdominal wall and then with Allis forceps outlines a rectangular flap, the base of which is placed near the greater curvature to ensure adequate blood supply **(Figure 7)**. Because the flap, when cut, contracts, it is made somewhat larger than would appear to be necessary to avoid subsequent interference with its blood supply when the flap is approximated about the catheter. The gastric wall is divided between Allis clamps near the lesser curvature, and a rectangular flap is developed by extending the incision on either side toward the Allis clamps on the greater curvature. To prevent soiling from the gastric contents and to control bleeding, long, straight enterostomy clamps may be applied to the stomach both above and below the operative site. The flap of gastric wall is pulled downward, and the catheter is placed along the inner surface of the flap **(Figure 9)**. The mucous membrane is closed with a continuous suture of catgut or interrupted 0000 silk sutures, starting at the lesser curvature, to approximate the mucous membrane of the rectangular flap over the catheter **(Figure 9)**. The outer layer, which includes the serosa and submucosa, is also closed either with continuous catgut sutures or preferably by a series of interrupted silk sutures **(Figure 11)**. When this cone-shaped entrance to the stomach has been completed about the catheter, the anterior gastric wall is attached to the peritoneum at the suture line with additional sutures of 00 silk **(Figure 11)**.

CLOSURE. After the pouch of gastric wall is lifted to the skin surface, the peritoneum is closed about the catheter. The catheter may be brought out through a small stab wound to the left of the major incision. The layers of the abdominal wall are closed about this, and the mucosa is anchored to the skin with a few sutures **(Figure 12)**. Catheters are anchored to the skin with strips of adhesive tape in addition to a suture that has included a bite in the catheter.

POSTOPERATIVE CARE. When the temporary Stamm type of gastrostomy is used in lieu of prolonged nasogastric suction, the usual principles of gastric decompression and fluid replacement are adhered to. Usually, the tube is clamped off as soon as normal bowel function returns. The temporary gastrostomy provides an invaluable method of fluid and nutritional replacement; compared to the more tedious and less efficient intravenous route, it is the method of choice, especially in the elderly patient.

The temporary gastrostomy should not be removed for at least seven to ten days to ensure adequate peritoneal sealing. In addition, it should not be removed until alimentary function has returned to normal and all postoperative gastric secretory studies have been completed.

When a permanent gastrostomy is done because of esophageal obstruction, liquids such as water and milk may be safely injected into the catheter within 24 hours, while intravenous hyperalimentation continues. Liquids of a high-calorie and high-vitamin value are added gradually. After a week or more the catheter may be removed and cleaned but should be replaced immediately, because of the tendency toward too rapid closure of the sinus tract in the Janeway type of gastrostomy.

PLATE IX   GASTROSTOMY

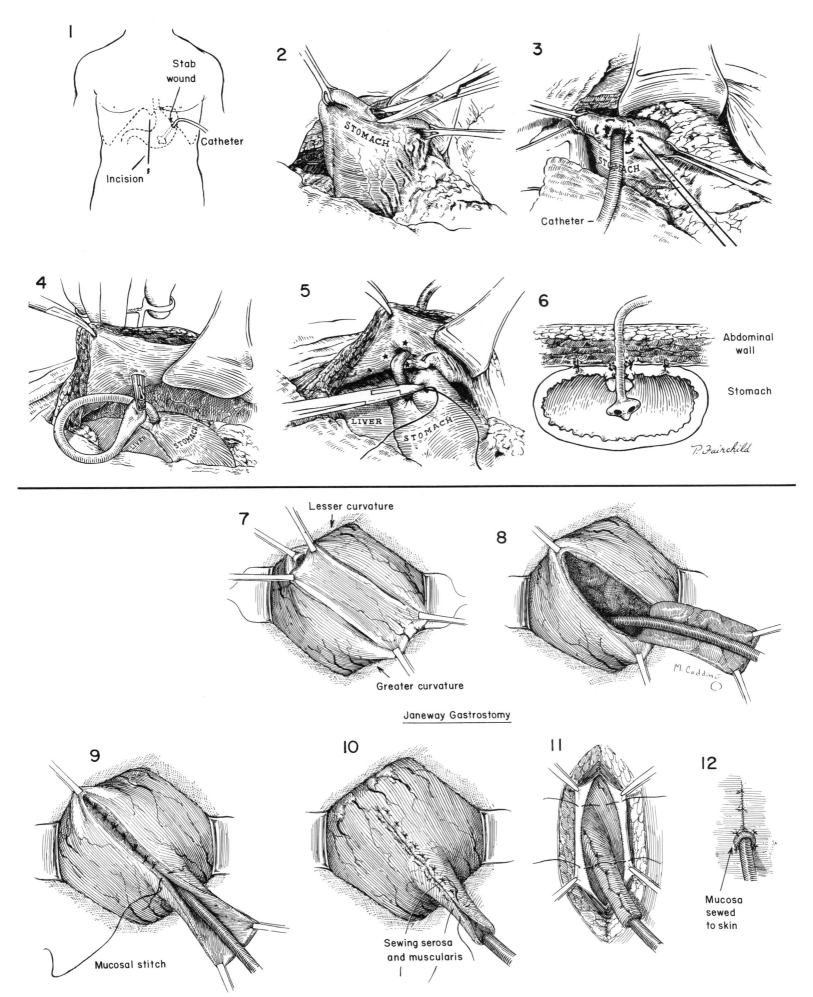

1. Stab wound / Catheter / Incision

3. Catheter —

6. Abdominal wall / Stomach

P. Fairchild

7. Lesser curvature / Greater curvature

8. M. Codding

Janeway Gastrostomy

9. Mucosal stitch

10. Sewing serosa and muscularis

12. Mucosa sewed to skin

PLATE X · CLOSURE OF PERFORATION—SUBPHRENIC ABSCESS

A. Closure of Perforation

INDICATIONS. Perforation of an ulcer of the stomach or duodenum is a surgical emergency; however, before performing the operation, sufficient time should be allowed for the patient to recover from the initial shock (rarely severe or prolonged) and for the restoration of the fluid balance.

PREOPERATIVE PREPARATION. A narcotic is used to control pain only after the diagnosis is established. The intravenous administration of saline, glucose, and whole blood or plasma may be necessary, depending upon the patient's general condition and the length of time that has elapsed since perforation. The parenteral administration of antibiotics and the institution of constant gastric suction are routine.

ANESTHESIA. General endotracheal anesthesia combined with muscle relaxants is preferred. In the poor-risk patient or patients with severe respiratory infection, local infiltration anesthesia is substituted.

POSITION. The patient is placed in a comfortable supine position with the feet slightly lower than the head to assist in bringing the field below the costal margin and to keep gastric leakage away from the subphrenic area.

OPERATIVE PREPARATION. The skin is prepared in the usual manner.

INCISION AND EXPOSURE. Since the majority of perforations occur in the anterior superior surface of the first portion of the duodenum, a small, high, right rectus midline or right paramedian incision is made. A culture of the peritoneal fluid is taken, and as much exudate as possible is removed by suction. The liver is held upward with retractors, exposing the most frequent sites of perforation. The site may be walled off with omentum if the perforation has been present several hours; therefore, care is exercised in approaching the perforation to avoid unnecessary soiling.

DETAILS OF PROCEDURE. The easiest method of closure consists of placing three sutures of fine silk or catgut through the submucosal layer on one side and extending through the region of the ulcer and out a corresponding distance on the other side of the ulcer **(Figure 1)**. Starting at the top of the ulcer, the sutures are tied very gently to prevent laceration of the friable tissues. The long ends are retained **(Figure 2)**. The closure is reinforced with omentum by separating the long ends of the three previously tied sutures and placing a small portion of omentum along the suture line. The ends of these sutures are loosely tied, anchoring the omentum over the site of the ulcer **(Figure 3)**.

The tissue may be so indurated that the ulcer cannot be closed successfully, making it necessary to seal the perforation by anchoring omentum directly over the ulcer.

In the presence of a perforated gastric ulcer, a small biopsy of the margin of the perforation is taken because of the possibility of malignancy **(Figures 4 and 5)**. The omentum may be anchored over the suture line **(Figure 6)**. Closure of a gastric ulcer may be reinforced with a layer of interrupted silk serosal sutures, since there is little danger of obstruction.

In the presence of perforation of an obvious carcinoma, it is usually safer to close the perforation, to be followed upon recovery by resection. If the patient's general condition is good and the perforation has lasted only a few hours, a gastric resection may be justified. Vagotomy and pyloroplasty or antrectomy for an early perforated duodenal ulcer in a good-risk patient is preferred by some surgeons.

CLOSURE. All exudate and fluid are removed by suction. Repeated irrigation of the peritoneal cavity with saline should be considered when there is gross contamination by food particles. The wound is closed without drainage. A temporary Stamm gastrostomy (Plate IX) should be considered since prolonged obstruction of the pylorus may occur.

POSTOPERATIVE CARE. The patient, when conscious, is placed in Fowler's position. Constant gastric suction is continued for several days until there is reasonable assurance that the pylorus is not occluded by edema. When a temporary gastrostomy has been performed, repeated studies should be made of the volume of the overnight 12-hour secretion. The tube is removed when the stomach is emptying satisfactorily. The fluid balance is maintained by intravenous infusions. Antibiotics are continued.

After three to four days, the patient is started on a strict ulcer diet regimen. Simple closure of the perforation has not cured the patient of his ulcer nor of his tendency to form another. It must be remembered that a subphrenic or a pelvic abscess may complicate the postoperative period.

B. Subphrenic Abscess

INDICATIONS. The commonest origins of a subphrenic abscess are perforation of a peptic ulcer, perforation of the appendix, or acute infection of the gallbladder. It is to be suspected in an unsatisfactory recovery from any of these conditions. Intensive antibiotic therapy may mask the systemic reaction to the infection.

PREOPERATIVE PREPARATION. The clinical data combined with roentgenologic studies usually indicate the location of the abscess. Subphrenic abscesses occur much more frequently on the right side. Antibiotics, blood transfusions, and intravenous fluids are usually necessary because of the prolonged sepsis.

ANESTHESIA. Local anesthesia by direct infiltration of the site of the incision is preferable for the poor-risk patient. Spinal or inhalation anesthesia also may be used, depending upon the patient's general condition.

POSITION. For an anterior abscess the patient is placed supine with the head of the table elevated. For a posterior abscess the patient is placed on his side with the arm on his affected side pulled forward.

OPERATIVE PREPARATION. The skin is prepared in the usual manner.

1. ANTERIOR ABSCESS

INCISION AND EXPOSURE. The incision is placed one fingerbreadth below the costal margin and extended from the midrectus region laterally **(Figure 7)**. The free peritoneal cavity is not opened.

DETAILS OF PROCEDURE. The surgeon inserts the index finger upward between the peritoneum and diaphragm until the abscess cavity is encountered; extraperitoneal drainage is thus established **(Figure 8)**.

2. POSTERIOR ABSCESS

INCISION AND EXPOSURE. It is desirable to drain the subphrenic abscess by the extraperitoneal route without rib resection whenever possible. On occasion it may be desirable to approach the abscess through the bed of the twelfth rib **(Figure 9, Incision A)**. The entire twelfth rib is resected as in thoracostomy (Plate CLII). The erector spinae are retracted toward the midline, and a transverse incision is made at right angles to the vertebrae across the periosteal bed of the resected rib, opposite the transverse process of the first lumbar vertebra **(Figure 9, Incision B)**.

DETAILS OF PROCEDURE. The location of the abscess cavity is approached by the index finger of the surgeon, who separates the peritoneum from the undersurface of the diaphragm, thus ensuring dependent drainage without contamination of the peritoneal cavities **(Figure 10)**. Once pus has been obtained, the abscess cavity can be entered and thoroughly evacuated, and rubber tissue drains or mushroom catheters can be inserted. Several cultures are taken routinely, and the sensitivity of the offending organism is determined. Some organisms, such as staphylococcus, require isolating the patient to prevent spread of the organism to others.

The cavity is opened adjacent to the aspiration needle, which serves as a guide into the abscess cavity **(Figure 11)**.

CLOSURE. Drains are inserted into the abscess cavity in numbers indicated by the size of the abscess. There is no further closure.

POSTOPERATIVE CARE. The abscess cavity is carefully irrigated with normal saline each day and the capacity of the cavity measured from time to time. The external opening is maintained until obliteration of the cavity occurs. Antibiotics may be indicated parenterally as well as instilled locally into the abscess cavity, the choice depending upon the sensitivities of the organisms grown from the pus. A high-protein, high-calorie, high-vitamin diet is given. Repeated blood transfusion may be indicated.

PLATE X   CLOSURE OF PERFORATION—SUBPHRENIC ABSCESS

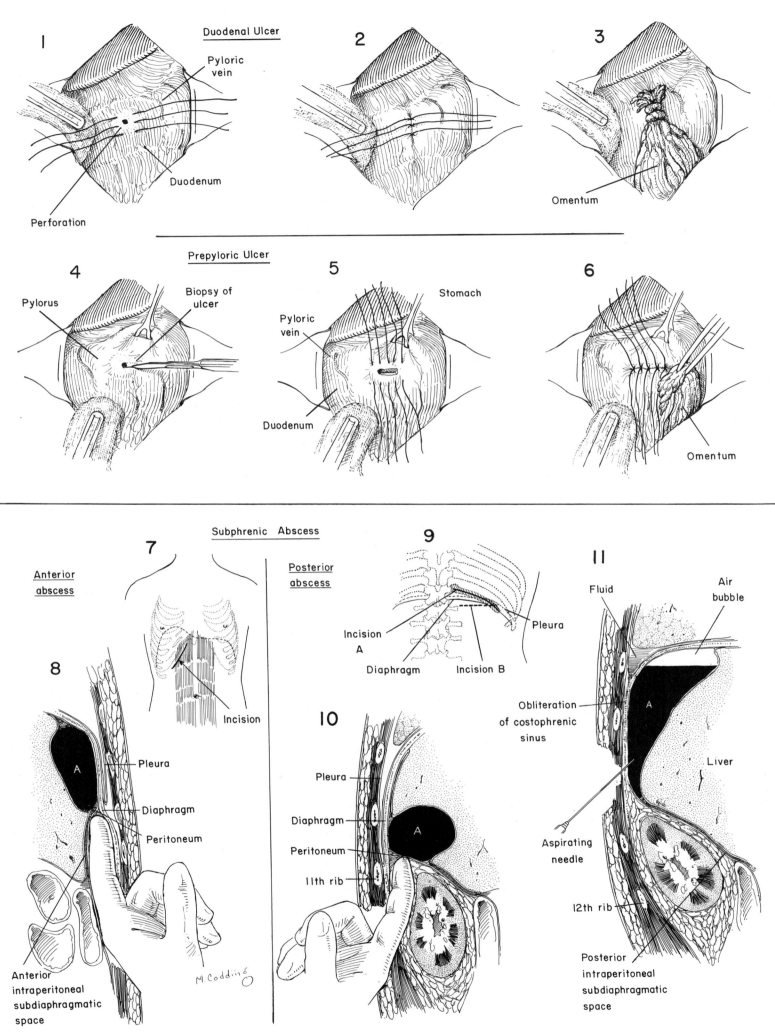

Duodenal Ulcer

1 Pyloric vein / Duodenum / Perforation

2

3 Omentum

Prepyloric Ulcer

4 Pylorus / Biopsy of ulcer

5 Pyloric vein / Stomach / Duodenum

6 Omentum

Subphrenic Abscess

Anterior abscess

7 Incision

Posterior abscess

9 Incision A / Diaphragm / Incision B / Pleura

8 Pleura / Diaphragm / Peritoneum / Anterior intraperitoneal subdiaphragmatic space

10 Pleura / Diaphragm / Peritoneum / 11th rib

11 Fluid / Air bubble / Obliteration of costophrenic sinus / Liver / Aspirating needle / 12th rib / Posterior intraperitoneal subdiaphragmatic space

M. Codding

PLATE XI · GASTROJEJUNOSTOMY

INDICATIONS. Gastrojejunostomy is indicated for certain elderly patients with duodenal ulcer complicated by pyloric obstruction and low acid value. It is indicated also if technical difficulties prevent resection or make it hazardous, if the patient is such a poor operative risk that only the safest possible surgical procedure should be carried out, or if vagus resection has been performed. It is occasionally indicated for the relief of pyloric obstruction in the presence of nonresectable malignancies of the stomach, duodenum, or head of the pancreas.

PREOPERATIVE PREPARATION. The preoperative preparation must be varied, depending upon the duration and severity of the pyloric obstruction, the degree of secondary anemia, and the protein depletion. The restoration of blood volume is especially important in patients who have lost considerable weight. Low values of sodium chloride and potassium must be corrected, and the carbon dioxide combining power and blood urea nitrogen returned to normal before operation. Secondary anemia and protein and vitamin deficiencies should be corrected insofar as possible before operation. Their correction aids healing and contributes to the proper emptying of the stomach after operation. The large atonic stomach is emptied by constant gastric suction for several days before operation. The stomach is emptied by gastric lavage, usually the night preceding operation, to make certain that all coarse particles of food have been removed and that gastric tension is relieved. The lavage is repeated one to two hours before operation. Constant gastric suction with a Levine tube is maintained. Blood must be available for transfusion during the operation.

ANESTHESIA. General anesthesia combined with endotracheal intubation is usually satisfactory. Muscle relaxants may be employed to avoid the deeper planes of anesthesia. Spinal or continuous spinal anesthesia provides profound muscle relaxation and a contracted bowel. Local infiltration is sometimes advisable in poor-risk patients.

POSITION. The patient is placed in a comfortable supine position with the feet at least a foot lower than the head. In patients with an unusually high stomach, a more upright position may be of assistance. The optimum position can be obtained after the abdomen is opened and the exact location of the stomach is determined.

OPERATIVE PREPARATION. The lower thorax and abdomen are prepared in the routine manner.

INCISION AND EXPOSURE. As a rule, a midline epigastric incision is made. If it is certain that gastrojejunostomy alone is to be performed, a left paramedian incision is made, opening the left rectus sheath about 2 to 3 cm. lateral to the midline. This permits closure with two fascial layers. The incision is extended upward to the xiphoid or to the costal margin and downward to the umbilicus. With the abdomen opened, a self-retaining retractor may be utilized; but, since most of the structures involved in this operation are mobile, it is usually unnecessary to use any great amount of traction for adequate exposure.

DETAILS OF PROCEDURE. The stomach and duodenum are visualized and palpated to determine the type and extent of the pathologic lesion present. A short loop of jejunum is utilized for gastrojejunostomy, with the proximal portion anchored to the lesser curvature. The stoma is made on the posterior gastric wall and extends from the lesser to the greater curvature, about two fingers in length. It is located at the most dependent part of the stomach **(Figure 1, A).**

When the gastroenterostomy is performed with vagotomy in the treatment of duodenal ulcer, the location and size of the stoma are very important. In order to ensure adequate drainage of the paralyzed antrum and keep postoperative side effects to a minimum, a small stoma parallel to the greater curvature and near the pylorus is indicated **(Figure 1, B).** Special effort is required as a rule to ensure placement of the stoma within 3 to 5 cm. of the pylorus. Because of the fixation of the pylorus associated with duodenal ulceration, it is too impracticable to attempt to bring the site of the anastomosis outside the abdominal wall, as shown in the accompanying diagrams.

The location of the stoma is first outlined on the anterior gastric wall with Babcock forceps. The greater omentum may be brought outside the wound so that the contour of the stomach is not distorted, and the most dependent portion of the greater curvature may be more accurately determined **(Figure 2).** The Babcock forceps are left in place as the greater omentum is reflected upward over the stomach and the inferior aspect of the mesocolon is visualized **(Figure 3).** The transverse colon is held firmly by an assistant as the surgeon invaginates the Babcock forceps on the anterior gastric wall. This produces a bulge in the mesentery of the colon at the point through which the stomach is to be drawn **(Figure 3).** The mesocolon is carefully incised to the left of the middle colic vessels and near the ligament of Treitz, great care being taken to avoid any of the large vessels in the arcade. Four to six guide sutures (sutures a, b, c, d, e, and f) are placed in the margins of the incised mesocolon to be utilized after the anastomosis to the stomach at the proper level. The presenting posterior wall of the stomach is grasped with a Babcock forceps adjacent to the lesser and greater curvatures, and opposite the points of counterpressure from the similarly placed forceps on the anterior gastric wall **(Figure 4).** A portion of the gastric wall is pulled through the opening. In many instances the inflammatory reaction associated with the duodenal ulcer may anchor the posterior surface of the antrum to the capsule of the pancreas. Sharp and blunt dissection may be required to mobilize the stomach in order to ensure placement of the stoma sufficiently near the pylorus. Some surgeons prefer to anchor the mesocolon to the stomach at this time. The forceps on the greater curvature is swung toward the operator on the patient's right side, while the forceps on the lesser curvature is rotated to a position opposite the first assistant.

The ligament of Treitz is identified, and a loop of jejunum 10 to 15 cm. distal to this fixed point is delivered into the wound. The jejunum at this point is held with Babcock forceps as the enterostomy clamp is applied. The midsection of the portion of jejunum to be included in the enterostomy clamp may require fixation with thumb forceps to assure an even inclusion of the bowel in the clamp **(Figure 5).** The clamp should be applied near the mesenteric border, with the handle of the clamp toward the patient's right side and with the proximal jejunal loop in the toe end of the clamp **(Figure 5).**

Spring clamps are best used without rubber covers, because covers make them bulky and so slippery that more pressure is likely to be used than is necessary, especially at either end of the clamp. A clamp of fine spring steel holds its position well without great pressure and leaves no deleterious effects.

With the clamp in position, a piece of gauze is laid next to the jejunum. Then the stomach is grasped in a similar enterostomy clamp, placed with the handle of the clamp toward the patient's head, to include the selected oblique portion of the posterior gastric wall **(Figure 6).** Now the two enterostomy clamps are brought side to side, so that the distal end of the jejunal opening will be at the greater curvature of the stomach. The portion of the jejunum toward the ligament of Treitz, i.e., the proximal portion, is anchored to the lesser curvature of the stomach **(Figure 6).** At times the stomach cannot be sufficiently mobilized for the application of clamps as shown in **Figure 6,** and the anastomosis is made without a clamp on either side.

PLATE XI   GASTROJEJUNOSTOMY

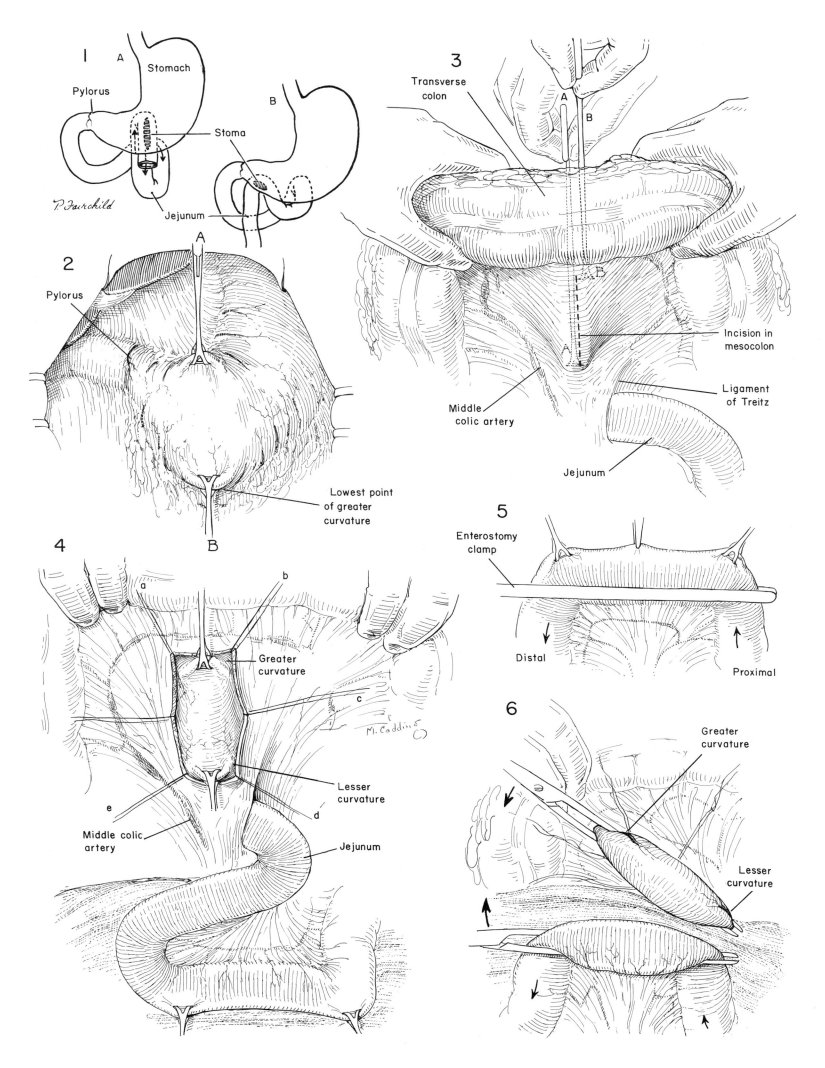

1

Pylorus

Stomach

A

Stoma

B

Jejunum

P. Fairchild

2

A

Pylorus

Lowest point
of greater
curvature

B

3

Transverse
colon

A

B

Incision in
mesocolon

Ligament
of Treitz

Middle
colic artery

Jejunum

4

a

b

Greater
curvature

c

Lesser
curvature

e

d

Middle colic
artery

Jejunum

M. Codding

5

Enterostomy
clamp

Distal

Proximal

6

Greater
curvature

Lesser
curvature

PLATE XII · GASTROJEJUNOSTOMY

DETAILS OF PROCEDURE (*Continued*). The enterostomy clamps applied to the stomach and the jejunum are held in apposition by ligatures or rubber bands **(Figures 7,** x and y**).** The large intestine and omentum are returned within the abdomen above the stomach. The clamps and the anastomotic site usually can be delivered outside the peritoneal cavity, which should be entirely protected with gauze. Retraction on the edges of the abdominal wound is discontinued while the anastomosis is being performed. This mobilization is usually impossible when the stoma must be made within 3 to 5 cm. of the pylorus following vagotomy. Under these circumstances the anastomosis must be made within the peritoneal cavity, lest the stoma be made too far to the left, with recurrent ulcer difficulties due to hormone stimulation from the distended antrum inducing gastric hypersecretion.

The posterior serosal sutures are now begun by placing a mattress suture of fine silk at either angle **(Figure 7).** The surgeon depresses the presenting portions of the stomach and jejunum with his index and middle fingers as the posterior row of interrupted mattress sutures in the serosa, parallel with the enterostomy clamp, is completed **(Figure 8).** Alternate bites of jejunum and stomach are taken; these include the submucosa but do not enter the lumen of the bowel. Each suture is taken close to the preceding one to ensure a complete closure. It is best to tie them after all have been placed.

When the posterior serosal layer is completed, fresh moist toweling is laid on both sides of the field; the only instruments left on this toweling are those to be used for opening the stomach and jejunum, for cleaning the lumen, and for closing the bowel with the mucosal sutures.

Short, lengthwise incisions in the stomach and jejunum are made by depressing the bowel and incising with a scalpel several millimeters from the serosal suture and not in the middle of the presenting contents of the clamp **(Figure 9).** If this incision is too far from the serosal layer, too large a cuff of inverted bowel may result. In making these incisions, the operator should be careful to cut the bowel wall perpendicular to its surface, since there is always a tendency to incise the intestine obliquely, thereby leaving an irregular and unequalized mucosal layer for the next suture line **(Figure 10).** The larger vessels in the stomach wall are then ligated with 0000 transfixing sutures of silk. The contents of the bowel are wiped out with a small piece of gauze moistened with saline, and the mucosal incision is completed with straight scissors. The incision in the jejunum is made slightly shorter than that made in the stomach **(Figure 11).** With the stomach and intestine opened and cleaned, a continuous suture of fine catgut on straight needles is started in the midportion of the posterior mucosal layers **(Figure 12).** As the operator sews away from himself, he uses a simple over-and-over suture or a lock stitch which pulls together the mucosal layers **(Figure 13).** Since this suture is also used to control the blood supply, it must be kept under a tension sufficient for accurate approximation and prevention of hemorrhage, yet not completely strangulating the blood supply and hindering healing. This is a critical step. The amount of tension is adjusted by the surgeon, who should hold the suture in his left hand while he works with his right. The first assistant exposes the point to be sutured and pulls the needle through. Interrupted sutures are placed to secure any bleeding points which have not been controlled by the continuous suture. When the operator reaches the angle of the wound, a Connell suture, which allows inversion of the structures as they are sewn, is substituted **(Figure 14).** In **Figure 14,** for example, the needle has just entered the gastric side. It comes out on the gastric side 2 or 3 mm. from its point of entrance **(Figure 15).** It is then crossed over, inserted through the jejunal wall from outside as in **Figure 16,** and comes back out through the jejunal wall before being reinserted through the gastric wall **(Figure 17).** After this angle has been closed, the other end, B, of the continuous suture is used to close the opposite angle in a similar fashion

(Figure 18). The continuous sutures, A and B, finally meet along the anterior surface. The final bite of each suture brings it to the inner wall of the stomach and jejunum **(Figure 19).** The two ends are tied together with the final knot on the inside. The clamps may then be released to see if there is any bleeding. If slight oozing persists, additional interrupted sutures may be taken to supplement the anterior mucosal layer.

Some surgeons prefer to do the anastomosis without clamps and tie each individual bleeding point before approximating the mucosa. Others prefer interrupted fine 0000 silk sutures for the mucosa instead of a continuous suture. The interrupted sutures on the anterior surface are tied with the knot on the inside. This series of interrupted Connell-type sutures ensures an even inversion of the mucosa.

The special toweling and the instruments used for the preceding stage of the operation are discarded; the gloves are changed, or gloved hands are thoroughly washed in an antiseptic solution, and approximation of the anterior serosal layer is carried out with interrupted fine silk sutures **(Figure 20).** These are placed very close together. Additional interrupted sutures of fine silk are placed at the angles of the anastomosis for reinforcement so that any strain at this point avoids the original suture line **(Figure 21).** The patency and size of the stoma should be determined by palpation. A secure anastomosis is desirable with a stoma approximately the size of the end of the thumb or two fingers.

A stoma about one half the size illustrated is indicated when vagotomy is performed. The lumen should not be larger in diameter than the adult thumb in order to reduce the incidence and severity of postoperative complaints. The stomach is anchored to the mesocolon, with sutures b, c, and d adjacent to the anastomosis in order to close the opening and thus prevent a potential internal hernia **(Figure 22).** This also prevents any torsion of the jejunum near the anastomosis, which might result if the stoma retracts above the mesocolon.

Occasionally, in the presence of extensive inflammation about the pylorus, marked obesity, or extensive malignancy, it may be impossible to mobilize the posterior gastric wall sufficiently for an anastomosis that allows adequate drainage of the antrum. Under these circumstances anterior gastrostomy or enterostomy should be considered following vagotomy to ensure adequate drainage of the antrum or proximal drainage of an inoperable gastric malignancy. In order to avoid the possibility of poor emptying following anterior gastrojejunostomy, the thick omentum should be divided to permit the upper jejunum to be easily brought up over the transverse colon. Some prefer to clear the greater curvature near the pylorus for 5 to 8 cm. and place the gastrojejunal stoma in this area. A Stamm-type gastrostomy should be considered to ensure patient comfort and provide an efficient and readily available method of gastric decompression until gastric emptying is satisfactory.

CLOSURE. The wound is closed in the routine manner. It is not drained.

POSTOPERATIVE CARE. Constant gastric suction is maintained for several days until it is evident that the stomach is emptying satisfactorily. The use of fluids, glucose, vitamins, blood, plasma, and parenternal alimentation depends upon daily clinical and laboratory evaluation. The patient may be permitted out of bed on the first day after operation. Water in sips is given within 24 hours, and the fluid and food intake is increased gradually thereafter. Six small feedings per day are gradually replaced by a full diet as tolerated. Twelve-hour overnight secretion studies should be made to evaluate the completeness of the vagotomy when the latter procedure has been performed in the treatment of duodenal ulcer. If a gastrostomy has been done, the tube can be withdrawn usually in ten days unless there is evidence of a delay in gastric emptying.

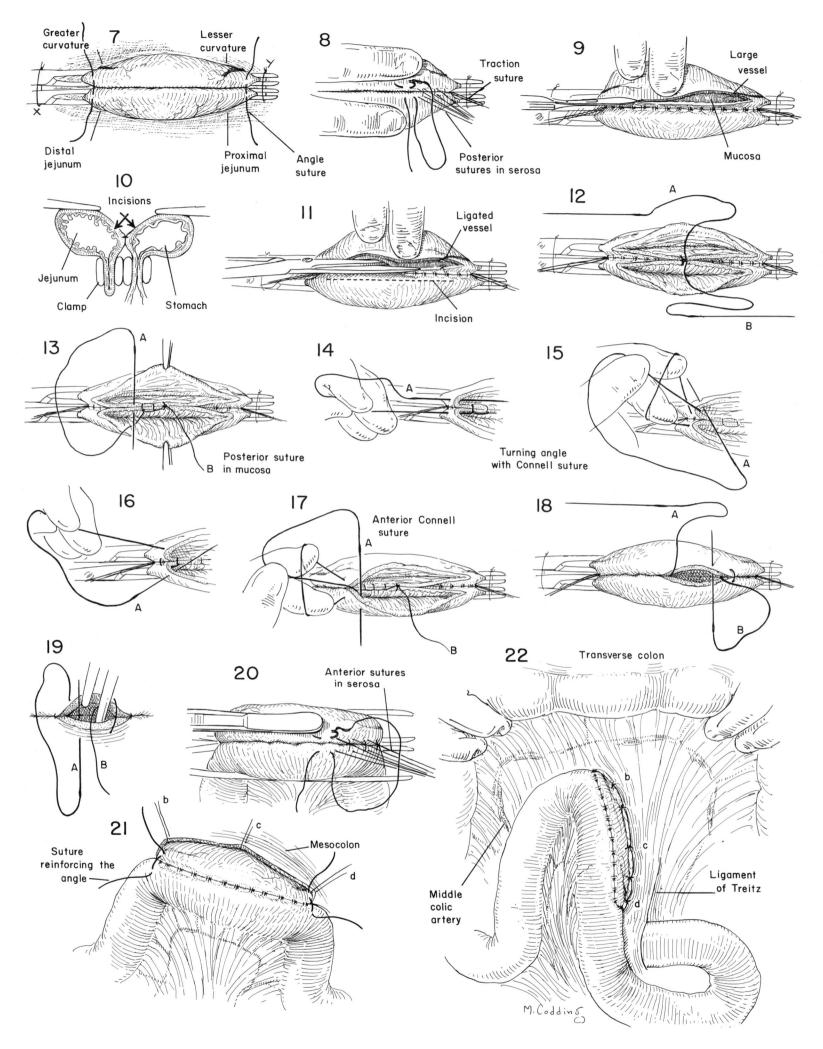

7 Greater curvature, Lesser curvature, Distal jejunum, Proximal jejunum, Angle suture

8 Traction suture, Posterior sutures in serosa

9 Large vessel, Mucosa

10 Incisions, Jejunum, Clamp, Stomach

11 Ligated vessel, Incision

12 A, B

13 A, Posterior suture in mucosa, B

14 A

15 Turning angle with Connell suture, A

16 A

17 Anterior Connell suture, A, B

18 A, B

19 A, B

20 Anterior sutures in serosa

21 Suture reinforcing the angle, b, c, Mesocolon, d

22 Transverse colon, Middle colic artery, b, c, d, Ligament of Treitz

M. Codding

PLATE XIII · PYLOROPLASTY—GASTRODUODENOSTOMY

INDICATIONS. These procedures may be used when the vagus innervation of the stomach has been interrupted either by truncal vagotomy, selective vagotomy, or division of the vagus nerves associated with esophagogastric resection and reestablishment of esophagogastric continuity. The pyloroplasty ensures drainage of the gastric antrum following vagotomy and therefore partially eliminates the antral phase of gastric secretion. It does not alter the continuity of the gastrointestinal tract and decreases the possibility of marginal ulceration occasionally seen after gastrojejunostomy. Pyloroplasty carries a low surgical morbidity and mortality rate because of its technical simplicity. Two types of pyloroplasty are commonly used, the Heineke-Mikulicz pyloroplasty **(Figure A)** and the Finney pyloroplasty **(Figure B).** Pyloroplasty should be avoided in the presence of a marked inflammatory reaction or severe scarring and deformity on the duodenal side of the gastric outlet. Under these circumstances the Jaboulay procedure **(Figure C)** should be considered, or a gastroenterostomy located within 3 cm. of the pylorus on the greater curvature.

Heineke-Mikulicz Pyloroplasty (Figure A)

The pylorus is identified with the pyloric vein as the landmark. A Kocher maneuver (Plate XVII) is then carried out to mobilize the duodenum for good exposure and relaxation of tension on the subsequent transverse suture line. Traction sutures of 00 silk are placed and tied at the superior and inferior margins of the pyloric ring for anatomical orientation. Efforts should be made to include the pyloric vein in these sutures, in order to partially control the subsequent bleeding. A longitudinal incision is made approximately 2 to 3 cm. on each side of the pyloric ring through all layers of the anterior wall **(Figure 1).** In the presence of marked deformity it may be advisable to incise the midportion of the duodenum and then, with a hemostat directed up through the constricted pyloric canal as a guide, make the incision in the midportion of the pylorus, across the midportion of the anterior duodenal wall, and across the midpoint of the pyloric wall into the gastric side. Bleeding may be partially controlled by noncrushing clamps across the antrum and distal to the anastomosis across the duodenum, unless the induration and fixation associated with the ulcer are too marked.

Traction on the angle sutures draws the longitudinal incision apart until it becomes first diamond-shaped **(Figures 1 and 2)** and then transverse **(Figure 3).** All bleeding points are ligated with 0000 silk which includes the full thickness of gastric or duodenal wall. Active bleeders tend to occur in the divided duodenal wall and in the region of the divided pyloric sphincter. Inverting sutures of interrupted 0000 silk are passed through all layers to approximate the mucosa. Some prefer a one-layer closure in order to minimize the encroachment on the pyloric lumen resulting from the inversion that follows a two-layer closure. Usually, a second row of V-sutures of 00 silk is placed with the open end of the V on the gastric side **(Figure 3).** After the closure is completed, the thumb and index finger are used to palpate the newly formed lumen by invaginating the gastric and duodenal walls on each side of the transverse closure. A Cushing silver clip is placed to mark either end of the suture line to serve as a marker of the gastric outlet during subsequent barium studies. A temporary gastrostomy may be performed (Plate IX).

Finney U-Shaped Pyloroplasty (Figure B)

The pylorus is identified by noting the overlying pyloric vein. Freeing all interfering adhesions and mobilizing the pyloric end of the stomach, the pylorus, and the first and second portions of the duodenum by use of an extensive Kocher maneuver are essential (Plate XVII). A traction suture is placed in the superior margin of the midpylorus, and a second suture joins a point approximately 5 cm. proximal to the pyloric ring on the greater curvature of the stomach to a point 5 cm. distal to the pyloric ring on the duodenal wall **(Figure B).** The walls of the stomach and duodenum are sutured together with interrupted 00 silk. These sutures should be placed as near the greater curvature margins of the stomach and the inner margin of the duodenum as possible, to ensure adequate room for subsequent closure. A U-shaped incision is then made into the stomach from a point just above the traction suture around through the pylorus and down a similar distance on the duodenal wall adjacent to the suture line. If an ulcer is present on the anterior wall, it may be excised. Bleeding points are clamped and tied with 0000 silk. A wedge of the pyloric sphincter may be removed from either side to facilitate the mucosal closure. The posterior mucosal septum between the stomach and duodenum is united with interrupted 0000 silk sutures. These sutures run from the superior aspect and include all layers of the septum **(Figure 4).** The anterior mucosal layer is approximated with inverting interrupted sutures of 0000 silk.

As seen in **Figure 5,** a second layer of sutures using a mattress overlapping stitch starts superiorly and brings together the seromuscular layers of the anterior walls of the stomach and duodenum. A portion of the omentum may be sutured over the anastomosis. A temporary gastrostomy may be performed (Plate IX) or constant nasogastric suction maintained a few days or until the stomach empties satisfactorily.

Jaboulay Gastroduodenostomy (Figure C)

It is advisable to carry out a very extensive Kocher maneuver (Plate XVII) with thorough mobilization of the second and third parts of the duodenum. When this procedure is carried out, it is wise to visualize the middle colic vessels, which sometimes tend to swing down over the duodenum and appear rather unexpectedly during the dissection. It is also advisable to attempt a limited mobilization of the inner surface of the duodenum without interference with its blood supply. The gastric wall, however, adjacent to the pylorus and downward for 6 to 8 cm. may be freed of its blood supply and tested for mobility over to the duodenal wall. A suture is taken between the gastric wall and duodenum as near the pylorus as practical, and a second suture is taken between the gastric wall and the second part of the duodenum as near the inner duodenal border as possible, to provide for approximation of 6 to 8 cm. of the gastric wall and duodenum **(Figure C).**

The procedure varies little from that described for pyloroplasty. Sutures of 00 interrupted silk are used on the serosa. Noncrushing clamps should be applied across the gastric wall to avoid gross contamination and at the same time partially control the tendency to bleeding. An incision is made in the gastric wall as well as in the duodenal wall adjacent to the serosal suture line. The pylorus is left intact **(Figure 6).** All active bleeding points on both the gastric and duodenal sides should be carefully ligated with 0000 silk or similar small-caliber suture material. The mucosa is approximated with either interrupted sutures of 0000 silk or a continuous catgut layer. Interrupted mattress sutures of 00 silk are placed to approximate the seromuscular coat as a second layer **(Figure 7).** Silver clips are applied to mark the site of anastomosis. The inferior angle between the second part of the duodenum and greater curvature of the stomach may require several additional interrupted sutures of 00 silk to assure complete sealing of the angle. Either prolonged nasogastric suction should be instituted or a temporary gastrostomy performed (Plate IX), particularly if vagotomy has been carried out.

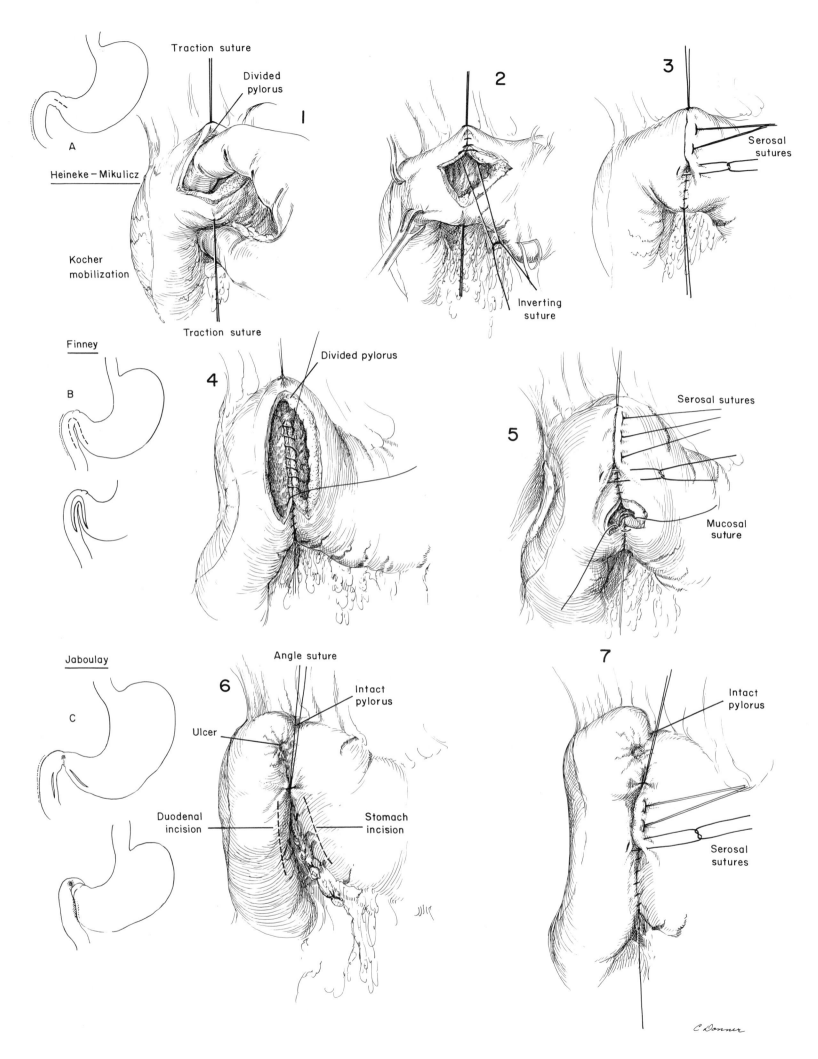

Heineke—Mikulicz

Kocher mobilization

A

Finney

B

Jaboulay

C

Traction suture

Divided pylorus

1

Traction suture

2

Inverting suture

3

Serosal sutures

Divided pylorus

4

5

Serosal sutures

Mucosal suture

Angle suture

Intact pylorus

Ulcer

6

Duodenal incision

Stomach incision

7

Intact pylorus

Serosal sutures

C Donner

PLATE XIV · VAGOTOMY

Bilateral resection of segments of the vagus nerves in the region of the lower esophagus is a key component in treating intractable duodenal or gastrojejunal ulcers. The motor paralysis and resultant gastric retention that follow vagotomy alone make it mandatory that a concomitant gastric resection or drainage procedure, such as pyloroplasty or an antrally placed gastroenterostomy, be performed. Gastrojejunal or stomal ulcers following a previous gastrectomy or gastrojejunostomy show a favorable response to vagotomy. The use of vagotomy to control the cephalic phase of secretion is preferred when it is desirable to retain as much gastric capacity as possible because of the preoperative nutritional status of the patient with duodenal ulcer. In females and in those individuals below their ideal weight preoperatively, controlling the acid factor by vagotomy followed by pyloroplasty, posterior gastroenterostomy, or hemigastrectomy should be seriously considered. Controlling the acid factor by vagotomy has been used in combination with other procedures in managing chronic recurrent pancreatitis.

There are two vagal trunks—the anterior or left vagus nerve, which lies along the anterior wall of the esophagus, and the posterior or right vagus nerve, which is sometimes overlooked since it is more easily separated from the esophagus. The vagus nerves may be divided several centimeters above the esophageal junction (truncal vagotomy), divided below the celiac and hepatic branches (selective vagotomy), or divided so that only the branches to the upper two-thirds of the stomach are interrupted, while the nerves of Latarjet, innervating the antrum or lower one-third, as well as the celiac and hepatic branches, are retained (superselective vagotomy).

Truncal Vagotomy

A good exposure of the lower end of the esophagus is essential and sometimes requires removal of the xiphoid as well as mobilization of the left lobe of the liver. The vagal nerves should be identified and divided as far from the esophagogastric junction as possible **(Figure 1)**. Sections of these trunks should be sent to the pathologist for microscopic evidence that at least two vagus nerves have been divided. Whether silver clips or ligatures are applied to both ends of each nerve is the choice of the individual surgeon. It may be advisable to ligate the posterior nerve to control possible oozing that may take place in the mediastinum. The esophagus should be carefully inspected, and the area behind the esophagus in particular should be searched as the esophagus is retracted upward to make sure that the posterior vagus nerve is not overlooked. In most instances the cephalic phase of secretion will not be controlled if vagotomy has been incomplete. Some prefer to combine the vagotomy with a hemigastrectomy in order to control the gastric phase of secretion as well as the cephalic phase. Drainage of the antrum is essential by pyloroplasty, gastroenterostomy, or gastroduodenostomy (see Plate XIII). The increased incidence of recurrent ulceration following vagotomy and antral drainage by pyloroplasty or gastroenterostomy must be weighed against a somewhat higher mortality following vagotomy and hemigastrectomy.

Selective Vagotomy

Selective vagotomy has been suggested as a means of decreasing the incidence of dumping by maintaining the vagal innervation of the liver and small intestine. The vagus nerves are carefully isolated from the esophagus and divided beyond the point where they give off branches to the liver and to the celiac ganglion **(Figure 2)**. It is necessary to visualize clearly the lower end of the esophagus and to follow the anterior nerve down over the esophagogastric junction with identification of the hepatic branch. The nerve is divided beyond the hepatic branch, as shown in

Figure 2. The posterior vagus nerve is likewise very carefully identified as it courses down over the esophagogastric junction, and the branch going to the celiac ganglion is identified. The nerve is divided beyond that point in order to make certain that the vagus nerve supply to the small intestine has not been interrupted. Following this, some type of decompression procedure or resection is done.

Superselective Vagotomy

Superselective vagotomy, also known as highly selective vagotomy, selective proximal vagotomy, or parietal cell vagotomy, is illustrated in **Figure 3**. This procedure attempts to control the cephalic phase of secretion while maintaining the celiac branch, the hepatic branch, and the anterior and posterior nerves of Latarjet to the distal antrum **(Figure 3)**. In this procedure the vagal denervation is confined to the upper two-thirds of the stomach, while innervation is left intact to the lower third as well as to the biliary tract and small intestine. With superselective vagotomy it is anticipated that a drainage procedure will not be required, since the pyloric sphincter retains its normal function. As a result, the incidence of disagreeable side effects associated with dumping should be decreased.

It has been pointed out that the nerves of Latarjet send out branches in a crow's-foot pattern over the terminal 6 or 7 cm. of the antrum. All other branches of the vagus nerves on either side of the lesser curvature are divided up to and around the esophagus **(Figure 3)**. This may be a time-consuming and difficult technical procedure, particularly when the exposure is limited and the patient obese. Some prefer to identify the anterior and posterior vagus nerves at the lower end of the esophagus and place them under traction with carefully placed sutures or nerve hooks that serve as retractors, thus ensuring that the vagal nerve trunks will not be damaged and at the same time helping define the branches going to the stomach. The dissection is usually started about 6 cm. from the pylorus on the anterior wall of the stomach **(Figure 4A)**. Small hemostats are used in pairs to carefully clamp and divide the blood vessels and vagal branches as the dissection progresses up the anterior surface of the gastric wall along the lesser curvature **(Figure 4B)**.

Special care must be taken as the dissection reaches the area where the left gastric artery reaches the lesser curvature of the stomach. The anterior nerve of Latarjet must be identified frequently as the dissection approaches the esophagogastric junction. The peritoneum over the lower end of the esophagus is carefully divided to permit identification of the vagal branches as the dissection is carried around the anterior portion of the esophagogastric junction. Finger dissection may be used to push gently both the anterior as well as the posterior vagus nerves away from the esophageal wall. After the finger has encircled the esophagus, a rubber tissue drain or a rubber catheter is introduced around the esophagus to provide traction. Upward traction on the esophagus provides easier identification of the top branches of the posterior nerve of Latarjet as they course over to the lesser curvature to provide innervation to the posterior gastric wall **(Figure 5)**. The lower 5 cm. of the esophagus should be completely cleared to avoid overlooking small fibers. The posterior branches are carefully identified and divided between pairs of small curved hemostats, similar to the procedure utilized on the anterior wall. A rubber tissue drain can be passed around the mobilized lesser omentum, including the nerves of Latarjet, to provide better exposure of the divided lesser curvature. A final search is made for any overlooked vagal branches, incomplete hemostasis, or possible injury to the nerves of Latarjet. Since the innervation to the antrum is retained, it is unnecessary to provide antral drainage by either pyloroplasty or gastroenterostomy, provided the duodenal outlet is not obstructed by scarring or a marked inflammatory reaction.

PLATE XIV VAGOTOMY

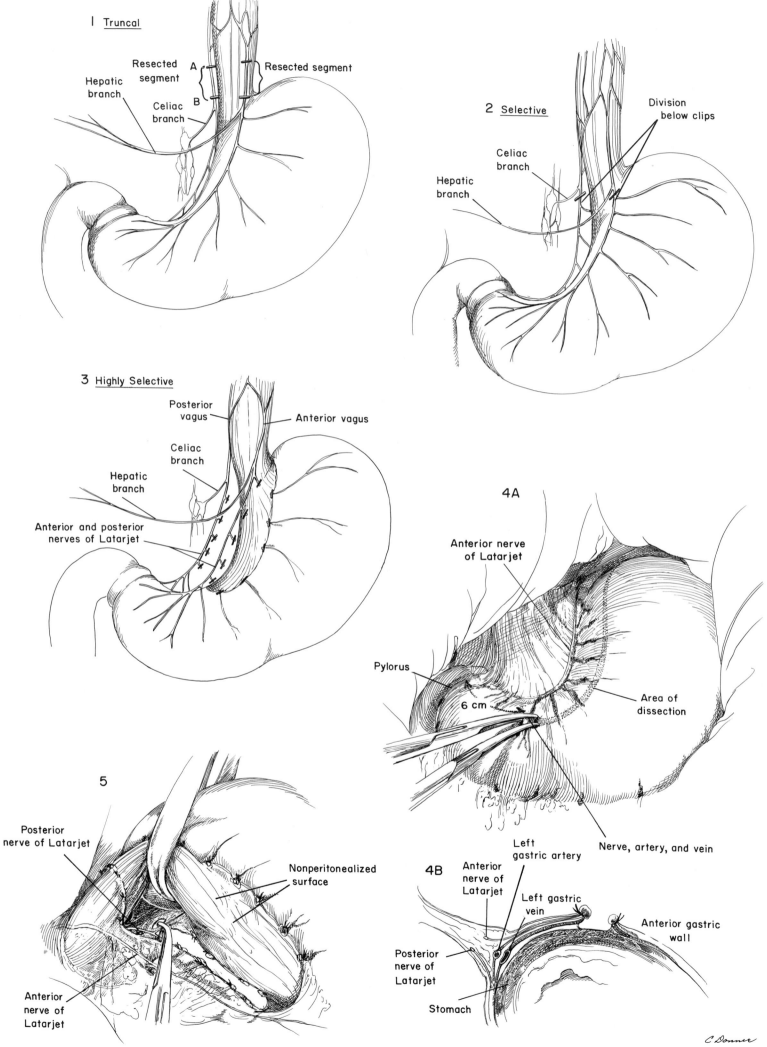

1 <u>Truncal</u>

Hepatic branch

Resected segment

Celiac branch

A

B

Resected segment

2 <u>Selective</u>

Division below clips

Celiac branch

Hepatic branch

3 <u>Highly Selective</u>

Posterior vagus

Anterior vagus

Celiac branch

Hepatic branch

Anterior and posterior nerves of Latarjet

4A

Anterior nerve of Latarjet

Pylorus

6 cm

Area of dissection

Nerve, artery, and vein

5

Posterior nerve of Latarjet

Nonperitonealized surface

Anterior nerve of Latarjet

4B

Anterior nerve of Latarjet

Left gastric artery

Left gastric vein

Anterior gastric wall

Posterior nerve of Latarjet

Stomach

C Donner

PLATE XV · VAGOTOMY, SUBDIAPHRAGMATIC APPROACH

INDICATIONS. The long-term results of vagotomy are closely related to the completeness of the vagotomy and to efficient drainage or resection of the antrum (see Plate XIV). This operation should not be employed in psychoneurotic individuals with no proved organic lesion or in those that suffer from some type of gastric neurosis.

OPERATIVE PREPARATION. A careful evaluation of the adequacy and extent of the medical management is made. A 12-hour night secretion determination with continuous suction is done to ascertain the gastric secretory status of the patient. Fasting serum gastrin levels may be indicated. Proof of the presence of a duodenal ulcer and determination of the amount of gastric retention are established by a barium meal, by fluoroscopy and roentgenologic studies, and by fasting aspirations through a stomach tube. Constant nasogastric suction is maintained during the operation.

ANESTHESIA. General anesthesia, supplemented with curare for relaxation, is satisfactory. The insertion of an endotracheal tube provides smoother operating conditions for the surgeon and easy control of the airway for the anesthesiologist.

POSITION. The patient is placed flat on the operating table, with the foot of the table lowered to permit the contents of the abdomen to gravitate toward the pelvis.

OPERATIVE PREPARATION. The skin is prepared in the usual manner.

INCISION AND EXPOSURE. A high left paramedian incision is extended up over the costal margin adjacent to the xiphoid and down to the region of the umbilicus. In some patients the exposure is greatly enhanced by removal of the xiphoid process. A thorough exploration of the abdomen is carried out, including visualization of the site of the ulcer. The location of the ulcer, especially if it is near the common duct, the extent of the inflammatory reaction, and the patient's general condition should all be taken into consideration in evaluating the risk of gastric resection in comparison to a more conservative drainage procedure.

The next step is to mobilize the left lobe of the liver. If the operator stands on the right side of the patient, it is usually easier to grasp the left lobe of the liver with the right hand and with the index finger to define the limits of the thin, relatively avascular left triangular ligament of the left lobe of the liver. In many instances the tip of the left lobe extends quite far to the left **(Figure 2)**. By downward traction on the left lobe of the liver, and with the index finger beneath the triangular ligament to define its limits and to protect the underlying structures, the triangular ligament is divided with long, curved scissors. The assistant stands on the patient's left side and can usually do this more easily than the surgeon **(Figure 3)**. It should be unnecessary to tie any bleeding points; however, occasionally the tip of the left lobe may require several ties to control slight oozing on the liver side. The left lobe of the liver is then folded either downward or upward so that the region of the esophagus is clearly exposed **(Figure 4)**. A moist, warm gauze pad is placed over the liver, and an S retractor is inserted to maintain even pressure throughout the rest of the procedure **(Figure 5)**. In many instances the exposure is adequate without mobilization of the left lobe of the liver.

DETAILS OF PROCEDURE. The region of the esophagus is palpated. The peritoneum immediately over the esophagus is grasped with toothed forceps, and an incision is made in the peritoneum at right angles to the long axis of the esophagus **(Figure 5)**. The incision may be extended laterally to ensure mobilization of the fundus of the stomach. Curved scissors are then directed gently upward to free the anterior surface of the esophagus from the surrounding tissue. This can be done by blunt dissection, using the index finger which has been covered with a piece of gauze **(Figure 6)**. Traction sutures of fine silk may be introduced into this peritoneal cuff to assist in visualizing the area. After one inch or more of the anterior wall of the esophagus has been freed from the surrounding structures, the index finger should be introduced beneath the esophagus from the left side. It is frequently necessary to loosen some adhesions in this area by sharp dissection. Usually, little difficulty is encountered in gently passing the index finger beneath the esophagus and its indwelling nasogastric tube and completely freeing it from the surrounding structures. Just to the right of the esophagus, the index finger will usually encounter resistance from the uppermost limit of the hepatogastric ligament **(Figure 7)**. This portion of the structure should be divided, since its division affords more mobilization of the esophagus and tends to provide exposure of the posterior or right vagus nerve. The major portion of the hepatogastric ligament in this area is quite avascular and thin, so that it can be perforated easily with scissors or the index finger. A pair of right-angle clamps is then applied to the uppermost portion of the ligament, and the contents of these clamps divided with long, curved scissors **(Figure 8)**. This exposes the region posterior to the esophagus and ensures adequate exposure of the hiatal region.

PLATE XV   VAGOTOMY, SUBDIAPHRAGMATIC APPROACH

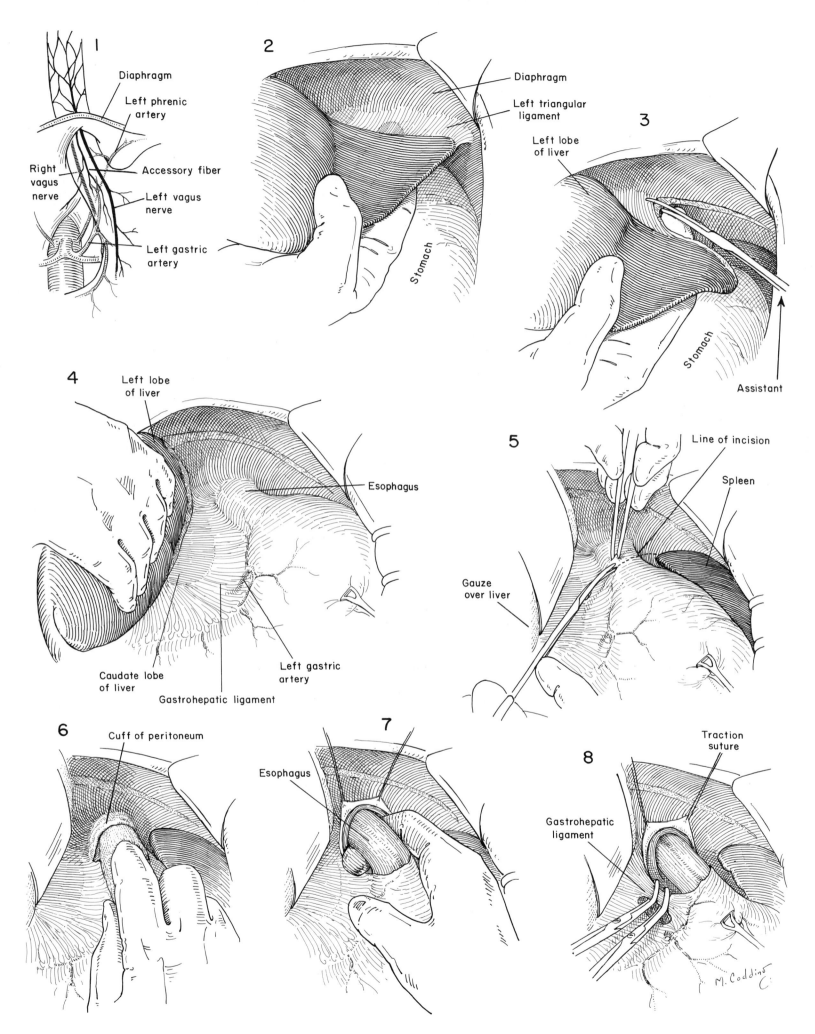

1

Diaphragm

Left phrenic artery

Right vagus nerve

Accessory fiber

Left vagus nerve

Left gastric artery

2

Diaphragm

Left triangular ligament

Stomach

3

Left lobe of liver

Stomach

Assistant

4

Left lobe of liver

Esophagus

Caudate lobe of liver

Gastrohepatic ligament

Left gastric artery

5

Line of incision

Spleen

Gauze over liver

6

Cuff of peritoneum

7

Esophagus

8

Traction suture

Gastrohepatic ligament

M. Coddino

PLATE XVI · VAGOTOMY, SUBDIAPHRAGMATIC APPROACH

DETAILS OF PROCEDURE (*Continued*). The contents of these clamps are then ligated with 00 silk sutures. Downward traction is maintained on the esophagus while it is further freed from the surrounding structures by blunt dissection with the index finger. The vagus nerves are not always easily identified, but their location is more quickly discovered by palpation **(Figure 9)**. As the tip of the index finger is passed over the esophagus, the tense wirelike structure of the nerve is easily identified. It should be remembered that one or more smaller nerves may be found, both anteriorly and posteriorly, in addition to the large left and right vagus nerves. Additional small filaments may be seen crossing over the surface of the esophagus in its long axis. The left vagus nerve is usually located on the anterior surface of the esophagus, a little to the left of the midline, while the right vagus nerve is usually located a little to the right of the midline, posteriorly **(Figures 10 and 10A)**. The left vagus is then grasped with a blunt nerve hook, such as the de Takats nerve dissector, and with curved scissors is dissected free from the adjacent structures **(Figure 11)**. The nerve can be separated from the esophagus easily by blunt dissection with the surgeon's index finger. It is usually possible to free at least 6 cm. of the nerve **(Figure 12)**. The nerve is divided with long, curved scissors as high as possible. It is unnecessary to ligate the ends of the vagus nerve unless bleeding occurs from the gastric end **(Figure 13)**. The use of silver clips at the point where the vagus nerves divide minimizes bleeding and serves to identify the procedures on subsequent roentgenograms. After the left vagus nerve has been resected, the esophagus is rotated slightly, and the traction is directed more to the left. It is usually not difficult to dissect free the right or posterior vagus nerve with the index finger or nerve hook **(Figure 14)**. In some instances it has been found that the nerve has been separated from the esophagus at the time it was initially freed from the surrounding structures. The nerve, in such instances, appears to be resting against the posterior wall of the esophageal hiatus. The tendency to displace the right vagus nerve posteriorly during the blind process of freeing the esophagus no doubt accounts for the fact that this large nerve may be overlooked while all filaments about the esophagus are meticulously divided. This is the nerve most commonly found to be intact at the time of secondary exploration for a clinical failure of the vagotomy. A careful search should be made for additional nerves, since it is not uncommon to find more than one. A minimum of 6 cm. of the right or posterior vagus nerve should be resected **(Figure 15)**. Although the nerves may be clearly identified, the surgeon should not be satisfied until another careful search has been made completely around the esophagus. By traction on the esophagus and by direct palpation, any constricting band should be freed and resected, and a careful inspection should be made throughout the circumference of the esophagus. The operator will find that many of the little filaments that he dissects, in the belief that they are nerves, will prove to be small blood vessels which will require ligation. A final survey should always be made to be absolutely certain that the large right vagus nerve has not been displaced posteriorly, thus escaping division. In order to correct esophageal reflux associated with an incompetent lower esophageal sphincter, it may be wise to perform fundoplication around the lower esophagus. The mobilized fundus is approximated by four or five sutures about the lower end of the esophagus with a large stomach tube in place to prevent excessive constriction.

Traction should be released and the esophagus allowed to return to its normal position. The area should be carefully inspected for bleeding. No effort is made to reapproximate the peritoneal cuff over the esophagus to the cuff of peritoneum at the junction of the esophagus with the stomach. Finally, the esophagus is retracted upward and to the left by a narrow S retractor in order to expose the crus of the diaphragm. Two to three sutures of No. 1 silk are placed to approximate the crus of the diaphragm as in the repair of a hiatus hernia if the hiatus appears patulous **(Figures 16 and 17)**. Sufficient space about the esophagus to admit one finger must be retained. All packs are removed from the abdomen, and the left lobe of the liver is returned to its normal position. It is not necessary to reapproximate the triangular ligament of the left lobe.

Vagotomy must always be accompanied either by a gastric resection or a drainage of the antrum by posterior gastroenterostomy or division of the pylorus by pyloroplasty. Since gastric emptying may be unduly delayed following vagotomy, efficient gastric drainage by gastrostomy should be considered.

POSTOPERATIVE CARE. Constant gastric suction is maintained for four to five days until it has been determined that the stomach is emptying satisfactorily. If evidence of gastric dilatation develops, constant gastric suction is instituted. The volume and acidity of the 12-hour (7 P.M. to 7 A.M.) night secretion should be determined before the suction is discontinued to test the completeness of the vagotomy. The problems associated with vagotomy are minimized by the use of gastrostomy (Plate IX). The tube is removed at the end of ten days or when gastric juice studies have been completed and the overnight residual is low. Occasionally, a moderate diarrhea will develop, which may be temporarily troublesome. The general care is that of any major upper abdominal procedure. Inability to swallow solid food because of temporary cardiospasm may occur for a few days in the early postoperative period. Six small feedings consistent with an ulcer diet should be recommended in order to combat the distention that may occur with an atonic stomach. The return to an unrestricted diet is determined by the patient's progress.

The completeness of the vagus resection may be determined by the volume and acidity response of the gastric secretion to an induced hypoglycemia (40 mg. blood sugar per 100 ml.). Apparently, one overlooked vagus fiber can nullify the beneficial effect of the procedure.

PLATE XVI   VAGOTOMY, SUBDIAPHRAGMATIC APPROACH

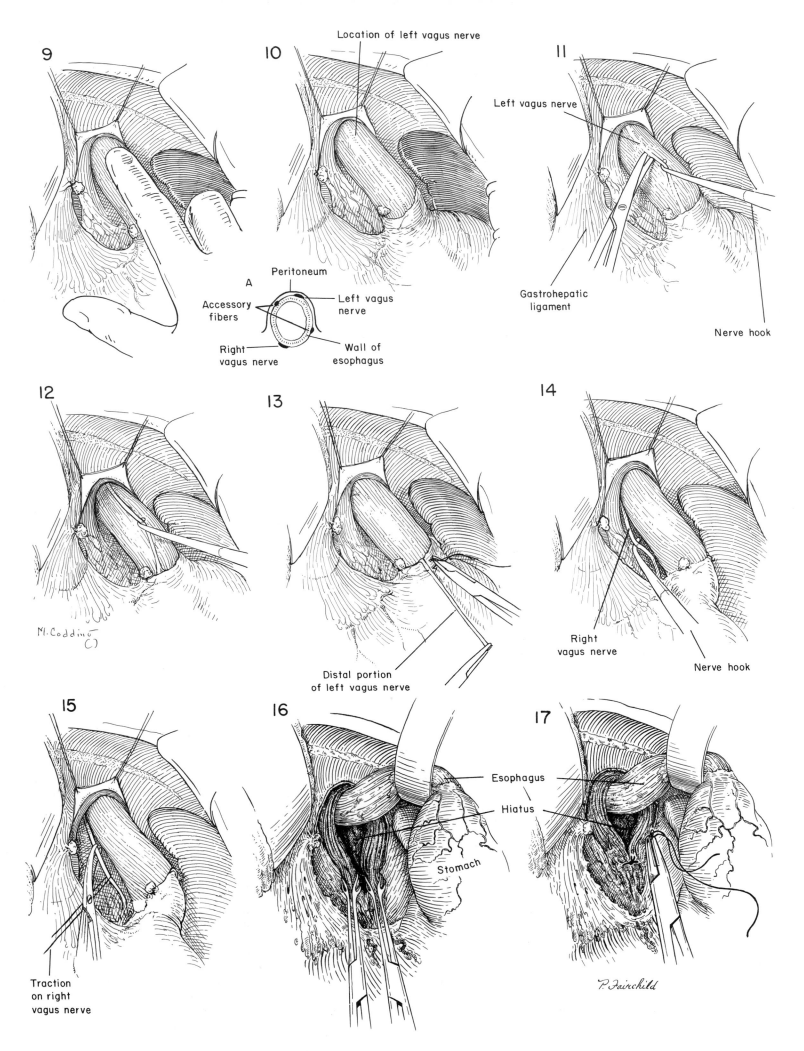

9

10

Location of left vagus nerve

11

Left vagus nerve

Gastrohepatic
ligament

Nerve hook

A

Peritoneum

Accessory
fibers

Left vagus
nerve

Right
vagus nerve

Wall of
esophagus

12

M. Codding
C

13

Distal portion
of left vagus nerve

14

Right
vagus nerve

Nerve hook

15

Traction
on right
vagus nerve

16

Esophagus

Hiatus

Stomach

17

Esophagus

Hiatus

P. Fairchild

PLATE XVII · HEMIGASTRECTOMY, BILLROTH I METHOD

INDICATIONS. The Billroth I procedure for gastroduodenostomy is the most physiologic type of gastric resection, since it restores normal continuity. While long preferred by some in the treatment of gastric ulcer or antral carcinoma, its use for duodenal ulcer has been less popular. Control of the acid factor by vagotomy and antrectomy has permitted retention of approximately 50 per cent of the stomach while ensuring the lowest ulcer recurrence rate of all procedures **(Figure 1).** This allows an easy anastomosis without tension, providing both stomach and duodenum have been thoroughly mobilized. Furthermore, the poorly nourished patient, especially the female, has an adequate gastric capacity for maintaining a proper nutritional status postoperatively. Purposeful constriction of the gastric outlet to the size of the pylorus tends to delay gastric emptying and decrease postgastrectomy complaints. A temporary gastrostomy provides comfortable gastric decompression for as long as desired in addition to providing long-term studies of the overnight secretion to determine the completeness of the vagotomy.

PREOPERATIVE PREPARATION. The patient's eating habits should be evaluated, and the relationship between his preoperative and ideal weight should be determined. The retention of an adequate gastric capacity as well as reestablishment of a normal continuity tends to give the best assurance of a satisfactory nutritional status in undernourished patients, especially females.

ANESTHESIA. Intratracheal anesthesia is used rather routinely.

POSITION. The patient is laid supine on the flat table, the legs being slightly lower than the head. If the stomach is high, a more erect position is preferable.

OPERATIVE PREPARATION. The skin is prepared in a routine manner.

INCISION AND EXPOSURE. A midline or left paramedian incision is usually made. If the distance between the xiphoid and the umbilicus is relatively short, or if the xiphoid is quite long and pronounced, the xiphoid is excised. Troublesome bleeding in the xiphocostal angle on either side will require transfixing sutures of fine silk and bone wax applied to the end of the sternum. Sufficient room must be provided to extend the incision up over the surface of the liver, because vagotomy is routinely performed with hemigastrectomy and the Billroth I type of anastomosis, especially in the presence of duodenal ulcer.

DETAILS OF PROCEDURE. The Billroth I procedure requires extensive mobilization of the gastric pouch as well as the duodenum. This mobilization should include an extensive Kocher maneuver for mobilization of the duodenum. In addition, the greater omentum should be detached from the transverse colon, including the region of the flexures. In many instances the splenorenal ligament is divided, as well as the attachments between the fundus of the stomach and the diaphragm. Additional mobility is gained following the division of the vagus nerves and the uppermost portion of the gastrohepatic ligament. The stomach is mobilized so that it can be readily divided at its midpoint. The halfway point can be estimated by selecting a point on the greater curvature where the left gastrohepatic artery most nearly approximates the greater curvature wall **(Figure 1).** The stomach on the lesser curvature is divided just distal to the third prominent vein on the lesser curvature.

Extensive mobilization of the duodenum is essential in the performance of the Billroth I procedure. Should there be a marked inflammatory reaction, especially in the region of the common duct, a more conservative procedure, such as a pyloroplasty or gastroenterostomy and vagotomy, should be considered. If it appears that the duodenum, especially in the region of the ulcer, can be well mobilized, the peritoneum is incised along the lateral border of the duodenum and the Kocher maneuver is carried out. Usually it is unnecessary to ligate any bleeding points in this peritoneal reflection. With blunt finger and gauze dissection the peritoneum can be swept away from the duodenal surface as the duodenum is grasped in the left hand and reflected medially **(Figure 2).** It is important to remember that the middle colic vessels tend to course over the second part of the duodenum and are many times encountered rather suddenly and unexpectedly. For this reason the hepatic flexure of the colon should be directed downward and medially and the middle colic vessels identified early **(Figure 2).** As the posterior wall of the duodenum and head of the pancreas are exposed, the inferior vena cava readily comes into view. The firm, white, avascular ligamentous attachments between the second and third parts of the duodenum and the posterior parietal wall are divided

with curved scissors, down through and almost including the region of the ligament of Treitz **(Figure 2).** This extensive mobilization is carried downward in order to ensure a very thorough mobilization of the duodenum. Following this, the omentum is separated from the colon, as described in Plate XXIII. In obese patients it is usually much easier to start the mobilization by dividing the attachment between the splenic flexure of the colon and the parietes **(Figure 3).** An incision is made along the superior surface of the splenic flexure of the colon as the next step in freeing up the omentum. This should be done in an avascular cleavage plane. The lesser sac is entered from the left side. Care should be taken not to apply undue traction upon the tissues extending up to the spleen, since the splenic capsule may be torn, and troublesome bleeding, even to the point of requiring splenectomy, may be encountered. The omentum is then dissected free throughout the course of the transverse colon.

The left lobe of the liver is then mobilized, and a vagotomy carried out as described in Plate XV. At this point considerable distance can be gained if the peritoneum attaching the fundus of the stomach to the base of the diaphragm is divided up to and around the superior aspect of the spleen. If the exposure appears difficult, it is advisable for the surgeon to retract the spleen downward with his right hand and, using long curved scissors in his left hand, divide the avascular splenorenal ligament (Plate CII, **Figures 8** and **9).** It must be admitted that sometimes troublesome bleeding does occur, which requires an incidental splenectomy, but in general great mobilization of the stomach is accomplished by this maneuver. The benefits gained from such mobilization far exceed the disadvantage of the occasionally necessary splenectomy.

So far, the surgeon is not committed to any particular type of gastric resection but has ensured an extensive mobilization of the stomach and duodenum. The omentum should be reflected upward and the posterior wall of the stomach dissected free from the capsule of the pancreas, should any adhesions be found in this area. In the presence of a gastric ulcer, penetration through to the capsule of the pancreas may be encountered. These adhesions can be pinched off between the thumb and index finger of the surgeon and the ulcer crater allowed to remain on the capsule of the pancreas. A biopsy for frozen section study should be taken if there is a suspicion of malignancy. The colon is returned to the peritoneal cavity. The right gastric and gastroepiploic arteries are doubly ligated (Plates XX and XXI, **Figures 12** through **16),** and the duodenum distal to the ulcer divided.

At least 1 cm. or 1.5 cm. of the superior as well as the inferior margins of the duodenum must be thoroughly cleared of fat and blood vessels adjacent to the Potts vascular clamp in preparation for the angle sutures. This is especially important on the superior side in order to avoid a diverticulum-like extension from the superior surface of the duodenum with an inadequate blood supply for a safe anastomosis. After the duodenal stump has been well prepared for anastomosis, the end that has been closed with the Potts clamp is covered with a moist, sterile gauze while the site of resection of the stomach is decided upon **(Figure 4).**

In many instances, especially in the obese patient, it is advisable to further mobilize the stomach by dividing the thickened, lowermost portion of the gastrosplenic ligament without dividing the left gastroepiploic vessels. Considerable mobilization of the greater curvature of the stomach without traction on the spleen can be obtained if time is taken to divide carefully this extra heavy layer of adipose tissue, which is commonly present in this area. Following this further mobilization of the greater curvature, a point is selected where the left gastroepiploic vessel appears to come nearer the gastric wall. This is the point in the greater curvature selected for the anastomosis, and the omentum is divided up to this point with freeing of the serosa of fat and vessels for the distance of the surgeon's finger **(Figure 4).** Traction sutures are applied to mark the proposed site of anastomosis. A site on the lesser curvature is selected just distal to the third prominent vein on the lesser curvature **(Figure 1).** Again, two traction sutures are applied, separated by the width of the surgeon's finger. This distance of about a centimeter on both curvatures assures a good serosal surface for closure of the angles.

It makes little difference how the stomach is divided, although there is some advantage to using a Von Petz sewing clamp. Regardless of the crushing clamp that is to be applied, the curvatures of the stomach should be fixed by the application of Babcock forceps to prevent rotation of the tissues when the clamp is closed. Before the stomach is divided, a row of interrupted 0000 silk sutures on French needles is placed almost through the entire gastric wall in order to (1) control the bleeding from the subsequent cut surface of the gastric wall; (2) fix the mucosa to the seromuscular coat; and (3) pucker and constrict the end of the stomach **(Figure 5).**

PLATE XVII   HEMIGASTRECTOMY, BILLROTH I METHOD

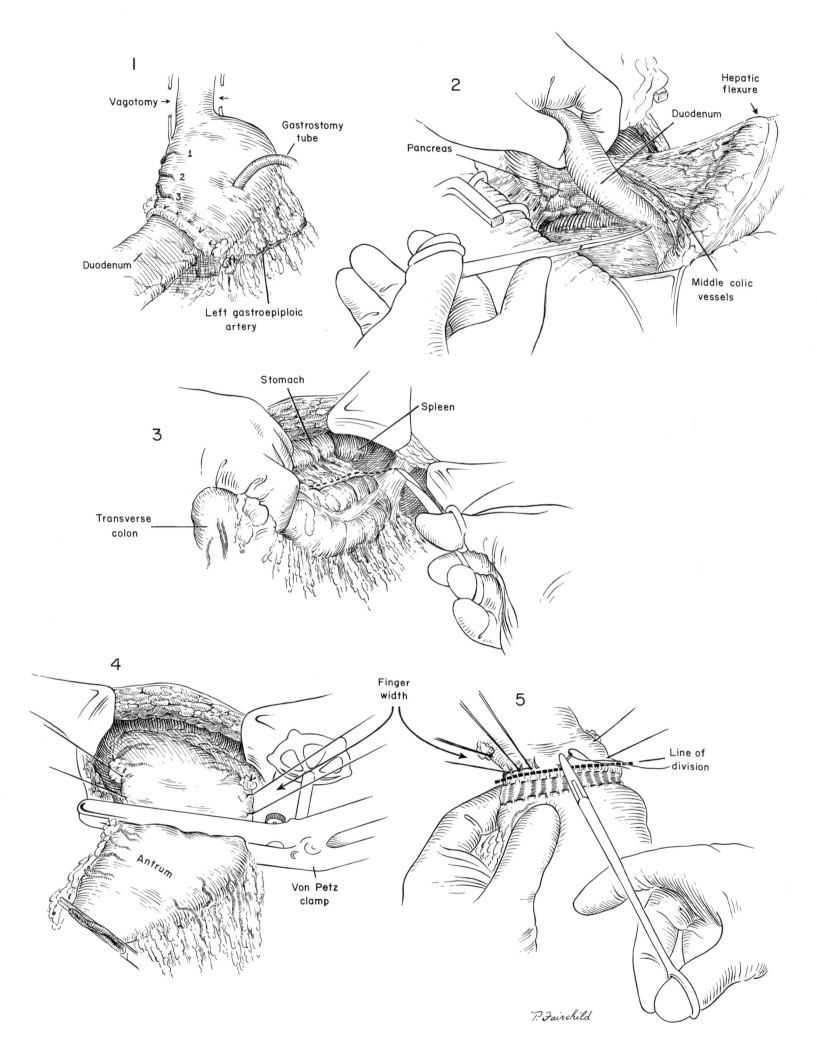

P. Fairchild

PLATE XVIII · HEMIGASTRECTOMY, BILLROTH I METHOD

DETAILS OF PROCEDURE (*Continued*). Additional sutures of fine silk are taken around the edge of the mucosal opening until the end of the stomach has been puckered to fit relatively snugly around the surgeon's index finger. This opening should be approximately 2.5 to 3 cm. wide **(Figure 6)**. These sutures are then cut in anticipation of a direct end-to-end anastomosis with the duodenum **(Figure 7)**. If the margins of the lesser and greater curvatures of the stomach as well as the superior and inferior margins of the duodenum have been properly prepared, it is relatively easy to insert angle sutures of 00 silk. Successful closure of the angles depends upon starting the suture on the anterior gastric as well as the anterior duodenal wall rather than more posteriorly. Interrupted sutures of 00 silk are then taken to close the stomach and duodenum together. Slightly bigger bites are necessary on the gastric side as a rule rather than on the duodenal side, depending upon the discrepancy in size between the two openings **(Figure 8)**. The sutures should be tied, starting at the lesser curvature and progressing downward to the greater curvature. The angle sutures are retained while additional 0000 silk sutures are placed to approximate the mucosa **(Figure 9, A-A' and B-B')**. No clamps are applied to the stomach or duodenum to control bleeding, since the sutures on the gastric side, if properly placed, should provide complete hemostasis as far as the stomach is concerned. Bleeding from the duodenal side is controlled by placing interrupted 0000 silk sutures. The anterior mucosal layer is closed with a series of interrupted sutures of 0000 silk with the knots tied on the inside. The seromuscular coat is then approximated to the duodenal wall with a layer of interrupted mattress sutures **(Figure 10)**. It has been found that a cuff of gastric wall can be brought over the duodenum, resulting in a "pseudo-pylorus," if two bites are taken on the gastric side and one bite on the duodenal side. When this suture is tied **(Figure 10)**, the gastric wall is pulled over the initial mucosal suture line.

The vascular pedicles on the gastric side are anchored to the ligated right gastric pedicle along the top surface of the duodenum as well as the ligated right gastroepiploic artery pedicle **(Figure 10, A and B)**. A and B are then tied together to seal the greater curvature angle **(Figure 11)**. A similar type of approximation is effected along the superior surface in order to seal the angle and remove all tension from the anastomosis **(Figure 11)**. Cushing silver clips placed at the site of anastomosis will aid in identifying this area when future X-rays are obtained. The stoma should admit one finger relatively easily. There should be no tension whatsoever on the suture line.

The upper quadrant is inspected for oozing and thoroughly irrigated with saline.

A gastrostomy (Plate XVII, **Figure 1**) is routinely added and the gastric wall anchored to the anterior parietes at a point where it reaches easily and without undue tension. The fixation of the gastric wall should be at a point where there is no tension on the spleen or the anastomosis. In fact, the tissue between the gastrostomy and the gastroduodenostomy should be loose and flaccid.

POSTOPERATIVE CARE. Two liters of 5 per cent glucose and water are given and the blood volume restored during the first 24 hours. The gastrostomy tube is allowed to drain by gravity or is attached to low-pressure suction. Frequent irrigations of the tube with small amounts of saline are necessary to avoid obstruction and resultant gastric distention. Losses from the gastrostomy tube are accurately recorded. Usually, the fluid requirements will include sodium chloride and potassium by the second or third day after operation.

When bowel activity has resumed, clear liquids are given by mouth and the gastrostomy tube is clamped. Four hours after each of the first several meals the tube is unclamped and gastric residual measured. If there is no evidence of retention, a progressive feeding regimen is begun. This consists of five or six small feedings per day of soft food, moderately restricted in volume, high in protein, and relatively low in carbohydrate. Although many patients after gastric surgery dislike dairy products, the majority will tolerate milk, eggs, custards, toast, and cream soups, as the first step of the diet. Other soft foods are added as rapidly as the tolerance of the individual will permit. By the tenth day, a feeling of fullness may develop caused by mild retention and a tendency to overeat. Self-restriction of the dietary intake for a few days is indicated.

Several 12-hour night secretion studies are made to determine the volume as well as milliequivalents of free hydrochloric acid present. Evidence to support or deny complete vagotomy is thereby assured. The gastrostomy tube is usually removed within eight to ten days, unless there is evidence of pyloric obstruction. The gastrostomy tube adds comfort to the postoperative period, provides good gastric drainage as long as necessary, and helps provide a more accurate management of the patient.

The patient's weight is recorded daily. The progressive regimen forms a basis for the discharge diet. Instructions are given to the patient to eat frequently, avoid concentrated carbohydrates, and to add "new" foods, including spices, and other foods restricted preoperatively, one at a time. Eventually, the only limitations to the individual's diet are those imposed by his own intolerance.

Intermittent and regular follow-up discussions are essential over a long period of time to answer the many problems encountered by patients before the operation can be considered a complete success. Return to an unlimited diet and maintenance of ideal weight with freedom from gastrointestinal complaints are the goals.

PLATE XVIII   HEMIGASTRECTOMY, BILLROTH I METHOD

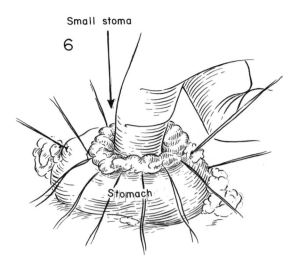

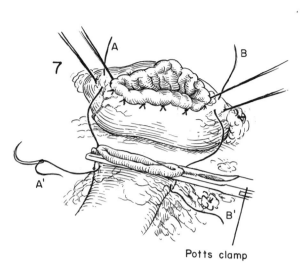

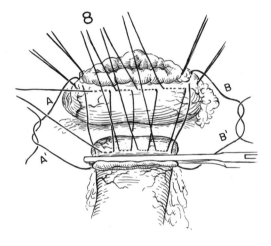

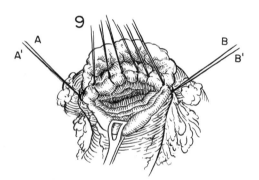

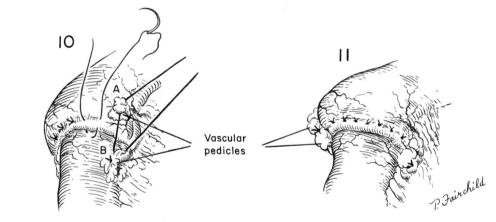

P. Fairchild

PLATE XIX · GASTRECTOMY, SUBTOTAL

INDICATIONS. Subtotal gastrectomy is indicated in the presence of malignancy; in the presence of gastric ulcer that persists despite three weeks of intensive medical therapy; in the presence of antacidity, pernicious anemia, suspicious cells by gastric washings, or equivocal evidence for and against malignancy by repeated barium studies or fiberoptic gastroscopic observation with direct biopsy. It is most commonly utilized to control the acid factor in cases of intractable duodenal ulcer. A more conservative procedure should be considered in underweight patients with duodenal ulcer, especially females. Likewise, block excision of a gastric ulcer with multicentric frozen section studies should be made for proof of malignancy before performing a radical resection on the assumption the lesion may be malignant. This special effort for proof is especially important in all females as well as underweight males.

PREOPERATIVE PREPARATION. The preoperative preparation will be determined largely by the type of lesion presented and by the complication it produces. After surgery has been definitely planned, the patient without pyloric obstruction is encouraged to substitute a high-protein, high-carbohydrate, and high-vitamin diet for the rigid regimen, to prepare for the postoperative period of limited caloric intake. Sufficient time should be taken to improve the nutrition if possible, especially if there has been considerable weight loss in patients with pyloric obstruction. The fluid and electrolyte balance must be established by the intravenous injection of a 5 to 10 per cent solution of dextrose in isotonic saline solution. Potassium deficiencies are corrected. Anemia and hypoproteinemia should be corrected as nearly as possible by transfusion of whole blood and plasma or by hyperalimentation. The increased incidence of pulmonary complications associated with upper abdominal surgery makes it imperative that elective gastric surgery be carried out only in the absence of respiratory infection, and active pulmonary physiotherapy with possible bronchodilators, expectorants, and positive-pressure breathing exercises should be started in patients with chronic lung diseases.

If there is any degree of pyloric obstruction, the electrolyte balance, which includes potassium and sodium chloride; blood urea nitrogen levels; blood pH; and pCO_2, or carbon dioxide combining power, must be returned to normal by the appropriate replacement therapy. Repeated gastric lavage, including several days of constant gastric suction, may be indicated until a satisfactory balance is attained. Constant gastric suction by means of a Levine tube is instituted before operation and maintained during and after operation unless a gastrostomy is performed following the resection. Whole blood in the amount of 1,000 to 2,000 ml. should be available for transfusion during the operation.

ANESTHESIA. General anesthesia with endotracheal intubation should be used. Excellent muscular relaxation without deep general anesthesia can be attained by utilizing muscle relaxants. Spinal anesthesia, either continuous or single-injection technic, provides excellent relaxation; however, supplementation with intravenous sedatives may be indicated to prevent nausea during visceral manipulation.

POSITION. As a rule, the patient is laid supine on a flat table, the feet being slightly lower than the head. If the stomach is high, a more erect position is preferable.

OPERATIVE PREPARATION. The skin is prepared in the routine manner.

INCISION AND EXPOSURE. A midline incision extending from the xiphoid to the umbilicus may be used. Additional exposure can be obtained by excising the xiphoid. Bone wax is applied to the sternal end to control bleeding. Active arterial bleeding on either side of the xiphoid is ligated with a transfixing suture of 00 silk. Further exposure can be obtained by splitting the sternum with a sternal knife. If preferred, a paramedian incision can be made to the left of the midline. The left paramedian incision is preferable to the right, since the most difficult part of the procedure may be the gastrojejunal anastomosis following a high resection. Either of these incisions will give adequate exposure without great traction, but either a self-retaining retractor or a broad-bladed, fairly deep retractor placed against the liver down to the gastrohepatic ligament will aid in visualization.

DETAILS OF PROCEDURE. The surgeon should focus his attention on the arterial blood supply **(Figure 1).** While the stomach will retain viability despite extensive interference with its blood supply, the duodenum lacks such a liberal anastomotic blood supply, and great care must be exercised in the latter instance to prevent postoperative necrosis in the duodenal stump. The blood supply to the lesser curvature of the stomach can be destroyed entirely, and the retained fundus will be nourished by the small vessels in the gastrosplenic ligament in the region of the fundus. Likewise, if it is desirable to mobilize the stomach into the chest, its viability can be retained if only the right gastric artery is left intact. In such instances, however, the gastrocolic ligament should be divided some distance from the greater curvature to prevent interference with the right and the left gastroepiploic vessels.

The blood supply may also be used as landmarks in designating the extent of the gastric resection. Approximately 50 per cent of the stomach is resected where the line of division extends from the region of the third large vein on the lesser curvature down from the esophagus to a point on the greater curvature where the left gastroepiploic vessels most nearly approach the gastric wall. Approximately 75 per cent resection can be assumed when the line of resection includes most of the lesser curvature with extra gastric ligation of both the left gastric and left gastroepiploic vessels.

The surgeon likewise should be familiar with the major lymphatic drainage of the stomach in determining the presence or absence of metastasis if malignancy is suspected. Under such circumstances it is advisable to keep the dissection as far away as possible from both curvatures in order to retain all involved lymph nodes with the specimen. There is a tendency for metastases to involve distant nodes of the lesser curvature, or the lymph nodes beneath the pylorus, as well as those of the greater omentum. Chances for prolonged survival in the presence of malignant disease are greatly enhanced if consideration is given to lymphatic drainage in planning the extent of removal necessary **(Figure 1).** In the presence of malignancy it is desirable to remove the greater omentum, the lesser curvature to the esophagus, about 2.5 cm. the duodenum (including the subpyloric lymph nodes), and the greater curvature up to and at times including the spleen.

If the operation is undertaken because a tumor exists, the extent of nodular involvement, as well as possible metastases to the liver and pelvis, should be noted immediately upon exposure. It must also be determined whether there have been direct extension and fixation to adjacent structures, such as the pancreas, liver, or spleen. Additional information may be obtained as to the extent and fixation of the tumor mass by exploring the lesser omental cavity through an opening made in the relatively avascular gastrohepatic ligament **(Figure 2).** Evidence of fixation of the posterior gastric wall with the pancreas or involvement of the tissues about the middle colic vessels should be sought. However, in the absence of visible or palpable distant metastases, it may be feasible to excise the stomach, *en masse,* along with the spleen and portions of the left lobe of the liver, or tail and body of the pancreas, if the involvement is by direct extension of the tumor. If there is widespread metastatic involvement with impending pyloric obstruction, it may be wiser to avoid radical surgery and to carry out the simple procedure of anterior or posterior gastrojejunostomy.

After evaluation indicates that a subtotal gastrectomy is practicable, it has been found that preliminary mobilization of the duodenum by the Kocher maneuver may facilitate some of the subsequent steps necessary in the procedure **(Figures 3, 4, and 5).** The duodenum is grasped with Babcock forceps in the region of the pylorus, and traction is sustained downward **(Figure 3).** Any avascular adhesive bands that appear to be fixing the duodenum in the region of the hepatoduodenal ligament should be severed. The common duct is exposed so that it can be identified easily from time to time as the duodenum is divided and the stump is inverted **(Figure 6).**

After the duodenum and region of the pylorus have been mobilized by freeing all the avascular attachments, the index finger of the right hand is passed through an avascular portion of the gastrohepatic ligament above the pylorus to facilitate the introduction of a Penrose drain or gauze tape, which is brought up through an avascular space along the greater curvature and is used for traction **(Figure 7).**

PLATE XIX   GASTRECTOMY, SUBTOTAL

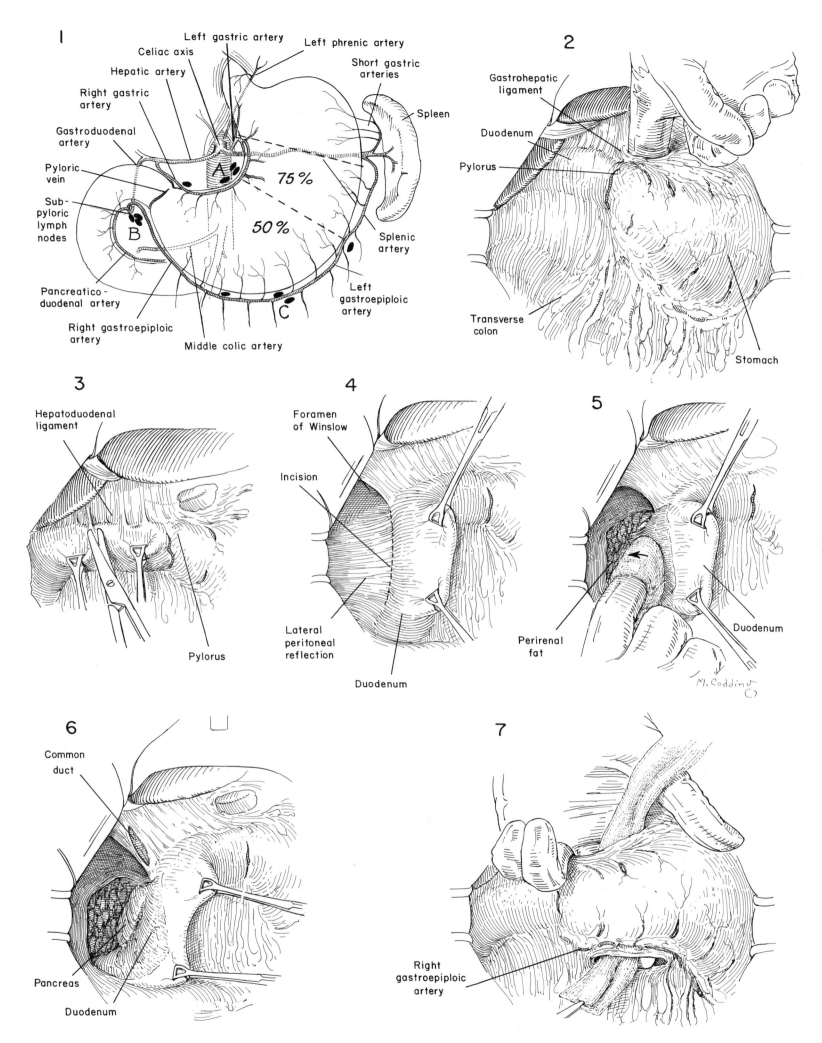

1
Left gastric artery
Celiac axis
Hepatic artery
Right gastric artery
Gastroduodenal artery
Pyloric vein
Sub-pyloric lymph nodes
Pancreatico-duodenal artery
Right gastroepiploic artery
Middle colic artery
Left phrenic artery
Short gastric arteries
Spleen
Splenic artery
Left gastroepiploic artery
75 %
50 %
A
B
C

2
Gastrohepatic ligament
Duodenum
Pylorus
Transverse colon
Stomach

3
Hepatoduodenal ligament
Pylorus

4
Foramen of Winslow
Incision
Lateral peritoneal reflection
Duodenum

5
Perirenal fat
Duodenum
M. Codding

6
Common duct
Pancreas
Duodenum

7
Right gastroepiploic artery

PLATE XX · GASTRECTOMY, SUBTOTAL

DETAILS OF PROCEDURE (*Continued*). The gastrocolic ligament is divided near the epiploic vessels along the greater curvature, if there is no evidence of malignancy. The stomach is retracted upward, and the surgeon's left hand is introduced behind the stomach to avoid the possibility of damaging the middle colic vessels when the gastrocolic ligament is divided, since these vessels may be very near **(Figure 9).** Furthermore, by spreading the fingers apart beneath the gastrocolic ligament along the greater curvature, it is easier to identify the individual vessels so that they can be more accurately clamped and divided between pairs of small curved clamps **(Figure 8).** The dissection is carried around to the region of the gastrosplenic ligament, and a portion of this structure may also be removed, depending upon the amount of stomach to be resected. It is necessary to free the greater curvature to this extent to accomplish a 75 to 80 per cent resection of the stomach. This usually demands the sacrifice of the left gastroepiploic artery and one or two of the short gastric arteries in the gastrosplenic ligament. The nutrition of the remaining fundus of the stomach depends upon the remaining short gastric arteries **(Figure 10)** when the left gastric artery has been ligated at its base. When hemigastrectomy is planned, the greater curvature is divided in the area where the left gastroepiploic artery most nearly approximates the gastric wall. On the lesser curvature the third large vein on the anterior gastric wall is used as the approximate point of division to ensure a hemigastrectomy.

In the obese patient the gastrosplenic ligament may be quite thickened and the identification of the vessels for ligation more difficult than elsewhere. However, fewer vessels require ligation if the omentum is removed, as in Plate XXIII, rather than repeatedly clamping and tying the blood vessels in the gastrocolic ligament near the greater curvature. The division of the usual attachments of the omentum to the lateral abdominal wall about the splenic flexure of the colon will further mobilize the greater curvature of the stomach. Undue traction on the stomach or omentum may result in troublesome bleeding from the spleen, especially if the small strands of tissue extending up to the anterior margin are torn along with some of the splenic capsule. Under such circumstances splenectomy may be safer than depending on a hemostatic sponge to control the troublesome and persistent bleeding. The greater curvature can be further mobilized into the field of operation if the relatively avascular splenocolic ligament is divided **(Figure 10).** Indeed, the spleen may be quite extensively mobilized by dividing the splenorenal ligament laterally, permitting it, along with the fundus of the stomach, to be presented into the field of operation. This procedure ensures an easier exposure for the gastro-jejunal anastomosis following a very high gastric resection. Any bleeding points in the splenic bed should be carefully ligated.

At this time it is desirable to prepare the greater curvature for subsequent anastomosis. The serosa should be dissected free of fat for approximately the width of the index finger. A transfixing silk suture is placed in the greater curvature in this area to serve as a guide suture at the time the clamps are finally applied for division of the stomach (Plate XXII, **Figure 30).** In addition, such a transfixing suture tends to prevent damage to the adjacent blood supply from subsequent manipulation of the stomach while preparing it for anastomosis **(Figure 11).**

Upward retraction of the stomach is maintained as the gastrocolic ligament is divided up to the region of the pylorus. If there is a possibility of malignancy within the area, care should be taken to stay about 3 to 5 cm. from the pylorus in order to include the subpyloric nodes with the specimen. At the same time large, blind bites with hemostats in the neighborhood of the inferior portion of the duodenum should be avoided because of possible damage to the pancreaticoduodenal artery. It should be remembered that since the duodenum does not have a rich anastomotic blood supply but is supplied by end arteries, it is necessary to guard its blood supply carefully. The right gastroepiploic vessels should be carefully isolated from the surrounding fat and securely ligated **(Figure 12).**

After the blood supply of the greater curvature of the stomach has been divided and tied, the vascular supply and ligamentous attachments to the superior portion of the first part of the duodenum can be divided. Freeing the pylorus and the upper portion of the duodenum may be one of the most difficult steps in the operation, especially in the presence of a large, penetrating ulcer. One cannot state beforehand whether the attack should begin at the upper or lower border of the duodenum. In the presence of gastric malignancy extending to the pylorus, it is essential to remove at least 3 cm. of the duodenum because of the possibility of infiltration of carcinoma for some distance within the wall of the duodenum itself. The most medial portion of the hepatoduodenal ligament, which includes the right gastric artery, is divided. It is better to take small bites in this area with a small curved hemostat and reapply the clamps repeatedly than to attempt mass ligation **(Figure 13).** The location of the common duct and adjacent vessels within the hepatoduodenal ligament should be accurately identified before these clamps are applied. The mobilization of the duodenum is facilitated by the division and ligation of the contents of these clamps. The vascular pedicles from the duodenal side of the anastomosis are clearly defined.

PLATE XX   GASTRECTOMY, SUBTOTAL

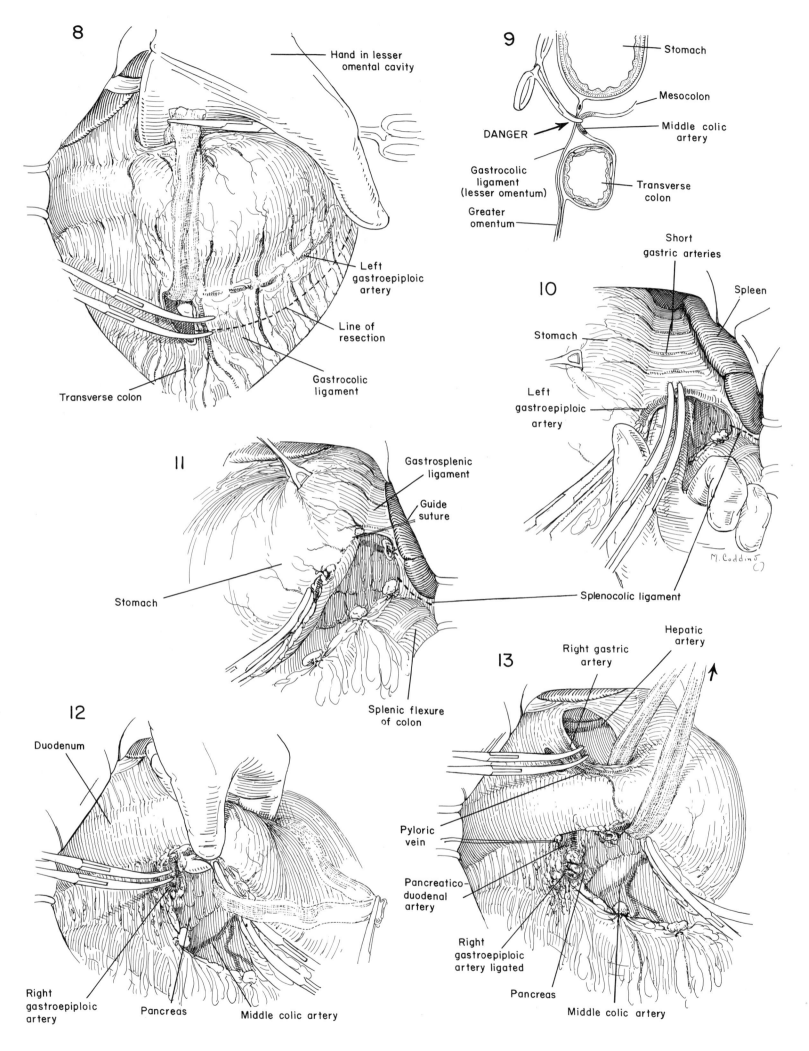

8

Hand in lesser
omental cavity

Left
gastroepiploic
artery

Line of
resection

Gastrocolic
ligament

Transverse colon

9

Stomach

Mesocolon

DANGER

Middle colic
artery

Gastrocolic
ligament
(lesser omentum)

Transverse
colon

Greater
omentum

Short
gastric arteries

Spleen

10

Stomach

Left
gastroepiploic
artery

Splenocolic ligament

11

Gastrosplenic
ligament

Guide
suture

Stomach

Splenic flexure
of colon

M. Coddins
C

12

Duodenum

Right
gastroepiploic
artery

Pancreas

Middle colic artery

13

Right gastric
artery

Hepatic
artery

Pyloric
vein

Pancreatico-
duodenal
artery

Right
gastroepiploic
artery ligated

Pancreas

Middle colic artery

PLATE XXI · GASTRECTOMY, SUBTOTAL

DETAILS OF PROCEDURE. (*Continued*). Transfixing silk traction sutures are applied to the superior and inferior borders of the duodenum adjacent to its retained blood supply. These traction sutures are helpful when the narrow crushing large vascular clamp is applied to the duodenum, as well as in the subsequent closure of the duodenal stump **(Figure 14)**. After the blood supply about the pylorus has been divided and tied, the stomach is held upward in order to free any adhesions between the first portion of the duodenum and the pancreas **(Figure 14)**. At this time the transverse colon can be returned to the abdomen and retracted out of the operating field. The field is then walled off by several warm, moist sponges.

A thin-bladed, noncrushing clamp of the vascular type (Pott's) is then applied across the duodenum at the prepared level **(Figure 15)**. A Kocher clamp is applied to the gastric side. There should be at least 1 cm. of cleansed serosal surface at either border of the duodenum, between the noncrushing clamp and the traction sutures. This amount of prepared duodenal wall is necessary to ensure a safe subsequent closure of the duodenal stump. If the adjacent ligature does not permit 1 cm. of cleared serosa between it and the margin of the clamp, small curved clamps should be applied to the interfering vascular attachments, and such attachments should be divided and ligated. The duodenum is divided with a knife. The clamp applied to the gastric side is covered with a piece of gauze, and the stomach is retracted to one side. The duodenal stump is then retracted laterally in order to determine if a sufficient amount of the serosa of the posterior wall has been cleared away to permit a safe closure of the duodenal stump. At least 1 cm. distal to the clamp, the duodenum should be freed from the pancreas in order that subsequent sutures in the serosa may be placed under full vision. Individual clamping and subsequent ligation of the small vascular attachments must be carried out without damaging the gastroduodenal artery **(Figure 16)**. Placing deep sutures to control bleeding should be rigorously avoided in this area because of the potential danger of pancreatitis.

There are many ways of closing the duodenal stump. However, it should be remembered that a very firm closure is necessary, since blowing-out of the duodenal stump is not an uncommon fatal complication of gastric surgery caused by failure to clear a sufficient amount of duodenum, especially along the upper border. The tendency of the "cloverleaf" deformity associated with the ulcer to produce a diverticulum-like extension beyond the superior margin must be corrected in many instances to ensure a closure of the stump in this area. Failure to free up and excise this deformity tends to make inversion of the mucosal layer very difficult. The superior margin as well as the inferior margin of the duodenum adjacent to the clamp may be grasped with Babcock forceps preliminary to removal of the noncrushing clamp **(Figure 17)**. As the noncrushing clamp is removed, the bleeding margin of the duodenal stump is grasped with two or three Babcock or Allis forceps **(Figure 18)**. The duodenum is then closed with interrupted 0000 silk sutures or a continuous fine catgut suture **(Figure 18 and 19)**. The mucosal suture line should then be inverted by applying a row of interrupted mattress sutures of 00 silk, which tends to pull the anterior wall downward toward the pancreas **(Figure 20)**. A cleaned serosal surface should be available at both the superior and inferior margins when this layer of interrupted serosal sutures is finally inverted.

As a final safety measure to reinforce the closure, interrupted sutures may be taken in the anterior wall of the duodenum and, superficially, in the capsule of the pancreas **(Figures 21 and 22)**. While the duodenal stump is being closed, the common duct should be visualized and its relationship determined from time to time, so that there is no possibility of its accidental angulation, injury, or obstruction as a result of inverting the duodenal stump. The gallbladder, if present, should be compressed to provide evidence of a nonobstructed common duct.

PLATE XXI   GASTRECTOMY, SUBTOTAL

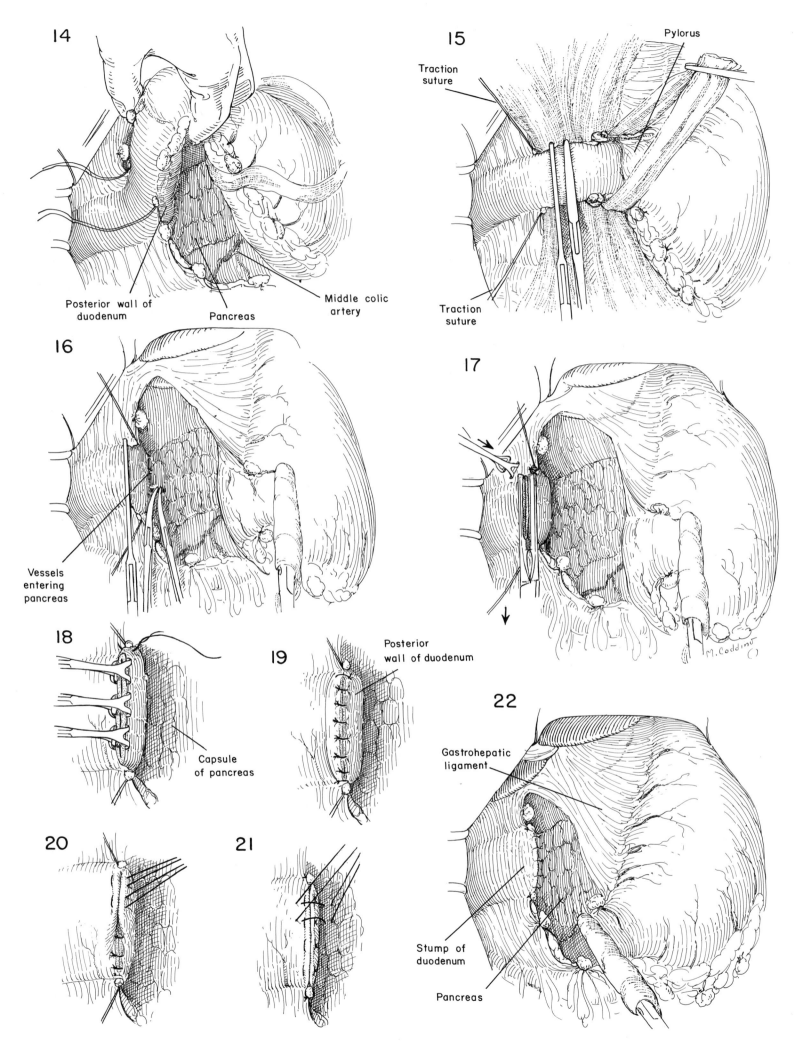

14

Posterior wall of duodenum   Pancreas   Middle colic artery

15

Pylorus

Traction suture

Traction suture

16

Vessels entering pancreas

17

18

Capsule of pancreas

19

Posterior wall of duodenum

20

21

22

Gastrohepatic ligament

Stump of duodenum

Pancreas

M. Codding

PLATE XXII · GASTRECTOMY, SUBTOTAL

DETAILS OF PROCEDURE (*Continued*). One of the important steps in gastric resection is the preparation of the lesser curvature. Frequently, the gastrohepatic ligament is quite thin and avascular at some distance from the lesser curvature. It is divided between pairs of small curved forceps **(Figure 23).** In the presence of malignancy the division of the gastrohepatic ligament should be as near the liver as possible and carried up almost to the esophagus to make certain that all involved nodes along the lesser curvature are removed. The uppermost portion of the gastrohepatic ligament must be clamped before division, since it contains a sizeable artery that requires ligation. The division of the gastrohepatic ligament does not involve a division of the left gastric artery, which comes up from the celiac axis directly to the stomach **(Figures 24 and 25).** Whether the left gastric artery is ligated depends upon how extensive a resection is indicated. A radical gastric resection is usually interpreted as one in which the left gastric artery has been ligated and the stomach divided at this level or higher. Attempts at mass ligation, especially in the obese, of the fat and blood vessels along the lesser curvature are dangerous and do not ensure a lesser curvature properly prepared for closure or anastomosis, as the case may be. The left gastric vessels divide as they reach the stomach, extending paired branches to either side of the curvature to enter the gastric wall **(Figure 24).** An effort should be made to pass a right-angle clamp beneath an individual vessel before its division and ligation **(Figure 25).** The main vessels on either side of the curvature should be ligated as well as the individual tributaries that run down over the gastric wall **(Figures 26 and 27).** In a thin patient a mass ligation may be carried out without difficulty by passing a small curved clamp from front to back, being careful to avoid the blood vessels extending downward over both anterior and posterior surfaces of the stomach. Following this, a transfixing suture, A **(Figure 27),** is placed to approximate the serosa of the anterior gastric wall to the serosa of the posterior gastric wall, so that when it is tied, a firm peritonealized surface is provided for the important

subsequent sutures to be placed in this area. The lesser curvature should be freed of attached fat for several centimeters, and the larger blood vessels should be clamped and tied on the gastric wall. A smooth serosal surface is essential for a safe anastomosis **(Figure 27).**

When a very high resection is indicated, especially in the presence of malignancy, it is desirable to divide the left gastric artery as far away from the lesser curvature as possible **(Figure 28).** Care should be taken to isolate the surrounding tissue from the pillar that includes the left gastric vessels. Since these are large vessels, they are doubly clamped on the proximal side and transfixing sutures are used. It is frequently much simpler to ligate the left gastric artery near its point of origin rather than to attempt to ligate its individual branches as they divide along the lesser curvature. When the left gastric artery has been ligated, it is essential that the lesser curvature be prepared for anastomosis relatively near the gastroesophageal junction **(Figure 29).** It is possible to mobilize the small gastric pouch into the field by dividing the vagus nerves and incising the peritoneal attachments to the fundus as well as to the splenorenal ligament. The blood supply to the remaining stomach will be adequate through the short gastric vessels. Such mobilization facilitates the anastomosis when the exposure is otherwise difficult.

Regardless of the method used, it is important that the serosa be properly cleansed for about the width of the index finger adjacent to the traction sutures, A and B, on either curvature **(Figure 30).** One or more additional sutures are usually required to adequately approximate the serosal surfaces along the lesser curvature. The stomach is now ready for the application of a Von Petz sewing clamp, or Payr, Schoemaker, or similar crushing instrument, preparatory to division of the stomach. It is important to stabilize the lesser as well as the greater curvature of the stomach by means of either Allis or Babcock forceps, lest the gastric wall be distorted as the crushing or sewing clamps are applied across the areas of both curvatures which have been previously prepared **(Figure 30).**

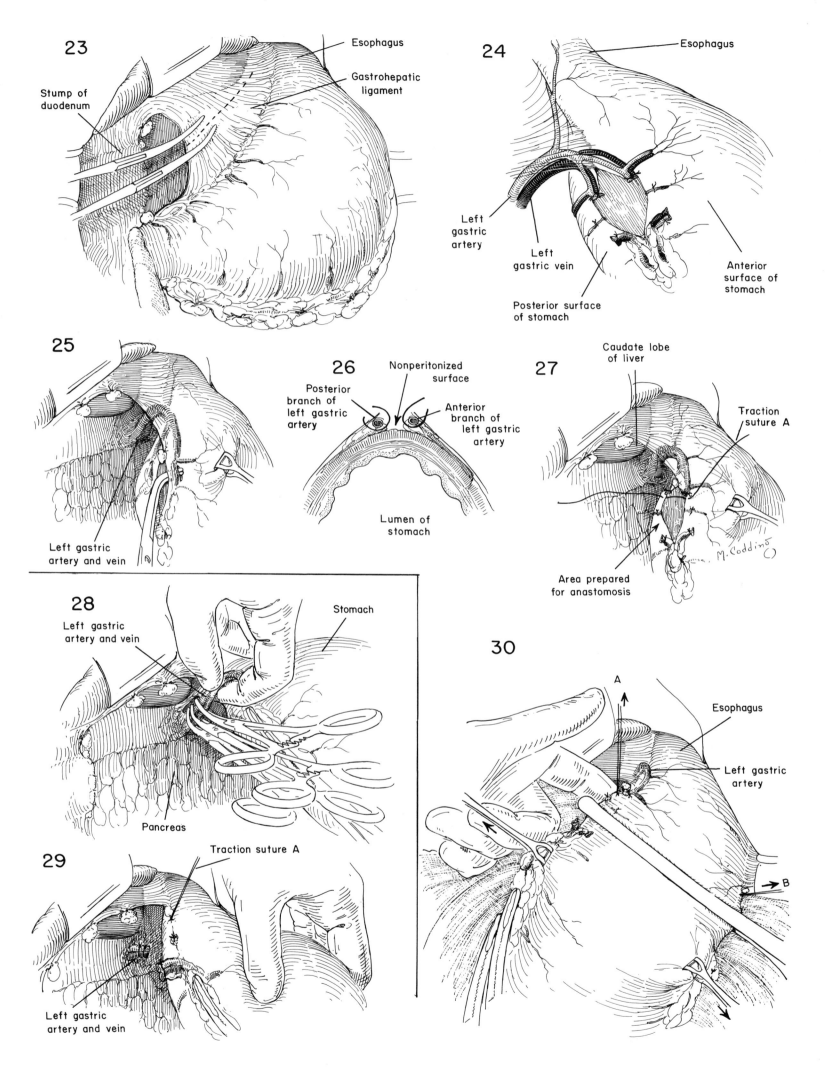

23
Stump of duodenum
Esophagus
Gastrohepatic ligament

24
Esophagus
Left gastric artery
Left gastric vein
Posterior surface of stomach
Anterior surface of stomach

25
Left gastric artery and vein

26
Posterior branch of left gastric artery
Nonperitonized surface
Anterior branch of left gastric artery
Lumen of stomach

27
Caudate lobe of liver
Traction suture A
Area prepared for anastomosis
M. Codding

28
Left gastric artery and vein
Stomach
Pancreas

29
Traction suture A
Left gastric artery and vein

30
A
Esophagus
Left gastric artery
B

PLATE XXIII · GASTRECTOMY, SUBTOTAL—OMENTECTOMY

Removal of Omentum

DETAILS OF PROCEDURE. In cases of malignancy of the stomach, it is desirable to resect the greater omentum because of the possibility of metastatic implants in this structure. Removing the omentum is not difficult and can commonly be effected with less technical effort than dividing the gastrocolic ligament adjacent to the greater curvature of the stomach. For this reason some prefer to use this procedure rather routinely regardless of the indication for subtotal gastrectomy. The transverse colon is brought out of the wound, and the omentum is held sharply upward by the operator and assistants **(Figure1).** Using scissors of the Metzenbaum type, dissection is started at the right side, adjacent to the posterior taenia of the colon. In many instances the peritoneal attachment can be more easily divided with a scalpel than with scissors. A thin and relatively avascular peritoneal layer can be seen, which can be rapidly divided **(Figures 1, 2, and 3).** Upward traction is maintained on the omentum as blunt gauze dissection is utilized to sweep the colon downward, freeing it from the omentum **(Figure 2).** As the dissection progresses, a few small blood vessels in the region of the anterior taenia of the colon may require division and ligation. Finally, the thin, avascular peritoneal layer can be seen above the colon. This is incised, giving direct entrance into the lesser omental sac **(Figures 4 and 5).** In the obese individual it may be easier to divide the attachments of the omentum to the lateral abdominal wall just below the spleen as a preliminary step. If the upper margin of the splenic flexure can be visualized clearly, the splenocolic ligament is divided and the lesser sac entered from the left side rather than from above the transverse colon, as shown in **Figure 6.** The surgeon should be on guard constantly to avoid injuring the middle colic vessels, since the mesentery of the transverse colon may be intimately attached to the gastrocolic ligament, especially on the right side. As the dissection progresses toward the left, the gastrocolic omentum is divided, and the greater curvature of the stomach is separated from its blood supply to the desired level **(Figure 6).** In some instances it may be easier to ligate the splenic artery and vein along the superior surface of the pancreas and remove the spleen, especially if there is a malignant growth in this location. It should be remembered that if the left gastric artery has been ligated proximal to its bifurcation, and the spleen has been removed, the blood supply to the stomach has been so compromised that the surgeon is committed to total gastrectomy.

In the presence of malignancy the omentum over the head of the pancreas is removed as well as the subpyloric lymph nodes **(Figure 7).** Small, curved clamps should be utilized as the wall of the duodenum is approached, and the middle colic vessels, which may be adherent to the gastrocolic ligament in this location, should be carefully visualized and avoided before the clamps are applied. Unless care is exercised, troublesome hemorrhage and a compromised blood supply to the colon may result.

PLATE XXIII   GASTRECTOMY, SUBTOTAL—OMENTECTOMY

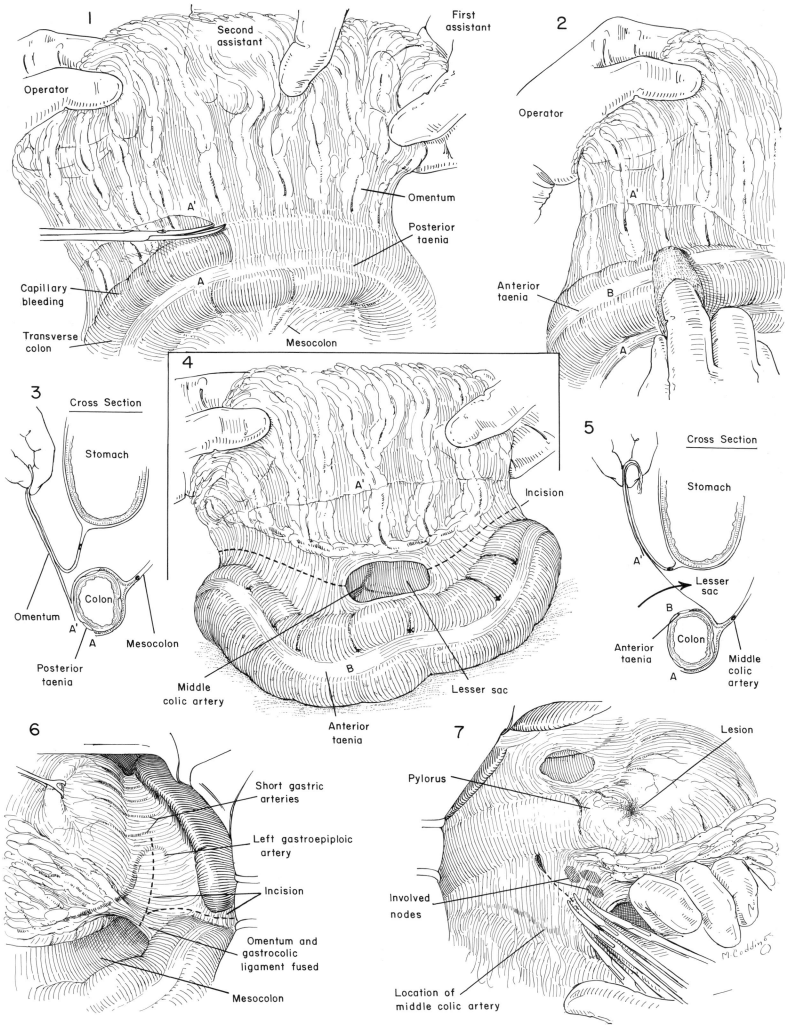

1

Operator

Second assistant

First assistant

Omentum

Posterior taenia

A'

A

Capillary bleeding

Transverse colon

Mesocolon

2

Operator

A'

Anterior taenia

B

A

3

Cross Section

Stomach

Omentum

A'

A

Posterior taenia

Colon

Mesocolon

4

A'

Incision

Middle colic artery

Lesser sac

Anterior taenia

B

5

Cross Section

Stomach

A'

Lesser sac

B

Anterior taenia

Colon

A

Middle colic artery

6

Short gastric arteries

Left gastroepiploic artery

Incision

Omentum and gastrocolic ligament fused

Mesocolon

7

Lesion

Pylorus

Involved nodes

Location of middle colic artery

M. Codding

PLATE XXIV · GASTRECTOMY, POLYA METHOD

INDICATIONS. The Polya procedure, or a modification of it, is one of the safest and most widely used repairs after extensive gastric resections have been performed, whether for ulcer or cancer.

DETAILS OF PROCEDURE. The schematic drawing **(Figure 1)** shows the position of the viscera after this operation is completed, which in principle consists of uniting the jejunum to the open end of the stomach. The jejunum may be anastomosed either behind or in front of the colon. In the retrocolic anastomosis, a loop of jejunum is brought through a rent in the mesentery of the colon to the left of the middle colic vessels and near the ligament of Treitz **(Figure 2)**. In the antecolic anastomosis a longer loop must be used in order to pass in front of the colon. If the resection has been done for ulcer to control the acid factor, it is important that the jejunal loop be made reasonably short, since long loops are more prone to subsequent marginal ulceration. The jejunum is grasped with Babcock forceps and brought up through the opening made in the mesocolon, with the proximal portion in juxtaposition to the lesser curvature of the stomach **(Figure 2)**. The abdomen is then completely walled off with warm, moist sponges. The jejunal loop is grasped in an enterostomy clamp and approximated to the posterior surface of the stomach adjacent to the gastric crushing clamp by a layer of closely placed, interrupted 00 silk mattress sutures **(Figure 3)**. This posterior row should include both the greater curvature and the lesser curvature of the stomach. Otherwise, subsequent closure of the angles may be insecure. The ends of the sutures are cut, except those at the lesser and greater curvatures, A, B, which are retained for purposes of traction **(Figure 4)**. Following this, an enterostomy clamp is placed across the stomach at least 2 cm. proximal to the suture line, and the gastric crushing clamp is removed. The crushed border of the stomach may be cut away with scissors, if desired. An opening is made lengthwise in the jejunum, approximating in size the opening in the stomach. The fingers hold the jejunum down flat, and the incision is made close to the suture line **(Figure 5)**.

The mucous membranes of the stomach and jejunum are approximated by a continuous mucosal suture of fine catgut as the opposing surfaces are approximated by Allis clamps applied to either angle **(Figure 6)**. A continuous suture on the straight needles is started in the middle and is carried toward either angle as a running suture or as an interlocking continuous suture, if preferred. The corners are inverted with a Connell-type suture which is continued anteriorly, and the final knot is tied on the inside of the midline **(Figure 7)**. Some prefer to approximate the mucosa with multiple interrupted 0000 silk sutures on French needles. The anterior layer is closed with the knots on the inside by using an interrupted Connell-type suture. The enterostomy clamps are released to inspect the anastomosis for any leakage or bleeding. Additional sutures may be required. The anterior serosal layers are then approximated with interrupted 00 silk mattress sutures on either straight milliner's needles or small French needles **(Figure 8)**. Finally, at the upper and lower angles of the new stoma, additional mattress sutures are placed so that any strain exerted on the stoma is met by these additional reinforcing serosal sutures and not by the sutures of the anastomosis **(Figure 9)**. In the retrocolic anastomosis the new stoma is anchored to the mesocolon with interrupted mattress sutures, care being taken to avoid blood vessels in the mesocolon **(Figure 10)**.

If sufficient stomach remains, a temporary Stamm gastrostomy is performed (Plate IX). The gastric wall must reach the anterior abdominal wall without tension. Mobilization of the fundus of the stomach and the spleen may be indicated to ensure adequate mobility, especially of a small gastric pouch, to permit suturing of the gastric wall to the peritoneum about the gastrostomy tube without undue tension.

CLOSURE. The closure is performed in a routine manner without drainage.

POSTOPERATIVE CARE. The patient is placed in a semi-Fowler's position when conscious. Any deficiencies resulting from the measured blood loss during surgery should be corrected by whole blood transfusions. Chemotherapy and/or antibiotics may be used as prophylaxis against peritoneal sepsis, especially in the presence of achlorhydria.

The fluid intake is maintained daily at approximately 2,000 ml. by the intravenous administration of 5 to 10 per cent dextrose in water and/or saline. The amount of saline given will depend in part upon the volume of fluid recovered by gastric suction. Accurate records of the intake and output from all sources are mandatory. Parenteral vitamins may be given.

Pulmonary complications are anticipated, and frequent changes are made in position. The patient is encouraged to cough, etc. If the patient's condition warrants, he may be out of bed on the first day after operation. Water in sips is allowed 24 hours after operation. Constant gastric suction is maintained during the procedure and for several days after operation. It may be discontinued when the tube can be clamped for at least 12 hours without symptoms of gastric distention appearing. After the nasal tube is removed or the gastrostomy tube clamped off for 24 hours, the patient may be placed on a postgastrectomy diet regimen that progresses gradually from bland liquids to six small feedings per day. Fruit juices may be diluted in half and milk added cautiously as tolerated. Beverages containing caffeine, excessive sugar, or carbonation should be avoided. The gastrostomy tube is removed within seven to ten days. A diet consistent with an ulcer regimen should gradually be replaced by an unlimited diet. An additional daily intake of fats should be encouraged for those patients well below their ideal body weight. All carbohydrates may not be tolerated well, especially in the morning, for a long time after operation. Smoking should be prohibited until the patient's weight has returned to a satisfactory level. Frequent evaluation of the patient's dietary intake and weight trends is strongly advised during the first year after surgery and at longer intervals thereafter for at least five years.

PLATE XXIV   GASTRECTOMY, POLYA METHOD

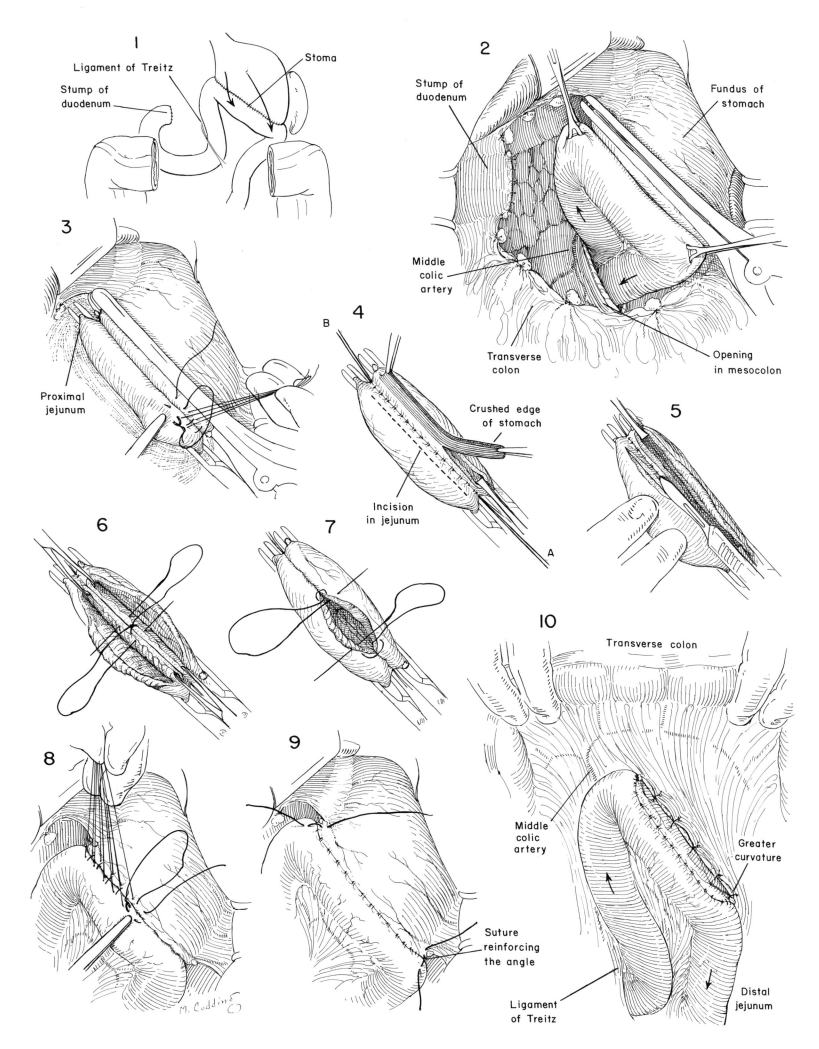

1
Ligament of Treitz
Stoma
Stump of duodenum

2
Stump of duodenum
Fundus of stomach
Middle colic artery
Transverse colon
Opening in mesocolon

3
Proximal jejunum

4
B
Crushed edge of stomach
Incision in jejunum
A

5

6

7

8

9
Suture reinforcing the angle

10
Transverse colon
Middle colic artery
Greater curvature
Ligament of Treitz
Distal jejunum

M. Codding

PLATE XXV · GASTRECTOMY, HOFMEISTER METHOD

DETAILS OF PROCEDURE. The schematic drawing shows the position of the viscera after this operation is completed. In principle, this consists of closing about one-half of the gastric outlet adjacent to the lesser curvature and performing a gastrojejunal anastomosis adjacent to the greater curvature, with approximation of the jejunum to the entire end of the gastric remnant **(Figure 1).** This operation is favored when very high resections are indicated, because it provides a safer closure of the lesser curvature. It also may retard sudden overdistention of the jejunum after eating. The jejunum may be brought up either anterior to the colon or through an opening in the mesocolon to the left of the middle colic vessels (Plate XXIV, **Figure 2).**

There are many ways of closing the opening of the stomach adjacent to the lesser curvature. Some surgeons use a sewing clamp of the Von Petz type; others prefer Payr, Schoemaker, or similar crushing clamps. If Payr clamps are used, the procedure can be accomplished safely by separating them for at least 1 cm. as they are applied and dividing the stomach against the distal clamp **(Figure 2).** This provides a protruding cuff of gastric wall. This method has the disadvantage of having to turn in crushed gastric wall; however, it does permit closure of the gastric opening adjacent to the lesser curvature with a minimal amount of blood loss and contamination.

The protruding mucosa adjacent to the greater curvature is grasped with Babcock forceps to ensure a stoma approximately two fingers wide. A continuous suture is started in the mucosa, which protrudes beyond the crushing clamp in the region of the lesser curvature, and is carried downward toward the greater curvature until the Babcock forceps defining the upper end of the stoma is encountered **(Figure 3).** Some prefer to approximate the mucosa with interrupted 0000 silk sutures. The crushing clamp is then removed, and an enterostomy clamp is applied to the gastric wall. A layer of interrupted mattress sutures of 00 silk is placed to invert not only the mucosal suture line but the crushed gastric wall as well **(Figure 4).** It should be carefully ascertained that a good serosal surface approximation has been effected at the very top of the lesser curvature. The threads are not cut but may be retained and subsequently utilized to anchor the jejunum to the anterior gastric wall along the closed end of the gastric pouch.

A loop of jejunum adjacent to the ligament of Treitz is brought up anterior to the colon or posteriorly through the mesocolon in order to approximate it to the remaining stomach. The jejunal loop should be as short as possible but must reach the line of anastomosis without tension when the anastomosis is completed. An enterostomy clamp is applied to the portion of jejunum to be used in making the anastomosis. The proximal portion of the jejunum is anchored to the lesser curvature of the stomach. An enterostomy clamp is maintained on the gastric remnant unless this is impossible because of its high location. Under these circumstances it is necessary to make the anastomosis without applying clamps to the stomach.

The posterior serosal layer of interrupted mattress sutures of 00 silk anchors the jejunum to the entire remaining end of the stomach. This is done to avoid undue angulation of the jejunum; it removes strain from the site of the stoma and reinforces the closed upper half of the stomach posteriorly **(Figure 5).** Following this, the crushed cuff of gastric wall still retained in the Babcock forceps is excised with scissors, and any active bleeding points are tied **(Figure 6).** The contents of the stomach are aspirated by suction, unless it has been possible to apply an enterostomy clamp on the gastric side. The mucosa of the stomach and of the jejunum toward the greater curvature are approximated by a continuous fine catgut suture on a straight atraumatic needle **(Figure 7).** Some prefer interrupted sutures of 000 silk. A Connell-type stitch is used to invert the angles and the anterior mucosal layer **(Figure 8).** A layer of interrupted mattress sutures is continued anteriorly from the closed portion to the margin at the greater curvature. Both the angles of the lesser and greater curvatures are reinforced with additional interrupted sutures. The long threads retained from closing the upper portion of the stomach are rethreaded **(Figure 9).** These sutures are utilized to anchor the jejunum to the anterior gastric wall and buttress the closed end of the stomach anteriorly, as was previously done on the posterior surface. The stoma is tested for patency as well as for the degree of tension placed on the mesentery of the jejunum. The transverse colon is adjusted behind the jejunal loops going to and from the anastomosis. If a retrocolic anastomosis has been performed, the margins of the mesocolon are anchored to the stomach about the anastomosis (Plate XXIV, **Figure 10).**

CLOSURE. The wound is closed in the routine manner. Retention sutures should be used in emaciated or cachectic patients.

POSTOPERATIVE CARE. See Postoperative Care, Plate XXIV.

PLATE XXV   GASTRECTOMY, HOFMEISTER METHOD

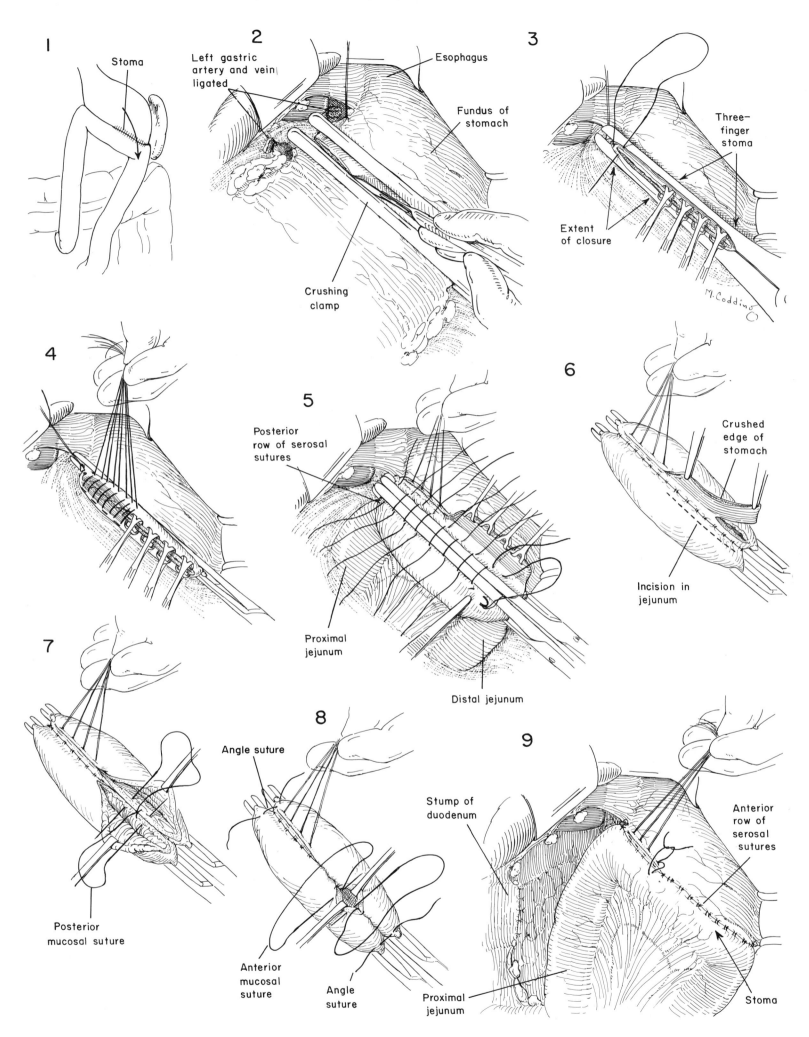

1

Stoma

2

Left gastric
artery and vein
ligated

Esophagus

Fundus of
stomach

Crushing
clamp

3

Three-
finger
stoma

Extent
of closure

M. Codding

4

5

Posterior
row of serosal
sutures

Proximal
jejunum

Distal jejunum

6

Crushed
edge of
stomach

Incision in
jejunum

7

Posterior
mucosal suture

8

Angle suture

Anterior
mucosal
suture

Angle
suture

9

Stump of
duodenum

Anterior
row of
serosal
sutures

Proximal
jejunum

Stoma

PLATE XXVI · TOTAL GASTRECTOMY

INDICATIONS. Total gastrectomy may be indicated in treating extensive stomach malignancies. This radical procedure is not performed when carcinoma with distant metastasis to the liver or pouch of Douglas or seeding throughout the peritoneal cavity is present. It may be performed in association with the extirpation of adjacent organs, such as the spleen, body and tail of the pancreas, a portion of the transverse colon, etc. It is also the procedure of choice in controlling the intractable ulcer diathesis associated with non-beta islet cell tumors of the pancreas that are multiple or proved to be malignant with multiple hepatic metastases.

PREOPERATIVE PREPARATION. The blood volume should be restored and antibiotics given in the presence of achlorhydria. If colonic involvement is anticipated, appropriate antibacterial agents should be administered. Four to six units of blood should be readily available for transfusion.

ANESTHESIA. General anesthesia with endotracheal intubation.

POSITION. The patient is placed in a comfortable supine position on the table with the feet slightly lower than the head.

OPERATIVE PREPARATION. The area of the chest from above the nipple downward to the symphysis is shaved. The skin over the sternum, lower chest wall, and entire abdomen is cleansed with the appropriate antiseptic solution. Preparation should extend sufficiently high and to the left on the chest for a midsternal or left thoracoabdominal incision if necessary.

INCISION AND EXPOSURE. A limited incision is made in the midline (**Figure 1,** A—A₁) between the xiphoid and umbilicus. The initial opening is only to permit inspection of the stomach and liver and to introduce the hand for general exploration of the abdomen. Because of the high incidence of metastases, a more liberal incision extending up to the region of the xiphoid and down to the umbilicus, or beyond it on the left side, is not made until it has been determined that there is no contraindication to total or subtotal gastrectomy **(Figure 1).** Additional exposure is allowed by removal of the xiphoid. Active bleeding points in the xiphocostal angle are transfixed with 00 silk sutures, and bone wax is applied to the end of the sternum. Some prefer to split the lower sternum in the midline and extend the incision to the left into the fourth intercostal space. Adequate exposure is mandatory for a safe anastomosis between the esophagus and jejunum.

DETAILS OF PROCEDURE. Total gastrectomy should be considered for malignancy high on the lesser curvature if there is no metastasis to the liver or seeding over the general peritoneal cavity, particularly in the pouch of Douglas **(Figure 2).** Before the surgeon is committed to a total gastrectomy, he must have a clear view of the posterior relationship of the stomach to determine if the growth has extended into the adjacent structures—i.e., pancreas, mesocolon, or the major vessels **(Figure 3).** This can be determined by reflecting the greater omentum upward, withdrawing the transverse colon from the peritoneal cavity, and searching the transverse mesocolon for evidence of invasion. By palpation the surgeon should determine that there is free mobility of the growth without involvement of fixation to the underlying pancreas or major vessels, especially in the region of the left gastric vessels **(Figure 4).**

The entire transverse colon, including the hepatic and splenic flexures, should be freed from the omentum and retracted downward. As the omentum is retracted upward and the transverse colon downward, the venous branch between the right gastroepiploic and middle colic veins is visualized and ligated to avoid troublesome bleeding. The greater omentum in the region of the head of the pancreas and the hepatic flexure of the colon should be freed by sharp and blunt dissection so that it can be entirely mobilized from the underlying head of the pancreas and duodenum. In very thin patients the surgeon may prefer to carry out a Kocher maneuver, with incision of the peritoneum lateral to the duodenum, in order to eventually test whether an anastomosis between the duodenum and esophagus can be performed without tension. This is occasionally possible in thin patients having great mobility of the abdominal viscera.

When the lesser sac has been explored, the surgeon proceeds with further mobilization of the stomach. If the growth appears to be localized, even though it is large and involves the tail of the pancreas, colon, and kidney, a very radical extirpation may be carried out. Resection of the left lobe of the liver may occasionally be necessary.

To ensure complete removal of the neoplasm, at least 2.5 to 3 cm. of duodenum distal to the pyloric vein should be resected **(Figure 2).** Since it is not uncommon to have metastasis to the infrapyloric lymph nodes, they should be included in the resection. The right gastroepiploic vessels are doubly ligated as far away from the inferior surface of the duodenum as possible, to ensure removal of the infrapyloric lymph nodes and adjacent fat **(Figure 5).**

PLATE XXVI   TOTAL GASTRECTOMY

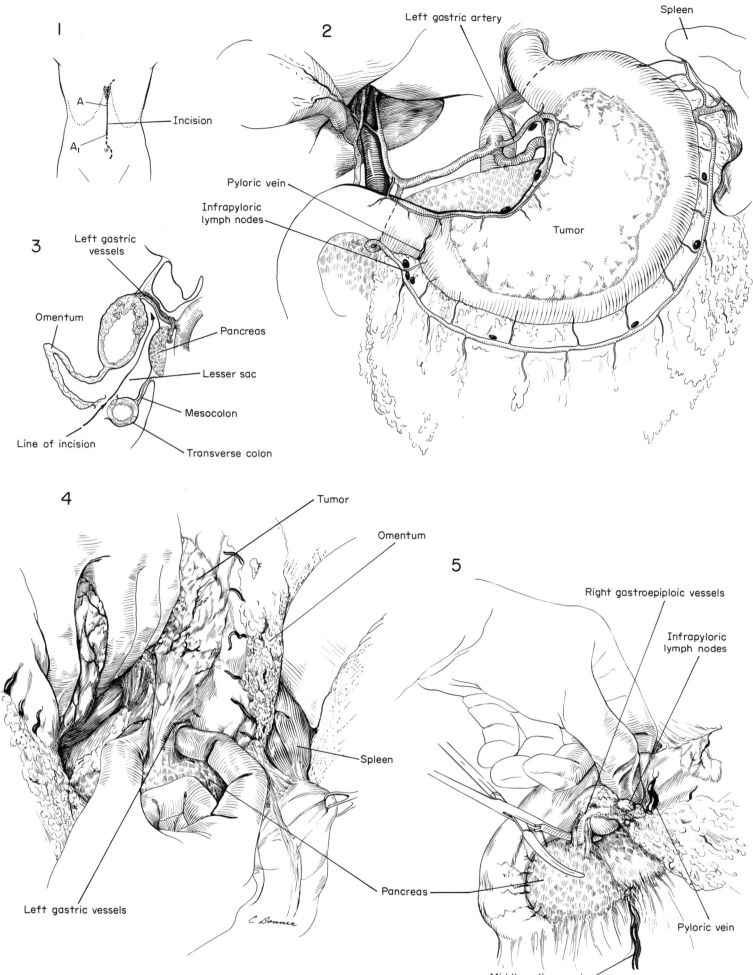

1

A

A₁

Incision

2

Left gastric artery

Spleen

Pyloric vein

Infrapyloric
lymph nodes

Tumor

3

Left gastric
vessels

Omentum

Pancreas

Lesser sac

Mesocolon

Line of incision

Transverse colon

4

Tumor

Omentum

Spleen

Left gastric vessels

Pancreas

C Donner

5

Right gastroepiploic vessels

Infrapyloric
lymph nodes

Pancreas

Pyloric vein

Middle colic vessels

PLATE XXVII · TOTAL GASTRECTOMY

DETAILS OF PROCEDURE (*Continued*). The right gastric vessels along the superior margin of the first part of the duodenum are isolated by blunt dissection and doubly ligated some distance from the duodenal wall **(Figure 6).** The thinned-out gastrohepatic ligament is divided as near the liver as possible up to the thickened portion, which contains a branch of the inferior phrenic artery.

The duodenum is then divided with noncrushing straight forceps on the duodenal side and a crushing clamp, such as a Kocher, on the gastric side **(Figure 7).** The duodenum is divided with a scalpel. A sufficient amount of the posterior wall of the duodenum should be freed from the adjacent pancreas, especially inferiorly, where a few vessels may enter the wall of the duodenum **(Figure 8).** The duodenal stump should not be closed until it has been determined that it cannot be easily mobilized sufficiently to extend up to the esophagus.

The region of the esophagus and fundus is next exposed and mobilized medially. The avascular suspensory ligament supporting the left lobe of the liver is first divided. The surgeon grasps the left lobe with his right hand and defines the limits of the avascular suspensory ligament from underneath by upward pressure with his index finger **(Figure 9).** This procedure is facilitated if the ligament is divided with long curved scissors held in the left hand. Occasionally, a suture will be required to control oozing from the very tip of the mobilized left lobe of the liver. The left lobe should be carefully palpated for evidence of metastatic nodules deep within the substance of the liver. The mobilized left lobe of the liver is folded upward and covered with a moist pack, over which a large S retractor is placed. At this time the need for upward extension of the incision, or removal of additional sternum, is considered. The uppermost portion of the gastrohepatic ligament, which includes a branch of the inferior phrenic vessel, is isolated by blunt dissection. Two right-angle clamps are applied to the thickened tissues as near the liver as possible. The tissues between the clamps are divided and the contents of the clamps ligated with transfixing sutures of 00 silk **(Figure 10).** The incision in the peritoneum over the esophagus and between the fundus of the stomach and base of the diaphragm is outlined in **Figure 10.**

PLATE XXVII   TOTAL GASTRECTOMY

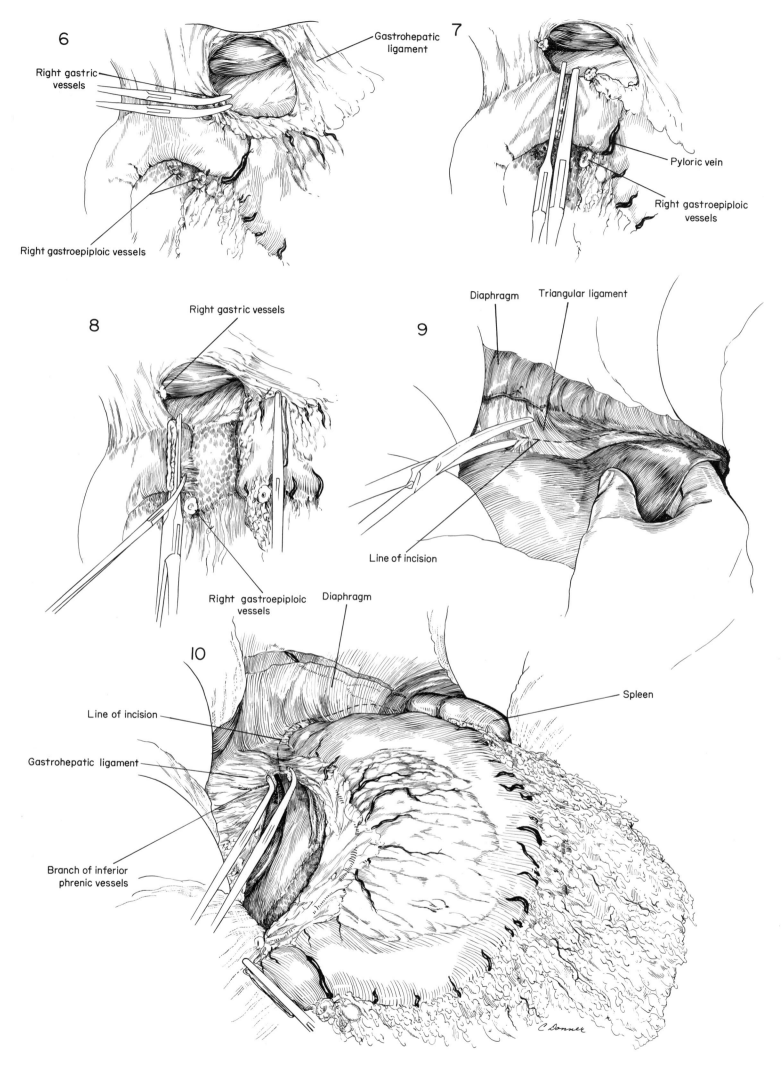

6

Right gastric vessels

Gastrohepatic ligament

Right gastroepiploic vessels

7

Pyloric vein

Right gastroepiploic vessels

8

Right gastric vessels

Right gastroepiploic vessels

9

Diaphragm   Triangular ligament

Line of incision

10

Diaphragm

Line of incision

Gastrohepatic ligament

Branch of inferior phrenic vessels

Spleen

C Donner

PLATE XXVIII · TOTAL GASTRECTOMY

DETAILS OF PROCEDURE. (*Continued*). The peritoneum over the esophagus is divided, and all bleeding points are carefully ligated. Several small vessels may require ligation when the peritoneum between the gastric fundus and base of the diaphragm is separated. The lower esophagus is freed by finger dissection similar to the technic of vagotomy (Plates XV and XVI). The vagus nerves are divided to further mobilize the esophagus into the peritoneal cavity. By blunt and sharp dissection the left gastric vessels are isolated from adjacent tissues **(Figure 11)**. These vessels should be encircled with the surgeon's index finger and carefully palpated for evidence of metastatic lymph nodes. A pair of clamps, such as curved half-lengths, should be applied as close as possible to the point of origin of the left gastric artery, and a third clamp applied nearer the gastric wall. The contents of these clamps are first ligated and then transfixed distally. Likewise, the left gastric vessels on the lesser curvature should be ligated to enhance the subsequent exposure of the esophagogastric junction. When the tumor is near the greater curvature in the midportion of the stomach, it may be desirable to remove the spleen and tail of the pancreas to assure a block dissection of the immediate regional lymphatic drainage zone. The location and extent of the capsule, as well as the presence or absence of adhesions or tears in the capsule, determine whether the spleen should be removed. If the spleen is to remain, the gastrosplenic ligament is divided as described for splenectomy (Plates CII and CIII). The blood vessels on the gastric side are ligated with 00 silk sutures, transfixed to the gastric wall. The left gastroepiploic vessel is doubly tied. The greater curvature is freed up to the esophagus. Several vessels are usually encountered entering the posterior wall of the fundus near the greater curvature.

The anesthetist should aspirate the gastric contents from time to time to prevent possible regurgitation from the stomach as it is retracted upward, as well as peritoneal soiling when the esophagus is divided.

In the very emaciated patient it may be possible to approximate the duodenum to the esophagus by an extensive Kocher maneuver, which includes mobilizing the second and third parts of the duodenum. If it is determined that this cannot be done with confidence and safety owing to lack of mobility, the duodenum is closed in two layers (see Plate XXI). The walls of the duodenum are closed with a first layer of interrupted 0000 silk sutures, Connell-type. These are invaginated with a second layer of 00 silk mattress sutures.

One of the numerous methods that have been devised for reconstructing gastrointestinal continuity following total gastrectomy is selected.

The surgeon should keep in mind certain anatomic differences of the esophagus, which make its management more difficult than the rest of the gastrointestinal tract. First, since the esophagus is not covered by serosa, the longitudinal and circular muscle layers tend to tear when sutured. Second, the esophagus, while at first appearing to extend well down into the abdominal cavity, tends to retract up into the thorax when divided from the stomach, leaving the surgeon hard-pressed for adequate length. It should be mentioned, however, that if the exposure is inadequate the surgeon should not hesitate to remove more of the xiphoid or to split the sternum with extension into the left fourth intercostal space. A common approach is to extend the upper portion of the incision across the cartilages into the appropriate intercostal space, creating a thoracoabdominal incision. Adequate and free exposure must be obtained to secure a safe anastomosis.

The wall of the esophagus can be lightly anchored to the crus of the diaphragm on both sides, as well as anteriorly and posteriorly **(Figure 12)**, to prevent rotation of the esophagus or upward retraction. These sutures must not enter the lumen of the esophagus. Two or three 00 silk sutures are placed posterior to the esophagus to approximate the crus of the diaphragm **(Figure 12)**.

Many methods have been devised for facilitating the esophagojejunal anastomosis. Some prefer to leave the stomach attached as a retractor until the posterior layers have been completed. The posterior wall of the esophagus may be divided and the posterior layers closed before the stomach is removed by dividing the anterior esophageal wall. In another method a noncrushing vascular clamp of the modified Pace-Potts type can be applied to the esophagus. Because the esophageal wall tends to tear easily, it is helpful to give substance to the wall of the esophagus and prevent fraying of the muscle layers by fixing the mucosa to the muscle coats proximal to the point of division. A series of encircling mattress sutures of 0000 silk can be inserted and tied, using a surgeon's knot **(Figure 13)**. These sutures include the full thickness of the esophagus **(Figure 14)**. The angle sutures, A and B, are used to prevent rotation of the esophagus when it is anchored to the jejunum **(Figure 14)**.

The esophagus is then divided between this suture line and the gastric wall itself **(Figure 15)**. Soiling should be prevented by suction on the Levin tube as it is withdrawn up into the lower esophagus and a clamp is placed across the esophagus on the gastric side. In the presence of a very high tumor that reaches the gastroesophageal junction, several centimeters of esophagus should be resected above the tumor. If 2.5 cm. or more of esophagus does not protrude beyond the crus of the diaphragm, the lower mediastinum should be exposed in order to ensure a secure anastomosis without tension.

PLATE XXVIII   TOTAL GASTRECTOMY

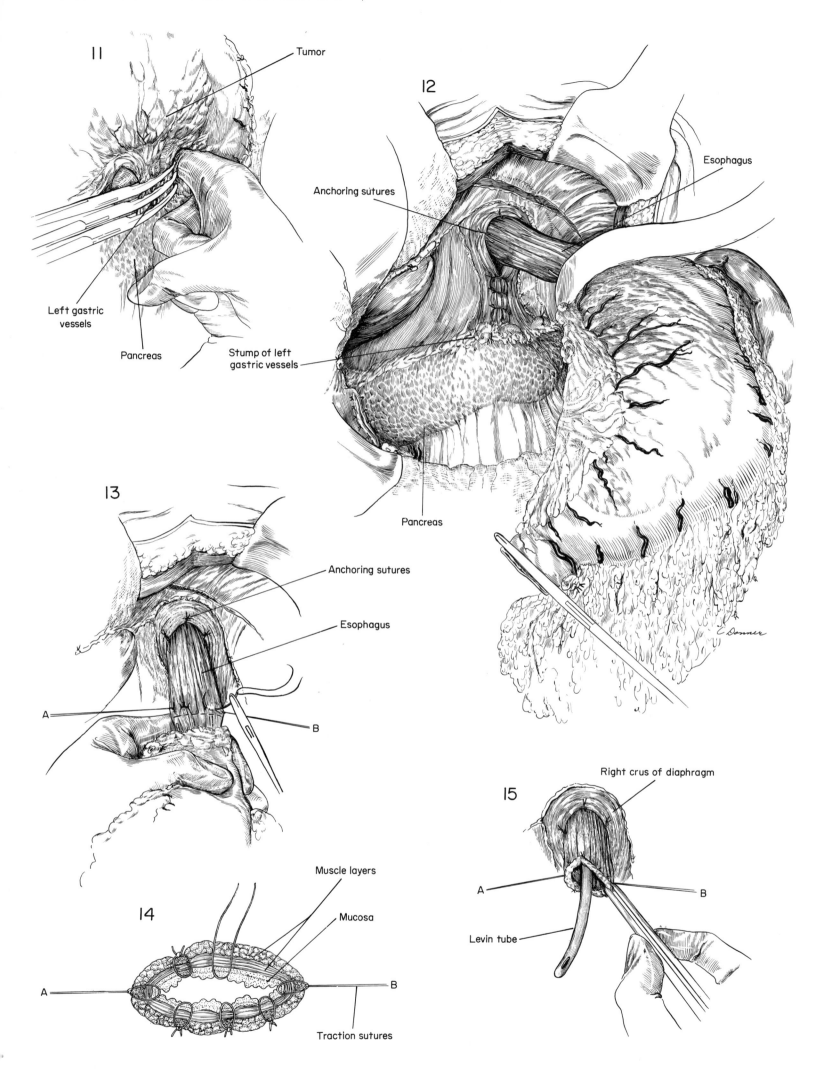

11

Tumor

Anchoring sutures

12

Esophagus

Left gastric vessels

Pancreas

Stump of left gastric vessels

Pancreas

13

Anchoring sutures

Esophagus

A

B

15

Right crus of diaphragm

A

B

Levin tube

Muscle layers

Mucosa

14

A

B

Traction sutures

PLATE XXIX · TOTAL GASTRECTOMY

DETAILS OF PROCEDURE (*Continued*). The next step consists of mobilizing a long loop of jejunum, redundant enough so that it extends easily to the open esophagus. The jejunal loop is brought up through an opening in the mesocolon just to the left of the middle colic vessels. The region about the ligament of Treitz may need to be mobilized to ensure that the jejunum will reach to the diaphragm for easy approximation with the esophagus. The surgeon should be sure that the mesentery is truly adequate for the completion of all the layers of the anastomosis.

Various methods have been used to assure better postoperative nutrition and fewer symptoms following the complete removal of the stomach. A large loop of jejunum with an enteroenterostomy has been commonly used. Regurgitation esophagitis may be lessened by the Roux-en-Y procedure. Interposition of jejunal segments between the esophagus and duodenum, including reversed short segments, has been found to be very satisfactory.

The Roux-en-Y procedure can be used after division of the jejunum at approximately 15 cm. beyond the ligament of Treitz. With the jejunum held outside the abdomen, the arcades of blood vessels can be more clearly defined by transillumination with a portable light **(Figure 16).** Two or more arcades of blood vessels are divided and a short segment of devascularized intestine resected **(Figure 17).** The arm of the distal segment of jejunum is passed through the opening made in the mesocolon to the left of the middle colic vessels. Additional mesentery is divided if the end segment of the jejunum does not easily extend up to and parallel with the crus of the diaphragm behind the esophagus. When the adequate length has been assured, the decision must be made whether it is safer and easier to do an end-to-end anastomosis or an end-to-side anastomosis with the esophagus. If the end-to-side anastomosis is selected, the end of the jejunum is closed with two layers of 0000 silk **(Figures 18** and **19).** The end of the jejunum is then pulled through the opening made in the mesocolon to the left of the middle colic vessels **(Figure 20).** Care must be taken to avoid angulating or twisting the mesentery of the jejunum as it is pulled through. The jejunal wall is anchored about the margins of the hole in the mesocolon. All openings in the mesocolon should be occluded to avoid the possibility of an internal hernia. The opening created beneath the free margin of the mesentery and the posterior parietes should be obliterated by interrupted sutures placed superficially, avoiding injury to blood vessels.

The length of jejunum should again be tested to make certain that the mesenteric border can be approximated easily for 5 to 6 cm. or more to the base of the diaphragm behind the esophagus **(Figure 21).** The closed end of the jejunum is shown directed to the right, but more commonly it is directed toward the left.

PLATE XXIX   TOTAL GASTRECTOMY

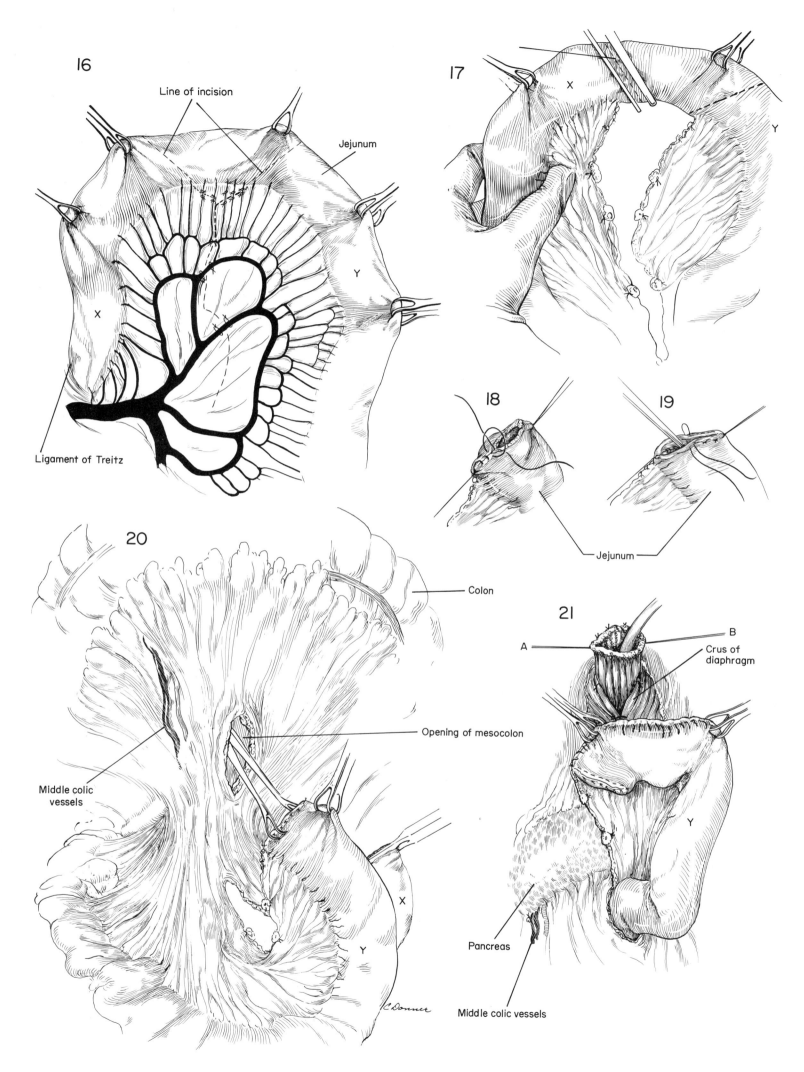

16

Line of incision

Jejunum

X

Ligament of Treitz

17

X

Y

18

19

Jejunum

20

Colon

Opening of mesocolon

Middle colic vessels

X

Y

21

A

B

Crus of diaphragm

Y

Pancreas

Middle colic vessels

C Donner

PLATE XXX · TOTAL GASTRECTOMY

DETAILS OF PROCEDURE (*Continued*). A row of interrupted 00 silk sutures is placed to approximate the jejunum to the diaphragm on either side of the esophagus, as well as directly behind it **(Figure 22)**. It is necessary to emphasize that the arm of jejunum is anchored to the diaphragm to remove tension from the subsequent anastomosis of the esophagus. After these anchor sutures are tied, angle sutures are placed in either side of the esophagus and jejunum **(Figure 23, C, D)**. The esophageal wall should be anchored to the upper side of the jejunum. An effort should be made to keep the interrupted sutures close to the mesenteric side of the jejunum, since there is a tendency to use all the presenting surface of the jejunum in the subsequent layers of closure. Three or four additional interrupted 00 silk mattress sutures, which include a bite of the esophageal wall with the serosa of the bowel, are required to complete the closure between the angle sutures, C and D **(Figure 24)**. A small opening is then made into the adjacent bowel wall with the jejunum under traction so that during the procedure there is no redundancy of the mucosa from too large an incision.

There is a tendency to make too large an opening in the jejunum with prolapse and irregularity of the mucosa, making an accurate anastomosis with the mucosa of the esophagus rather difficult. A layer of interrupted 0000 silk sutures is used to close the mucosal layer, starting at either end of the jejunal incision with angle sutures **(Figure 25, E, F)**. The posterior mucosal layer is closed with a row of interrupted 0000 silk sutures **(Figure 26)**. The Levin tube may be directed downward into the jejunum **(Figure 27)**. The presence of the tube within the lumen tends to facilitate the placement of the interrupted Connell-type sutures closing the anterior mucosal layer **(Figure 27)**. A larger lumen is assured if the Levin tube is replaced by an Ewald tube of a much larger diameter. This tube is replaced by the Levin tube when the anastomosis is completed. An additional layer will be added as carried out posteriorly. Therefore, when the jejunum is anchored to the diaphragm, the wall of the esophagus, and the mucosa of the esophagus, a three-layered closure is provided **(Figure 28)**.

PLATE XXX   TOTAL GASTRECTOMY

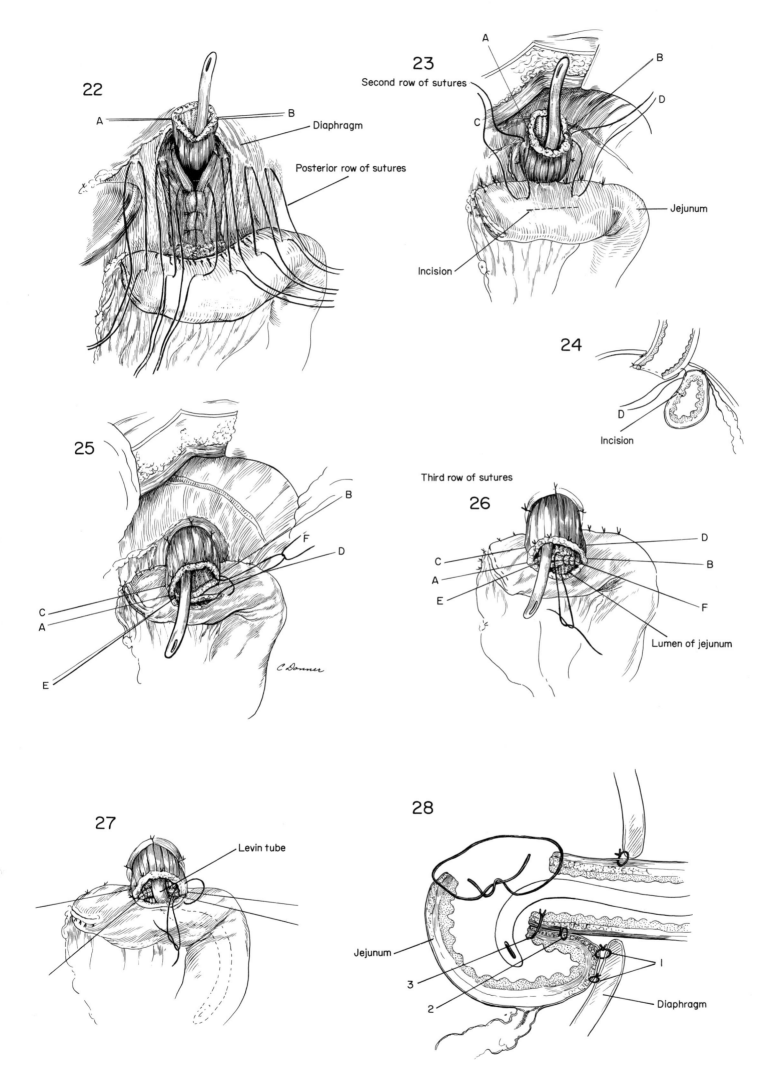

22

A

B — Diaphragm

Posterior row of sutures

23

A

Second row of sutures

B

D

C

Jejunum

Incision

24

D

Incision

25

B

F

D

C

A

E

C Donner

Third row of sutures

26

C

A

E

D

B

F

Lumen of jejunum

27

Levin tube

28

Jejunum

3

2

I

Diaphragm

PLATE XXXI · TOTAL GASTRECTOMY

DETAILS OF PROCEDURE (*Continued*). The second layer of interrupted 00 silk sutures is completed anteriorly **(Figure 29).** Next, the peritoneum, which has been initially incised to divide the vagus nerve and mobilize the esophagus, is brought down to cover the anastomosis and anchored with interrupted 00 silk sutures to the jejunum **(Figure 30).** This ensures a third layer of support which extends all the way anteriorly around the esophageal anastomosis and takes any tension off the delicate line of anastomosis **(Figure 31).** The catheter can be extended well down the jejunum through the opening in the mesocolon to prevent angulation of the bowel. A number of superficially placed fine sutures are taken to anchor the edge of the mesentery to the posterior parietes to prevent angulation and interference with the blood supply **(Figure 31).** These sutures should not include pancreatic tissue or vessels in the margin of the jejunal mesentery. The color of the arm of the jejunum should be checked from time to time to make sure the blood supply is adequate. The open end of the proximal jejunum **(Figure 32,** Y**)** is then anastomosed at an appropriate point in the jejunum **(Figure 32,** X**)** with two layers of 0000 silk, and the opening into the mesentery beneath the anastomosis is closed with interrupted sutures to prevent any possibility of subsequent herniation. A tube jejunostomy placed beyond the anastomosis may be considered in emaciated patients. **Figure 32A** is a diagram of the completed Roux-en-Y anastomosis.

PLATE XXXI   TOTAL GASTRECTOMY

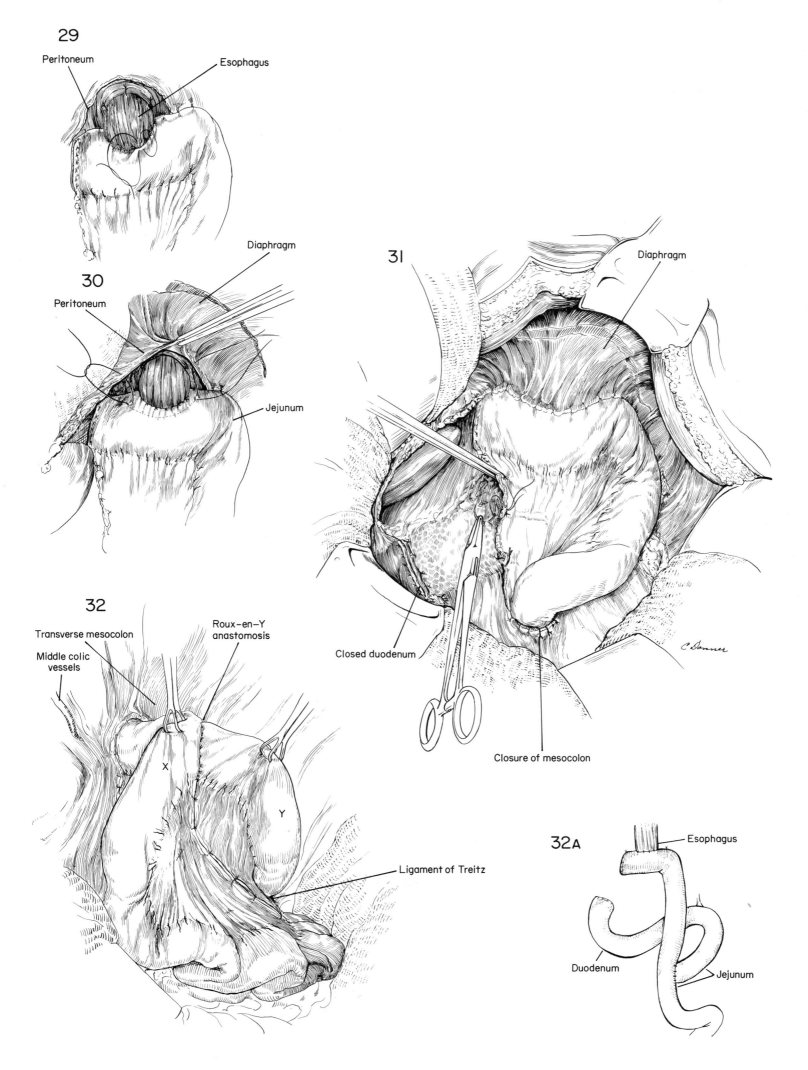

29

Peritoneum

Esophagus

30

Peritoneum

Diaphragm

Jejunum

31

Diaphragm

Closed duodenum

Closure of mesocolon

32

Transverse mesocolon

Middle colic vessels

Roux-en-Y anastomosis

X

Y

Ligament of Treitz

32A

Esophagus

Duodenum

Jejunum

C Danner

PLATE XXXII · TOTAL GASTRECTOMY

DETAILS OF PROCEDURE (*Continued*). The long jejunal loop anastomosis is shown in **Figures 33** and **33A**. The loop is first anchored to the diaphragm posterior to the esophagus, and the three-layered posterior and anterior closure shown in **Figure 28,** Plate XXX is carried out. To take tension off the suture line and to avoid acute angulation of the loop, two or three interrupted sutures may be required to "round out" the attachment to the diaphragm. The opening in the mesocolon is closed about the jejunum with interrupted sutures to avoid rotation of the loops and prevent any possible herniation through the opening **(Figure 34)**. An enteroenterostomy is made near the base of the loop. A stoma two to three fingers wide is all that is required. Some prefer a very long enteroenterostomy, which may include most of the loop, in an effort to provide a pouch with an increased absorptive potential.

Some attempts to improve postoperative nutrition and ensure fewer gastrointestinal symptoms have resulted in procedures that interpose segments of jejunum between the esophagus and duodenum. A segment of jejunum 12 to 15 cm. long may be used to bridge this gap **(Figure 35A)**. The blood supply to this isolated loop, AA^1, can be improved if the major arcades are not divided, but the jejunum proximal and distal to the selected segment is resected close to the mesenteric border **(Figure 35)**. The bowel on either side of the retained segment, AA^1, is resected to a point below the opening in the mesocolon, leaving a wide mesentery to supply for a short distance **(Figure 36)**. A two-layered, end-to-end anastomosis is made to the esophagus and duodenum. The jejunum should be anchored to the diaphragm behind the esophagus and to the peritoneal reflection anteriorly as the third layer of support. The color of the bowel and the presence of active arterial pulsations in the mesentery should be checked repeatedly.

Regardless of the type of pouch that has been reconstructed, the continuity of the jejunum must be reestablished. In preparation for anastomosis the jejunal loops below the mesocolon are freed of their blood supply for a short distance **(Figure 37)**. A two-layered, end-to-end anastomosis is carried out **(Figure 38)**. Any openings remaining beneath the anastomosis are sealed by interrupted sutures of fine silk. A final evaluation should be made to see that there is no tension at the anastomotic sites and that the color of the mobilized segments definitely indicates that the blood supply is not compromised. Improved nutrition with few symptoms may result from using two arms of jejunum for the interposition between the esophagus and duodenum **(Figure 39)**. One 25-cm. segment, YY^1, is anastomosed to the esophagus while the other segment, XX^1, is reversed with one end anastomosed to the duodenum. A large enteroenterostomy is made between the two loops. Approximately 5 cm. of the reversed segment extends beyond the enteroenterostomy and the anastomosis with the jejunum **(Figure 39)** (Poth).

CLOSURE. The wound is closed in the routine manner. In the obese or severely debilitated patient it may be wise to use retention sutures. No drainage is necessary.

POSTOPERATIVE CARE. Constant suction is maintained through the nasojejunal tube which has been threaded through and beyond the anastomosis. During this period alimentation is maintained with intravenous fluids and supplemental vitamins. The patient is ambulated on the first postoperative day, and a gradual increase in activity is encouraged. Early return of peristaltic activity to the bowels is stimulated by injecting 30 ml. of mineral oil through the jejunal tube at regular intervals during the first few postoperative days. When intestinal peristalsis has been established, the suction may be discontinued. At this time the caloric intake can be maintained by tube feedings through the jejunal tube. A slow administration of feedings low in fat and carbohydrate content will avoid diarrhea. Usually, only water followed by skim milk is given in 30- to 60-ml. amounts as tolerated. Oral feedings can be instituted as soon as there is complete assurance that no fistula has formed at the sites of anastomosis. These patients, of course, will need frequent small feedings, and adequate caloric intake will be a problem. The family will require instructions regarding diet. This calls for careful collaboration between surgeon and dietitian. In addition, supplemental vitamin B$_{12}$ will be necessary at monthly intervals, as well as iron.

Scheduled readmissions to the hospital at intervals of 6 to 12 months are advisable to reevaluate caloric intake. Stenosis of the suture line may require dilatations. The blood volume may need to be restored and numerous dietary corrections made.

When total gastrectomy has been performed to control the hormonal effects of an islet cell tumor of the pancreas, serum gastrin levels are taken to evaluate the presence and progress of residual tumor or metastasis. Blood calcium levels are also advised to document the status of the parathyroids. The possibility of familial multiple endocrine adenomatosis should be investigated in all members of the patient's family. Long-term follow-up studies should include serial serum gastrin levels following administration of secretin or calcium over a period of one to four hours. Normal fasting serum gastrin levels may become elevated following these tests if residual gastrin-producing tumor is present.

PLATE XXXII   TOTAL GASTRECTOMY

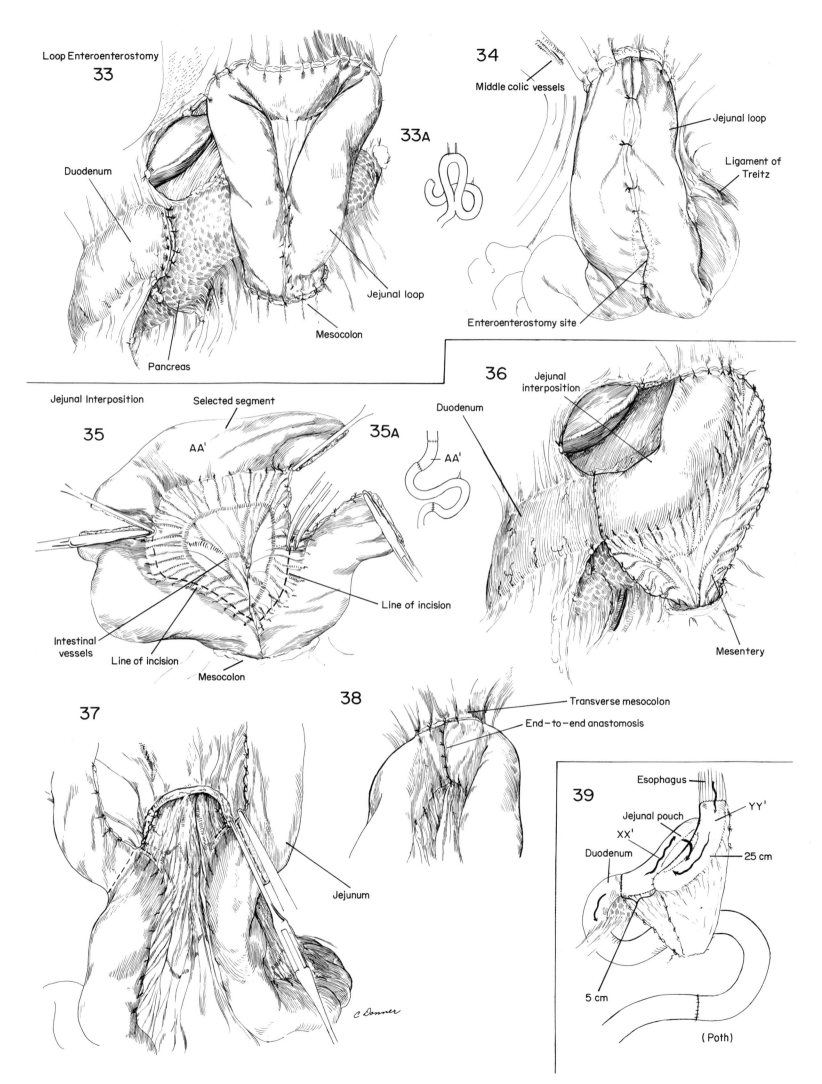

Loop Enteroenterostomy
33

33A

Duodenum

Jejunal loop

Mesocolon

Pancreas

34

Middle colic vessels

Jejunal loop

Ligament of Treitz

Enteroenterostomy site

Jejunal Interposition

Selected segment

35

AA'

35A

AA'

36

Jejunal interposition

Duodenum

Intestinal vessels

Line of incision

Line of incision

Mesocolon

Mesentery

37

38

Transverse mesocolon

End-to-end anastomosis

Jejunum

39

Esophagus

Jejunal pouch

YY'

XX'

Duodenum

25 cm

5 cm

(Poth)

C Donner

PLATE XXXIII · ESOPHAGOCARDIOMYOTOMY

INDICATIONS. The relief of dysphagia associated with megaesophagus secondary to cardiospasm (achalasia) may be corrected by an extensive extramucosal myotomy of the esophagogastric junction. Initial trial of dilatation by hydrostatic dilators may be carried out, providing the patient does not have a widely dilated esophagus with a sigmoidal configuration. The diagnosis of achalasia should be confirmed by roentgenographic examination as well as esophagoscopy. Roentgenography is utilized in differentiating achalasia from organic obstruction. Motility studies are useful in differentiating an organic lesion from achalasia. Both associated benign and malignant lesions of the esophagus must be ruled out by appropriate studies.

The entire gastrointestinal tract should be X-rayed, with particular emphasis on evidence supporting gastric hypersecretion and duodenal deformity due to ulcer. Overnight gastric secretion studies are indicated in the presence of esophagitis to accumulate evidence for possible control of the hypersecretion by vagotomy combined with pyloroplasty.

PREOPERATIVE PREPARATION. Although some patients are in relatively good nutritional status, others will require a period of high-protein, high-caloric, low-roughage feedings preoperatively or intravenous hyperalimentation. A nasogastric feeding tube may be used to supplement an inadequate oral intake. The blood volume is restored by the administration of whole blood, and supplemental liquid vitamins, including ascorbic acid, are provided.

On the day before surgery a large-bore rubber tube is passed into the lower esophagus to facilitate esophageal lavage. After thorough cleansing, this tube is replaced with a smaller-bore plastic nasogastric tube, positioned above the constriction. Instillation of several ounces of nonabsorbable antibiotic solution is carried out at four- to six-hour intervals. Suction is placed on the tube overnight before surgery to completely empty the dilated esophagus, and it is left in place during the operation.

Since these patients not infrequently have recurrent aspiration while recumbent, the pulmonary status should be completely evaluated preoperatively. Intermittent positive pressure aerosol, sputum culture, and systemic antibiotics may be necessary.

ANESTHESIA. General endotracheal anesthesia is preferred.

POSITION. The patient is placed flat on the table with the feet slightly lower than the head.

OPERATIVE PREPARATION. Preoperative gastrointestinal studies should include esophagoscopy, overnight gastric analysis, and gastroduodenal barium studies. If esophagitis is suspected on the basis of the barium swallow or esophagoscopy, if preoperative gastric secretions show high acid and volume, or if coincidental ulcer disease is present, the patient and surgeon should be prepared for vagotomy, pyloroplasty, and gastrostomy. The skin is prepared from the nipples to well below the umbilicus. Adherent plastic drapes may be used.

INCISION AND EXPOSURE. The type of incision utilized must be varied depending upon the patient's body build. If the midline incision is used, the xiphoid may be excised to further enhance the exposure. A long left paramedian incision dissecting the left xiphocostal region extending below the umbilicus on the left side provides a good exposure **(Figure 1).**

The extramucosal myotomy of the esophagogastric junction by the abdominal approach permits abdominal extirpation of associated lesions and facilitates the performance of drainage procedures such as pyloroplasty or gastroenterostomy with or without vagotomy. This exposure is similar to that carried out for vagotomy (Plate XV).

DETAILS OF PROCEDURE. After general exploration of the abdomen with particular attention to the region of the duodenal wall for evidence of ulcerative deformity or scarring, the lower end of the esophagus is exposed by mobilizing the left lobe of the liver. The triangular ligament to the left lobe is divided; the left lobe is retracted upward and held medially by gauze pads upon which is placed a large S retractor **(Figure 2).** Any small bands extending between the stomach and the free edge of the spleen should be divided, lest the capsule of the spleen be torn and splenectomy become necessary. A small pack may or may not be placed above the spleen to maintain downward traction. The xiphoid may be excised and the lower end of the sternum divided if exposure does not appear to be adequate. The peritoneum over the esophagus is divided as the upper end of the stomach is retracted downward with Babcock forceps **(Figure 2).** The avascular gastrohepatic ligament above the lesser curvature is divided, and the thick and uppermost portion of the gastrohepatic ligament containing a branch of the inferior phrenic artery is clamped **(Figure 3).** This provides increased mobilization of the esophagogastric junction with improved exposure, especially anteriorly. The esophagus may be further mobilized by dividing the peritoneum and attachments along the uppermost portion of the fundus of the stomach **(Figure 4).** There are vessels in this area that may need to be ligated. The surgeon's index finger is then passed around the esophagus, and the lower end of the esophagus is further freed from the adjacent structures **(Figure 5).** Usually, the constricted area of the esophagus becomes apparent. At first it may appear that the lower end of the esophagus will be insufficiently mobilized and for that reason additional finger dissection upward around the lower portion of the dilated esophagus may be indicated.

If there has been evidence of esophagitis or gastric hypersecretion, and particularly if there has been a history of duodenal ulcer or evidence of scarring of the duodenal wall, then both vagus nerves should be divided. Division of both vagus nerves greatly increases the mobility of the lower end of the esophagus and commits the surgeon to a gastric drainage procedure such as a pyloroplasty **(Figure 5).**

PLATE XXXIII   ESOPHAGOCARDIOMYOTOMY

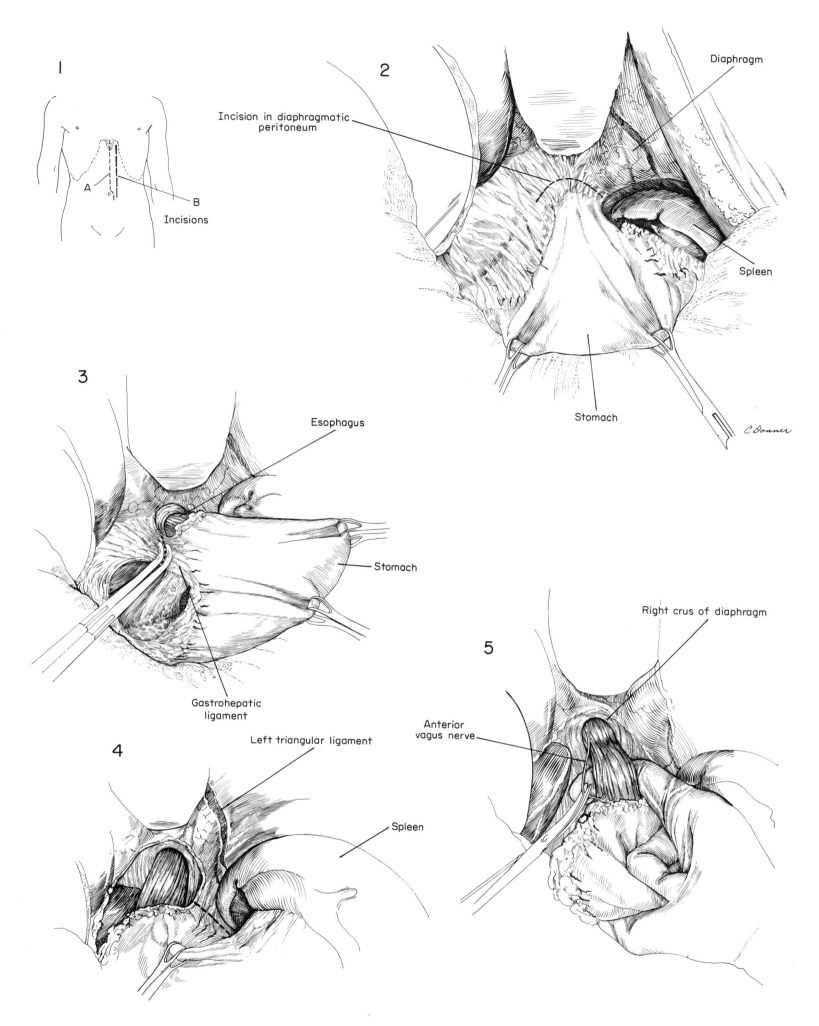

1

Incisions

2

Incision in diaphragmatic peritoneum

Diaphragm

Spleen

Stomach

C. Donner

3

Esophagus

Stomach

Gastrohepatic ligament

4

Left triangular ligament

Spleen

5

Right crus of diaphragm

Anterior vagus nerve

PLATE XXXIV · ESOPHAGOCARDIOMYOTOMY

DETAILS OF PROCEDURE (*Continued*). After the vagus nerves have been divided and an additional length of the esophagus is brought into the abdomen, the tissues about the anterior surface of the esophagogastric junction are cleared in anticipation of an incision through the muscle layers as part of the procedure **(Figure 6).** Right-angle clamps may be utilized to clear this area of all blood vessels and adipose tissue and their contents clamped and ligated with 00 silk. During this procedure the stomach tube, which has been left in place, is aspirated repeatedly by the anesthetist to minimize any contamination should an opening in the dilated esophagus develop.

A variety of procedures have been recommended for dividing the muscle layers of the esophagus. It is desirable to divide the muscles well above the point of apparent constriction and extend the division well down over the gastric wall. This requires a separation of the muscles for at least 8 cm.

In order to assist in the safe division of the muscles and at the same time to ensure a complete severance of all fibers and proof of the development of an adequate lumen, a distensible balloon on the end of a catheter has been found to be useful **(Figure 7).** A small incision is made on the anterior gastric wall between two Babcock clamps, and a small Foley catheter, which is not inflated, is easily passed up into the esophagus. It is then inflated with 5 or 10 ml. of sterile saline, depending upon the size of the esophagus and the degree of constriction encountered **(Figure 8).** An incision is made at the esophagogastric junction through the muscles in the midline anteriorly **(Figure 8).** Small curved clamps are utilized to develop a cleavage plane between the underneath gastric mucosa and the overlying muscle layers. Great care is taken to gently divide all constricting fibers and at the same time to avoid making an incision entirely through the mucosa **(Figure 9).** The balloon may be moderately deflated as the incision is carried through the point of apparent constriction and up over the dilated portion of the lower esophagus. With the esophagus moderately distended with the balloon, any constricting points can be determined by gently palpating the thinned-out remaining mucosal wall with the index finger **(Figure 10).** The incision is further extended well up over the point of constriction **(Figure 11).**

The surgeon must make certain that the incision extends well down over the anterior gastric wall and well up into the dilated wall of the esophagus above the point of constriction. Following this, the balloon is distended with saline until it produces obvious distention of the mucosa to a diameter considerably greater than normal **(Figure 12).** As the balloon is gently pulled through into the stomach, it is partly deflated, and the procedure repeated several times. Additional constricting fibers high up on the esophageal wall as well as down over the stomach may require division.

Following satisfactory dilatation and division of the muscle layers, a careful search is made for any possible small rents or openings that may have been made in the mucosa, and these are closed with fine silk sutures. When vagotomy has been performed, a pyloroplasty or a posterior gastroenterostomy in the region of the antrum is carried out. Some prefer to carry out a pyloroplasty regardless of whether a vagotomy has been performed.

The opening in the anterior gastric wall through which the Foley catheter has been inserted is now utilized as a temporary gastrostomy. The Foley catheter is then directed downward toward the region of the antrum; several sutures are taken through the gastric wall on either side of the catheter, and the gastric wall is inverted about the catheter. The catheter is then brought out through a stab wound to the left of the incision, and the gastric wall is anchored to the parietes to seal off this area as described for gastrostomy (Plate IX).

CLOSURE. The wound is routinely closed with interrupted sutures.

POSTOPERATIVE CARE. The end of the nasogastric tube may be left in place above the point of operation to provide decompression of the dilated esophagus for 48 to 72 hours. This may or may not be necessary, especially when a gastrostomy has been carried out. Fluid and electrolyte balance is maintained and antibiotics given if there has been evidence of gross contamination.

Within 48 to 72 hours the patient is started on clear liquids and then gradually progressed to a soft diet. Late postoperative barium studies of the esophagus may not show improvement consistent with the patient's relief of dysphagia. Occasionally, subsequent hydrostatic dilatations may be indicated.

PLATE XXXIV   ESOPHAGOCARDIOMYOTOMY

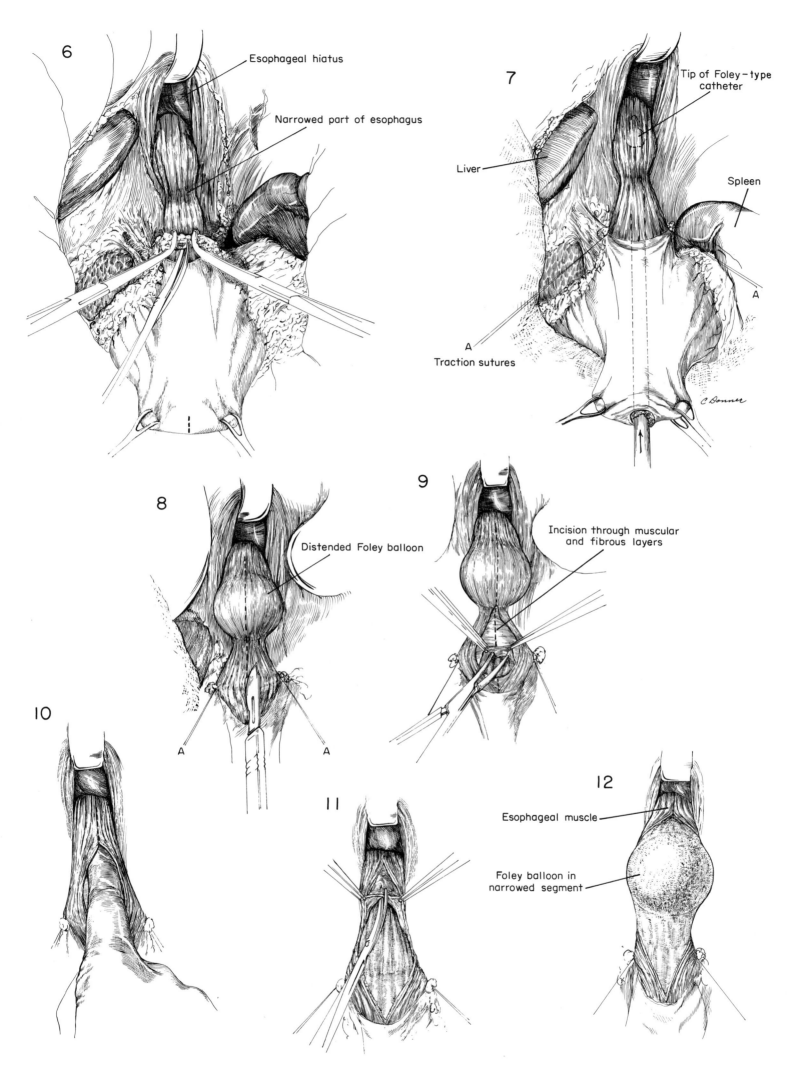

6

Esophageal hiatus

Narrowed part of esophagus

7

Tip of Foley-type catheter

Liver

Spleen

A

Traction sutures

A

C Donner

8

Distended Foley balloon

9

Incision through muscular and fibrous layers

A   A

10

11

12

Esophageal muscle

Foley balloon in narrowed segment

PLATE XXXV · RESECTION OF SMALL INTESTINE

INDICATIONS. This resection is usually an emergency procedure utilized in the presence of sudden obstruction, such as gangrenous intestine in a strangulated hernia, or from volvulus. Less frequently, it is used in mesenteric thrombosis and obstruction by tumor. Since the end-to-end anastomosis restores more accurately the natural continuity of the bowel, it is usually preferable to a lateral anastomosis; however, the surgeon should also be familiar with the side-to-side anastomosis, which is favored when there is marked disparity between the sizes of the ends of bowel to be anastomosed.

PREOPERATIVE PREPARATION. Since resection and anastomosis of the small intestine usually constitute an emergency procedure, preoperative measures are necessarily limited. However, before operation is attempted, the stomach is emptied and constant gastric suction maintained. Fluid and electrolyte balance, including normal sodium, chloride, and potassium levels, should be established in accordance with the degree of fluid depletion, the age, and the cardiac status of the patient. Whole blood and plasma are indicated if the obstruction is marked, the pulse elevated, or gangrenous intestine suspected. Chemotherapy and/or antibiotic therapy should be instituted if gangrenous intestine is suspected. The pulse should be slowed and a good output of urine established as evidence of adequate blood volume expansion before surgery. Constant bladder drainage may be necessary to determine accurately the urinary output in the elderly or seriously ill patient.

ANESTHESIA. General anesthesia with an endotracheal tube and cuff, which permits complete sealing of the trachea, is recommended and is the best prophylaxis against possible aspiration pneumonia. Spinal, either single injection or continuous technic, may be used. However, the threat of sudden regurgitation of large volumes of upper gastrointestinal juices from the obstructed intestine must be anticipated by readily available competent suction equipment. The danger of aspiration is ever-present.

POSITION. The patient is placed in a comfortable supine position.

OPERATIVE PREPARATION. The skin is prepared routinely.

INCISION AND EXPOSURE. The incision is placed over the suspected site of the lesion. If the location of the small bowel obstruction is not known, a lower midline or right rectus incision is often used since the lower ileum is most frequently involved. The incision is made preferably to one side of an old abdominal scar, if present, because the site of the obstruction will most likely be near this point, especially if the scar was tender before operation. A culture of the peritoneal fluid is taken, the amount, color, and consistency being noted. Bloody fluid indicates vascular obstruction. The dilated loops of intestine are retracted or removed carefully from the peritoneal cavity to a warm, moist surface and covered with gauze packs soaked in warm saline solution. When strangulation is present, the surgeon must determine the viability of the involved intestine by taking into consideration these factors: (1) a cadaveric odor; (2) the presence of bloody fluid indicating venous thrombosis; (3) failure of peristalsis to progress over the involved intestine; (4) loss of the normal luster and color of the serosal coat; and, most important of all, (5) absence of arterial pulsation. What may at first appear to be nonviable intestine requiring resection will often return to viability when the cause of the obstruction has been relieved and when the bowel has been packed for a time in warm, moist gauze. There is also a prompt change in the color of viable bowel when 100 per cent oxygen is inhaled. Infiltration of the mesentery with 1 per cent procaine hydrochloride solution may also overcome vascular spasm and bring about arterial pulsations in questionable cases.

In the presence of tumor the mesentery should be explored for metastatic nodes. If there is any doubt as to the site of the obstruction, the surgeon should not hesitate to eviscerate the patient until the offending lesion is adequately exposed and to pass the bowel between his fingers, section by section, from the ligament of Treitz to the cecum. The surgeon must be certain no secondary lesion or distal cause of obstruction exists.

DETAILS OF PROCEDURE. The intestinal wall should be resected 5 to 10 cm. beyond the grossly involved area, even if it means sacrificing several feet of small intestine **(Figure 1)**. The bowel and mesentery are divided, preferably the mesentery first **(Figure 2)**. The surgeon must be certain: (1) that clamps are not applied too far downward toward the base of the mesentery, since the blood supply to a long segment of bowel may be accidentally divided; (2) that the resection extends into the base of the mesentery only in the presence of malignant disease; and (3) that a sizable pulsating vessel is preserved to nourish the bowel adjacent to the

point of resection. The bowel should be cleaned of mesentery for at least 1 cm. beyond the proposed line of resection **(Figure 2)** to ensure the safe application of serosal sutures along the mesenteric border. A pair of narrow, straight clamps with five atraumatic teeth is applied to the intestine. The clamp on the viable portion is placed obliquely, ensuring not only a better blood supply to the antimesenteric border but also a larger lumen for anastomosis **(Figure 3)**. The bowel is divided on both sides of the lesion, and the retained bowel is covered with warm, moist sponges.

The color of the intestine is again observed to assure that the blood supply to the bowel adjacent to the clamp is adequate and that there is sufficient serosa exposed at the mesenteric border for the placement of sutures. If the intestine appears bluish, or if there is no pulsation in the mesenteric vessels, the intestine is resected until the circulation is adequate.

After the bowel ends have been prepared for anastomosis and mobilized distally and proximally far enough to prevent any tension on the suture line of the anastomosis, the clamps are rotated to present the posterior serosal surfaces for approximation. Enterostomy clamps are placed along the intestine 5 to 8 cm. from the crushing clamps to prevent leakage of intestinal contents after the clamps are removed. Silk mattress sutures are taken in the serosa at the mesenteric and antimesenteric borders. The mesenteric border must have been cleaned far enough so that the sutures include serosa only and no mesenteric fat. A layer of interrupted Halsted 00 silk sutures is placed in the serosa, using curved or straight needles **(Figure 4)**. The posterior mucosa is then closed either by a continuous lock stitch of fine catgut on a straight needle or interrupted 0000 silk on French needles **(Figure 5)**. The antimesenteric angle and anterior mucosa are closed by changing to a Connell inverting stitch **(Figures 5 and 6)**. The anterior serosal layer is then closed with interrupted Halsted sutures of 00 silk **(Figure 7)**. The mesentery is approximated with interrupted 0000 silk sutures placed to avoid injury to the vessels. Invaginating the bowel against the thumb with the finger verifies the patency of the anastomosis **(Figure 8)**.

Alternate Method

The method of lateral anastomosis may be used. After the bowel is divided in accordance with the procedure explained above, the severed ends are closed with a continuous inversion suture of fine catgut over the clamp **(Figure 9)**. The wall of the intestine is inverted, and smooth serosa is approximated as the clamp is withdrawn **(Figure 10)**. When the clamp is removed, the suture is pulled just tight enough to control the bleeding and occlude the lumen, and is tied at the mesenteric border. The end of the intestine may be closed by interrupted 0000 silk sutures. The bowel end is closed with a serosal row of interrupted 00 silk mattress sutures which must not include fat or mesentery **(Figure 11)**. In order to avoid interference with the blood supply, the final suture may pull the edge of the mesentery up to the point of closure but should not invert or include it.

Straight intestinal noncrushing clamps are applied to the intestine close to the mesenteric border and near the closed ends to avoid a blind segment beyond the anastomosis. The bowel is held in position with Allis, Babcock, or thumb forceps as the clamps are applied **(Figure 12)**. The clamps are tied together, and the field is covered with fresh towels. Traction sutures are placed at either angle of the anastomosis **(Figure 13)**. A row of interrupted 00 silk sutures is placed in the serosa. The bowel wall is incised with a knife on either side close to the suture line **(Figure 13)**. The incision is lengthened with straight scissors until a stoma about two or three fingers wide is assured. The posterior mucosa is closed with a continuous fine catgut lock stitch or interrupted 0000 fine silk sutures **(Figure 14)**. The anterior layer of mucosa is closed with a Connell inverting stitch and the anterior serosal layer with interrupted 00 silk mattress sutures **(Figure 15)**. The angles may be reinforced with several interrupted 00 silk sutures until the closed ends of intestine are securely anchored to the adjacent bowel **(Figure 16)**. The mesentery is approximated using interrupted 0000 silk sutures placed in such a way as to avoid major blood vessels **(Figure 16)**. A temporary gastrostomy should be considered if the stomach is readily accessible.

CLOSURE. Retention sutures may be added.

POSTOPERATIVE CARE. The fluid balance is established and maintained by the use of intravenous glucose and saline. Whole blood transfusions are usually indicated until the pulse rate has returned to normal. Antibiotic therapy is used. Constant decompression by continuous gastric suction or temporary gastrostomy is maintained until normal emptying of the intestinal tract begins. An enterostomy (Plate XXXVI) proximal to the anastomosis in low obstructions with considerable dilation of the intestine should be considered.

PLATE XXXV   RESECTION OF SMALL INTESTINE

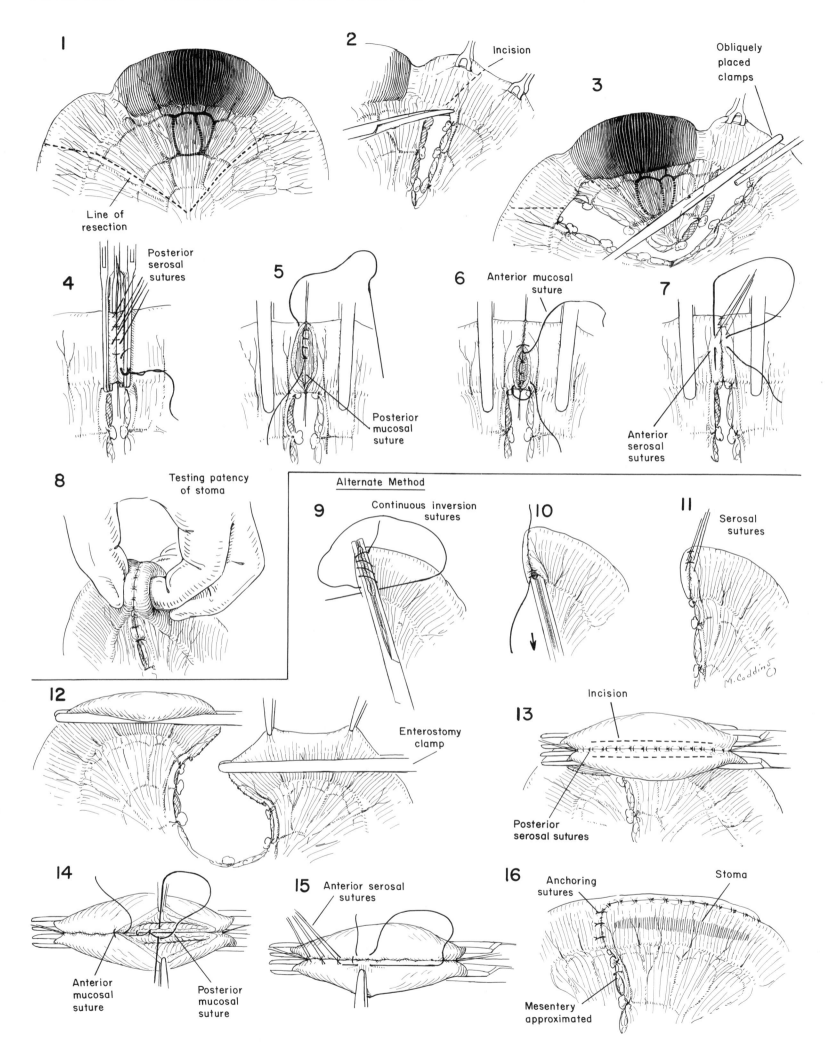

1 Line of resection

2 Incision

3 Obliquely placed clamps

4 Posterior serosal sutures

5 Posterior mucosal suture

6 Anterior mucosal suture

7 Anterior serosal sutures

8 Testing patency of stoma

Alternate Method

9 Continuous inversion sutures

10

11 Serosal sutures

12 Enterostomy clamp

13 Incision
Posterior serosal sutures

14 Anterior mucosal suture
Posterior mucosal suture

15 Anterior serosal sutures

16 Anchoring sutures
Stoma
Mesentery approximated

M. Codding

PLATE XXXVI · ENTEROSTOMY

INDICATIONS. Enterostomy in the high jejunum may be utilized for feeding purposes in malnourished patients, either before or after major surgical procedures. Enterostomy in the low ileum may be clinically indicated in the presence of adynamic ileus when intubation and other methods of bowel decompression have failed to relieve the obstruction, or when the patient's condition will not permit the removal of the cause. Enterostomy may also be done to decompress the gastrointestinal tract proximal to the point of major resection and anastomosis, or to decompress the stomach indirectly after gastric resection by directing a long tube in a retrograde fashion back into the stomach. Bile, pancreatic juice, as well as gastric juice lost from intubation or a fistula, can be refed through the tube. Intravenous hyperalimentation is usually used initially except in the presence of obstruction or severe and persistent paralytic ileus.

PREOPERATIVE PREPARATION. The preoperative preparation is determined by the underlying conditions found preoperatively. Often an enterostomy is done in conjunction with another major surgical procedure on the gastrointestinal tract.

POSITION. The patient is placed in a comfortable supine position.

OPERATIVE PREPARATION. The skin is prepared routinely.

INCISION AND EXPOSURE. As a rule, a paramedian incision is placed close to the umbilicus. If the enterostomy is performed for adynamic ileus in the presence of peritonitis, the incision should be so small that few sutures are necessary in the closure. When the procedure is part of a major intestinal resection or for feeding purposes, the enterostomy tube is brought out through a stab wound, preferably some distance away from the original incision. If the enterostomy is primarily for feeding purposes, or for draining the stomach, the incision should be made in the region of the ligament of Treitz in the left upper quadrant.

A. Stamm Enterostomy

INDICATIONS. When used for feeding purposes, either preliminary, complementary, or supplementary to a major resection, a Stamm enterostomy should be made close to the ligament of Treitz in the jejunum. When intended to relieve distention in adynamic ileus, the first presenting dilated loop may be utilized.

DETAILS OF PROCEDURE. In the enterostomy used as a means of feeding, a loop of jejunum close to the ligament of Treitz is delivered into the wound, and the proximal and distal ends of the bowel are identified. The bowel is stripped of its contents, and enterostomy clamps are applied. Two concentric purse-string sutures of 00 silk are taken in the submucosa of the antimesenteric surface **(Figure 1)**. The outer suture is taken in a soft rubber catheter (16F) about 15 cm. from the tip of the catheter. A small stab wound is made through the intestinal wall in the center of the inner purse-string suture **(Figure 2)** through which the catheter is slipped into the lumen of the distal portion of the intestine. The clamps are removed. The inner purse-string suture is tightened about the catheter. The outer purse-string suture is pulled snug to anchor the catheter to the intestinal wall and serves to invert a small cuff of intestine about the catheter **(Figure 3)**.

CLOSURE. The proximal end of the catheter is brought out through a stab wound in the abdominal wall. The intestine adjacent to the catheter is anchored to the overlying peritoneum with four fine silk sutures **(Figure 4)**. The catheter is anchored to the skin with a silk suture **(Figure 5)**.

B. Witzel Enterostomy

INDICATIONS. The Witzel enterostomy may be preferred when a long-term need for a small bowel enterostomy is clearly indicated. This procedure provides a valve-like protection to the opening into the jejunum.

DETAILS OF PROCEDURE. The loop of small bowel selected for the enterostomy is stripped of its contents and noncrushing clamps applied **(Figure 6)**. A purse-string suture of 00 silk is placed opposite the mesenteric border. A modest-sized soft rubber catheter with several openings is then placed on the gastric wall while interrupted sutures are placed about 1 cm. apart, incorporating a small bite of the intestinal wall on either side of the catheter **(Figure 7)**. When these sutures are tied, the catheter is buried within the wall of the small intestine for 6 to 8 cm. Following this, an incision is made into the bowel in the midportion of the purse-string suture, and the end of the catheter is inserted into the small intestine **(Figure 8)** and threaded the desired distance into the lumen, after which the purse-string suture is tied. The remaining exposed portion of the catheter and the area of the purse-string suture are further buried with three or four interrupted 00 silk sutures **(Figure 9)**. A stab wound is made in the abdominal wall and a clamp inserted as a guide to the placement of sutures between the small intestine and the peritoneum adjacent to the suture line **(Figure 10)**. A broad-based attachment is desirable to avoid twisting or angulating the small intestine. After the first layer of sutures is tied, the catheter is withdrawn through the stab wound, permitting the anterior layer or sutures to be placed between the peritoneum and the small intestine, which completely seals off the area of the catheter. It is advisable to attach the small intestine to the parietes for 5 to 8 cm. in order to avoid volvulus of the small intestine around a small fixed point. The intestine should be anchored to the peritoneum in the direction of peristalsis.

CLOSURE. The abdomen is closed routinely. The catheter is anchored to the skin with a silk suture and with an additional adhesive dressing.

POSTOPERATIVE CARE. When the enterostomy is performed to relieve an adynamic ileus, the catheter is attached to a drainage bottle, and approximately 30 ml. of sterile water or saline may be injected over two to four hours to assure adequate drainage through the tube. If the enterostomy is used for feeding, the patient's fluid and calorie requirements can be partially met by homogenized milk and glucose in water or saline, which may be started through the enterostomy tube by continuous gravity drip at the rate of 50 ml. per hour. The calorie intake should be increased slowly because of the common complication of diarrhea and abdominal discomfort. Enterostomy feeding should not be continued during the night because of the possibility that distress and/or diarrhea may develop. The catheter usually is removed within 10 to 14 days unless it is required for feeding purposes, or if the obstruction has not been relieved, as proved by recurrent symptoms after clamping of the catheter.

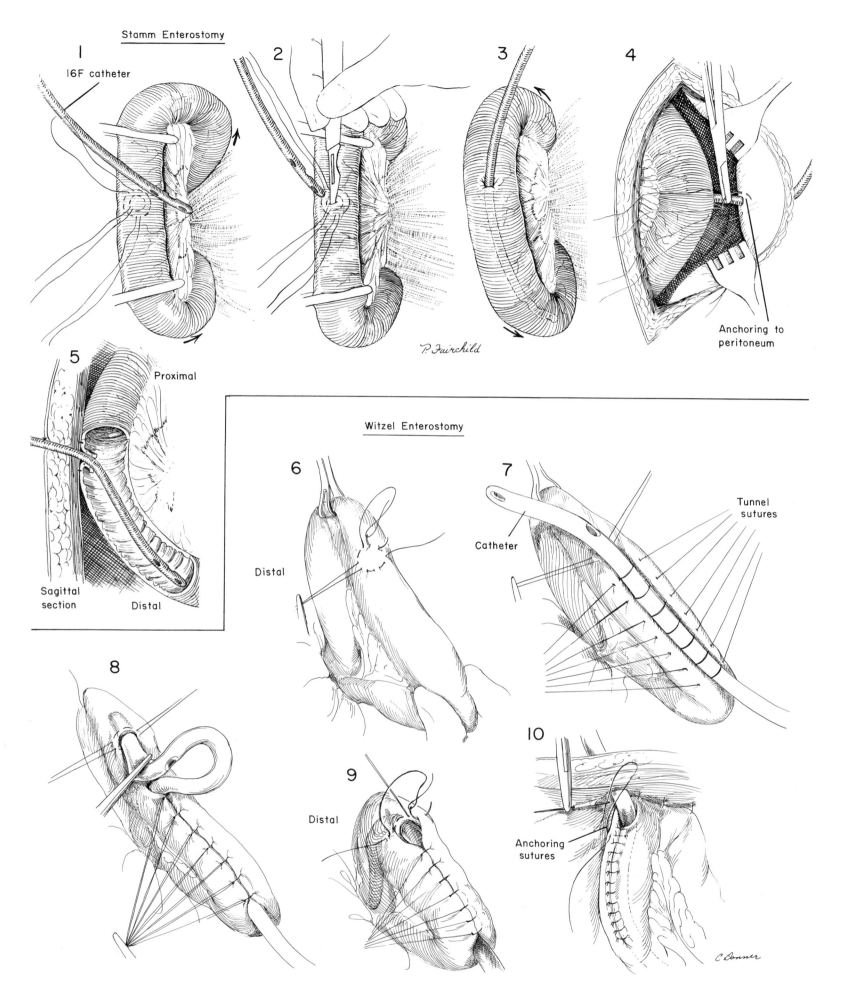

Stamm Enterostomy

1   16F catheter

2

3

4   Anchoring to peritoneum

P. Fairchild

5   Proximal

Sagittal section   Distal

Witzel Enterostomy

6   Distal

7   Catheter   Tunnel sutures

8

9   Distal

10   Anchoring sutures

C. Denner

PLATE XXXVII · PYLOROMYOTOMY—INTUSSUSCEPTION

A. Pyloromyotomy

INDICATIONS. Pyloromyotomy (the Fredet-Ramstedt operation) is done in infants with congenital hypertrophic pyloric stenosis.

PREOPERATIVE CARE. The correction of dehydration and acid-base imbalance by adequate parenteral fluid therapy is as important as surgical skill in lowering the mortality rate. Although prolonged gastric intubation is to be avoided, 6 to 12 hours of preparation with intravenous hydration plus suction may be necessary to restore the baby to good operative condition. Oral feedings are discontinued as soon as the diagnosis is made, and an intravenous infusion is started in a scalp vein. Ten ml. per kilogram of 5 per cent glucose in normal saline is administered rapidly. This is followed by a solution of one part 5 per cent dextrose in normal saline to one part 5 per cent dextrose in water (one half normal saline with 5 per cent D/W) given at the rate of 150 ml./kg. per 24 hours. The baby should be reevaluated every eight hours with respect to his state of hydration, weight, and evidence of edema. Ordinarily, this solution is continued for 8 to 16 hours. After adequate urinary output is established, potassium should be added to the intravenous solutions. In the baby who is moderately or severely dehydrated, it is wise to determine the serum electrolyte values before initiating replacement therapy and to check the values in 8 to 12 hours.

ANESTHESIA. Atropine sulfate 0.0001 Gm. without the addition of a narcotic is sufficient preoperative medication. Endotracheal intubation on the conscious infant is the safest anesthetic technic, followed by general anesthesia.

POSITION. A hot-water bottle partially filled with warm water or a temperature-controlled blanket is placed under the infant's back to help compensate for the loss of body heat and to arch the abdomen slightly to improve the operative exposure. To prevent heat loss through the arms and legs, they are wrapped with sheet wadding, and the intravenous site is carefully protected.

OPERATIVE PREPARATION. The skin is prepared in the routine manner.

INCISION AND EXPOSURE. A gridiron incision placed below the right costal margin, but above the inferior edge of the liver, is used. The incision is 3 cm. long and extends laterally from the outer edge of the rectus muscle. The omentum or the transverse colon usually presents in the wound and is easily identified. By gentle traction on the omentum, the transverse colon is delivered and, in turn, traction on the transverse colon will deliver the greater curvature of the stomach easily into the wound. The anterior wall of the stomach is held with a moistened gauze sponge and, by upward traction on the antral portion of the stomach, the pylorus is delivered into the wound.

DETAILS OF PROCEDURE. The anterosuperior surface of the pylorus is not very vascular and is the region selected for the pyloromyotomy **(Figure 2).** As the pylorus is held between the surgeon's thumb and index finger, a longitudinal incision 1 to 2 cm. long is made **(Figure 3).** The incision is carried down through the serosal and muscle coats until the mucosa is exposed, but the mucosa is left intact **(Figure 4).** Great care must be taken at the duodenal end of the incision, for here the pyloric muscle ends abruptly, in contrast with the gastric end, and the mucosa of the duodenum may be perforated (see Danger Point, **Figure 1**). The cut muscle is now spread apart with a straight or a half-length hemostat until the mucosa pouts up to the level of the cut serosa **(Figures 4 and 5).** Usually, hemorrhage can be controlled by applying a sponge wet with saline, and only rarely is a ligature or stitch necessary to control a bleeding vessel. The surgeon must ascertain that no perforation of the mucous membrane exists.

CLOSURE. The peritoneum and transversalis fascia are closed with a running suture of 0000 chromic catgut. The remaining fascial layers are closed with interrupted sutures of 00000 silk. The skin margins are approximated with running 000000 silk sutures.

POSTOPERATIVE CARE. Six hours following operation, the Wangensteen suction is discontinued and the nasogastric tube removed. Fifteen ml. of dextrose and water is offered to the infant at this time. Following this the infant is offered 30 ml. of an evaporated milk formula every two hours until the morning after operation. Thereafter, the infant is fed progressively more formula on a three-hour schedule.

B. Intussusception

INDICATIONS. Intussusception occurs most commonly in infants from the age of a few months to two years. Time must be taken to correct dehydration or debility by administering parenteral fluids. A stomach tube should be passed to deflate the stomach and to reduce to a minimum the danger of aspirated vomitus. If the intussusception has been of considerable duration and there is evidence of bleeding, as in the characteristic mahogany stools in infants, blood and plasma should be administered with the operating room alerted and hydration established satisfactory for operation. The child is taken to the X-ray department, and here hydrostatic reduction by barium enema is attempted, utilizing a pressure of no more than three feet. As much as one hour may be spent in this procedure as long as manipulation of the abdomen is avoided and the exposure to fluoroscopy limited as much as possible. If the intussusception is going to reduce, it will progressively do so. If this method fails, surgery follows immediately.

ANESTHESIA. Atropine sulfate alone in a dose of 0.0001 Gm. is sufficient for preanesthetic medication in infants of six months or less. Meperidine or morphine should be added in appropriate doses in older infants and children. Endotracheal intubation on the conscious infant is the safest anesthetic technic, followed by general anesthesia.

POSITION. The patient is placed in a dorsal recumbent position. Feet and hands are held flat to the operating table by straps or pinned wrappings.

OPERATIVE PREPARATION. The skin is prepared in the routine manner.

INCISION AND EXPOSURE. In most instances a transverse incision made in the right lower quadrant provides adequate exposure. The lateral third of the anterior rectus fascia and the adjacent aponeurosis of the external oblique are incised transversely. The lateral edge of the rectus muscle may then be retracted medially and the internal oblique and transversalis muscles divided in the direction of their fibers. If more exposure is required, the incision in the anterior rectus fascia may be extended, and a portion or all of the right rectus muscle may be transected.

DETAILS OF PROCEDURE. The major portion of the reduction is done intra-abdominally by milking the mass back along the descending colon, transverse colon, and ascending colon. When reduction has proceeded thus far, the remainder can be delivered out of the abdominal cavity. The mass is pushed back along the descending colon by squeezing the colon distal to the intussusception **(Figure 7).** If traction is applied, it should be extremely gentle to avoid rupturing the bowel. The discolored and edematous bowel may not at first appear to be viable, but the application of warm saline solution may improve its tone and appearance. Unless the intestine is necrotic, it is better to persist in attempts at reduction than to resort to early and unnecessary resection, required in less than 5 per cent of the cases. An etiologic factor, such as an inverted Meckel's diverticulum or intestinal polyp, is found in only 3 or 4 per cent of childhood cases of intussusception. It is unnecessary to tack down the terminal ileum or to anchor the mesentery. Recurrences are not common, and such preventive procedures only prolong the operation. Intussusception is uncommon in adults. It may occur at any level of the small or large intestine. After the intussusception in adults has been reduced, a search should be made for the initiating cause, i.e., tumors (especially intrinsic), adhesive bands, Meckel's diverticulum, etc.

CLOSURE. The peritoneum is closed with a continuous suture of 0000 chromic catgut. The remainder of the incision is closed with interrupted sutures of 00000 silk.

POSTOPERATIVE CARE. Nasogastric suction is continued until peristaltic activity is audible or until a stool is passed. Antibiotics and colloid replacement are not necessary in an uncomplicated intussusception, but again are most valuable adjuncts in the case requiring resection. About 5 ml. per kilogram of colloid, using either blood, plasma, or 5 per cent albumin solution, provides an invaluable daily supportive measure for the seriously ill child who has had resection of a gangrenous intussusception. Recurrence in the adult should suggest a cause overlooked initially but probably amenable to surgical correction, such as removal of a polyp or adhesive band.

PLATE XXXVII   PYLOROMYOTOMY—INTUSSUSCEPTION

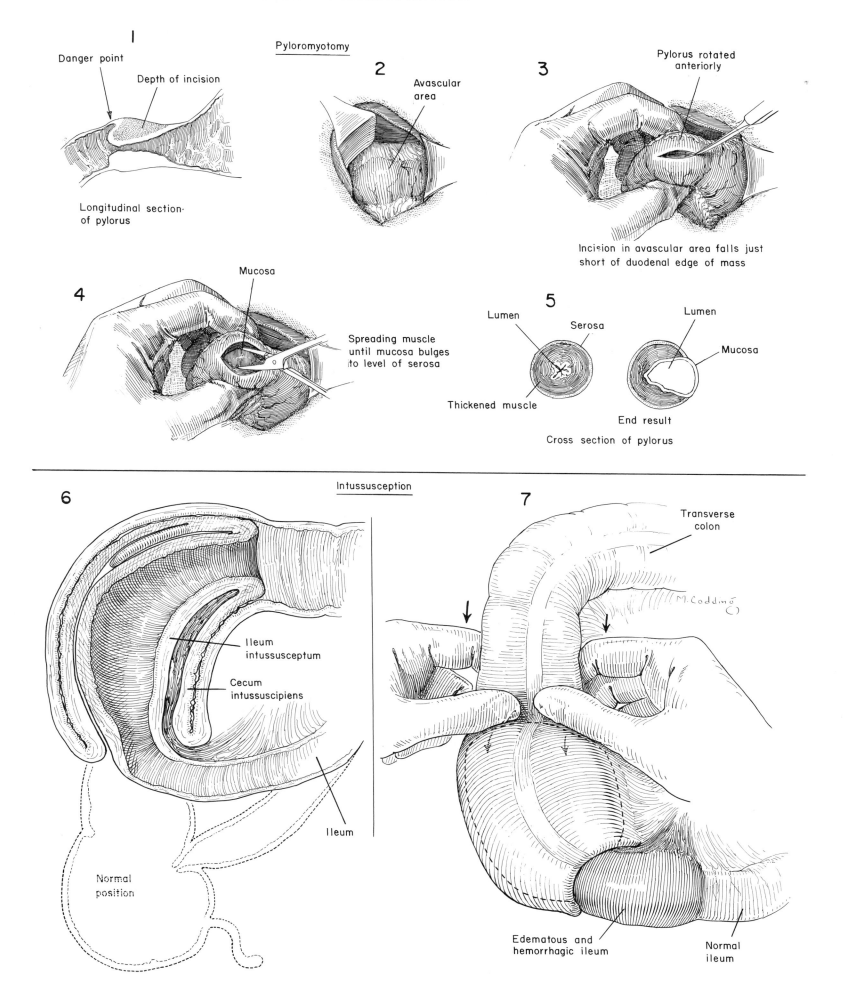

1
Danger point
Depth of incision
Longitudinal section of pylorus

Pyloromyotomy

2
Avascular area

3
Pylorus rotated anteriorly
Incision in avascular area falls just short of duodenal edge of mass

4
Mucosa
Spreading muscle until mucosa bulges to level of serosa

5
Lumen
Serosa
Thickened muscle
Lumen
Mucosa
End result
Cross section of pylorus

Intussusception

6
Ileum intussusceptum
Cecum intussuscipiens
Ileum
Normal position

7
Transverse colon
M. Codding
Edematous and hemorrhagic ileum
Normal ileum

PLATE XXXVIII · MECKEL'S DIVERTICULECTOMY

INDICATIONS. Excision of a Meckel's diverticulum is performed when the diverticulum is found to cause an acute abdominal condition. More frequently excision is a benign incidental procedure during a laparotomy for other causes. The majority of these diverticula cause no symptoms, but a diseased one can successfully mimic many other intestinal diseases, any of which would require exploratory laparotomy.

The presence of gastric mucosa in the diverticulum can produce ulceration with massive intestinal hemorrhage with brick-red stools, inflammation, or a free perforation with peritonitis, particularly in children. While similar complications can occur in adults, intestinal obstruction caused by fixation of the tip of the diverticulum or a connecting band running to the umbilicus is not uncommon. The diverticulum may become inverted and form the starting point of an intussusception. Benign diverticula should be removed as incidental procedures unless contraindicated by a potentially complicating disease elsewhere in the abdomen. These congenital anomalies are remnants of the embryonic omphalomesenteric duct arising from the midgut, are found in 1 to 3 per cent of patients, principally males, and are located usually 20 to 35 cm. above the ileocecal valve. The terminal ileum should be routinely examined for a Meckel's diverticulum as part of a thorough abdominal exploration.

PREOPERATIVE PREPARATION. Preoperative preparation is devoted chiefly to the restoration of blood, fluids, and electrolytes. Nasogastric suction is advisable in the presence of obstruction or peritonitis, which may require additional blood, plasma, and antibiotics.

ANESTHESIA. General inhalation anesthesia is preferred; however, spinal or local anesthesia may be indicated under special circumstances.

POSITION. The patient is placed in a comfortable supine position.

OPERATIVE PREPARATION. The skin is prepared with antiseptic, then draped with towels or an adhesive plastic drape. A large sterile laparotomy sheet completes the draping.

INCISION AND EXPOSURE. A right lower paramedian or midline incision is preferred because of its maximum flexibility. However, incidental excision of a Meckel's diverticulum may be performed through any incision that exposes it.

DETAILS OF PROCEDURE. The segment of the terminal ileum involved with the Meckel's diverticulum is delivered into the wound by Babcock forceps for stabilization. The Meckel's diverticulum may be as far as 20 to 35 cm. back from the level of the ileocecal valve. If a mesodiverticulum is present, it should be freed, divided between hemostats, and ligated as a mesoappendix **(Figure 1)**. If the diverticulum has quite a wide neck, it may be excised by either oblique or cross clamping of the base; by wedge or V-shaped excision of the base; or by segmental resection of the involved ileum with end-to-end anastomosis **(Figure 2)**. The base is doubly clamped with noncrushing Potts-type clamps in a direction transverse or diagonally across to the bowel. The specimen is excised with a scalpel. Traction sutures, A and B, of 00 silk are placed to approximate the serosal surface of the intestinal wall just beyond either end of the incision **(Figure 3)**. When tied, these sutures, A and B, serve to stabilize the intestinal wall during the subsequent closure. Sutures of 00 silk are placed at either end of the incision, and a row of interrupted 0000 silk horizontal mattress sutures is placed beneath the clamp **(Figure 4)**. The clamp is then removed, the sutures tied, and any excess intestinal wall excised. Then an inverting layer of interrupted 0000 silk horizontal mattress sutures is placed **(Figures 5 and 6)**. The patency of the lumen is then tested between the surgeon's thumb and index finger **(Figure 7)**.

CLOSURE. The usual laparotomy closure is performed.

POSTOPERATIVE CARE. Postoperative care is similar to that for appendectomy or small bowel anastomosis. Fluid and electrolyte balance is maintained intravenously until intestinal motility returns. The nasogastric tube is then removed and progressive alimentation begun. Any subsiding inflammation, peritonitis, or drained abscess is treated with the appropriate systemic antibiotics plus blood and plasma replacement. The major postoperative complications are obstruction, peritonitis, and wound infection, which may require further appropriate surgical therapy.

PLATE XXXVIII   MECKEL'S DIVERTICULECTOMY

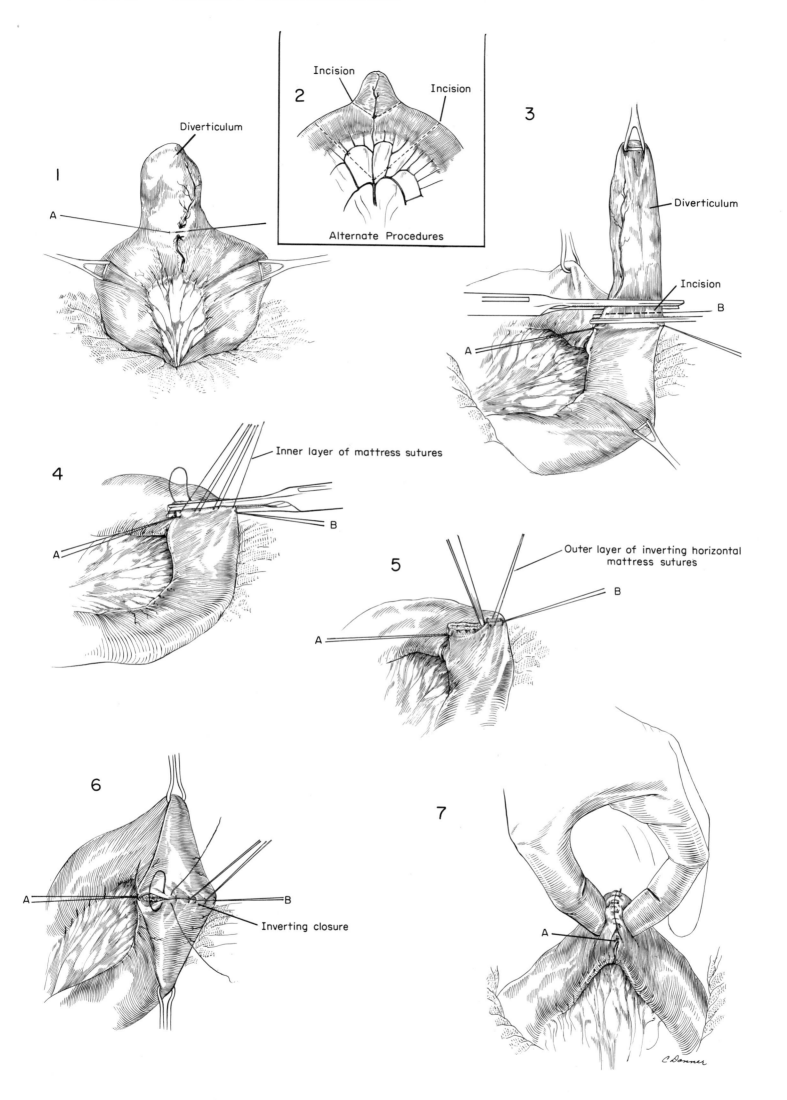

1

Diverticulum

A

2

Incision

Incision

Alternate Procedures

3

Diverticulum

Incision

B

A

4

Inner layer of mattress sutures

B

A

5

Outer layer of inverting horizontal
mattress sutures

B

A

6

A

B

Inverting closure

7

A

C. Donner

PLATE XXXIX · APPENDECTOMY

INDICATIONS. If acute appendicitis has been diagnosed, prompt operation is almost always indicated. Delay for administration of parenteral fluids may be advisable in toxic patients and in children or elderly persons. If there is evidence of generalized peritonitis of some duration with marked distention and toxemia, some surgeons prefer expectant treatment, with the patient in a semisitting position, continuous gastric suction, parenteral feedings including blood, and massive therapy with antibiotic and chemotherapeutic agents. Localization of abscesses, particularly in the pelvis, right lower quadrant, and subphrenic region is then carefully watched so that they can be drained at the appropriate time. This practice of conservation is rarely indicated if the symptoms have lasted less than four days.

If the patient has a mass in the right lower quadrant when first seen, several days of preparative treatment are usually advisable; occasionally, such a mass will recede, but an appendectomy at a later date is always indicated. If the abscess requires drainage, appendectomy is carried out at the same time if it can be easily accomplished, but not otherwise. Appendectomy must then be carried out at a later date. If the diagnosis is so-called chronic appendicitis, other possible causes of pain and sources of pathology should be ruled out.

PREOPERATIVE PREPARATION. The preoperative preparation is devoted chiefly to the restoration of the fluid balance, especially in very young and aged persons. Administration of antibiotics, chemotherapy, and whole blood in the presence of peritonitis is usually an adjunct to an uneventful recovery by the patient. Continuous gastric suction is advisable if peritonitis is present or if the patient has been vomiting.

ANESTHESIA. Inhalation anesthesia is preferred; however, spinal anesthesia is satisfactory. Local anesthesia may be indicated in the very ill patient.

POSITION. The patient is placed in a comfortable supine position.

OPERATIVE PREPARATION. The skin is prepared in the usual manner.

INCISION AND EXPOSURE. In no surgical procedure has the practice of standardizing the incision proved more harmful. There can be no incision that should always be utilized, since the appendix is a mobile part of the body and may be found anyplace in the right lower quadrant, in the pelvis, up under the ascending colon, and even rarely on the left side of the peritoneal cavity **(Figures 2 and 3).** The surgeon determines the location of the appendix, chiefly from the point of maximum tenderness by physical examination, and makes the incision best adapted for exposing this particular area. The great majority of appendices are reached satisfactorily through the right lower muscle-splitting incision, which is a variation of the original McBurney procedure **(Figure 1,** Incision A**).** If the patient is a woman, many surgeons prefer the routine use of the right rectus incision **(Figure 1,** Incision B**)** or a midline one to permit exposure of the pelvis unless there is evidence of abscess formation. Then the incision should be made directly over the site of the abscess.

Wherever the incision is, it is deepened first to the aponeurosis of the outer layer of muscle. In the muscle-splitting incision the aponeurosis of the external oblique is split from the edge of the rectus sheath out into the flank parallel to its fibers **(Figure 4).** With the external oblique held aside by retractors, the internal oblique muscle is split parallel to its fibers up to the rectus sheath **(Figure 5)** and laterally toward the iliac crest **(Figure 6).** Sometimes the transversalis fascia and muscle are divided with the internal oblique, but a stouter structure for repair results if the transversalis fascia is opened with the peritoneum. The rectus sheath may be opened for 1 or 2 cm. to give additional exposure **(Figure 7).** The peritoneum is picked up between forceps, first by the operator and then by the assistant **(Figure 8).** The operator drops his original bite, picks up again close to the forceps of the first assistant, and compresses the peritoneum between the forceps with the handle of the scalpel to free the underlying intestine. This maneuver to safeguard the bowel is important and should always be carried out before opening the peritoneum. As soon as the peritoneum is opened **(Figure 8),** its edges are clamped to the moist gauze sponges already surrounding the wound **(Figure 9).** Cultures are taken of the peritoneal fluid.

DETAILS OF PROCEDURE. As a rule, if the cecum presents almost immediately, it is better to pull it into the wound, to hold it in a piece of moist gauze, and to deliver the appendix without feeling around blindly in the abdomen **(Figure 10).** The peritoneal attachments of the cecum may require division to facilitate the removal of the appendix. Once the appendix is delivered, its mesentery near the tip may be seized in a clamp, and the cecum may be returned to the abdominal cavity. Following this, the peritoneal cavity is walled off with moist gauze sponges **(Figure 11).** The mesentery of the appendix is divided between clamps, and the vessels are carefully ligated **(Figure 12).** It is better to apply a transfixing suture rather than a tie to the contents of the clamps, for when structures are under tension, the vessels not infrequently retract from the clamp and bleed later into the mesentery. With the vessels of the mesentery tied off, the stump of the appendix is crushed in a right-angle clamp **(Figure 13).**

PLATE XXXIX   APPENDECTOMY

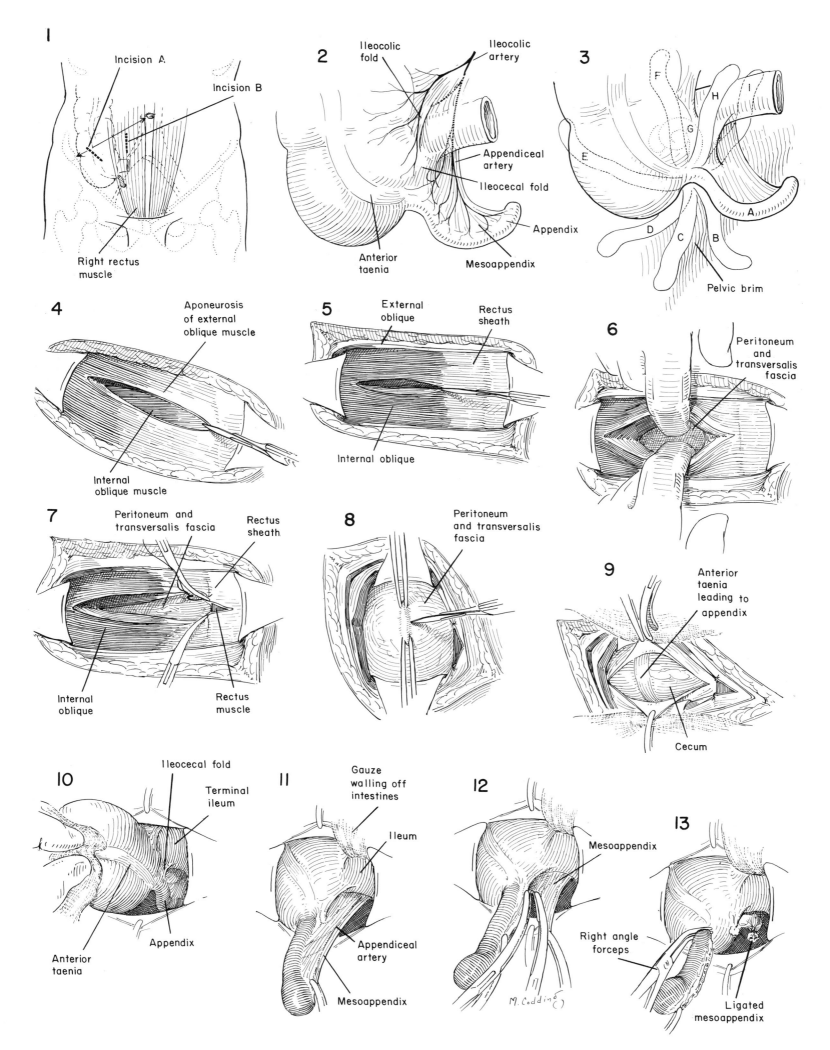

1   Incision A
    Incision B
    Right rectus muscle

2   Ileocolic fold
    Ileocolic artery
    Appendiceal artery
    Ileocecal fold
    Appendix
    Mesoappendix
    Anterior taenia

3   F
    H
    I
    G
    E
    A
    D
    C
    B
    Pelvic brim

4   Aponeurosis of external oblique muscle
    Internal oblique muscle

5   External oblique
    Rectus sheath
    Internal oblique

6   Peritoneum and transversalis fascia

7   Peritoneum and transversalis fascia
    Rectus sheath
    Internal oblique
    Rectus muscle

8   Peritoneum and transversalis fascia

9   Anterior taenia leading to appendix
    Cecum

10 Ileocecal fold
    Terminal ileum
    Appendix
    Anterior taenia

11 Gauze walling off intestines
    Ileum
    Appendiceal artery
    Mesoappendix

12 Mesoappendix
    M. Codding

13 Mesoappendix
    Right angle forceps
    Ligated mesoappendix

PLATE XL · APPENDECTOMY

DETAILS OF PROCEDURE (*Continued*). The right-angle clamp is moved 1 cm. toward the tip of the appendix. Just at the proximal edge of the crushed portion the appendix is ligated **(Figure 14),** and a straight clamp is placed on the knot. A purse-string suture is laid in the wall of the cecum at the base of the appendix, care being taken not to perforate blood vessels where the mesentery of the appendix was attached **(Figure 15).** The appendix is held upward; the cecum is walled off with moist gauze to prevent contamination; and the appendix is divided between the ligature and clamp **(Figure 16).** The suture on the base of the appendix is cut and pushed inward with the straight clamp on the ligature of the stump to invaginate the stump into the cecal wall. The jaws of the clamp are separated, and the clamp is removed as the purse-string suture is tied. The wall of the cecum may be fixed with tissue forceps to aid in inverting the appendiceal stump **(Figure 17).** The cecum then appears as shown in **Figure 18.** The omentum is replaced over the site of operation **(Figure 19).** If there has been a localized abscess, or if there has been a perforation near the base so that a secure closure of the cecum is not possible, or if hemostasis has been poor, drainage may be advisable. Drains should be soft and smooth, preferably a rubber Penrose drain without gauze filler. On no occasion should dry gauze or heavy rubber tubing be used, since these may cause bowel injury. Some surgeons do not drain the peritoneal cavity in the presence of obvious peritonitis which is not localized, relying upon peritoneal irrigation, parenteral antibiotic or chemotherapy, and systemic antibiotic therapy to control it.

If the appendix is not obviously involved with acute inflammation, a more extensive exploration is mandatory. In the presence of peritonitis without involvement of the appendix, the possibility of a ruptured peptic ulcer or sigmoid diverticulitis must be ruled out. Acute cholecystitis, regional ileitis, and involvement of the cecum by carcinoma are not uncommon possibilities. In the female the possibility of bleeding from a ruptured graafian follicle, ectopic pregnancy, or pelvic infection is ever present. Inspection of the pelvic organs under these circumstances cannot be omitted. On occasion a Meckel's diverticulum will be found. Closure of the abdomen, with subsequent study and adequate preparation for bowel resection at a later date, may be indicated.

CLOSURE. The muscle layers are held apart while the peritoneum is closed with interrupted sutures of 00 silk **(Figure 19).** Transversalis fascia incorporated with the peritoneum offers a better foundation for the suture. Interrupted sutures are placed in the internal oblique muscle and in the small opening at the outer border of the rectus sheath **(Figure 20).** The external oblique aponeurosis is closed but not constricted with interrupted 00 silk sutures **(Figure 21).** The subcutaneous tissue and skin are closed in layers.

Alternate Method

In some instances, in order to avoid rupturing a distended acute appendix, it is safer to ligate and divide the base of the appendix before attempting to deliver the appendix into the wound. For example, if the appendix is adherent to the lateral wall of the cecum **(Figure 22),** it is occasionally simpler to pass a curved clamp beneath the base of the appendix in order that it may be doubly clamped and ligated **(Figure 23).** Following ligation of the base of the appendix, which is often quite indurated, it is divided with a knife **(Figure 24).** The base of the appendix is then inverted with a purse-string suture **(Figures 25 and 26).** The attachments of the appendix are divided with long, curved scissors until the blood supply can be clearly identified **(Figure 27).** Curved clamps are then applied to the mesentery of the appendix, and the contents of these clamps are subsequently ligated with 00 silk sutures.

When the appendix is not readily found, the search should follow the anterior taenia of the cecum, which will lead directly to the base of the appendix regardless of its position. When the appendix is found in the retrocecal position, it becomes necessary to incise the parietal peritoneum parallel to the lateral border of the appendix as it is seen through the peritoneum **(Figure 29).** This allows the appendix to be dissected free from its position behind the cecum and on the peritoneal covering of the iliopsoas muscle **(Figure 30).**

On occasion the cecum may be in the right upper quadrant or indeed on the left side of the abdomen when failure of rotation has occurred. A liberal increase in the size of the incision and even a second incision may be, on occasion, good judgment.

POSTOPERATIVE CARE. The fluid balance is maintained by the intravenous administration of 5 per cent glucose and saline. The patient is permitted to sit up for eating on the day of operation, and he may get out of bed on the first postoperative day. Sips of water may be given as soon as nausea subsides. The diet is gradually increased.

If there has been evidence of peritoneal sepsis, large and frequent doses of antibiotics and/or chemotherapy are administered. In addition to the usual fluids and electrolytes, whole blood transfusions may be included. Constant gastric suction is advisable until all evidence of peritonitis and abdominal distention have subsided. Accurate estimate of the fluid intake and output must be made.

Pelvic localization of pus is enhanced by placing the patient in a semi-sitting position. The patient is allowed out of bed as soon as his general condition warrants. Prophylaxis against deep venous thrombosis is instituted. In the presence of persistent signs of sepsis, wound infection and pelvic or subphrenic abscess should be considered. Repeated blood transfusions are usually necessary in the presence of prolonged sepsis.

PLATE XL   APPENDECTOMY

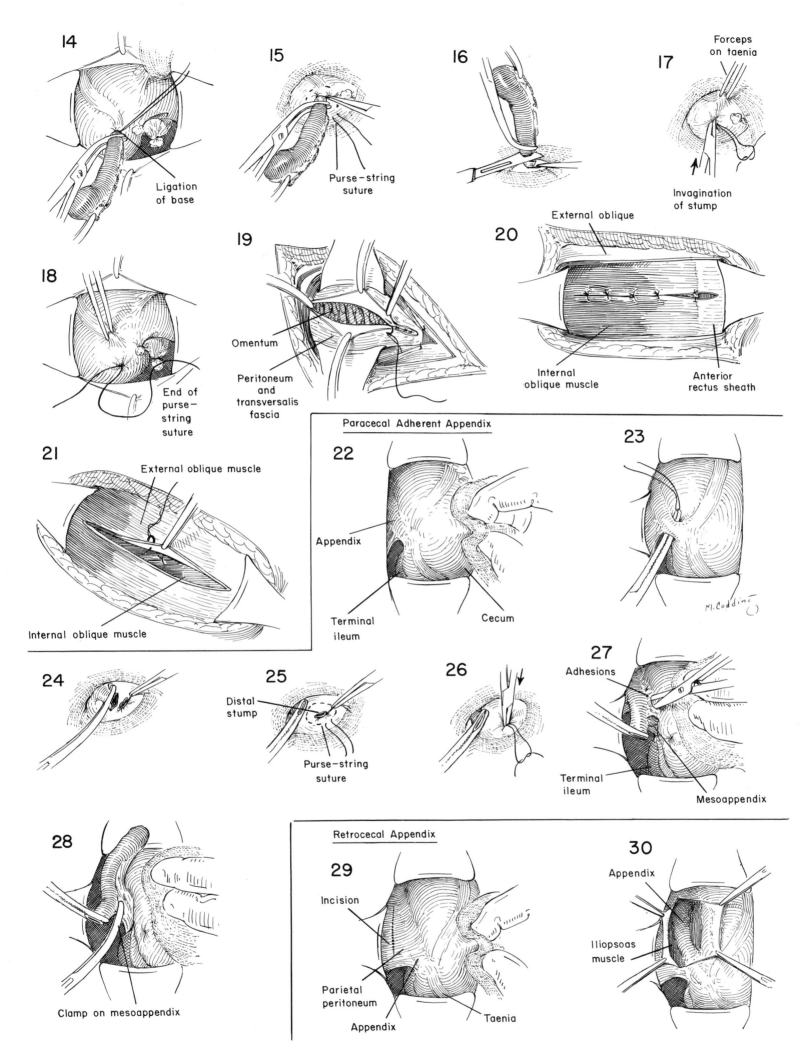

14 Ligation of base

15 Purse–string suture

16

17 Forceps on taenia / Invagination of stump

18 End of purse–string suture

19 Omentum / Peritoneum and transversalis fascia

20 External oblique / Internal oblique muscle / Anterior rectus sheath

21 External oblique muscle / Internal oblique muscle

Paracecal Adherent Appendix

22 Appendix / Terminal ileum / Cecum

23

24

25 Distal stump / Purse–string suture

26

27 Adhesions / Terminal ileum / Mesoappendix

28 Clamp on mesoappendix

Retrocecal Appendix

29 Incision / Parietal peritoneum / Appendix / Taenia

30 Appendix / Iliopsoas muscle

PLATE XLI · SURGICAL ANATOMY OF LARGE INTESTINE

Several important anatomic facts influence the technic of surgery in the large intestine. As a consequence of its embryologic development, the colon has two main sources of blood supply. The cecum, ascending colon, and proximal portion of the transverse colon are supplied with blood from the superior mesenteric artery, while the distal transverse colon, splenic flexure, descending colon, sigmoid, and upper rectum are supplied by branches of the inferior mesenteric artery (see figure).

Advantage may be taken of the free anastomotic blood supply along the medial border of the bowel by dividing either the inferior mesenteric artery or the middle colic artery and by depending upon the collateral circulation through the marginal artery of Drummond to maintain the viability of a long segment of intestine. The peritoneal reflection on the lateral aspect of the colon is practically bloodless, except at the flexures or in the presence of ulcerative colitis or portal hypertension, and may be completely incised without causing bleeding or jeopardizing the viability of the bowel. When the lateral peritoneum is divided and the greater omentum freed from the transverse colon, extensive mobilization is possible, including derotation of the cecum into the right or left upper quadrant. Care should be taken to avoid undue traction on the splenic flexure lest attachments to the capsule of the spleen be torn and troublesome bleeding occur. In the presence of malignancy of the transverse colon, the omentum is usually resected adjacent to the blood supply of the greater curvature of the stomach.

After the colon has been freed from its attachments to the peritoneum of the abdominal wall, the flexures, and the greater omentum, it can be drawn toward the midline through the surgical incision limited only by the length of its mesentery. This mobility of the colon renders the blood supply more accessible and often permits a procedure to be performed outside the peritoneal cavity. The most mobile part of the large bowel is the sigmoid, because it normally possesses a long mesentery, whereas the descending colon and right half of the colon are fixed to the lateral abdominal wall.

The lymphatic distribution of the large bowel conforms to the vascular supply. A knowledge of this is of great surgical importance, especially in the treatment of malignant neoplasm, because an adequate extirpation of potentially involved lymph nodes requires the sacrifice of a much larger portion of the blood supply than would at first seem essential. The lymphatic spread of carcinoma of the large intestine along the major vascular supply has been responsible for the development of classic resections. Local "sleeve" resection for malignancy may be indicated in the presence of metastasis or because of the patient's poor general condition.

When a curative resection is planned, the tumor and adjacent bowel must be sufficiently mobilized to permit removal of the immediate lymphatic drainage area.

Basically, the resections of the colon should include either the lymphatic drainage area of the superior mesenteric vessels or that of the inferior mesenteric vessels. While this would approach the ideal, experience has shown that approximately four types of resections are commonly performed: right colectomy, left colectomy, anterior resection of the rectosigmoid, and abdominoperineal resection. For years lesions of the cecum, ascending colon, and hepatic flexure have been resected by a right colectomy with ligation of the ileocolic, right colic, and all or part of the middle colic vessels (A). Lesions in the cecal area may be associated with involved lymph glands along the ileocolic vessels. As a result, a segment of the terminal ileum is commonly resected along with the right colon. Lesions in the region of the splenic flexure are in the one area where left colectomy by a sleeve resection may be performed. Extensive resections can be carried out with good assurance of an adequate blood supply, since the marginal vessels are divided nearer their points of origin. In addition to the marginal vessels, the left colic artery near its point of origin and the inferior mesenteric vein are ligated even before manipulation of the tumor is carried out to minimize the venous spread of cancer cells. End-to-end anastomosis without tension can be accomplished by freeing the right colon of its peritoneal attachments and derotating the cecum back to its embryologic position on the left side. The blood supply is sustained through the middle colic vessels and the sigmoidal vessels. While the veins tend to parallel the arteries, this is not the case with the inferior mesenteric vein. This vein courses to the left before it dips beneath the body of the pancreas to join the splenic vein (B).

Lesions of the lower descending colon, sigmoid, and rectosigmoid may be removed by an anterior resection. The inferior mesenteric artery is ligated at its point of origin from the aorta (C) or just distal to the origin of the left colic artery. The upper segment for anastomosis will receive its blood supply through the marginal arteries of Drummond from the middle colic artery. The viability of the rectosigmoid is more uncertain following the ligation of the inferior mesenteric artery. Accordingly, the resection is carried low enough to ensure a good blood supply from the middle and inferior hemorrhoidal vessels. This level is usually so low that the anastomosis must be carried out in the pelvis anterior to the sacrum. Here again the principle of mobilizing the flexures as well as the right colon may be required to ensure an anastomosis without tension.

The most extensive resection involves lesions of the low rectosigmoid, rectum, and anus. High ligation of the inferior mesenteric vessels and ligation of the middle and inferior hemorrhoidal vessels, along with wide excision of the rectum and anus, are required. Since the lymphatic drainage to the anus and lower rectum may drain laterally even to the inguinal region, wide lateral excision of low-lying rectal and anal neoplasms is mandatory.

In order to minimize the possibilities of tumor spread, the lesion should be covered with gauze as early in the procedure as possible. Further isolation should be provided by ligation of the colon above as well as below the tumor with gauze or umbilical tapes. Likewise, early ligation of the vascular supply should be performed before manipulation of the tumor is carried out.

Since bowel anastomosis must be performed in the absence of tension, it is imperative that considerable mobilization of the colon, especially of the splenic flexure, be carried out if continuity is to be restored following extensive resection of the left colon. The presence of pulsating vessels adjacent to the mesenteric margin, which has been cleared preparatory to the anastomosis, should be assured. Injection of 1 per cent procaine into the adjacent mesentery will sometimes enhance arterial pulsation. Occasionally, pulsations are not apparent since the middle colic artery is compressed as a result of the small bowel's being introduced into a plastic bag and displaced to the right and outside of the abdominal wall.

The large intestine bears an important relation to a number of vital structures. Thus, in operations on the right half of the colon, the right ureter and its accompanying vessels are encountered behind the mesocolon. The duodenum lies posterior to the mesentery of the hepatic flexure and is always exposed in mobilizing this portion of the bowel. The spleen is easily injured in mobilizing the splenic flexure. The left ureter and its accompanying spermatic or ovarian vessels are always encountered in operations on the sigmoid and descending colon. In an abdominoperineal resection of the rectum, both ureters are potentially in danger of injury. The surgeon not only must be aware of these structures, but he must positively identify them before dividing the vessels in the mesentery of the colon.

The anatomic arrangement of the colon which permits mobilization of low-lying segments sometimes tempts the surgeon to reconstruct the normal continuity of the fecal current without adequate extirpation of the lymphatic drainage zones. Extensive block excision of the usual lymphatic drainage areas, combined with excision of a liberal segment of normal-appearing bowel on either side of a malignant lesion, is mandatory. Primary anastomosis of the large intestine requires viable intestine, the absence of tension, especially when the bowel becomes distended postoperatively, and a bowel wall of near-normal consistency. Although the danger from sepsis has decreased substantially in recent years, the fact remains that the surgical problems concerned with the large intestine are often complex and require more seasoned judgment and experience than does almost any other field in general surgery.

PLATE XLI   SURGICAL ANATOMY OF LARGE INTESTINE

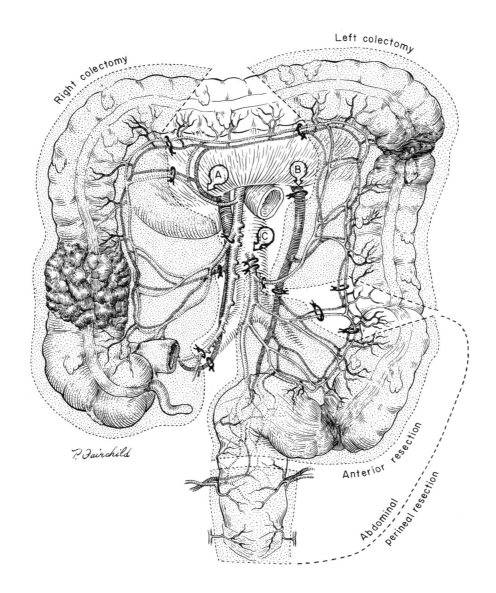

Right colectomy

Left colectomy

A

B

C

P. Fairchild

Anterior resection

Abdominal
perineal resection

PLATE XLII · TUBE CECOSTOMY—COLOSTOMY

A. Tube Cecostomy

INDICATIONS. Cecostomy may be performed as an emergency procedure in the presence of a closed-loop obstruction of the colon caused by a competent ileocecal valve; to provide emergency decompression of the cecum; or as a safety valve following distal anastomosis of the colon. A tube-type cecostomy is usually preferred **(Figure 1, A).** This procedure is not performed as elective preparation for contemplated surgery on the more distal colon, nor is it recommended in poor-risk patients with complete obstruction of the distal colon; under these conditions, a right transverse colostomy **(Figure 1,** B; see Plate XLIII) or a colostomy utilizing the mobile sigmoid **(Figure 1,** C) may be performed.

PREOPERATIVE PREPARATION. In the presence of acute obstruction of the large bowel at an undetermined level, flat and upright roentgenograms of the abdomen are of value. As a further aid a barium enema may be given; but barium should rarely be given by mouth in the presence of suspected intestinal obstruction, because it may produce a complete obstruction. If the obstruction is complete, surgery is carried out as soon as fluid balance is established. If distention is present, constant gastric suction and small-bowel decompression are maintained. Intravenous glucose in saline or lactated Ringer's solution is given to establish the fluid balance. Blood transfusions are usually indicated to correct the anemia and overcome the decreased plasma volume associated with the intestinal obstruction. Surgery is delayed until the pulse rate has been substantially lowered and normal electrolyte levels have been established. Proof of a satisfactory urinary output commonly requires the establishment of constant bladder drainage.

If the obstruction is not complete, the patient is placed on a low-residue diet with a high carbohydrate and high vitamin content for three to five days. The oral administration of chemotherapeutic agents is indicated to soften the bowel contents and lower the bacterial count. Chemotherapy and/or antibiotics administered parenterally may also be given preoperatively. In the absence of complete obstruction mild purgatives and enemas are used to prepare the bowel (see discussion of bowel preparation, Plate XLVII).

ANESTHESIA. General anesthesia is used. If the patient has been vomiting, an endotracheal tube with cuff should be used to prevent aspiration of regurgitated gastrointestinal contents.

POSITION. The patient is placed in a comfortable supine position with the proposed site for the incision presenting.

OPERATIVE PREPARATION. The skin is prepared in the routine manner. The surgeon stands on the patient's right side.

INCISION AND EXPOSURE. The temporary cecostomy shown in **Figures 2** through **5** is ordinarily carried out as part of a distal colon resection which has been performed through a midline or left paramedian incision. Only a small stab wound incision is required in the right lower quadrant, of sufficient size to permit the introduction of a clamp, through which a mushroom catheter (20 F) can subsequently be drawn when the tube has been placed within the right colon.

DETAILS OF PROCEDURE. If the appendix has not been removed, it is removed in a routine fashion **(Figure 2).** With a right-angle clamp on the base of the appendix, the adjacent bowel is encircled with a purse-string suture of 00 silk. If the cecum appears to be distended, it is advisable to place a noncrushing clamp across the tip of the cecum after milking the cecal contents upward into the ascending colon. Following this, a mushroom catheter or Foley-type catheter is introduced into the lumen through the base of the appendix for a distance of approximately 15 cm. The purse-string suture is tied snugly and the bowel inverted about the catheter **(Figure 3).** It is usually technically advantageous to make a short stab wound in the right lower quadrant and to introduce a long hemostat through the abdominal wall before the sutures are placed between the cecum and the parietes, in order to ensure a tight closure lateral to the tube. The right wall of the cecum is attached with interrupted sutures to the peritoneum in the right lower quadrant. The point of fixation should be consistent with the length and mobility of the cecum. The right lumbar gutter should be closed to avoid the possibility of subsequent internal herniation between the cecal wall and the parietes **(Figure 4).** Following tying of these sutures, the end of the catheter is grasped with the hemostat, and it is pulled through to the outside. The proper position of the tube in the ascending colon is ascertained, and the cecum is further attached to the parietes by a series of interrupted 00 silk sutures until the area of the catheter is completely sealed off. Additional sutures may be taken to

make certain that the cecum is attached to the peritoneum over a considerable distance, to avoid any possible subsequent angulation or rotation of the cecal wall **(Figure 5).** The patency of the ileocecal valve should be checked to prevent subsequent obstruction of the terminal ileum.

CLOSURE. After the abdominal wound has been closed, the drainage tube is connected to a bottle, and the tube is irrigated intermittently with normal saline to assure its patency.

POSTOPERATIVE CARE. Postoperative care is determined by the primary operation. When there is no longer any need for decompression, the tube is gently pulled out. Spontaneous closure is anticipated.

B. Colostomy

INDICATIONS. Colostomy is performed as an emergency procedure to relieve acute obstruction of the large intestine or following the repair of a traumatic wound of the colon. It may be carried out as an elective procedure before resection of the colon, or to form a permanent anus, either for inoperable lesions or after resection of the rectum and anus. It is also used infrequently to divert the fecal stream under certain circumstances associated with benign lesions of the colon such as diverticulitis, ulcerative colitis, etc.

The type of colostomy to be used and the selection of the site vary with the patient's condition, the location of the lesion, and the individual surgeon's choice. The common sites for colostomy are shown in **Figure 1,** B and C.

PREOPERATIVE PREPARATION. See Cecostomy.

ANESTHESIA. See Cecostomy.

POSITION. See Cecostomy.

OPERATIVE PREPARATION. The skin is prepared in the usual manner.

INCISION AND EXPOSURE. The incision for colostomy will depend upon the site selected for opening the large intestine. For obstruction well beyond the hepatic flexure, an upper right rectus incision is preferable, although a short transverse incision is preferred by many; for an obstruction in the rectum or anus or for a permanent colostomy, a left paramedian incision is made just below the umbilicus. An acutely distended colon must be handled with great care to avoid perforation, and accordingly, it is often wise to enlarge the incision to permit its presentation. If the bowel is greatly distended, it is essential to deflate it through a trocar or needle, since the collapsed bowel can be handled more safely.

1. LOOP COLOSTOMY

On rare occasions a loop colostomy may be utilized to ensure complete diversion of the fecal stream and to prevent retraction of the colostomy within the abdominal cavity. Failure to mobilize the colon adequately for a safe and efficient colostomy is a very common mistake.

DETAILS OF PROCEDURE. A loop of large intestine is drawn into the wound, and an opening is made in an avascular area of the mesentery. The opening in the mesentery is of sufficient size to permit approximation of the parietes beneath it, yet not large enough to interfere with the blood supply of the adjacent mesentery **(Figure 6).** The skin is closed around and between the two limbs of intestine so that the bowel bridges a portion of the skin **(Figure 7).** The bowel is opened for 2 or 3 cm. along a taenia and the contents of the colon aspirated by suction before the dressing is applied.

2. KNUCKLE COLOSTOMY

DETAILS OF PROCEDURE. A loop of large intestine is pulled into the wound and anchored securely to the peritoneum with interrupted sutures **(Figure 8)** and subsequently to the skin to prevent its recession into the abdominal cavity **(Figure 9).** If the wall of the bowel is extremely thin because of acute distention, the peritoneal sutures are omitted since leakage and peritonitis may result. Whenever possible, the fat tabs should be utilized to anchor the bowel wall to the peritoneum. The bowel is immediately decompressed by a short 3- to 4-cm. incision placed in the midportion of the presenting taenia. Gauze in petrolatum is applied to the intestine followed by a dry sterile dressing.

PLATE XLII   TUBE CECOSTOMY—COLOSTOMY

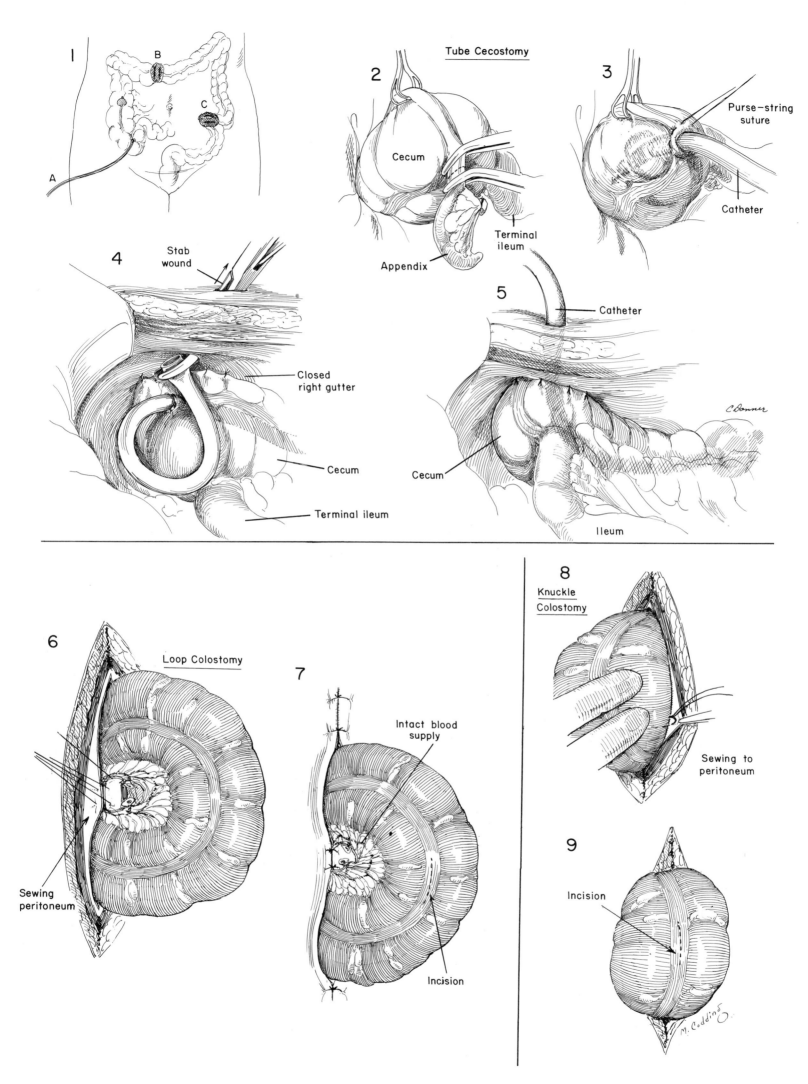

Tube Cecostomy

Cecum
Appendix
Terminal ileum

Purse-string suture
Catheter

Stab wound
Closed right gutter
Cecum
Terminal ileum

Catheter
Cecum
Ileum

Loop Colostomy
Sewing peritoneum

Intact blood supply
Incision

Knuckle Colostomy
Sewing to peritoneum

Incision

PLATE XLIII · TRANSVERSE COLOSTOMY

INDICATIONS. The right transverse colostomy is preferred by many over cecostomy for decompression of the obstructed colon due to a left-side lesion. This procedure completely diverts the fecal stream and permits an efficient cleansing and preparation of the obstructed colon proximal to the lesion.

PREOPERATIVE PREPARATION. Since this procedure is usually performed to relieve acute obstruction of the left colon, the preoperative preparation is limited to the correction of fluid and electrolyte imbalance as well as blood volume deficits. Flat and upright roentgenograms of the abdomen are made with a marker, such as a coin, on the umbilicus. When in doubt, emergency barium enema may be indicated to locate conclusively the left-sided point of obstruction.

ANESTHESIA. Usually, endotracheal anesthesia, which provides a cuff for secure closure of the trachea, is indicated to avoid aspiration of regurgitated gastrointestinal contents.

POSITION. The patient is placed in a comfortable supine position with the proposed site for the incision presenting.

INCISION AND EXPOSURE. The incision is placed in the right upper quadrant. A right rectus or a transverse incision can be made in a location over the distended colon as indicated from a study of the abdominal roentgenograms. When the transverse incision is used, the medial end may include a portion of the right rectus sheath and muscle, but complete division is usually unnecessary. The opening into the abdomen, while limited in length, must be large enough to permit easy identification and mobilization of the tightly distended transverse colon.

DETAILS OF PROCEDURE. A knuckle of transverse colon is delivered into the wound, and the omentum is retracted upward. If the intestine is tremendously distended, a large-bore needle attached to a syringe is inserted obliquely through its wall to allow gas to escape. Decompression through a small trocar attached to a suction apparatus may be indicated before the distended bowel can be safely mobilized. If necessary to avoid contamination, the small opening is closed with a purse-string suture. Under such circumstances the decompression of the bowel permits a safe delivery of a larger segment of the transverse colon through a smaller incision. The greater omentum, which is frequently more vascular than usual under these circumstances, should be dissected free of the colon that is to be used as a colostomy **(Figure 1).** All bleeding points should be ligated before replacing the omentum in the abdomen. The principle utilized is similar to that described in Plate XXIII, **Figures 1** and **2.** Some surgeons prefer to pass a curved clamp through an avascular portion of the omentum and transverse mesocolon beneath the colon, following which a finger is inserted as a guide **(Figure 2).** The omentum is divided over the presenting portion of the transverse colon and reflected to either side **(Figure 3).** It may be necessary to divide several small blood vessels where the omentum is attached to the colon above the anterior taenia. After an adequate through-and-through opening has been made beneath the transverse colon, a sterile solid glass rod is inserted as the finger is removed **(Figure 4).** Both ends of the glass rod are connected with a rubber tube **(Figure 5).** A liberal amount of transverse colon should be exteriorized to ensure a complete diversion of the fecal stream.

The Wangensteen method can be utilized; this consists of inserting a second glass rod through an avascular portion of the mesentery about 3 cm. from the first. By this method a sufficient amount of transverse colon is exteriorized to divert the fecal stream completely.

CLOSURE. The fat tags on the loop of bowel are now anchored to the adjacent peritoneum with fine silk sutures, great care being taken not to penetrate to the lumen of the bowel **(Figure 6).** The use of black silk sutures in anchoring the intestine to the parieties is advantageous, since these will serve as a guide to the individual layers when the colostomy is closed. In the presence of great distention where the intestinal wall is quite thin, it is wiser to depend upon the fixation of the intestine by the glass rod, since perforation of the intestine may take place with resultant leakage and peritonitis if sutures are taken to anchor the bowel to the abdominal wall.

If a very liberal incision was necessary to deliver the dilated intestine, the peritoneal opening may be partially closed by interrupted fine silk sutures **(Figure 7).** The peritoneal closure should not constrict the arms of the knuckle of the intestine but should permit the introduction of the index finger directly into the peritoneal cavity about the intestine. The fascia is approximated with interrupted 00 silk sutures **(Figure 7).** The subcutaneous tissue and skin are closed in a similar manner **(Figures 8** and **9).** Subcuticular interrupted sutures of 0000 silk may be used to provide a firm closure and a wound less likely to be irritated by the subsequent constant fecal soilage. The glass rod (or rods) is elevated from the underlying skin by several layers of dry sterile gauze to ensure that a sufficient amount of colon is exteriorized to divert the fecal stream.

POSTOPERATIVE CARE. It is usually better judgment to open the colostomy before the initial dressings are applied rather than to delay two or three days to avoid possible infection of the wound, since the dangers of unrelieved obstruction are greater than the possible complications of wound infection. A transverse incision in the taenia should not be made, for the bowel may be almost half divided, and subsequent closure of the colostomy thus may be made unnecessarily difficult. Invariably, the opening appears to increase in size after the colon returns to its normal size (see Plate XLIV).

A short incision should be made in the midportion of the presenting taenia **(Figure 8).** All bleeding points are transfixed and tied with fine suture material. When the bleeding is controlled, the surface of the presenting colon about the opening is covered with gauze in petrolatum. Some prefer to relieve the obstruction by inserting an open-end catheter proximally and sealing the opening with a purse-string suture **(Figures 9** and **10).** Frequent dressing changes are indicated for a few days.

In cases of acute obstruction it may be desirable to continue constant gastric suction for several days. Following this, the patient is given fluids the first day, a soft diet for the next few days, progressively increasing to a high-vitamin, high-calorie, high-protein, low-residue diet. Early ambulation is permitted. Irrigations of the proximal colon may be given through the colostomy opening in preparation for secondary surgical procedures or to establish regular emptying of the colostomy if the colostomy is to be permanent. Following diversion of the fecal stream, the reaction about the obstructing tumor tends to subside and the obstruction is relieved. Through-and-through irrigations for cleansing purposes may then be possible. Blood transfusions, high-calorie solutions, and glucose in saline or distilled water are given as required, depending on the degree of the patient's debility.

PLATE XLIII   TRANSVERSE COLOSTOMY

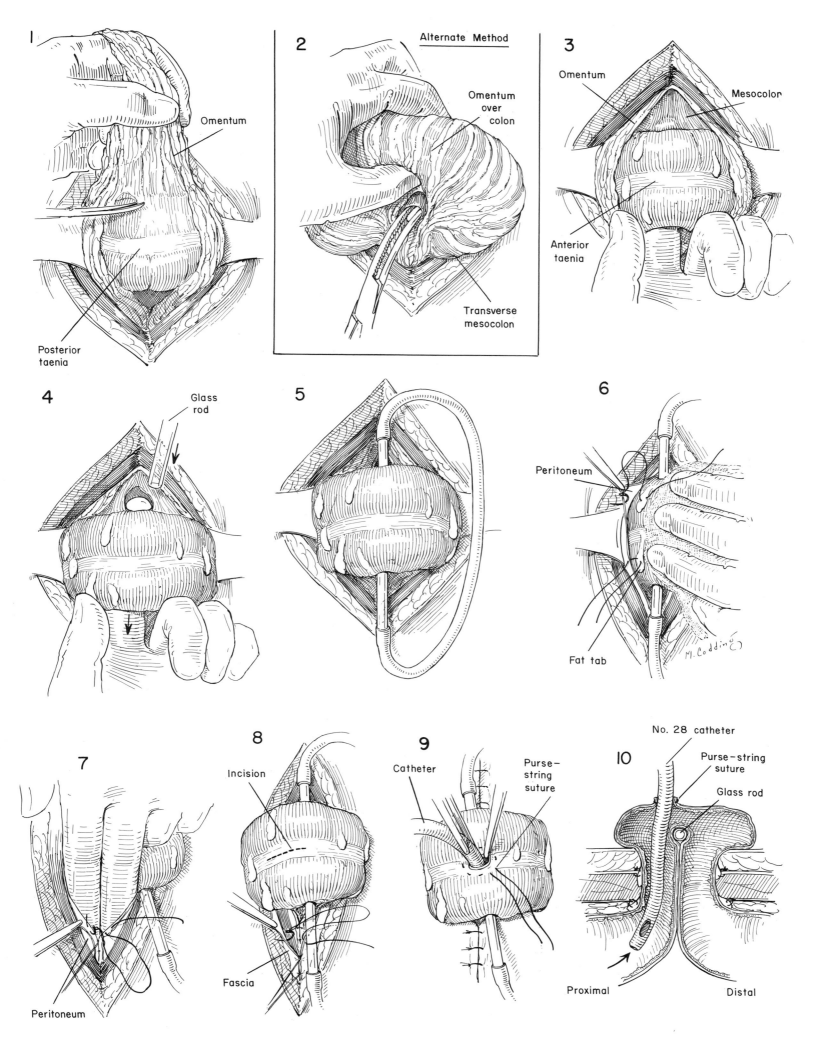

1

Omentum

Posterior taenia

2   Alternate Method

Omentum over colon

Transverse mesocolon

3

Omentum

Mesocolon

Anterior taenia

4   Glass rod

5

6

Peritoneum

Fat tab

M. Codding

7

Peritoneum

8

Incision

Fascia

9

Catheter

Purse-string suture

10

No. 28 catheter

Purse-string suture

Glass rod

Proximal

Distal

PLATE XLIV · CLOSURE OF COLOSTOMY

INDICATIONS. In every instance an interlude which may be as long as six weeks should be allowed between the performance of a colostomy and its closure. This enables the patient's general condition to improve, the site of the colostomy to become walled off, local immunity to the infected contents of the intestine to develop, any infection in the wound to subside, and the wounds from technical procedures carried out on the distal colon to heal. This time may be drastically shortened if the colostomy was performed to decompress or exteriorize a traumatized normal colon. Occasionally, the colostomy partially or completely closes itself after the obstruction has been removed, which permits the fecal current to return to its normal route through the site of the anastomosis. After a Mikulicz procedure the surgeon must make certain that the spur is removed before attempting to close the colostomy. Closure should be delayed until the edema and induration of the bowel about the colostomy opening have subsided and the intestine has resumed a normal appearance. The patency of any anastomosis of the intestine distal to the colostomy should be assured by barium studies.

PREOPERATIVE PREPARATION. The patient is placed on a low-residue diet with oral chemotherapy several days before operation, and the intestines are emptied as completely as possible. During the 24 hours preceding operation, repeated irrigations in both directions through the colostomy opening are done to empty the colon. Other preoperative preparation is in accordance with that given in Plate XLII.

ANESTHESIA. Spinal or general anesthesia may be used. Local anesthesia is contraindicated in the presence of infection about a wound.

POSITION. The patient is placed in a comfortable supine position.

OPERATIVE PREPARATION. Supplementary to the routine skin preparation, the skin about the artificial anus is shaved carefully, and a sterile gauze sponge is inserted into the colostomy opening.

INCISION AND EXPOSURE. Figure 2 shows the anatomy of the colostomy. While a piece of gauze is held in the lumen of the intestine, an oval incision is made through the skin and subcutaneous tissue about the colostomy **(Figure 1).**

DETAILS OF PROCEDURE. The operator's index finger is inserted into the colostomy to act as a guide to prevent incision through the intestinal wall or opening into the peritoneal cavity as the skin and subcutaneous tissue are divided by blunt and sharp dissection **(Figures 3 and 4).**

In the case of a colostomy that has been functioning for some time, the ring of scar tissue at the junction of mucous membrane and skin must be excised before proceeding with the closure **(Figure 5).** With the index finger still in the lumen of the intestine, the operator makes an incision with scissors around the margin of the mucosal reflection **(Figure 6).** This incision is carried through the seromuscular layer down to the submucosa in an effort to develop separate layers for closure **(Figure 6).**

CLOSURE. With its margin held taut with forceps, the mucous membrane is closed transversely to the long axis of the bowel. A continuous suture of fine catgut of the Connell type or interrupted sutures of fine 0000 silk on a French needle are used **(Figure 7).** Following closure of the mucosa, the previously developed seromuscular layer, which has been freed of any fat, is approximated with interrupted Halsted sutures of fine silk **(Figure 8).** The wound is irrigated repeatedly, and clean towels are applied around the wound. All instruments and materials are removed, gloves are changed, and the wound is closed only with clean instruments.

The closed portion of the bowel is held to one side while the adjacent fascia is divided with curved scissors. The detachment of the fascia from the bowel is facilitated by exposure of the silk sutures previously placed for fixation of the bowel at the time of colostomy **(Figure 9).** The peritoneal cavity is not opened in this method of closure.

The patency of the bowel is tested by the surgeon's thumb and index finger. If a small opening has been accidentally made in the peritoneum, it is carefully closed with interrupted sutures of fine silk. The wound is irrigated repeatedly with warm saline. The suture line is depressed with forceps, while the margins of the overlying fascia are approximated with interrupted sutures of 00 silk **(Figure 10).** A rubber tissue drain may be brought out at the lower angle of the wound. The subcutaneous tissue and skin are closed in layers in the routine manner **(Figure 11).**

Alternate Method

INCISION AND EXPOSURE. Instead of attempting to incise the ring of scar tissue at the junction of mucous membrane and the serosa of the bowel, some operators prefer to divide the full thickness of the bowel adjacent to the colostomy opening. After the bowel has been freed from the surrounding tissues, the surgeon's index finger may be inserted into the colostomy to serve as a guide while the bowel is being divided with curved scissors adjacent to the margin of the presenting mucous membrane **(Figure 12).** It may be necessary to free the intestine from the peritoneum and open into the peritoneal cavity in order to mobilize a sufficient amount of the bowel for a satisfactory closure.

DETAILS OF PROCEDURE. The intestinal wall is excised until the scarred edges of bowel around the colostomy opening are completely cut away, leaving normal-appearing intestinal wall to be closed. The bowel is closed transversely to the long axis of the intestine to prevent stenosis. The bowel wall is held taut with either Allis or Babcock forceps above and below the angles of the new opening. The mucous membrane of the intestine is closed on the inner side with a continuous fine catgut suture of the Connell type. Interrupted 0000 silk sutures on a French or straight milliner's needle are preferred by many **(Figure 13).** Interrupted mattress sutures of 00 silk are placed with straight or curved needles to invert the mucosal suture line and to approximate the seromuscular layer over it **(Figure 14).**

CLOSURE. The wound is irrigated with saline. All contaminated instruments, gloves, and towels are discarded, and clean materials are used if it is necessary to open the peritoneal cavity about the margin of the bowel in order to replace the closure within the peritoneal cavity **(Figure 15).** The patency of the lumen of the bowel is assured by palpation between the surgeon's thumb and index finger. If possible, the omentum is tucked over the site of the closure. The peritoneum is closed with interrupted sutures of 00 silk followed by a routine closure of the layers of the abdominal wall **(Figures 16 and 17).** A rubber tissue drain may be brought out of the lower angle of the wound. When gross contamination has occurred, some prefer to partially approximate the subcutaneous tissue and omit skin approximation by sutures. The wound is covered with a sterile dressing.

POSTOPERATIVE CARE. Parenteral fluids and antibiotics are administered for several days. A clear liquid diet is given for several days, followed by a low-residue diet; a regular diet can be resumed after bowel action has started. Hot applications to the wound may be beneficial if induration develops. Occasionally, a leak may occur at the closure site, but no immediate effort is made to repair the fistula because frequently closure is spontaneous. Early ambulation is permitted.

PLATE XLIV   CLOSURE OF COLOSTOMY

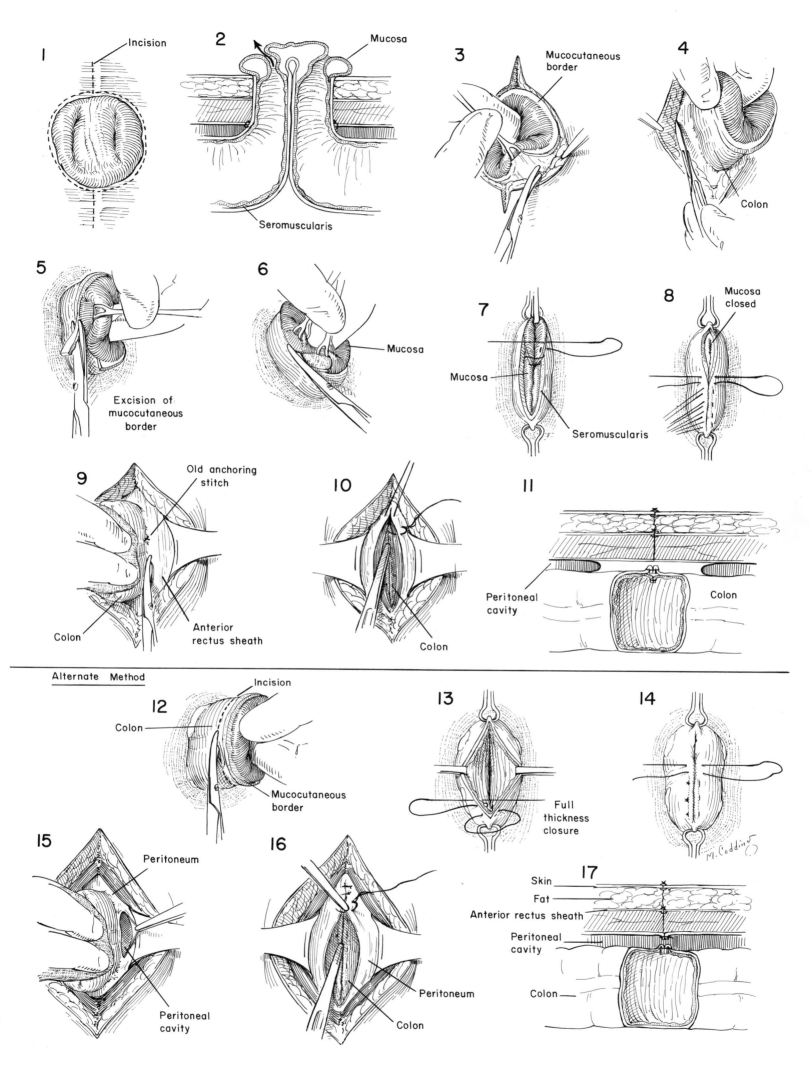

1 Incision

2 Mucosa
Seromuscularis

3 Mucocutaneous border

4 Colon

5 Excision of mucocutaneous border

6 Mucosa

7 Mucosa
Seromuscularis

8 Mucosa closed

9 Old anchoring stitch
Colon
Anterior rectus sheath

10 Colon

11 Peritoneal cavity
Colon

Alternate Method

12 Incision
Colon
Mucocutaneous border

13 Full thickness closure

14

15 Peritoneum
Peritoneal cavity

16 Peritoneum
Colon

17 Skin
Fat
Anterior rectus sheath
Peritoneal cavity
Colon

M. Codding

PLATE XLV · COLECTOMY, RIGHT

INDICATIONS. Resection of the right colon is commonly indicated for carcinoma, cicatrizing enteritis, and more rarely for tuberculosis, etc., of the cecum, ascending colon, or hepatic flexure.

PREOPERATIVE PREPARATION. Since tumors of the right colon rarely cause obstruction, the preparation for surgery need not be prolonged beyond five to seven days. Oral chemotherapy, saline purgatives, and daily enemas are used during the preoperative period. The patient is placed on a high-calorie, high-vitamin, low-residue diet. Since secondary anemia is commonly associated with neoplasms of the right colon, blood transfusions are advisable before operation. Normal blood volume and total protein levels should be established. Whole blood must be available during the operation. Steroid therapy should be continued when it has been used in the treatment of the disease requiring resection.

ANESTHESIA. Either general inhalation or spinal anesthesia is satisfactory.

POSITION. The patient is placed in a comfortable supine position. The surgeon stands on the patient's right side.

OPERATIVE PREPARATION. The skin is prepared in the routine manner and a sterile plastic drape applied.

INCISION AND EXPOSURE. A liberal right paramedian incision centered opposite the umbilicus is made about 2 or 3 cm. to the right of the midline. A transverse incision just above the level of the umbilicus also provides an excellent exposure. The lesion of the right colon is inspected and palpated to determine whether removal is possible. In the presence of malignancy the liver also is palpated for evidence of metastasis. If the lesion is inoperable or questionably so, a lateral anastomosis may be performed between the terminal ileum and the transverse colon. After the fecal current is short-circuited, the inflammation about the tumor often decreases; this permits a lesion that appears to be inoperable to be removed within several weeks at a second operation. In a poor-risk or completely obstructed patient, the two-stage procedure should be used. After resection has been decided upon, the small intestines are walled off with gauze, or replaced partially in a plastic bag, and the cecum is exposed. When possible, the lesion should be covered with gauze tied in place and the venous drainage ligated early to minimize the spread of malignant cells.

A right colectomy is also commonly indicated when the terminal ileum is involved with regional ileitis. When this lesion is found, the entire small intestine should be examined for "skip" areas. Several segments of small intestine may require resection in addition to the right colectomy. In poor-risk patients with extensive involvement, it may be advisable to perform a bypass around the terminal ileum by performing an entero-transverse colostomy. Cultures are taken if pus is encountered.

DETAILS OF PROCEDURE. An incision is made in the peritoneal reflection close to the lateral wall of the bowel from the tip of the cecum upward to the region of the hepatic flexure **(Figure 1)**. A liberal margin should be assured in the region of the tumor. Occasionally, the full thickness of the adjacent abdominal wall may require excision to include the local spread of tumor. Since the entire hepatic flexure is usually removed as part of a right colectomy, the hepatocolic ligament, which contains some small blood vessels, must be divided and ligated, but there will be no blood vessels of importance in the peritoneal attachments along the right gutter. With the lateral peritoneal attachment divided, the large bowel may be lifted mesially with the left hand, while the loose areolar tissue lying under it is dissected off with a moist gauze sponge over the right index finger **(Figure 2)**. In elevating the right colon toward the midline, the surgeon must positively identify the right ureter and be certain that it is not injured. Care is taken also toward the top of the ascending colon and near the hepatic flexure to avoid injury to the third portion of the duodenum which underlies the large bowel **(Figure 3)**. The raw surface remaining after the intestine has been freed and brought outside the peritoneal cavity is covered with warm, moist gauze pads. The mesentery of the large bowel is clamped and divided just distal to the hepatic flexure, or wherever the bowel is to be resected. Either the right branches or all of the middle colic vessels are divided and doubly ligated. This vessel is invariably included if the lesion is in the ascending colon or in the hepatic flexure. The bowel at the selected level for division is freed of all mesentery, omentum, and fat on both sides. All vessels must be carefully ligated. The right half of the greater omentum is divided near the greater curvature of the stomach and excised along with the right colon.

The terminal ileum is prepared for resection some distance away from the ileocecal valve, depending upon the amount of blood supply that must be sacrificed to ensure excision of the lymph node drainage area of the right colon. In the presence of regional ileitis the resection of the small intestine should extend 7 to 10 cm. or more proximal to the line of demarcation of involvement. After the small intestine has been prepared at its mesenteric border, a fan-shaped excision of the mesentery to the right colon is carried out. This usually includes all or part of the middle colic vessels and invariably the right colic and ileocolic vessels **(Figure 4)**. The blood vessels of the mesentery are doubly tied (see Plate XLI).

A straight vascular clamp, or some other type of straight clamp, is applied obliquely to the small intestine about 1 cm. from the mesenteric border to ensure a serosal surface for the placement of sutures for the subsequent anastomosis. Stone, Kocher, or Pace-Potts clamps are next applied across the large intestine, which is then divided between the clamps. The intervening section of bowel with its fan-shaped section of mesentery and nodes is excised. The divided proximal end of the small intestine is covered with gauze moistened with saline, and closure of the stump of the large bowel is started, unless an end-to-end or end-to-side anastomosis is planned.

PLATE XLV   COLECTOMY, RIGHT

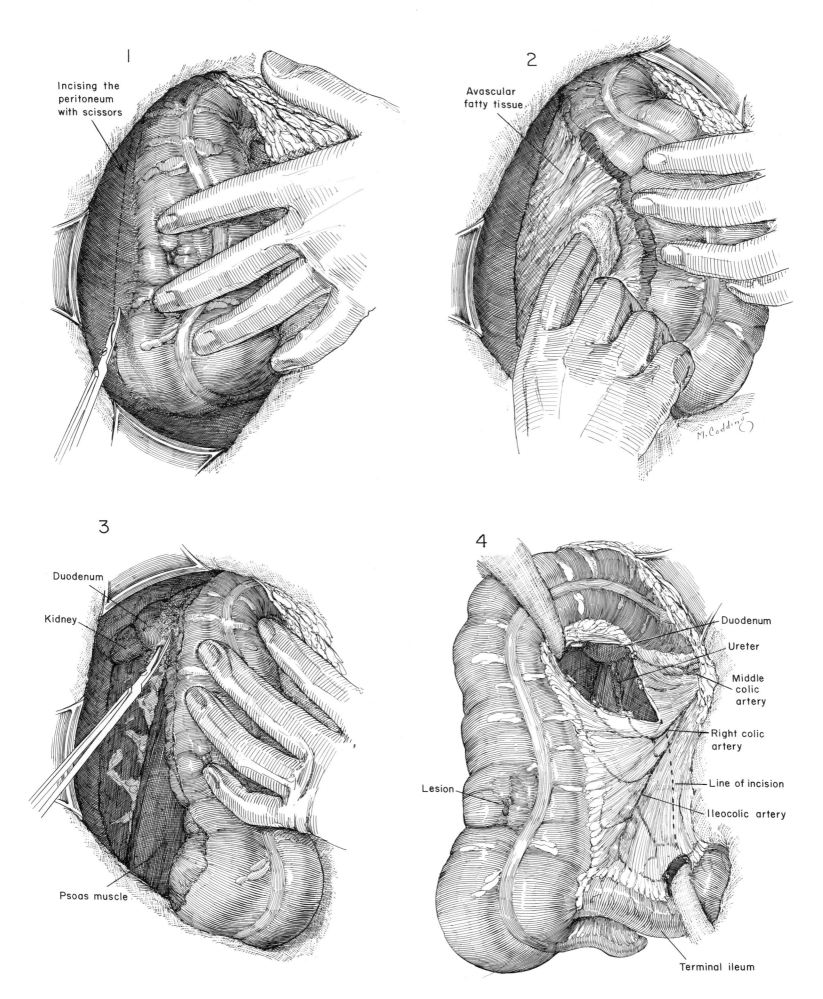

1

Incising the peritoneum with scissors

2

Avascular fatty tissue

M. Codding

3

Duodenum

Kidney

Psoas muscle

4

Duodenum

Ureter

Middle colic artery

Right colic artery

Line of incision

Ileocolic artery

Lesion

Terminal ileum

PLATE XLVI · COLECTOMY, RIGHT

DETAILS OF PROCEDURE (*Continued*). The end of the colon is closed by a continuous catgut suture on a small, straight, atraumatic needle and whipped loosely over a Pace-Potts or similar noncrushing clamp. Interrupted 0000 silk sutures placed beneath the clamp may be used **(Figure 5)**. The clamp is then opened and removed. If a continuous suture is used, it is pulled up snugly and tied. A single layer of 00 silk Halsted mattress sutures on straight or French needles is placed about 3 or 4 cm. from the original suture line, care being taken that no fat is included. As these sutures are tied, the original suture line is invaginated so that serosa meets serosa **(Figure 6)**. The surgeon must determine before closing the ends of the colon whether an end-to-end, end-to-side, or lateral anastomosis is to be carried out **(Figures 14, 16, 17, and 18)**.

The end-to-side approximation is physiologic, simple, and safe to perform, although most prefer the direct end-to-end anastomosis **(Figures 15 and 16)**. If an end-to-side repair is used, the small intestine, still held in its clamp, is brought up adjacent to the anterior taenia of the colon **(Figure 7)**. The small intestine should retain a good color and give evidence of adequate blood supply before the anastomosis is attempted. If its color indicates an inadequate blood supply, the surgeon should not hesitate to resect a sufficient length until its viability is unquestionable. Next, the omentum, if not previously excised, is retracted upward, and the anterior taenia of the transverse colon is grasped with Babcock forceps at the site chosen for anastomosis **(Figure 7)**. Following this, the edge of the mesentery of the small intestine should be approximated to the edge of that of the large intestine, so that herniation of the small intestine cannot occur beneath the anastomosis into the right gutter **(Figure 14)**. This opening is closed before the anastomosis is started, since on rare occasions the blood supply may be injured by the procedure and the viability of the anastomosis jeopardized. A small, straight crushing clamp is applied to the anterior taenia, including a small bite of the bowel wall **(Figure 8)**. Following this, the clamps on the terminal ileum, as well as on the anterior taenia of the transverse colon, are so arranged that a serosal layer of interrupted 00 silk mattress sutures can be placed, anchoring the terminal ileum to the transverse colon **(Figure 9)**. The two angle sutures are not cut and serve as traction sutures **(Figure 9)**. An opening is made into the large intestine by excising the protruding contents of the crushing clamp that has been applied to the anterior taenia **(Figure 10)**. An enterostomy clamp is then applied behind each of the crushing clamps. The crushing clamps are removed, and the terminal ileum is opened; likewise, the crushed contents of the transverse colon are separated. Sometimes it is necessary to enlarge the opening in the mucosa of the colon, since the previous excision of the contents of the crushing clamp did not provide a sufficiently large stoma for satisfactory anastomosis. The mucosa is then approximated with a continuous locked fine catgut suture on atraumatic needles, which is started in the midline, posteriorly. The sutures, A and B, are continued as a Connell inverting suture around the angles and anteriorly to ensure inversion of the mucosa **(Figures 11 and 12)**. Interrupted fine 0000 silk sutures on French needles are preferred by some for closing the mucosal layer. An anterior row of mattress sutures completes the anastomosis. Several additional mattress sutures may be placed to reinforce the angles **(Figure 13)**. The patency of the stoma is tested. It should permit introduction of the index finger. If the tension is not too great, the raw surface over the iliopsoas muscle may be covered by approximating the peritoneum of the lateral abdominal wall to the mesentery.

The second method, consisting of a direct end-to-end anastomosis, is commonly selected **(Figures 15 and 16)**. The discrepancy in the size of the terminal ileum and the transverse colon can be safely overcome by attention to certain technical details. Added luminal circumference can be provided by exaggerating the oblique division of the terminal ileum. During the anastomosis slightly larger bites are taken in the colonic side to compensate for the discrepancy between the two sides of the anastomosis. Following completion of the anastomosis, any remaining rent in the mesentery is approximated. The patency of the lumen is determined by palpation and the suture line marked by two or more Cushing silver clips. These serve as markers for subsequent identification of the suture line when barium follow-up studies are made.

If a side-to-end anastomosis is preferred by the surgeon, the stump of the small intestine is closed as previously described for the large intestine. The small intestine is then brought up to the open end of the large intestine **(Figure 17)**; the posterior row of serosal sutures is placed; the small intestine is opened; the continuous mucosal suture or the inverting sutures are placed and, finally, the anterior serosal sutures of interrupted 00 silk. Whenever this type of procedure is carried out, care should be taken that only a very small portion of small intestine protrudes beyond the suture line, since blind ends of bowel that are in the peristaltic line form a stagnant pouch against which peristalsis tends to work, increasing the chance of eventual breakdown.

By a fourth method the ends of the large and small intestines are closed, and a lateral anastomosis is carried out. This type of anastomosis is usually the end result of a two-stage resection, the lateral anastomosis between the ileum and transverse colon having been performed as the first stage in poor-risk patients or in the case of a tumor that appears inoperable. Only a small portion of small intestine should protrude beyond the suture line. The small intestine should be anchored to the colon with interrupted sutures of silk, including both angles of the stoma as well as the closed end of small bowel **(Figure 18)**.

CLOSURE. Drains are undesirable unless gross infection has been encountered. The advisability of performing a temporary gastrostomy should be considered, since gastrointestinal decompression for several days will be required. The site of anastomosis is covered with omentum. The abdominal wall is closed in routine fashion, and a sterile dressing is applied.

POSTOPERATIVE CARE. The patient should be in a comfortable position. Blood volume is returned to normal by whole blood transfusion. The stomach and small intestine should be decompressed by intubation for three to five days or by a temporary gastrostomy. Billiant blue dye introduced into the stomach will provide clear proof of patency of the anastomosis by passage of the dye marker eventually in the stool. The tube should not be removed until there is evidence that the fecal stream is passing the suture line, as demonstrated by the absence of abdominal distention after the tube has been clamped off for at least 12 hours. Diet is restricted to liquids for five to seven days, after which soft solids may be added. Diarrhea or frequent bowel movements may be satisfactorily controlled by medication and diet. The parenteral administration of chemotherapy and antibiotics should be continued until the danger of sepsis is past. The need for continued steroid therapy, particularly in patients with regional ileitis, should not be overlooked in the immediate postoperative period. When extensive resection of the small intestine has been required, it is essential to evaluate the patient's electrolyte and nutritional status at frequent intervals for a prolonged period of time.

PLATE XLVI   COLECTOMY, RIGHT

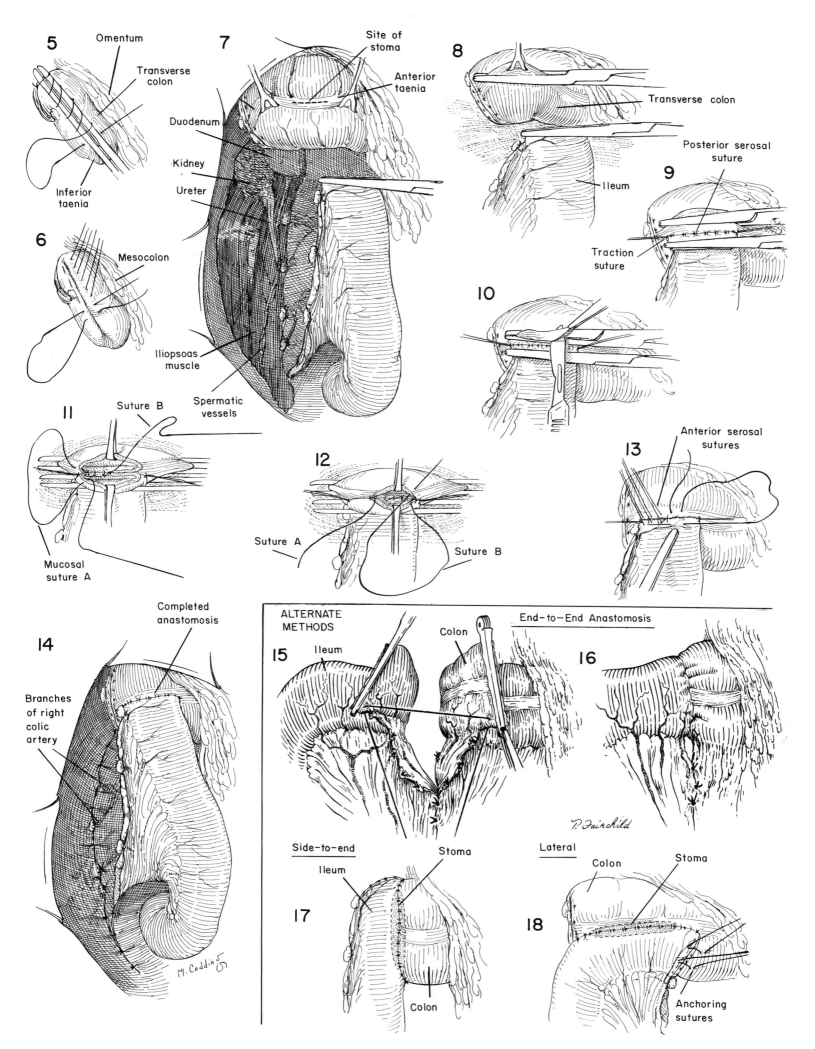

PLATE XLVII · COLECTOMY, LEFT, END-TO-END ANASTOMOSIS

INDICATIONS. The operation is performed chiefly for tumor of the left colon or a complication of diverticulitis.

PREOPERATIVE PREPARATION. Tumors of the left colon are frequently of the stenosing type. Patients with this condition often come to the surgeon with obvious signs of intestinal obstruction, and a preliminary colostomy or cecostomy may be necessary as a lifesaving procedure. This is best performed in the right side of the transverse colon, for cecostomy often leaves masses of impacted feces near the lesion and is an ordeal to the patient because of the liquid fecal stream from the ileum.

When obstruction is not complete, the bowel can best be prepared over a period of five to seven days by oral administration of the appropriate sulfonamides, an occasional saline purge, and a clear liquid diet for the last 48 to 72 hours. The frequency with which cathartics and cleansing agents are administered will vary depending upon the amount of obstruction and the type of oral chemotherapy. Blood volume and total protein values should be returned to normal by blood and plasma transfusions. Vitamins should be administered. A rectal tube and a nasogastric tube are inserted before surgery.

ANESTHESIA. Either general or spinal anesthesia is satisfactory.

POSITION. The patient is placed in a comfortable supine position and rotated slightly toward the operator. A slight Trendelenburg position may be used.

OPERATIVE PREPARATION. The skin is prepared in the routine manner.

INCISION AND EXPOSURE. The operator stands on the patient's left side. A liberal paramedian incision is made 2 to 3 cm. to the left of the midline opposite the umbilicus. Some surgeons prefer a transverse incision just below or above the level of the umbilicus, depending upon the location of the lesion. The liver, as well as other possible sites for metastasis, is explored. The small intestines are then packed away medially with warm, moist gauze sponges or placed in a plastic bag outside the abdomen on the right side. A gauze pack is placed toward the pelvis and another along the lateral wall up to the spleen. A plastic wound protector may be inserted.

DETAILS OF PROCEDURE. Precautions against possible spread of the tumor should include limited manipulation of the growth and application of a tightly tied tape or a clamp, such as a Kocher, above as well as below the tumor to avoid further seeding of the mucosal surfaces. As soon as possible the tumor should be covered with gauze and its major venous supply clamped.

With the bowel at the point of the lesion held in the left hand, the lateral peritoneal reflection of the mesocolon is incised close to the bowel, except in the region of the tumor, over as wide an area as seems essential for its free mobilization **(Figure 1).** Following this, the bowel is retracted toward the midline, and the mesentery is freed from the posterior abdominal wall by blunt gauze dissection. Troublesome bleeding may occur if the left spermatic or ovarian vein is torn and not ligated. Next to identify is the left ureter, which must not be drawn up with the mesentery of the intestine and accidentally divided. A fan-shaped incision of sufficient size is made so that the nodes in the mesentery along the left colic artery and vein are extirpated with the specimen **(Figure 2).** At least 15 to 20 cm. of margin from the gross border on either side of the lesion should be allowed. The contents of the clamps applied to the mesentery are tied. The mesenteric border of the bowel at the proposed site of resection is cleared of mesenteric fat in preparation for the anastomosis **(Figure 3).**

Paired crushing clamps of the Stone or similar type are placed obliquely across the bowel above the lesion within 1 cm. of the limits of the prepared mesentery **(Figure 4).** The field is walled off with gauze, and the bowel is divided. A pair of noncrushing clamps is then applied to the prepared area below the lesion, and the bowel is divided in a similar fashion. The ends of the large intestine are brought end to end to determine if the anastomosis can be carried out without tension; otherwise, one or both segments of the large bowel should be freed further. This can be accomplished by freeing up the splenic flexure, as well as freeing the transverse colon from the greater omentum. Indeed, the cecum can be mobilized into the left upper quadrant as it was before embryonic rotation occurred. When this has been accomplished, the clamps are approximated and so manipulated that the posterior serosal surface of the intestine is presented, to facilitate placement of a layer of interrupted mattress silk sutures **(Figure 5).** The mesenteric border should be free of fat to achieve accurate approximation of the serosa. The sutures at the angles are not cut and are utilized for traction **(Figure 6).**

Enterostomy clamps are placed several centimeters from the crushing clamps, and the crushing clamps are removed **(Figure 6).** The portions of excessive bowel that were beyond the clamps may be excised. The field is completely walled off with moist, sterile gauze packs, and a direct open anastomosis is carried out. Some operators prefer an aseptic type of anastomosis, which can be carried out at this point if desired. The mucosa is approximated with a continuous lock suture on an atraumatic needle starting in the middle of the posterior layer **(Figure 7).** At the angle the lock suture is changed to one of the Connell type to ensure inversion of the angle and the anterior mucosa **(Figures 8 and 9).** A second continuous suture is started adjacent to the first one and is carried out in a similar fashion **(Figure 10).** The mucosa may be approximated with interrupted 0000 silk sutures on French needles. After the mucosa has been accurately approximated, the two continuous sutures, A and B, are tied with the knot on the inside **(Figure 11).** A layer of interrupted 00 silk sutures is utilized to approximate the anterior serosal layer. Particular attention is given to either angle to ensure accurate and secure approximation.

PLATE XLVII   COLECTOMY, LEFT, END-TO-END ANASTOMOSIS

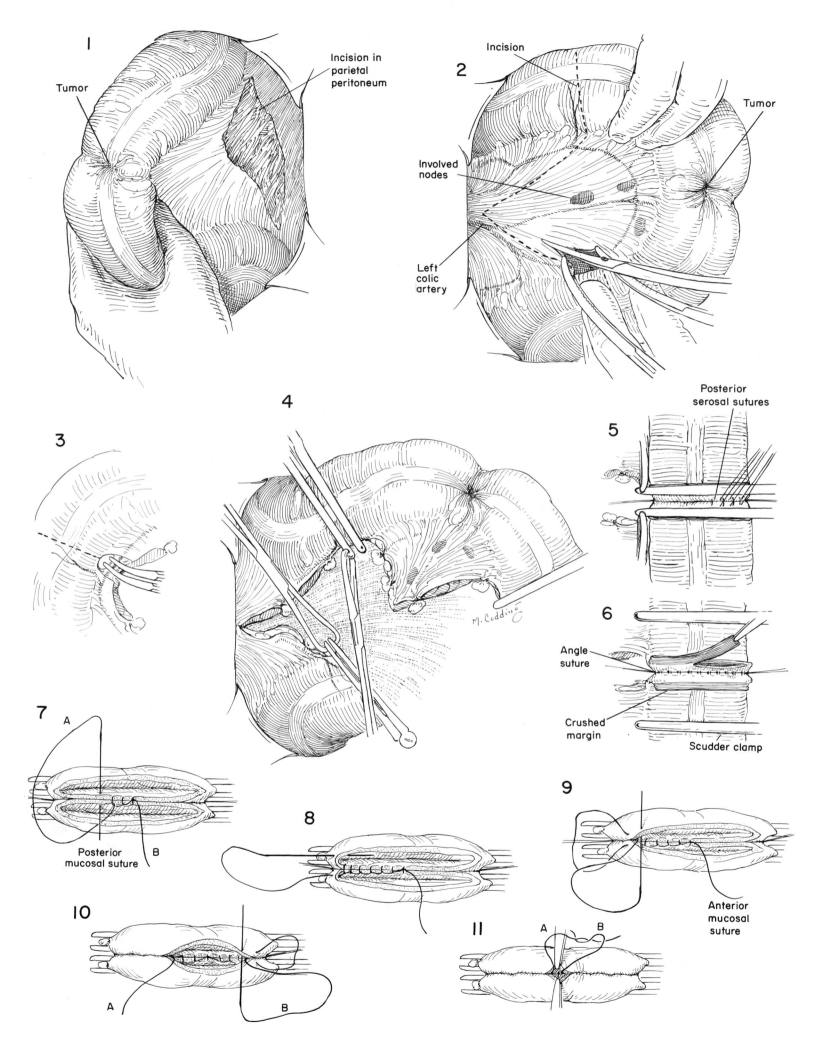

PLATE XLVIII · COLECTOMY, LEFT, END-TO-END ANASTOMOSIS

DETAILS OF PROCEDURE (*Continued*). Following the approximation of the mucosal layer, all contaminated instruments are discarded. The field is covered with fresh, moist, gauze sponges and towels. It is desirable for the members of the surgical team to change gloves. The anastomosis is further reinforced by an anterior serosal layer of interrupted 00 silk sutures **(Figure 12).** It is sometimes advisable to reinforce the mesenteric angle with one or two additional mattress sutures. To assist in localizing the site of the anastomosis by follow-up roentgenograms, several silver clips are placed about the suture line. Any remaining opening of the mesentery is then closed with interrupted sutures of fine silk. If there is a great deal of fat in the mesentery, which tends to hide the location of blood vessels, it is unwise to pass a needle blindly through it, lest a hematoma form between the leaves of the mesentery. It is safer to grasp the peritoneal margins of the mesentery with small, pointed clamps and effect a closure by simple ligation of their contents. Finally, adequacy of the blood supply to the site of the anastomosis should be inspected. Active, pulsating vessels should be present adjacent to the anastomosis on both sides **(Figure 13).** If the blood supply appears to be interfered with and the color of the bowel is altered, it is better to resect the anastomosis rather than to risk leakage and subsequent fatal peritonitis. The injection of several milliliters of procaine solution into the mesentery provides a temporary sympathectomy with an increase in arterial pulsations. The patency of the stoma is carefully tested by compression between the thumb and index finger **(Figure 14).** It is usually possible to obtain a two-finger stoma.

To assure easy approximation of the open ends of the large bowel, especially if the lesion is located near the splenic flexure, it is necessary to free the intestine from adjacent structures. The abdominal incision may have to be extended up to the costal margin, since exposure of the uppermost portion of the splenic flexure may be difficult. After the relatively avascular peritoneal attachments to the descending colon have been divided, it is necessary to free the splenic flexure from the diaphragm, spleen, and stomach. The splenocolic ligament is divided between curved clamps, and the contents are ligated to avoid possible injury to the spleen with troublesome hemorrhage **(Figure 15).** Following this, a pair of curved clamps is applied to the gastrocolic ligament for the necessary distance required to mobilize the bowel or remove sufficient intestine beyond the growth. Sometimes, in the presence of growths in this area, it is necessary to carry the division adjacent to the greater curvature of the stomach. The surgeon should not hesitate to remove a portion of the left gastroepiploic artery, if indicated, since the stomach has such a good collateral blood supply. In some instances a true phrenocolic ligament can be developed, which must be divided to free the splenic flexure **(Figure 16).**

If it is necessary to free a portion of the transverse colon, the omentum may be freed from the bowel by incising its avascular attachments adjacent to the colon **(Figure 17;** see Plate XXIII). In some instances omentum may be involved with the growth, and it may be desirable to remove all or part of the omentum. The splenic flexure is reflected medially following the division of its attachments, and care is taken to avoid the kidney and the underlying ureter. It is usually necessary to divide a portion of the transverse mesocolon **(Figure 18).** This should be done carefully, taking into consideration possible injury to the underlying jejunum in the region of the ligament of Treitz. The large inferior mesenteric vein will also require division and double ligation as it dips down under the inferior margin of the body of the pancreas to join the splenic vein. The bowel is freed of all fatty attachments at the site selected for anastomosis. Non-crushing clamps are applied, and the bowel is divided **(Figure 19).** The anastomosis is carried out as previously described. If it becomes necessary to ligate the middle colic artery, the entire transverse colon, including the hepatic and splenic flexures, may need to be resected to ensure an adequate blood supply at the site of anastomosis. In this situation the viability of the colon depends upon the right colic artery on one side and the left colic artery on the other. A temporary gastrostomy should be considered.

CLOSURE. The closure is made in the usual manner.

POSTOPERATIVE CARE. The patient should be kept in a comfortable position. The blood volume should be returned to normal by whole blood transfusion. The gastrostomy tube provides comfortable decompression until there is evidence that the fecal stream is passing the suture line. Fluid and electrolyte balance is maintained by intravenous administration for the first few days. The patient is then maintained on a restricted low-residue diet. A mild laxative may be given about the fourth day. The parenteral administration of chemotherapy and antibiotics should be considered if gross contamination has occurred. Elderly patients may be given fluid and nutritional supplements later through the gastrostomy tube. The tube is usually withdrawn by the tenth postoperative day.

PLATE XLVIII   COLECTOMY, LEFT, END-TO-END ANASTOMOSIS

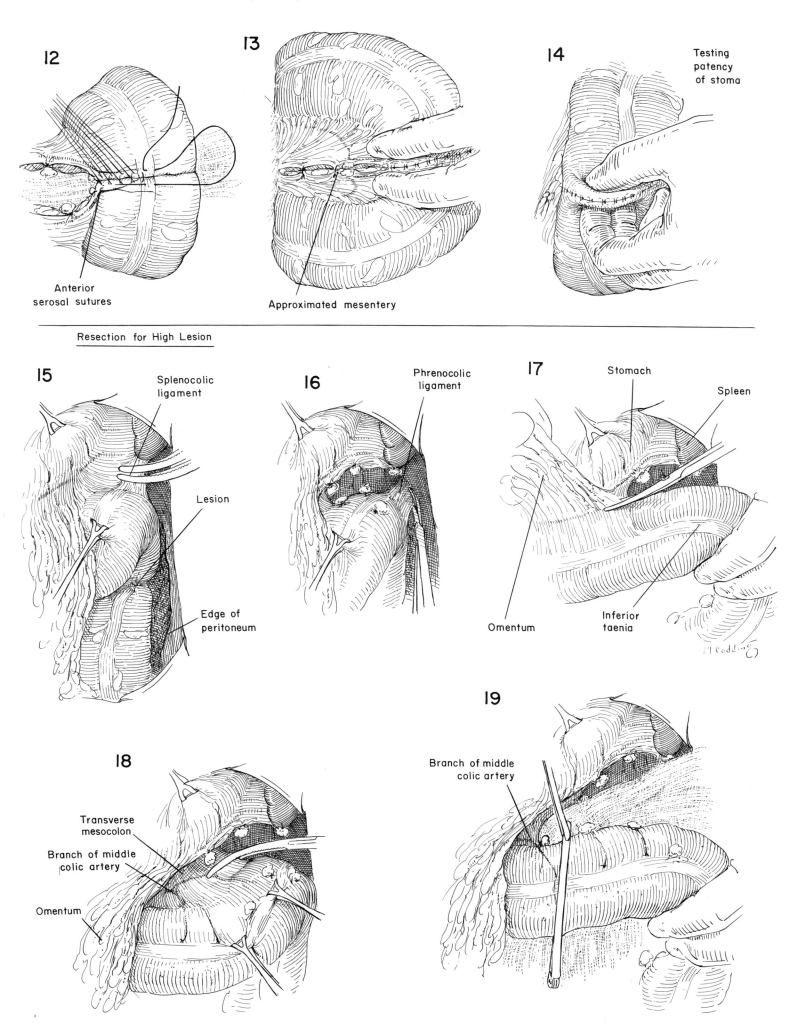

12

Anterior
serosal sutures

13

Approximated mesentery

14

Testing
patency
of stoma

Resection for High Lesion

15

Splenocolic
ligament

Lesion

Edge of
peritoneum

16

Phrenocolic
ligament

17

Stomach

Spleen

Omentum

Inferior
taenia

18

Transverse
mesocolon

Branch of middle
colic artery

Omentum

19

Branch of middle
colic artery

PLATE XLIX · COLECTOMY, LEFT, MIKULICZ PROCEDURE

INDICATIONS. Carcinoma is the most common indication for resection of the sigmoid. Occasionally, resection may be indicated in diverticulitis with stenosis, in benign tumors, and less commonly in the treatment of volvulus. The Mikulicz procedure is not ideal for treatment of cancer and the lymph-node-bearing area. But in the presence of long-standing and marked obstruction, the discrepancy in size between the proximal and distal loops and the urgency of relieving the obstruction make this procedure advisable if excision of the involved area is desirable at the time. In the hands of operators with limited experience in large-bowel surgery, it is much the safer procedure; however, improvement in preoperative and postoperative care makes primary resection with end-to-end anastomosis the procedure of choice in most cases. It is uncommon for this type of resection to be a planned procedure.

PREOPERATIVE PREPARATION. Unless the patient is obstructed, he is placed on a high-calorie, high-vitamin, low-residue diet and is given saline purgatives and enemas to prepare the intestinal tract. Oral chemotherapy is also given (see Plate XLVII).

ANESTHESIA. Spinal anesthesia is satisfactory, although general endotracheal anesthesia is preferred.

POSITION. The patient is placed in a moderate Trendelenburg position near the left side of the table.

INCISION AND EXPOSURE. The surgeon stands to the left of the patient. The incision may be midline or left paramedian. The abdomen, especially the liver and the pelvis, is carefully explored for evidence of metastases. Before the procedure continues, the small intestines are packed away with warm, moist gauze or placed in a plastic bag to which some warm saline is added.

DETAILS OF PROCEDURE. The loop of sigmoid with the lesion at its apex is drawn out of the wound, and a wedge of mesentery is divided between curved clamps along the dotted line shown in **Figure 1** to ensure removal of the lymph nodes most likely involved. The contents of the clamps are ligated with transfixing sutures of 00 silk on French needles. The tumor is covered with gauze which is secured by several 00 silk ties to avoid seeding of the tumor. Usually, to permit sufficient mobilization of the sigmoid, the peritoneum on the lateral wall must be divided for a considerable distance **(Figure 2)**. In some instances it may be necessary to free the splenic flexure to ensure adequate mobilization of the proximal segment of bowel (see Plate XLVIII). With traction on the sigmoid maintained by an encircling loop of gauze held by an assistant, a row of interrupted 00 silk sutures is placed some distance from the lesion between the proximal and distal arms, so that at least 8 to 10 cm. of the intestine are joined **(Figure 2, S1)**. It is most important that the intestinal loops be approximated in a parallel fashion without tension for a sufficient distance, so that the subsequent application of the crushing clamp will not cause a free perforation at the juncture of the loops **(Figure 2, X)**. The approximated area should not include the mesenteric border containing the blood vessels, since these might be injured by the crushing clamp applied 10 to 14 days later. When the row of interrupted sutures is completed, another row **(Figure 3, S2)** is similarly placed about 2 cm. lateral to the first row in order to have a broad, sealed surface for the eventual application of the crushing clamp **(Figure 3)**. This seals off the enclosed area between the two suture lines without interference with the blood supply of the intestine **(Figure 6)**.

CLOSURE. The loop of sigmoid containing the tumor and some of the attached mesentery are pulled out from the abdominal wall. With the loop of intestine drawn out on the skin, the operator should then close off the left lumbar gutter by a few sutures that approximate the proximal limb to the lateral wall **(Figure 5)**, in order to prevent the small intestine from being caught in this area. It is wise to anchor several fat tabs on each limb to the peritoneum after closure of the lumbar gutter **(Figure 4)**. It is important that these sutures do not enter the lumen of the intestine, because leakage and peritonitis may result. The wound is then closed loosely about the bowel, leaving sufficient space for the little finger to be inserted about each limb to avoid constriction of the blood supply. Crushing clamps are applied to each limb of the exteriorized bowel, and the portion of the intestine containing the tumor is removed. The retained viable intestine should extend at least 5 to 6 cm. beyond the skin level. A large rubber catheter can be inserted into the proximal lumen and anchored in place by an encircling suture of 00 silk. A clamp such as the Stone type may be left in place across the distal limb of bowel; within a few days the tube and clamp are removed. Some prefer to open the intestine immediately and anchor the mucosa to the adjacent skin. The mucosal margins of the two limbs of colon are sewed together and the margins anchored to the skin with interrupted catgut sutures **(Figure 6)**.

POSTOPERATIVE CARE. When the wound is well healed, usually after 10 to 14 days, a special clamp is passed into the colostomy, one blade in the distal end of the bowel and one in the proximal end, and gradually tightened **(Figures 7 and 8)**. A pair of heavy, straight clamps may be used for this purpose; but special clamps, arranged so that the blades always approach each other in a parallel manner, are far superior. The clamp is not fully tightened for the first 12 hours because of the discomfort produced and because a rapid slough may occur, resulting in a free perforation; after 12 hours the clamp may be tightened as much as possible, destroying the septum in another 48 to 72 hours. After sloughing has occurred, the fecal stream will not be deflected to the abdominal wall but will proceed through the area where the clamp has cut down the partition and pass along the distal bowel. After the crushing clamp has been removed, a digital examination determines whether the partition has been cut down sufficiently. If the partition is only partially divided and a spur exists, the crushing clamp is carefully reapplied to incorporate the desired amount of intestinal wall **(Figure 8)**. If the colostomy opening does not close spontaneously after several weeks, a routine colostomy closure is performed (Plate XLIV). Many times it is necessary to reapply the crushing clamp to remove a remaining spur when the patient returns before closure of the colostomy. General postoperative care is carried out as described for closure of colostomy (Plate XLIV).

PLATE XLIX   COLECTOMY, LEFT, MIKULICZ PROCEDURE

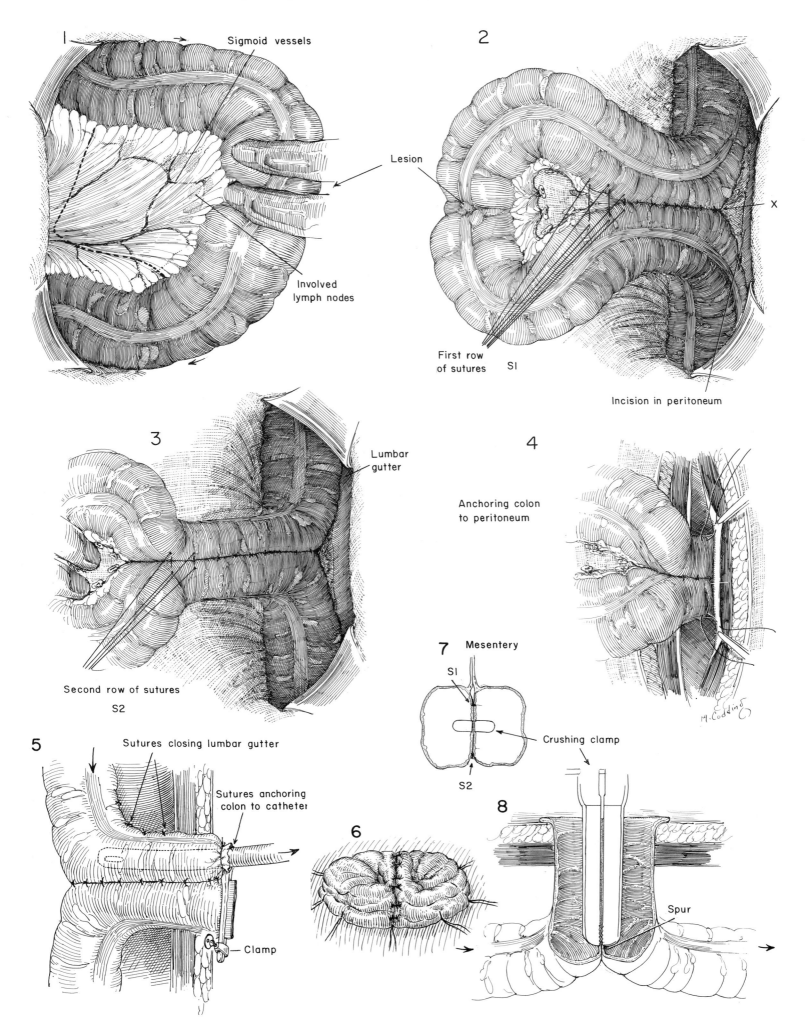

1

Sigmoid vessels

Lesion

Involved
lymph nodes

2

First row
of sutures   S1

Incision in peritoneum

X

3

Lumbar
gutter

Second row of sutures

S2

4

Anchoring colon
to peritoneum

7

Mesentery

S1

S2

Crushing clamp

5

Sutures closing lumbar gutter

Sutures anchoring
colon to catheter

Clamp

6

8

Spur

M. Codding

PLATE L · ABDOMINOPERINEAL RESECTION

INDICATIONS. Abdominoperineal resection of the lower bowel is the operation of choice for most rectal and lower rectosigmoid malignancies. It is preferably performed at a single session but, if the patient is markedly obstructed, a two-stage procedure with a preliminary colostomy may be desirable. The surgeon must be familiar with all methods, including resection of the tumor and anastomosis of the intestine within the hollow of the sacrum, and the several two-stage procedures.

PREOPERATIVE PREPARATION. The patient's general condition must be studied and improved as much as possible, since the operation is one of considerable magnitude. Unless there is evidence of acute or subacute obstruction, the patient is placed on a low-residue diet for several days. The appropriate chemotherapy or antibiotic therapy is given orally for two to five days to lower the fecal bacterial content as well as to change the consistency and decrease the bulk of the intestinal contents. The intestines are emptied by the occasional use of saline cathartics and enemas. If the lesion is near the anus, the bowels are further cleansed by irrigation through a catheter inserted beyond the tumor. Supplementary vitamin therapy should be given. The blood volume is restored to normal before operation, and several transfusions may be necessary if any degree of anemia is present. In addition to the routine intravenous pyelograms, in the presence of low-lying tumors, it may be advisable to evaluate by cystoscopy whether or not the bladder or other portions of the genitourinary tract are involved.

In males an indwelling catheter is inserted into the bladder the morning of operation to maintain complete urinary drainage throughout the procedure and to aid in identifying the membranous urethra. Indwelling catheter drainage of the bladder in females is likewise advisable. The rectum is emptied and a rectal tube inserted with a string attached to facilitate its easy removal when indicated during the operation. Suction is applied to the tube from time to time to remove any accumulated secretions before the bowel is divided.

ANESTHESIA. General anesthesia with endotracheal intubation and muscle relaxants is the preferred method. Spinal anesthesia is satisfactory.

Abdominal Resection

POSITION. Since the patient's position must be changed during the procedure, an operating table should be available that permits easy adjustment from a moderate Trendelenburg position to the lithotomy position. The patient is placed in a moderate Trendelenburg position. Before proceeding with the operation, the surgeon must make certain that the patient's general condition is satisfactory in this position. The surgeon stands on the patient's left side.

OPERATIVE PREPARATION. The lower abdomen is prepared in the usual manner.

INCISION AND EXPOSURE. A median or left paramedian suprapubic incision is made which is extended to the left and above the umbilicus. A Balfour self-retaining retractor is inserted.

DETAILS OF PROCEDURE. With his left hand the surgeon thoroughly explores the abdomen from above downward, palpating first the liver to ascertain the presence or absence of metastases, then the region of the aorta and common iliac and hemorrhoidal vessels for evidence of lymph gland involvement, and finally, by palpation and inspection, the extent and resectability of the growth itself **(Figure 1).** The inferior mesenteric artery and vein may be ligated distal to the origin of the left colic artery or at its point of origin from the aorta before the tumor is mobilized.

After the small intestine has been walled off in a plastic bag, the next procedure is the mobilization of the sigmoid, which is usually anchored in the left iliac fossa. The sigmoid is grasped with toothed forceps and reflected medially in order that the surgeon may obtain a clear view of the fibrous bands that anchor the sigmoid to the reflection of the peritoneum of the left pelvic wall **(Figure 2).** The adjacent adhesive bands are divided with long, curved scissors, and the peritoneal reflection is retracted laterally with forceps. Following this procedure, the sigmoid is usually mobilized easily toward the midline. The peritoneal surface on the left side of the colon is picked up with forceps and divided with long, curved, blunt-nosed Metzenbaum scissors, which are gently introduced downward beneath the peritoneum to separate the underlying structures, such as the left spermatic, or ovarian, vessels and ureter, from the peritoneum to avoid their accidental injury. The peritoneum is incised down to the cul-de-sac on the left side **(Figure 3).**

The next important step in the operation is the visualization of the left ureter throughout its course over the pelvic brim and down to the bladder. This is very important because on the left side the ureter may be in close proximity to the root of the mesentery of the rectosigmoid and may be included in the division of the latter structures, unless it is carefully retracted to the left side of the pelvis **(Figure 4).** The ureter will respond with peristaltic waves that progress along its length after it is pinched with forceps.

The next step involves the division of the peritoneum on the right side of the rectosigmoid. The same technic that has been described for the left side may be utilized, or the surgeon may mobilize the rectosigmoid over the pelvic brim from the left side by blunt finger dissection. The fingers of the surgeon's left hand can be passed completely behind the bowel toward the right side. With the fingers used as blunt dissectors, the right peritoneal reflection can be tented upward, separating it from the underlying structures, including the right ureter. This enables the surgeon to divide the peritoneum readily and safely with scissors **(Figure 5).**

PLATE L ABDOMINOPERINEAL RESECTION

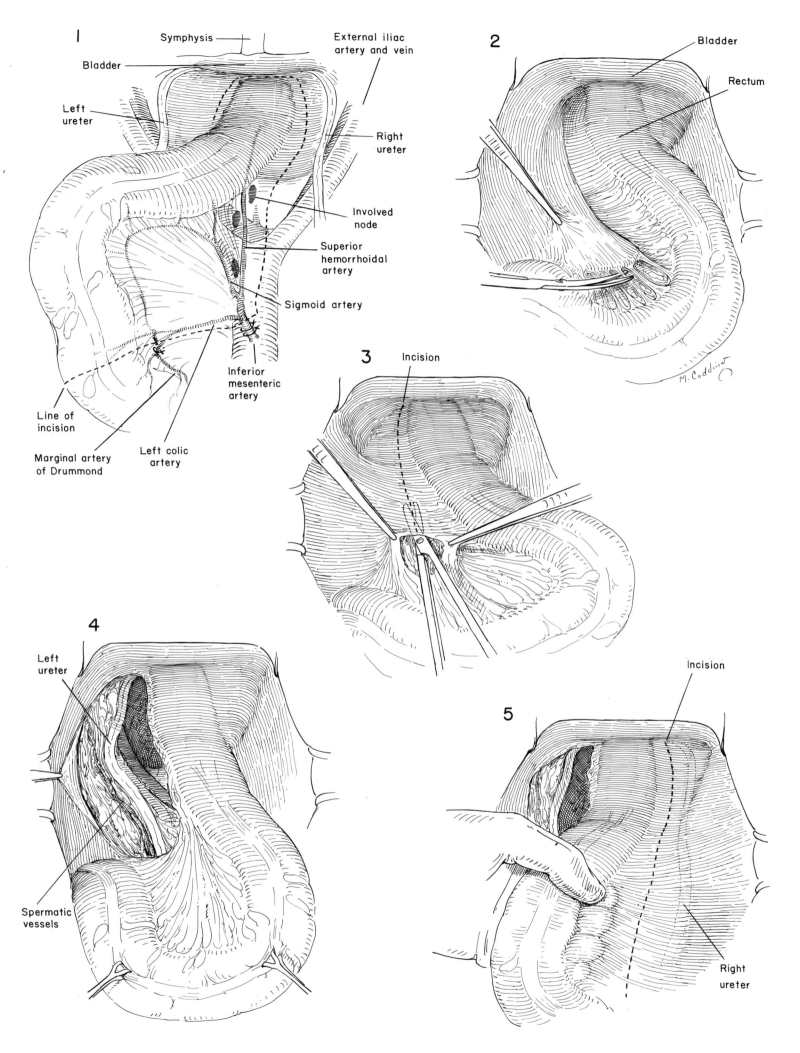

PLATE LI · ABDOMINOPERINEAL RESECTION

DETAILS OF PROCEDURE (*Continued*). After the peritoneal reflection on the right side has been divided adjacent to the superior hemorrhoidal vessels, the rectosigmoid and its blood supply can be completely encircled by the surgeon's left hand **(Figure 6).** The peritoneum is divided down to the level of the cul-de-sac on the right side, and the ureter, which may be attached to the reflected peritoneum on the right side, is freed by blunt gauze dissection throughout its course in the pelvis. The surgeon may pass a piece of gauze around the bowel and its blood supply to serve as a retractor instead of using his left hand **(Figure 7).** Some prefer to ligate the bowel with a tape proximal to the lesion.

The surgeon passes his right hand down into the hollow of the sacrum to free the rectum by blunt finger dissection **(Figure 8).** The hand should be kept as close to the bone as possible so that whatever loose areolar tissue is present will be removed with the bowel to be excised. The rectum can usually be free by blunt finger dissection as low as the sacrococcygeal junction **(Figure 9).** In the presence of large tumors that at first may appear to be immovable because of lateral fixation, it is important that the surgeon determine by this procedure that the tumor can be mobilized before proceeding to ligate the blood supply of this portion of the intestine.

After it has been determined that the rectum can be mobilized, it is necessary to divide three remaining points of fixation, i.e., the peritoneum in Douglas' pouch anterior to the rectum and the lateral suspensory ligaments containing the middle hemorrhoidal vessels. The peritoneum in Douglas' pouch anterior to the rectum is mobilized by blunt finger dissection and divided with long, curved scissors **(Figure 10).** The anterior wall of the rectum is further freed from the adjacent structures by blunt dissection. This is facilitated if the bladder in the male or the uterus in the female is retracted upward and forward by a large S-shaped retractor. In the male blunt dissection is carried down behind the prostate.

PLATE LI   ABDOMINOPERINEAL RESECTION

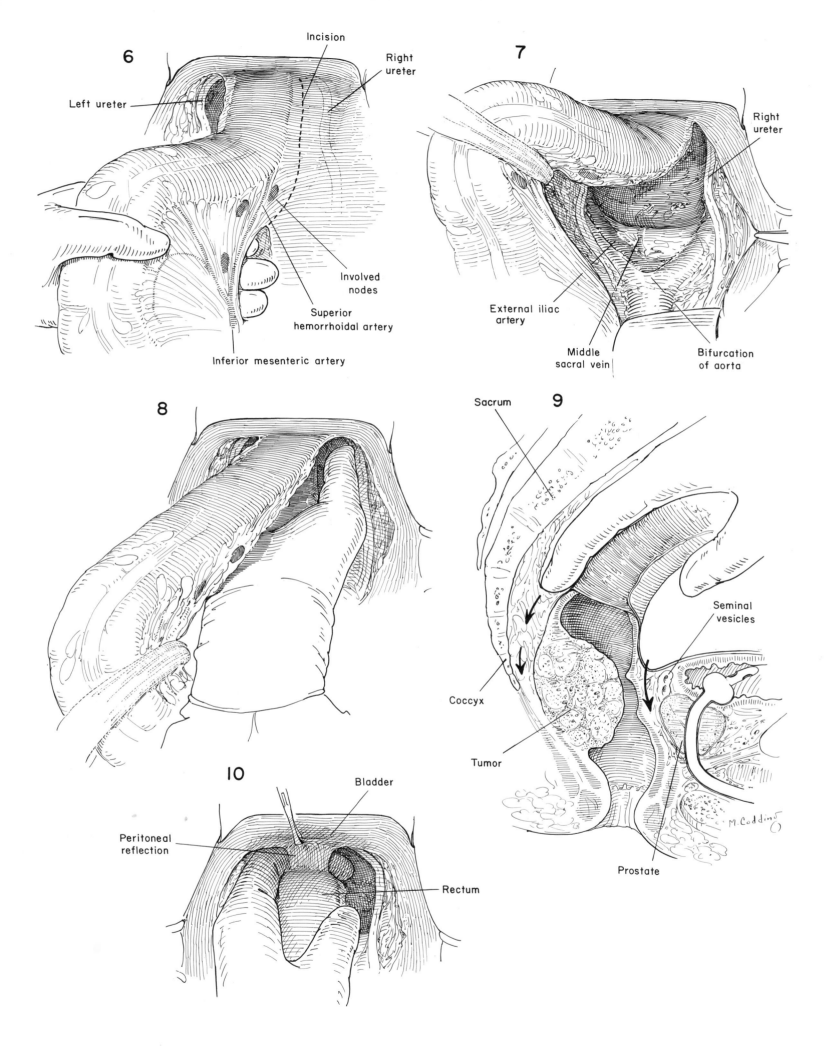

6

Left ureter

Incision

Right ureter

Involved nodes

Superior hemorrhoidal artery

Inferior mesenteric artery

7

Right ureter

External iliac artery

Middle sacral vein

Bifurcation of aorta

8

9

Sacrum

Seminal vesicles

Coccyx

Tumor

Prostate

M. Codding

10

Bladder

Peritoneal reflection

Rectum

PLATE LII · ABDOMINOPERINEAL RESECTION

DETAILS OF PROCEDURE (*Continued*). The hand is again introduced into the hollow of the sacrum, and blunt dissection is carried out laterally until the surgeon can hook his index finger around a tough structure, the lateral suspensory ligament of the rectum **(Figure 11)**. Since the middle hemorrhoidal vessels accompanying this structure may be of significant size, it is advisable to apply a long right-angle clamp before dividing the suspensory ligament. The contents of this clamp should be ligated. A similar procedure is carried out on the opposite side. Every effort should be made by means of finger as well as scissors dissection to free the lower segment of bowel to the lowest level possible in order to facilitate the subsequent perineal excision.

After it has been determined that the rectal tumor can be completely freed from the adjacent structures, the blood supply to the rectosigmoid is divided. The venous drainage should be ligated as early as possible to keep the vascular spread of tumor cells to a minimum. Although involved lymph nodes may not be evident in the mesentery over the bifurcation of the aorta, it is desirable to ligate the inferior mesenteric artery just distal to the origin of the left colic artery. The contents of the proximal clamps are tied, and the ligation is reinforced by a transfixing suture. Some prefer to ligate the inferior mesenteric artery as near its point of origin from the aorta as possible. Usually, this level is surprisingly near the ligament of Treitz. The blood supply to the sigmoid to be used as a colostomy is now derived from the middle colic artery through the marginal artery of Drummond.

Following this, the abdominal cavity and the pelvis are completely walled off with gauze as a preliminary to the application of a noncrushing Pace-Potts clamp to the region of the lower rectosigmoid **(Figure 13)**. The bowel may be divided between similar crushing clamps, either above or below the tumor. The bowel must be divided at a point sufficiently low to provide adequate room for it to be tucked down into the hollow of the sacrum and to permit subsequent closure of the pelvic peritoneum. The intestine is divided between the clamps. The sigmoid is covered with a warm, moist gauze pack and reflected upward **(Figure 13)**.

The lower segment of the bowel, which has been sealed with the crushing clamps, is closed with an over-and-over continuous suture of heavy No. 1 silk **(Figure 14)**. As the clamp is removed, this suture is pulled taut **(Figure 15)**. Some prefer to close the lower segment with several heavy interrupted No. 1 silk sutures. Following this, the closed end of the bowel is covered with a rubber glove or gauze sponge, which is secured in position by an encircling heavy silk suture **(Figure 16)**. The distal segment of bowel is then tucked down into the hollow of the sacrum as a preliminary to the construction of a new pelvic floor **(Figure 17)**.

The redundant sigmoid, which has been retracted upward over the abdominal wall, is inspected to determine the best site for dividing the bowel to serve as a permanent colostomy. The sigmoid is divided where it appears to be viable and will extend beyond the surface of the skin for 4 to 6 cm. without being under undue tension. Excessive fat tabs and thick fatty mesentery, if present, should be excised about the terminal end of the colon in anticipation of inversion of the mucosa with immediate fixation to the adjacent skin. Noncrushing clamps of the Pace-Potts type are applied obliquely, and the bowel is divided. The proximal clamp is left on the abdominal wall, while the peritoneal reflection is adequately mobilized for an easy closure.

PLATE LII   ABDOMINOPERINEAL RESECTION

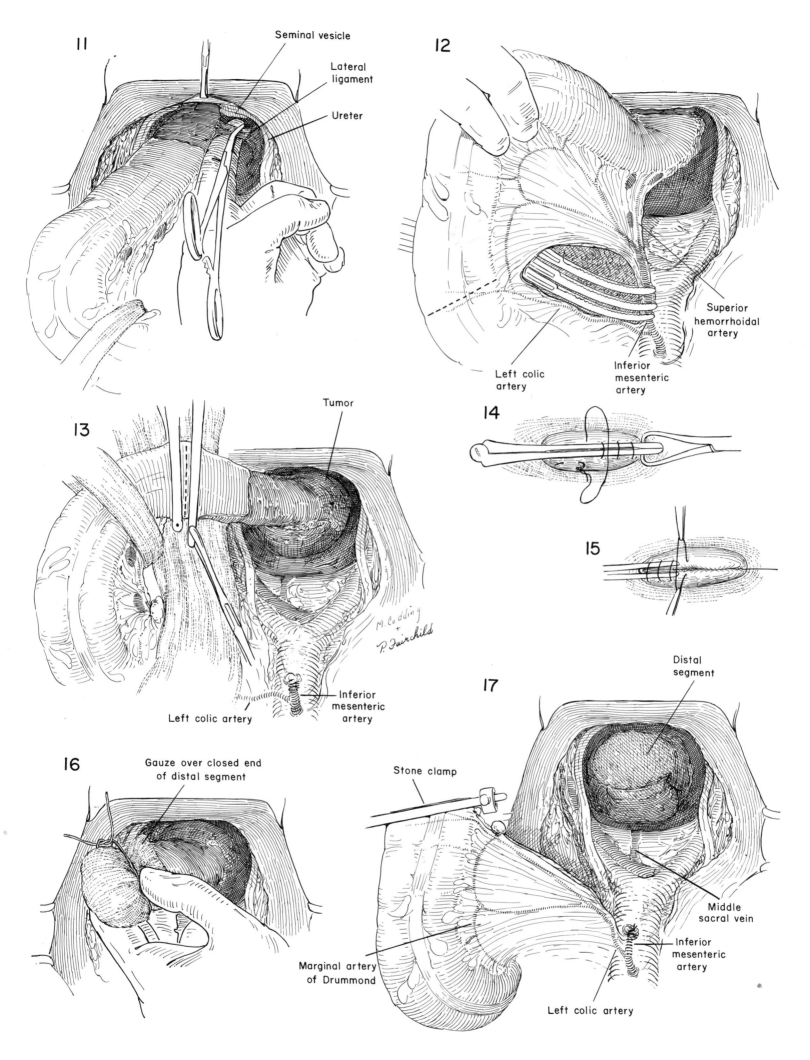

11

Seminal vesicle

Lateral
ligament

Ureter

12

Superior
hemorrhoidal
artery

Left colic
artery

Inferior
mesenteric
artery

13

Tumor

M. Codding
+
P. Fairchild

Left colic artery

Inferior
mesenteric
artery

14

15

Distal
segment

17

16

Gauze over closed end
of distal segment

Stone clamp

Middle
sacral vein

Inferior
mesenteric
artery

Marginal artery
of Drummond

Left colic artery

PLATE LIII · ABDOMINOPERINEAL RESECTION

DETAILS OF PROCEDURE (*Continued*). The margins of the peritoneum are mobilized in order to close the peritoneal floor securely. The peritoneum is grasped with toothed forceps and mobilized by the surgeon's hand or by blunt gauze dissection **(Figure 18)**. The peritoneum in the pouch of Douglas is mobilized as widely as possible to facilitate closing the pelvic floor. The location of the ureters is reaffirmed from time to time to avoid their accidental ligation or injury. In females the uterus and adnexa may be used, if necessary, to close the new pelvic floor. At times it may be possible to close the pelvic floor in a straight line, but, more frequently, a radial type of closure is necessary to avoid undue tension on the suture line **(Figure 19)**. All raw surfaces should be covered whenever possible. The omentum is placed over the peritoneal closure **(Figure 20)**.

Some surgeons prefer to anchor the sigmoid to the lateral parietal peritoneum in order to close the left lumbar gutter and to avoid the possibility of an internal hernia. Whenever possible, these sutures should include the fat tabs or mesentery to avoid possible perforation of the bowel. Before proceeding with the closure, the advantages of a gastrostomy should be weighed if the stomach is easily exposed.

CLOSURE. The colostomy is brought out of the upper angle of the wound or through a separate stab wound approximately midway between the umbilicus and the left anterior superior spine. The omentum is returned to the region of the new pelvic floor **(Figure 20)**. The operating table is leveled. The colostomy can be placed near the region of the umbilicus. The peritoneum is closed with interrupted mattress sutures up to the region of the exteriorized intestine. In order to avoid undue constriction of the bowel and interference with the blood supply, the surgeon introduces his index finger alongside the intestine as the final interrupted suture in the peritoneum is tied. This avoids too snug a closure of the peritoneum **(Figure 21)**. The bowel may be anchored to the abdominal wall by attaching several fat tabs to the peritoneum or fascia **(Figure 22)**. Sutures should not be taken through the bowel for this purpose, lest perforation and infection should result. The same general principles apply for anchoring the bowel to the abdominal wall if the colostomy is made through a separate incision. All bleeding points in the subcutaneous tissue are carefully ligated. An opening is made directly through the abdominal wall large enough to admit at least two fingers. Late herniation about a colostomy can be minimized by tailoring the opening on the abdominal wall to the size of the colon.

The abdominal wall is closed with interrupted 00 silk sutures. Subcuticular closure of the skin should be considered since this ensures a sealed wound about an area repeatedly contaminated from the adjacent colostomy. In patients with marked obesity or cachexia, etc., tension sutures may be utilized, or the fascia may be approximated with fine wire sutures. The exteriorized portion of the bowel is then inspected to make certain that active pulsation is present in its blood supply. Sufficient intestine should have been provided to ensure at least 4 to 6 cm. of viable bowel protruding above the skin level **(Figure 23)**.

Immediate opening of the colostomy after the remainder of the wound has been covered is becoming preferred to leaving a clamp on the exposed and completely obstructed intestine for several days. The Pace-Potts clamp is removed and the mucosa within the lumen of the bowel grasped with one or two Babcock forceps to provide fixation for the eversion of the mucosa **(Figure 23)**. It may be necessary to excise several large fat tabs and additional thickened mesentery, especially in the obese patient, to facilitate the eversion of the mucosa. The mucosa is anchored to the margin of the skin with interrupted sutures **(Figure 24)**. A sufficient number of sutures is taken to control bleeding as well as to seal off the subcutaneous tissue about the colostomy **(Figure 25)**. The mucosa should be pink in color to ensure viability. The surgeon should insert a gloved finger into the colostomy to make certain the lumen is free and adequate without undue constriction within the abdominal wall. Frequent dressing changes may be required, but compression dressings on the exposed mucosa should be avoided. A transparent disposable plastic bag tailored to fit the colostomy may be put on immediately after a protective film has been applied to the adjacent skin.

PLATE LIII   ABDOMINOPERINEAL RESECTION

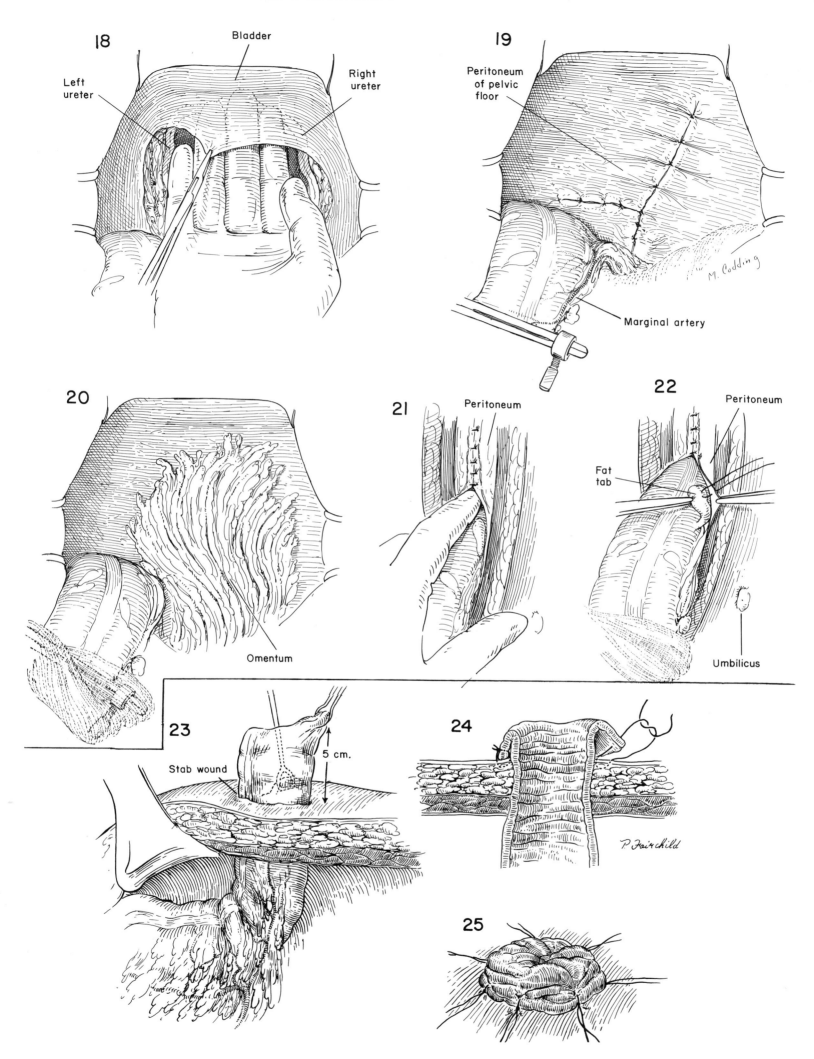

18

Bladder

Left ureter

Right ureter

19

Peritoneum of pelvic floor

Marginal artery

M. Codding

20

Omentum

21

Peritoneum

22

Peritoneum

Fat tab

Umbilicus

23

Stab wound

5 cm.

24

P. Fairchild

25

PLATE LIV · ABDOMINOPERINEAL RESECTION—PERINEAL RESECTION

Perineal Resection

The surgeon must be satisfied with the patient's condition before proceeding with the perineal excision of the rectosigmoid. The estimated blood loss from the abdominal procedure, often more than realized unless accurately determined by the anesthetist, should be replaced by whole blood transfusions, and the pulse and blood pressure should be established at a satisfactory level. Some prefer the two-team approach so that the perineal excision is carried out simultaneously with the abdominal procedure.

POSITION. Some surgeons prefer the patient on his left side in a modified Sims' position. Others change the patient to the lithotomy position by adjusting the stirrups to hold the legs. The change in position must be done gently and carefully; sudden shifts have been known to precipitate shock. The pulse and blood pressure should be stabilized after the change in position before the final resection is started.

OPERATIVE PREPARATION. To prevent possible subsequent contamination from blood and fecal material, the lower rectum is cleansed with gauze. Following this, the anus and adjacent skin surfaces are prepared with the usual skin antiseptics. The legs and buttocks are covered with sterile drapes.

INCISION AND EXPOSURE. The extent of the perineal excision is indicated in **Figure 3.** If the lesion is low and near the anus, a more radical excision is carried out. If the dissection has been carried down far enough from above, the perineal excision of the rectum and anus should be accomplished easily without undue loss of blood. To prevent contamination, the anus is sealed securely, either by several interrupted sutures of heavy silk or by a purse-string suture, and the skin is again cleansed with antiseptic solutions **(Figure 3).** An incision is outlined around the anus with anterior and posterior midline extensions **(Figure 2).** The skin in the region of the anal orifice is seized with several Allis forceps, and the incision is made through the skin and subcutaneous tissue at least 2 cm. away from the closed anal orifice **(Figure 4).** Some operators prefer to place the lateral incisions adjacent to the ischial tuberosities, especially for low-lying lesions. All blood vessels are clamped and tied to prevent further loss of blood as the operation progresses **(Figure 5).** The margins of the wound are retracted laterally to assist in the exposure.

DETAILS OF PROCEDURE. The posterior portion of the incision is extended backward over the coccyx, and the anus is tipped upward to enable its attachments to the coccyx to be severed more readily. After the anococcygeal raphe is severed, the rectum is separated by blunt dissection from the adjacent sacrum **(Figure 6).** Following this, the index finger is swept laterally to identify the levator ani muscles on either side. The levator muscle is exposed on one side and, with the finger held beneath it, is divided between paired clamps as far from the rectum as possible **(Figure 7).** Curved clamps should be applied to the levator ani muscles as they are divided to prevent the retraction of bleeding points. Following the ligation of all bleeding points on one side, a similar division of the levator ani muscles is carried out on the opposite side. Although the coccyx is not excised routinely to facilitate exposure, it may be advisable in the presence of large, low-lying tumors to remove it as well as the lower portion of the sacrum.

PLATE LIV   ABDOMINOPERINEAL RESECTION—PERINEAL RESECTION

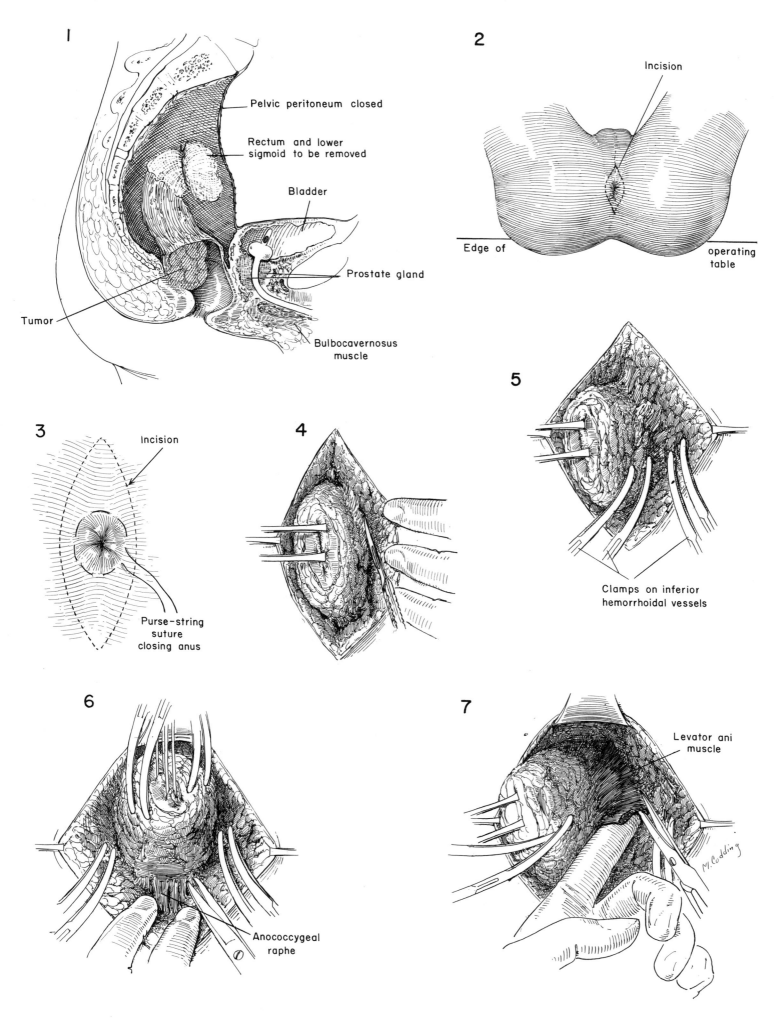

1

Pelvic peritoneum closed

Rectum and lower sigmoid to be removed

Bladder

Prostate gland

Tumor

Bulbocavernosus muscle

2

Incision

Edge of

operating table

3

Incision

Purse-string suture closing anus

4

5

Clamps on inferior hemorrhoidal vessels

6

Anococcygeal raphe

7

Levator ani muscle

M. Codding

PLATE LV · ABDOMINOPERINEAL RESECTION—PERINEAL RESECTION

DETAILS OF PROCEDURE (*Continued*). The procedure in the male is illustrated because the dissection between the rectum, membranous urethra, and prostate offers more problems than dissection in the female. Palpation of the inlying urethral catheter will facilitate the procedure by localizing the urethra and preventing accidental injury to the above-mentioned structures **(Figure 8)**. The skin and subcutaneous tissue of the perineum are retracted upward, while the anus is pulled downward and backward to assist in the exposure. The rectum is pulled down, the remaining attachments of the levator ani muscles and transversus perinea are divided, and all bleeding points are ligated. In the female the dissection between the rectum and vagina is more easily accomplished if counter-resistance is applied to the posterior vaginal wall by the surgeon's fingers. In the presence of extensive infiltrating growths it may be necessary to excise the perineal body as well as a portion of the posterior vaginal wall.

Any remaining attachments of the rectum are freed by the surgeon's hand introduced posteriorly and upward into the hollow of the sacrum **(Figure 9)**. As the finger dissection reaches the cleavage plane that has developed from above, there is usually a small gush of blood that has accumulated in the hollow of the sacrum. The upper end of the bowel segment is grasped with its enveloping gauze and delivered posteriorly over the coccyx **(Figure 10)**. A retractor is introduced anteriorly to assist in exposure, while any remaining anterior attachments of the rectum are divided **(Figure 11)**. The large pelvic space is thoroughly inspected under direct illumination in order to clamp and ligate any active bleeding points, since the patient cannot afford to lose blood unnecessarily in a procedure of this magnitude. The cavity is packed with warm, moist sponges until the field is free of oozing **(Figure 12)**. Some coagulant may be applied to control any oozing from raw surfaces.

CLOSURE. Although some surgeons prefer to fill the cavity in the hollow of the sacrum with several sponges introduced in a piece of sheet rubber or a thin pliable plastic sheet, especially if there is persistent oozing, the wound may be partially closed with interrupted sutures. It is sometimes possible to approximate the divided levator ani muscles in the midline **(Figure 13)**. Two or three large rubber drains are inserted into the hollow of the sacrum and brought out through the posterior portion of the wound. The subcutaneous tissue and skin are closed with interrupted sutures about these drains **(Figure 14)**.

Sterile multiperforated plastic suction catheters attached to long heavy metal needles can be inserted through the tissues on both sides of the wound directly into the hollow of the sacrum. The wound can be closed with absorbable sutures in layers, since drainage is ensured through the suction catheters.

POSTOPERATIVE CARE. Postoperative care is governed by the degree of shock present in the patient and the amount of blood lost. The blood loss must be replaced during the operation and postoperatively. Intravenous 5 or 10 per cent glucose in distilled water or saline is given to keep the patient in fluid balance. Large doses of chemotherapy and/or antibiotics can be administered.

The patient is maintained on constant bladder drainage for seven to ten days. In males the loss of bladder tone may result in one of the most distressing postoperative complications. Frequent and thorough evaluation of the patient's ability to empty the bladder is essential until good function has returned. The catheter should be clamped for several hours at a time to determine if the patient actually has retained the sensation arising from a full bladder. In many cases, especially in males, a cystometric study should be considered before removing the catheter. The catheter should be removed early in the morning to permit all-day observations on the patient's ability to void. Overdistention should be rigorously avoided by catheterizing the patient for residual urine every four to six hours, depending upon his fluid intake. Diuretic liquids, such as coffee and tea, should be withheld from the evening meal in an effort to avoid overdistention of the bladder during the night. On the day of the catheter removal the bladder residual should be determined at bedtime, unless the ability to void has been free and easy. Frequent urination of small amounts indicates retention, and reinsertion of the catheter for a few days should be considered. It is not uncommon for older males to require a transurethral resection to ensure a free flow of urine postoperatively. Rigid attention to the care of the bladder with assistance from the urologic surgeon pays rich dividends in the patient's postoperative progress.

The suction catheters are removed in a few days when the drainage output has markedly decreased.

When perineal drains are used, they are withdrawn a short distance within 48 to 72 hours and gradually withdrawn thereafter. The sinus tract resulting from the removal of the drains should be kept open by digital examination until the pelvic cavity has been obliterated. The patient is instructed in the care of a colostomy before being discharged from the hospital. This consists of the patient's giving himself an enema once daily through the colostomy opening. The colostomy is covered with gauze in petrolatum and a sterile dressing of some type supported by an elastic girdle 17.5 to 22.5 cm. in width. Complicated colostomy bags are not advisable.

Because of the proximity of the great veins in the pelvis to the structures affected by this procedure, daily evaluation of the signs and symptoms of deep venous thrombosis must be carried out.

PLATE LV   ABDOMINOPERINEAL RESECTION—PERINEAL RESECTION

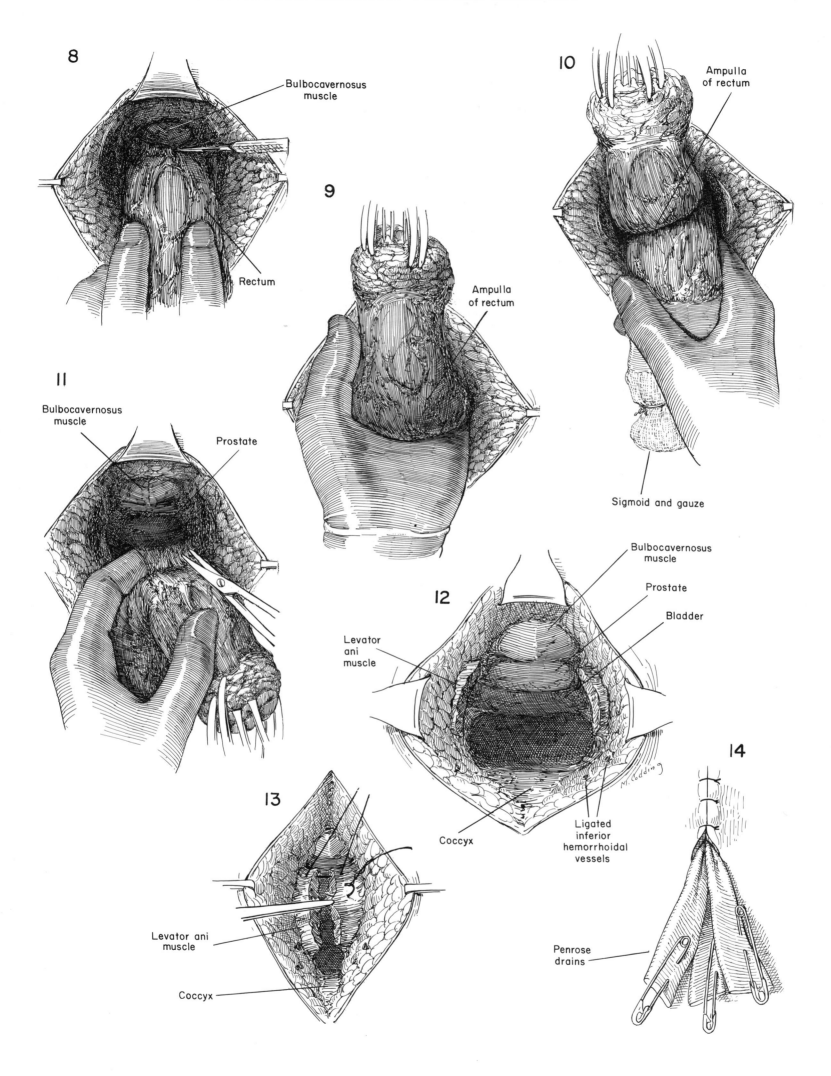

8

Bulbocavernosus muscle

Rectum

9

Ampulla of rectum

10

Ampulla of rectum

Sigmoid and gauze

11

Bulbocavernosus muscle

Prostate

12

Bulbocavernosus muscle

Prostate

Bladder

Levator ani muscle

Coccyx

Ligated inferior hemorrhoidal vessels

13

Levator ani muscle

Coccyx

14

Penrose drains

M. Codding

PLATE LVI · TOTAL COLECTOMY

INDICATIONS. The most common indications for total colectomy are ulcerative colitis and familial polyposis. In the very poor-risk patient with ulcerative colitis, particularly with a complication such as a free perforation, it is judicious to perform the operation in two stages. The removal of the rectum is delayed until the patient's condition is less critical. Although conservation of the anus and lower rectum by ileoproctostomy should be considered in congenital polyposis in the absence of proved rectal malignancy, it is controversial and is never indicated in ulcerative colitis. The polyps in the retained rectum that do not disappear spontaneously can be destroyed by repeated fulguration.

PREOPERATIVE PREPARATION. Unless total colectomy is done as an emergency procedure, efforts should be made to improve the patient's nutritional status with a high-protein, high-calorie diet. Intravenous hyperalimentation may be used. The blood volume is restored and supplemental vitamins provided. The surgeon must carefully evaluate the status of the steroid therapy. Nonabsorbable antibacterial agents, along with supplemental vitamin K, should be administered whenever possible for three to five days before surgery. The patient requires special psychologic preparation for the ileostomy. This should include a visit by an individual who can demonstrate successful rehabilitation following this procedure. The patient should be shown the permanent type of ileostomy appliance, and he should be encouraged to read the literature available from an ileostomy club to prepare him for postoperative management. In addition, the site of the ileostomy should be selected away from bony prominences and previous scars. A permanent type of appliance should be glued to the patient's skin for one to two days to allow him to move about with it in place and make any final adjustments in its eventual location. This point is marked with indelible ink to assure accurate placement of the stoma. Mechanical cleansing of the bowel should be kept to a minimum, since this would only enhance further blood loss and electrolyte imbalance. The male patient should be informed of the possibility of postoperative impotence.

ANESTHESIA. General endotracheal anesthesia is preferred.

POSITION. The patient is placed in a moderate Trendelenburg position near the left side of the table. For the perineal portion of the operation the patient is placed in the lithotomy position with the thighs widely extended.

OPERATIVE PREPARATION. The skin is prepared in the routine manner, and the ileostomy site just below the half-way mark between the right anterior iliac spine and the umbilicus is re-marked. A sterile plastic drape may be used.

INCISION AND EXPOSURE. The surgeon stands to the patient's left side. The incision must extend sufficiently high in the epigastrium to provide an easy exposure of the colonic flexures, lest undue traction of the friable bowel result in perforation and gross contamination **(Figure 1)**.

After general exploration of the abdomen, the small bowel is placed in a plastic bag. The dissection is started in the region of the tip of the cecum **(Figure 2)**. The right colon is retracted medially as the peritoneum in the right lumbar gutter is incised with curved scissors **(Figure 2)**. Because of the tendency to increased vascularity, it may be necessary to ligate a number of blood vessels in the free margin of the peritoneum along the right lumbar gutter.

The peritoneal attachments to the terminal ileum are divided and the cecum and terminal ileum mobilized well outside the wound **(Figure 3)**. The peritoneum is tented upward before it is incised to avoid injuring the underlying right spermatic vessels and ureter. Blunt gauze dissection is utilized to push these structures away from the adjacent mesentery. The right ureter should be identified throughout its course up to the right kidney and down to the pelvic brim. Any adhesions between gallbladder, liver, and hepatic flexure are divided. During the mobilization of the ascending colon and hepatic flexure, care must be taken to identify the retroperitoneal portion of the duodenum, which may come into view rather unexpectedly. Blunt gauze is utilized to sweep away the duodenum **(Figure 4)** from the overlying mesocolon. The thickened, contracted, and highly vascular greater omentum is divided between curved clamps and their contents ligated **(Figure 4)**. The greater omentum is retracted upward and the lesser omental sac entered from the right side.

PLATE LVI   TOTAL COLECTOMY

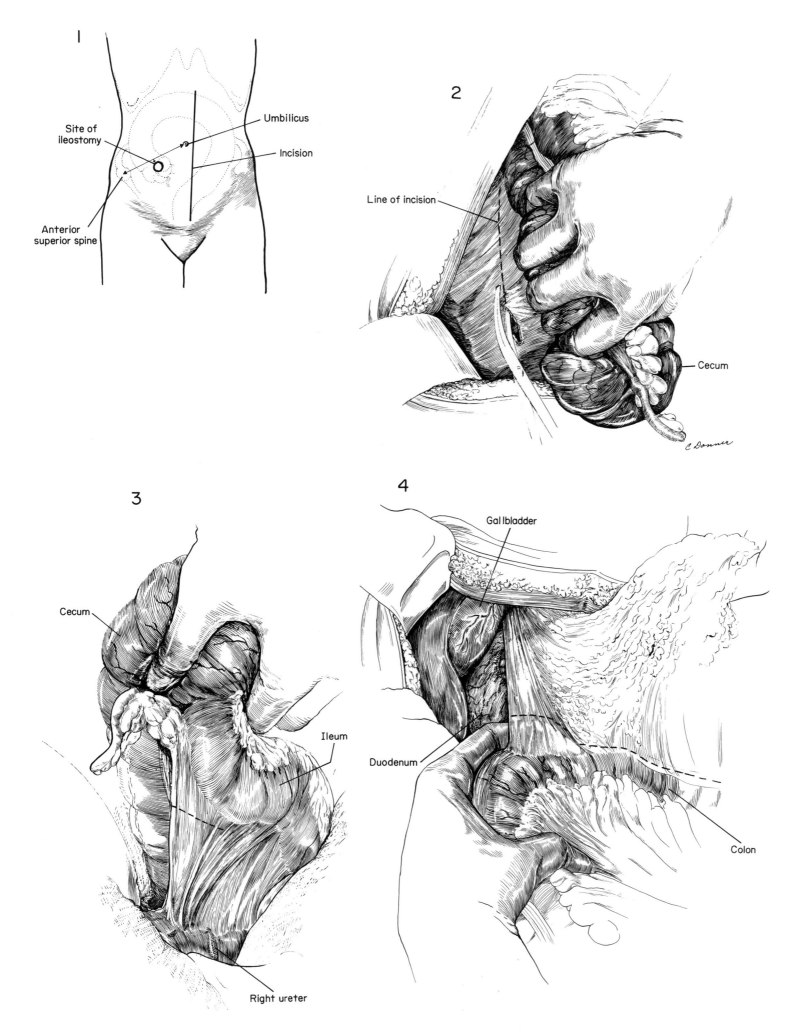

1

Site of
ileostomy

Umbilicus

Incision

Anterior
superior spine

2

Line of incision

Cecum

C Donner

3

Cecum

Ileum

Right ureter

4

Gallbladder

Duodenum

Colon

PLATE LVII · TOTAL COLECTOMY

DETAILS OF PROCEDURE (*Continued*). The thickened and vascular greater omentum is retracted upward in preparation for its separation from the transverse colon. An incision is made in the omental reflection along the superior surface of the colon **(Figure 5).** Since the omentum may be quite adherent to the colon, it may be easier to divide the gastrocolic omentum nearer the stomach than the transverse colon. This can be facilitated if the surgeon places his left hand, palm upward, in the lesser sac in order to better define the gastrocolic omentum. Paired curved clamps are applied and their contents ligated with 00 silk.

Special attention is required during the division of the thickened splenocolic ligament to avoid tearing the splenic capsule by undue tension **(Figure 6).** The splenocolic ligament is divided at some distance, if pos-
sible, from the inferior pole of the spleen **(Figure 7).** When the splenic flexure and descending colon have been partially freed down to the region of the sigmoid, the surgeon may wish to return to the region of the right colon and control the blood supply to the bowel before removing it in order to facilitate the eventual exposure of the pelvis for the exploration of the rectum. The mobilized right colon is drawn outside the peritoneal cavity, and the vessels in the mesentery can be easily identified **(Figure 8).** Enlarged lymph nodes often fill in the arcades about the mesenteric border. The blood supply can be ligated near the bowel wall as shown in **Figure 8.** Before the blood supply is ligated, the ureter is protected posteriorly by warm, moist packs.

PLATE LVII   TOTAL COLECTOMY

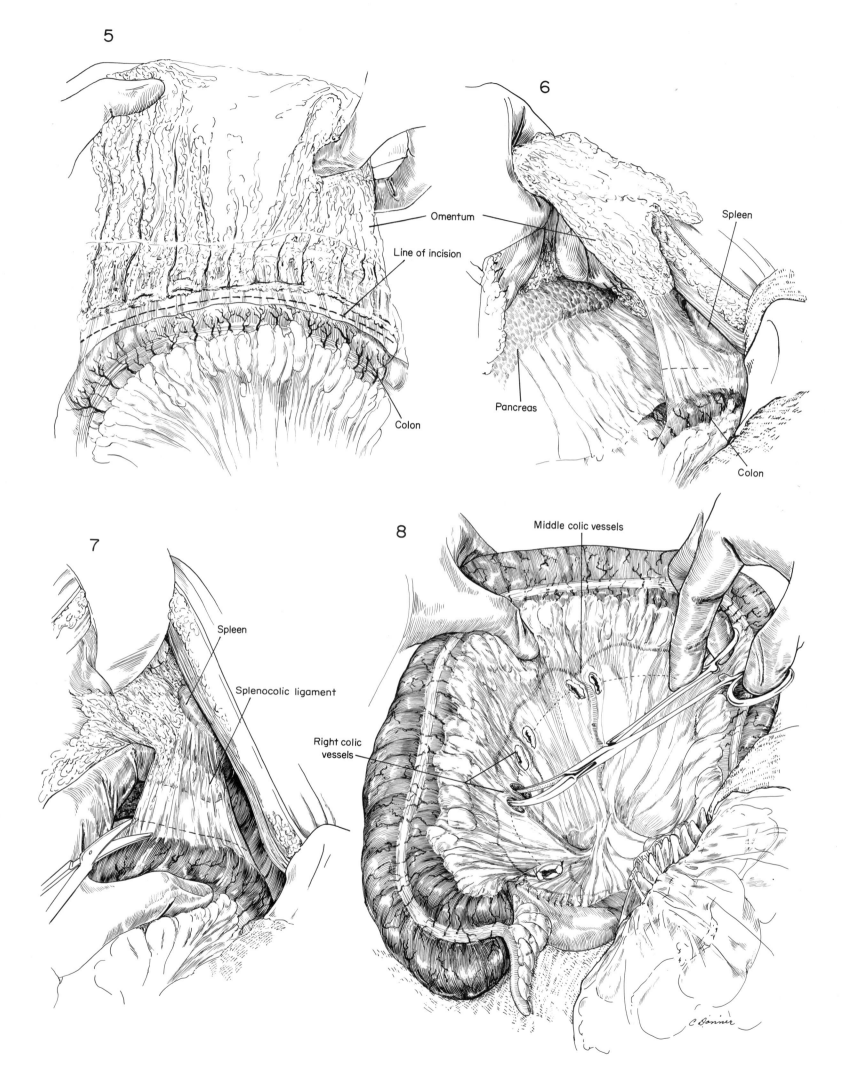

5

6

Omentum

Line of incision

Colon

Spleen

Pancreas

Colon

7

Spleen

Splenocolic ligament

8

Middle colic vessels

Right colic vessels

C. Donner

PLATE LVIII · TOTAL COLECTOMY

DETAILS OF PROCEDURE (*Continued*). After the blood supply to the region of the appendix and the right colon has been divided, the terminal ileum may be further mobilized. An incision is made into the mesentery of the terminal ileum with a clear view of the ureter at all times to avoid its injury. It is often necessary to remove a portion of the terminal ileum because of its possible involvement with the inflammatory process **(Figure 9).**

Considerable time is required to separate the blood supply proximally from the site where the ileum is to be divided. At least 7 cm. of ileum can be denuded of blood supply in preparation for the development of an ileostomy **(Figure 9).** The blood supply to this portion of the ileum should be divided very carefully, almost one vessel at a time, maintaining the large vascular arcade at some distance from the mesenteric border. A noncrushing vascular-type clamp is applied to the ileal side and a straight Kocher clamp to the cecal side in preparation for the division of the intestine **(Figure 10).** The contents of the Kocher clamp can be ligated with heavy silk or catgut to facilitate handling of the right colon **(Figure 11).** It is useful to cover this portion of the bowel with warm moist packs, tied in place with individual tapes or heavy ligatures.

The colon is then retracted medially, and the mesentery is divided up to the region of the middle colic vessel **(Figure 12).** Two half-length clamps should be applied proximally on the middle colic vessels because of their size and the increased vascularity in ulcerative colitis. The mesentery of the transverse colon is rather easily divided between pairs of clamps and the contents carefully ligated. This can be done at some distance from the inferior surface of the pancreas. As additional portions of colon are freed, they are incorporated in moist towels or gauze sponges to avoid tearing the bowel wall and possible gross contamination.

PLATE LVIII   TOTAL COLECTOMY

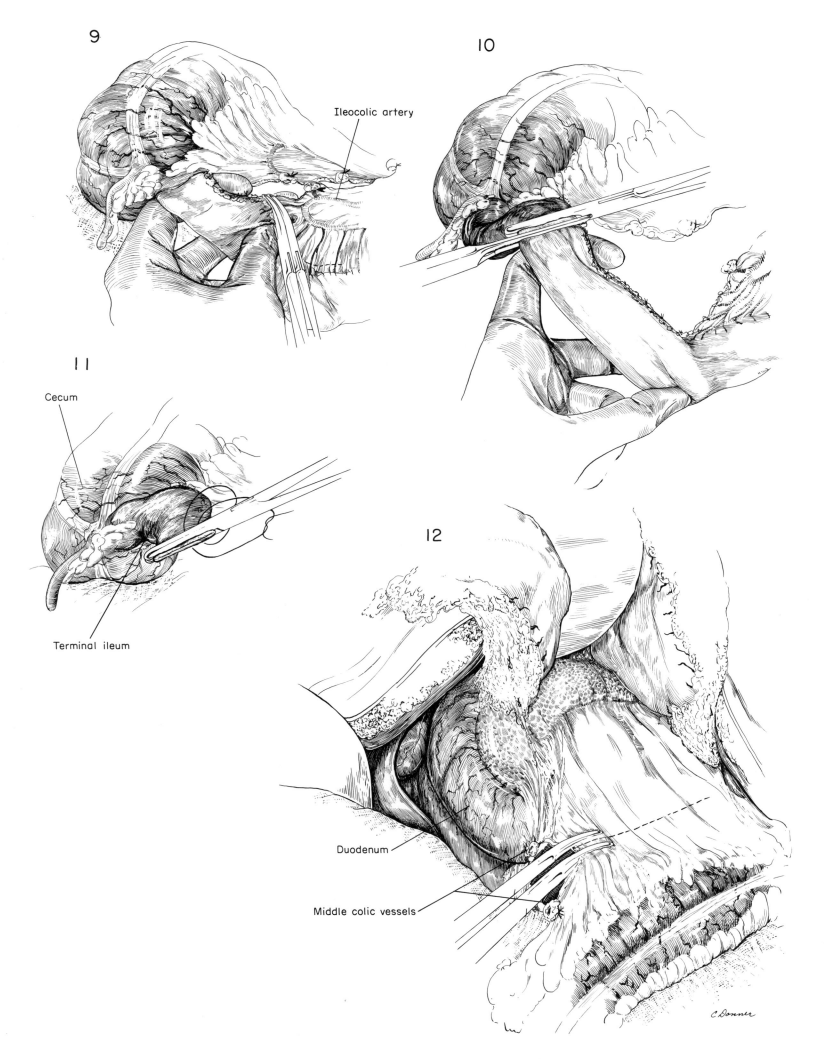

9

10

Ileocolic artery

11

Cecum

Terminal ileum

12

Duodenum

Middle colic vessels

C Donner

PLATE LIX · TOTAL COLECTOMY

DETAILS OF PROCEDURE (*Continued*). An incision is made down the left lumbar gutter, and because the thickened and vascular peritoneum has a tendency to contract, all bleeding points should be carefully ligated **(Figure 13).** The peritoneum is lifted up until the left gonadal vessels are identified. They should be identified throughout most of their course down over the brim of the pelvis **(Figure 14).**

As shown in **Figure 15,** the mesentery is divided adjacent to the rectosigmoid rather than up over the iliac artery bifurcation, as would be done in carcinoma. The rectum is gently separated from the hollow of the sacrum, and an effort is made, especially in very young male patients, to avoid interference with the sympathetic nerve supply to the bladder and genital organs. The peritoneum adjacent to the bowel is divided after identification of the ureters on either side. Blunt finger dissection is utilized, but it is not necessary to go as far laterally as in the presence of malignancy. Either a long special curved clamp or a modified noncrushing Pace-Potts clamp is applied low on the rectum **(Figure 16).** A clamp is applied to the bowel wall proximally to avoid contamination as the bowel is divided and the colon removed. At this time sharp and blunt dissection about the remaining rectal stump should be carried out to free it as low as possible to lessen the blood loss during the subsequent perineal excision of the involved rectum. In the presence of multiple polyposis a segment of rectum can be retained 5 to 8 cm. above the pouch of Douglas or at a distance that can be easily reached by the sigmoidoscope for subsequent fulguration of the multiple polyps. When this is done, the terminal ileum is anastomosed to the rectal pouch in a side-to-end manner.

The end of the rectal stump is closed with heavy silk sutures and buried beneath the peritoneum **(Figure 17).** Either silk or catgut sutures are used to close the peritoneal floor. The location of the ureters should be ascertained from time to time to avoid injury during the reconstruction of the pelvic floor.

PLATE LIX   TOTAL COLECTOMY

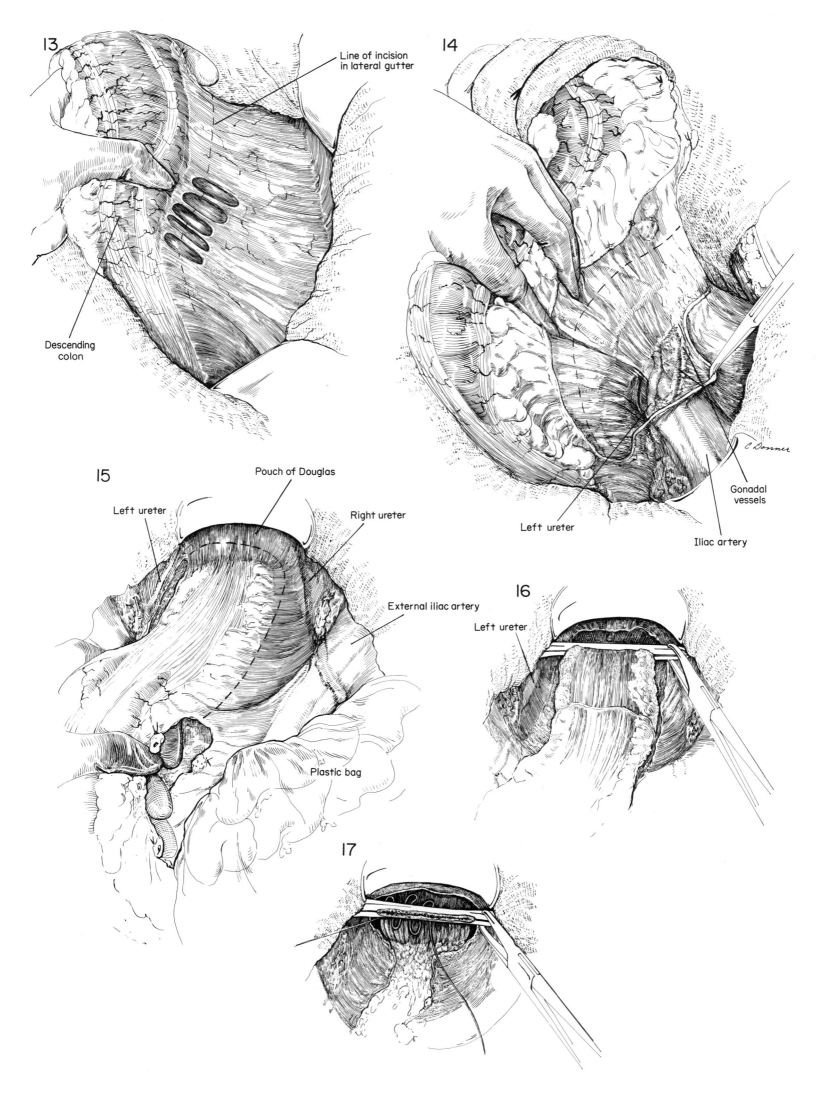

13

Line of incision
in lateral gutter

Descending
colon

14

Left ureter

Gonadal
vessels

Iliac artery

15

Pouch of Douglas

Left ureter

Right ureter

External iliac artery

Plastic bag

16

Left ureter

17

PLATE LX · TOTAL COLECTOMY

DETAILS OF PROCEDURE (*Continued*). After the pelvis has been reperitonealized, the raw surfaces in the left lumbar gutter also can be covered if the tissues are sufficiently lax **(Figure 18)**. Again, the sutures should be placed so as to avoid injuring the underlying ureters and gonadal vessels. Usually, it is impossible to peritonealize the raw surfaces up over the region of the left kidney and in the region of the spleen **(Figure 18)**.

The construction of the ileostomy is of major concern. The small intestine may be removed from the plastic bag and the site selected for ileostomy exposed. With half-length clamps applied to the peritoneal edge and the self-retaining retractor removed from the wound, the location of the previously marked ileostomy site is evaluated. The midway point between the umbilicus and anterior iliac spine is again verified by a sterilized ruler. The ileostomy site is placed a little below the midway point **(Figure 1, Plate LVI)**. A button of skin, about the size of a 50-cent piece, is excised in the lines of skin cleavage. After the button of skin and the underlying fat have been removed, all bleeding points are controlled with fine silk. Then, while applying traction against the abdominal wall from underneath with his left hand, the surgeon makes a stellate incision through the entire thickness of the abdominal wall. Occasionally, a segment of fascia is removed, and any bleeding that is encountered, especially in the rectus muscle, is clamped and ligated. An opening large enough to admit two fingers easily is usually sufficient.

Noncrushing vascular-type forceps are inserted through the ileostomy site and applied just proximal to the similar forceps on the terminal ileum **(Figure 19)**. The original forceps are removed, and the ileum is withdrawn through the abdominal wall with the mesentery cephalad. At least 5 or 6 cm. of mesentery-free ileum should be above the skin level so that an ileostomy of adequate length can be constructed. It may be necessary, especially in the obese patient, to free an additional several centimeters of ileum from its mesentery to attain this essential length. Some prefer to evert the mucosa of the terminal ileum before it is pulled through. This can be done as soon as the terminal ileum is divided; and after the remainder of the colon has been removed, the viability of the rim of mucosa which has been everted can be evaluated. This procedure also assures sufficient room to avoid constriction when the ileum is pulled through the opening previously described. The mesentery can be anchored to the abdominal wall or brought up into the subcutaneous tissue **(Figure 20)**. It may be advisable to anchor the mesentery of the ileum to the parietes laterally before constructing the ileostomy, because of the possibility of interfering with the blood supply to the terminal ileum. The right lumbar gutter should be closed off to avoid the potential of a postoperative internal hernia. At times it may be difficult to approximate the mesentery of the right colon and ileum to the right lumbar gutter and effect a closure **(Figures 20 and 21)**. The surgeon should palpate the right gutter repeatedly and make whatever sutures are necessary to completely close it. A pair of Babcock or Allis forceps is then inserted into the lumen of the ileum, and the ileum is everted on itself. The completed ileostomy should extend upward from the skin level at least 2.5 to 3 cm. The mucosa is anchored with interrupted fine catgut sutures to the skin **(Figure 21)**. No suture should be taken through the bowel wall because of the possibility of developing a fistula. Likewise, the mesentery may be anchored to the peritoneum, but no sutures should be taken between the seromuscular coat of the terminal ileum and the peritoneum. After this a temporary gastrostomy can be performed (see Plate IX).

CLOSURE. The abdominal wound is carefully closed with silk mattress sutures to the peritoneum and interrupted sutures to the fascia, subcutaneous tissue, and skin. In the presence of marked emaciation and prolonged steroid therapy, the use of retention sutures should be considered.

The anus is excised as described in the perineal section of abdominoperineal resection (Plates LIV and LV). The only exception is that it is not necessary to go wide on the levators, and a simple extirpation of the sphincter muscles and bowel wall itself is carried out. Likewise, because of the frequency of fistula-in-ano, etc., it is usually judicious to insert drainage rather than attempt primary closure. However, primary closure with constant sterile plastic catheter suction can be used in the absence of gross contamination during excision of the rectum.

POSTOPERATIVE CARE. Blood should be replaced as it is lost during the procedure. Additional blood or colloids are usually required on the afternoon of surgery and during the early postoperative period. Constant bladder drainage is maintained for at least a week. If the patient has been on steroid therapy, this is continued during the postoperative period. A transparent temporary-type ileostomy appliance is placed over the ileostomy before moving the patient to the recovery area. This permits frequent observations of the stoma to make sure it maintains a pink and viable color. A strict intake and output chart must be maintained at all times following an ileostomy. Likewise, daily electrolyte determinations are essential because of excessive losses of electrolyte-rich fluid. It may be necessary to insert the gloved small finger through the ileostomy if it does not begin to function properly within the first 24 hours. Excessive amounts of fluid are occasionally lost, and large amounts of intravenous fluids, electrolytes, and colloids will be required to maintain fluid balance. Antibiotic therapy is continued for five to seven days. Gradually, a liquid diet is replaced by a diet of choice. The drains, if used, should be removed slowly from the perineal wound, making certain that the skin opening is kept patent for several weeks to allow adequate drainage and healing from the inside out. These patients require frequent and prolonged observation because of the tendency to a variety of complications ranging from abscess formation to intestinal obstruction.

PLATE LX   TOTAL COLECTOMY

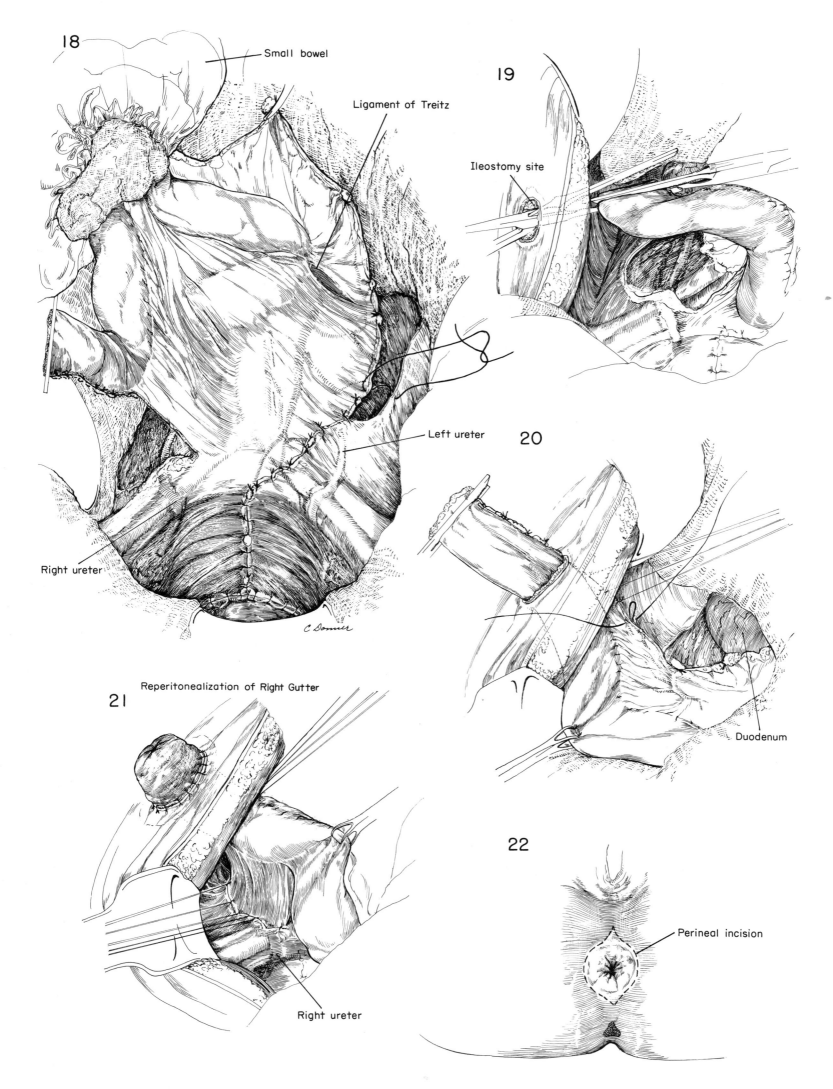

18 Small bowel

Ligament of Treitz

Left ureter

Right ureter

19 Ileostomy site

20

21 Reperitonealization of Right Gutter

Right ureter

Duodenum

22 Perineal incision

PLATE LXI · ANTERIOR RESECTION OF RECTOSIGMOID: END-TO-END ANASTOMOSIS

INDICATIONS. This may be the operation of choice in selected individuals with malignant lesions in the rectosigmoid or low sigmoid area in order to reestablish the continuity of the bowel and obviate a permanent colostomy. The operation is based on the premises (1) that the viability of the lower rectum can be sustained from the middle or inferior hemorrhoidal vessels, and (2) that carcinoma in this region as a rule metastasizes cephalad, only rarely metastasizing 3 to 4 cm. below the primary growth. It is questionable if an anterior resection should be advised for growths occurring much below the peritoneal reflection of the cul-de-sac. The ideal situation would appear to be a small tumor located at the junction of the rectum and the sigmoid. On some infrequent occasions this operation may be indicated if the patient refuses a colostomy, but it is considered routinely if there is evidence of metastasis to the liver or elsewhere. However, there are many times when the growth can be mobilized much more than anticipated, especially when the bowel is released down to the levator muscles. The exposure is another factor that may influence the surgeon for or against a low anastomosis. A low anastomosis is much easier and safer in the female than in the male, especially if the pelvic organs of the former have been previously removed. A catheter cecostomy or a transverse colostomy is sometimes done at the time to divert the fecal stream temporarily from the end-to-end anastomosis or to ensure decompression of an inadequately emptied colon. A side-to-end (Baker) anastomosis should be considered when there is considerable discrepancy between the sizes of the two lumina or an excess of fat that may encroach unduly upon the lumen of an end-to-end anastomosis.

PREOPERATIVE CARE. See Plate XLII.

ANESTHESIA. See Plate XLV.

POSITION. The patient is placed in the Trendelenburg position. The transverse position is useful while the splenic flexure is being mobilized.

OPERATIVE PREPARATION. The skin is prepared in the usual manner.

INCISION AND EXPOSURE. A left paramedian incision is made from the symphysis to a level above and to the left of the umbilicus. The liver and upper abdomen are carefully palpated to determine the existence of any metastases. The site of the tumor is examined with special consideration as to its size and location, the amount of dilation of the bowel proximal to the growth, and the ease of exposure. In many instances the type of resection cannot be determined until the lower segment of the bowel has been mobilized.

The small intestines are walled off in a plastic bag, and a self-retaining retractor is inserted into the wound. The peritoneum of the pelvic colon is freed from the region of the sigmoid downward on either side **(Figure 3)**. It is important at this point to identify and isolate both ureters and the spermatic or ovarian vessels. The peritoneum is divided anterior to the rectum at the level of the base of the bladder or cervix, as the sex determines. The growth can be further mobilized if the surgeon passes his right hand posteriorly down to the hollow of the sacrum (see Plate LI, **Figure 8**). After the peritoneal attachments have all been divided, and the rectum is freed both posteriorly and anteriorly by blunt finger dissection, it is possible to bring this growth up into the wound and gain considerable distance as a result of freeing and straightening the rectum **(Figures 1 and 2)**. The blood supply to the distal segment from the inferior hemorrhoidal vessels is adequate, should the middle hemorrhoidal vessels be ligated to ensure additional mobilization. The inferior mesenteric artery is ligated as it arises from the aorta **(Figure 3)**. The inferior mesenteric vein is also ligated. The blood supply to the colon must now come from the middle colic artery through the marginal vessels of Drummond.

The bowel should be prepared for division at least 4 cm. below the gross lower limits of the growth to assure removal of all adjacent lymph nodes. A Stone or a Pace-Potts anastomosis clamp is applied across the previously prepared site of division of the bowel, and a long, right-angle

kidney pedicle clamp may be utilized for the proximal clamp. The area is sealed off with gauze, and the bowel is divided between the clamps. The bowel containing the growth is then brought outside the wound, and clamps are applied to the previously prepared site well above the lesion **(Figure 5)**. The surgeon must now determine that the upper segment of the bowel is sufficiently mobile to be brought down for anastomosis without tension. In order to accomplish this, it may be necessary to divide the lateral peritoneal attachment of the left colon up to and including the splenic flexure. Unless the sigmoid is very redundant, the left half of the transverse colon along with the splenic flexure must be mobilized. The incision is extended at this point to ensure a good exposure, since undue traction on the colon may tear the capsule of the spleen with resultant hemorrhage. The lesser sac is entered after the splenic attachments to the colon have been divided. The greater omentum is freed from the transverse colon as shown in Plate XXI. Extra mobility and length of bowel are provided until repeated trials clearly demonstrate that the proximal segment will easily reach the site of anastomosis. The adequacy of the blood supply should be determined even when the bowel is extended down into the pelvis as a preliminary to the anastomosis.

The serosa along the mesenteric border of the upper segment should be cleared of fat for at least 1 cm. proximal to the Pace-Potts clamp **(Figure 5)**. Likewise, the margins and especially the posterior wall of the lower segment must be cleared of fat adjacent to the Pace-Potts clamp **(Figure 5)**. Careful dissection with repeated application of small clamps may be necessary to accomplish a clean serosal boundary of 1 cm. adjacent to the clamp in preparation for a safe anastomosis. Following this, the two ends of the clamps are approximated and then manipulated so that a posterior serosal layer of 00 silk can be placed easily **(Figure 6)**. The ends of these sutures are cut, except those at either angle, which are retained for traction. As a preliminary to removing the clamp, the field is walled off with gauze, and an enterostomy clamp is gently applied to the upper segment to prevent gross soiling **(Figure 6)**. The crushed contents of the clamps may be excised. The lower clamp is then removed, and the crushed margin of bowel is excised and opened **(Figure 7)**. Suction is instituted to avoid any gross contamination of the field. Fine silk sutures may be inserted for traction in the midportion of the lower opening and at either angle. These traction sutures tend to facilitate the anastomosis (see Plate XLV, **Figure 17**). The posterior mucosal layer is approximated with several Babcock forceps, and the mucosa is approximated with interrupted 0000 silk sutures **(Figure 8)**. The anterior serosal surface is closed with interrupted 0000 silk sutures of the Connell type, with the knot on the outside. Following this, the anterior serosal layer is carefully placed, using interrupted Halsted sutures of fine 00 silk. The peritoneum is anchored adjacent to the suture line. The patency of the anastomosis, as well as the lack of tension on the suture line, should be tested. The peritoneal floor is closed with interrupted silk sutures **(Figure 10)**. The raw surfaces are covered by approximating the mesenteric margin of the sigmoid to the right peritoneal margin **(Figure 10)**. The sigmoid is loosely attached to the left pelvic wall by anchoring the fat pads, not bowel cecostomy wall, to the left peritoneal margin to prevent subsequent tension on the anastomosis as well as to cover the raw surfaces. A transverse colostomy or a cecostomy should be considered if there is any suspicion regarding the technical perfection of the anastomosis. A drain may be inserted into the left side of the pelvis and brought out at the lower angle of the wound. Some operators prefer to have a rectal tube in place, which can be guided up beyond the anastomosis to assist in decompressing the bowel during the early postoperative period.

CLOSURE. Closure is performed in a routine manner.

POSTOPERATIVE CARE. The rectal tube is left in place for several days. Small irrigations can be carried out at this time, but regular enemas should be avoided. The patient is gradually allowed to resume a full diet. Mineral oil is given. If a transverse colostomy is used, the patency of the anastomosis may be previously tested by a barium enema before closure is effected several weeks after the anastomosis. See Postoperative Care, Plate LIII, for general postoperative care.

PLATE LXI   ANTERIOR RESECTION OF RECTOSIGMOID: END-TO-END ANASTOMOSIS

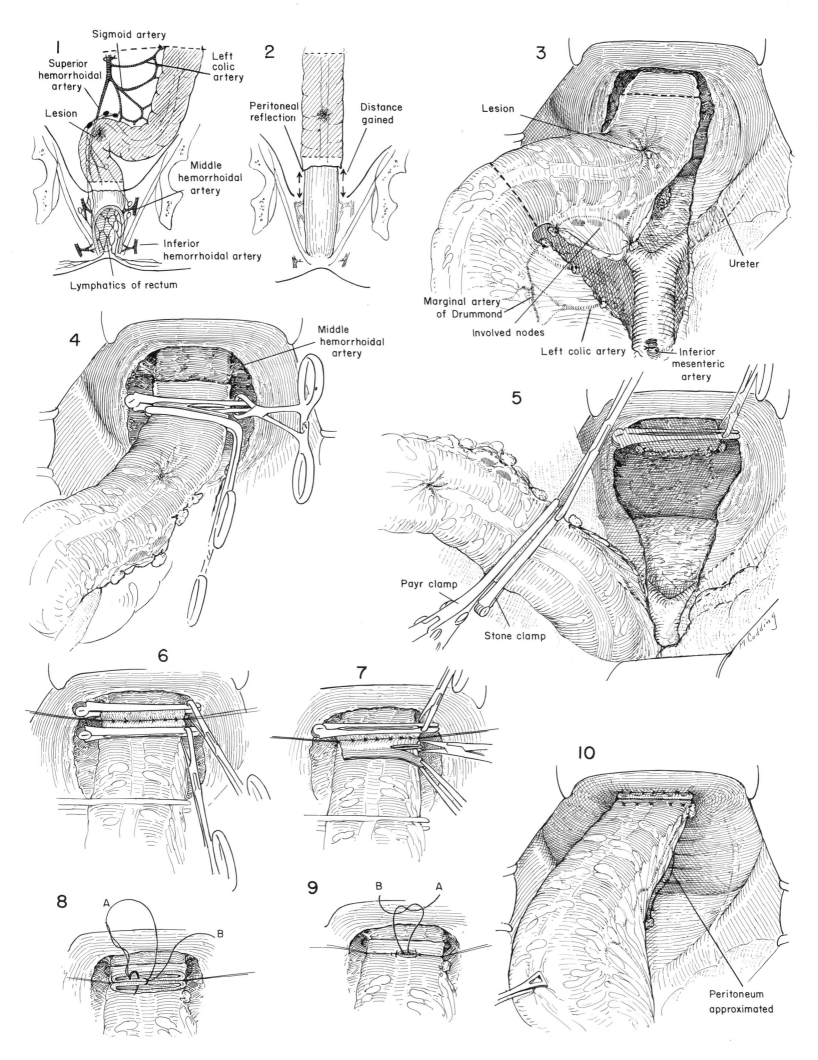

1

Sigmoid artery
Superior hemorrhoidal artery
Left colic artery
Lesion
Middle hemorrhoidal artery
Inferior hemorrhoidal artery
Lymphatics of rectum

2

Peritoneal reflection
Distance gained

3

Lesion
Ureter
Marginal artery of Drummond
Involved nodes
Left colic artery
Inferior mesenteric artery

4

Middle hemorrhoidal artery

5

Payr clamp
Stone clamp

6

7

8

A
B

9

B   A

10

Peritoneum approximated

M Codding

PLATE LXII · ANTERIOR RESECTION OF RECTOSIGMOID: SIDE-TO-END ANASTOMOSIS (BAKER)

INDICATIONS. The low-lying lesions of the rectum and rectosigmoid may be resected and bowel continuity established anterior to the sacrum in a variety of ways. While the end-to-end anastomosis (Plate LXI) can be used, side-to-end anastomosis is advantageous in cases with considerable discrepancy in size between the resected bowel and the rectal stump, particularly in obese patients. When the lesion is so low that abdominoperineal resection, with sacrifice of the rectum, would be ordinarily indicated, and in the presence of distant metastases, or when the patient refuses to give permission for a permanent colostomy, bowel continuity can be established by a very low side-to-end anastomosis.

The principles of cancer surgery should be observed, including bloc excision of the lymphatic drainage area and early ligation of the inferior mesenteric vessels near the point of origin **(Figures 1 and 2).** The blood supply to the sigmoid will be sustained through the marginal artery of Drummond via the middle colic artery arising from the superior mesenteric artery. The malignant lesion of the rectosigmoid should be at least 10 cm. above the anus unless the anterior resection is carried out for palliation alone. At least 5 cm. and preferably more of the bowel should be resected below the malignant tumor to assure removal of all adjacent lymph nodes. The continuity can be re-established after the descending colon, the splenic flexure, and the left portion of the transverse colon are mobilized **(Figure 3).**

The entire right colon can be freed from its lateral peritoneal attachments and rotated to its embryologic position on the left side of the abdomen, if more mobility is desired.

The advantages of the side-to-end anastomosis include assurance of a larger and more secure anastomosis than is possible by the end-to-end method.

PREOPERATIVE PREPARATION. After the lesion has been proved to be malignant by microscopic examination, and polyps or secondary lesions ruled out by appropriate sigmoidoscopic and barium studies of the colon, the patient is given nonabsorbable oral antibiotics. A low-residue diet, which may be shifted to a clear liquid diet for a day or so before surgery, is advisable. Any blood volume deficiency must be replaced, as patients with carcinoma of the large intestine, particularly with associated marked weight loss, often have a contracted blood volume with a deceptively normal hematocrit. A preliminary intravenous pyelogram will locate the courses of the ureters. This aids in evaluating kidney function and ensures the absence of ureteral obstruction.

The rectum is irrigated with soapsuds or saline enema. A rectal tube is introduced into the rectum for intermittent suction and subsequently directed on through the anastomosis, if desired. An indwelling urethral catheter ensures a collapsed bladder, providing better exposure of deep pelvic structures.

ANESTHESIA. General endotracheal anesthesia is satisfactory. Spinal anesthesia may be used.

POSITION. The patient is placed near the left side of the table and so immobilized that the Trendelenburg position can be assumed during the final anastomosis without difficulty.

OPERATIVE PREPARATION. The skin is prepared from the symphysis up to the epigastrium. Plastic drapes or sterile towels are applied.

INCISION AND EXPOSURE. A midline incision is made, starting just above the symphysis and extending down to the umbilicus and around it on the left side. The height to which the incision is carried in the epigastrium depends on the location of the splenic flexure, as seen on the barium enema. Because it will be necessary to detach the splenic flexure, easy exposure of this area must be provided. Undue tension of the left half of the colon and splenic flexure will tear the splenic capsule, causing blood loss and risking splenectomy.

After the abdomen is opened, a self-retaining retractor of the Balfour type is inserted, and the liver is palpated for evidence of metastasis. Palpation should be carried out well over the top of both lobes of the liver as well as on the undersurface. Likewise, lymph nodes along the course of the inferior mesenteric artery and at the bifurcation of the aorta are inspected for evidence of involvement. The position and fixation of the tumor are ascertained by palpation. In the presence of metastasis to the liver or seeding throughout the general peritoneal cavity, a sleeve type of segmental resection is indicated. When a palliative resection is carried out, wide dissection of the inferior mesenteric blood supply up to the point of origin in the region of the ligament of Treitz is not necessary.

DETAILS OF PROCEDURE. After it has been decided that the lesion is resectable, that an anterior resection is warranted, and that adequate bowel can be resected distal to the tumor, the small intestines are walled off in a plastic bag, and the transverse colon and splenic flexure are mobilized **(Figure 4).**

While the omentum is held upward, sharp dissection is used to divide the attachment of the omentum to the transverse colon. A few blood vessels may need to be ligated during this procedure. Opening into the lesser sac above the transverse colon ensures an easier and safer separation of the omentum from the splenic flexure of the colon, particularly in the obese patient. Again, great care must be exercised as the splenocolic ligament is divided in order to avoid tearing the splenic capsule. Clamps should be applied in this area so that the contents of the splenocolic ligament can be carefully divided and ligated **(Figure 5).**

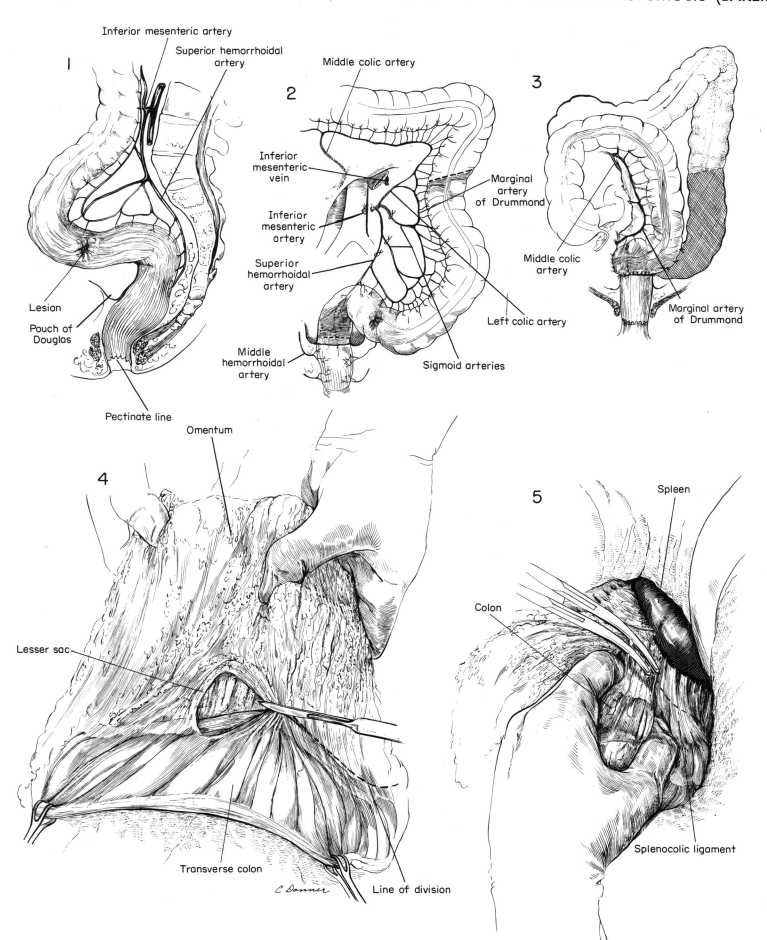

1

Inferior mesenteric artery

Superior hemorrhoidal artery

Lesion

Pouch of Douglas

Pectinate line

2

Middle colic artery

Inferior mesenteric vein

Inferior mesenteric artery

Superior hemorrhoidal artery

Middle hemorrhoidal artery

Marginal artery of Drummond

Left colic artery

Sigmoid arteries

3

Middle colic artery

Marginal artery of Drummond

4

Omentum

Lesser sac

Transverse colon

Line of division

C Donner

5

Spleen

Colon

Splenocolic ligament

PLATE LXIII · ANTERIOR RESECTION OF RECTOSIGMOID: SIDE-TO-END ANASTOMOSIS (BAKER)

DETAILS OF PROCEDURE (*Continued*). The peritoneum over the region of the left kidney is divided as gentle traction is maintained downward and medially on the splenic flexure of the colon. There is a tendency to grasp the colon and to encircle it completely with the fingers. This tends to puncture the thinned-out mesentery. Usually, rents can be avoided if a gauze pack is used to gently sweep the splenic flexure downward and medially **(Figure 6)**. Usually, it is unnecessary to divide and ligate any vessels during this procedure. If a tear in the splenic capsule causes bleeding that cannot be easily controlled by coagulant sponges, the spleen should be removed. The peritoneum in the left lumbar gutter is divided, and the entire descending colon is swept medially.

The rectosigmoid is freed from the hollow of the sacrum as shown in Plates LI and LII. The sigmoid is first separated from any attachments to the iliac fossa on the left side, and the left gonadal vessels and the ureter are identified throughout their course in the field of operation **(Figure 7)**. Then the surgeon passes his right hand down into the hollow of the sacrum to free the rectosigmoid by blunt finger dissection. Often, especially in the female, a very low-lying lesion can be mobilized and lifted up well into the wound (see Plate XLVII). The tumor is wrapped in gauze pads, and they are tied around the bowel as soon as sufficient mobilization has been provided.

After the bowel has been freed from the hollow of the sacrum, the fingers of the left hand should separate the right ureter from the overlying peritoneum by blunt disection **(Figure 8)**. The peritoneum is incised some distance from the tumor, and the rectum is freed further down to the region of the levator muscles. Division of the middle hemorrhoidal vessels with the suspensory ligaments may be necessary to ensure the needed length of bowel to be resected below the tumor. The surgeon should not hesitate to divide the peritoneal attachments in the region of the pouch of Douglas, to free the rectum from the prostate gland in the male and from the posterior wall of the vagina in the female. The rectum may be encircled by braided silk ligature below as well as above the tumor to limit the intraluminal spread of tumor cells **(Figure 9)**. The inferior mesenteric artery is freed from the underlying aorta to near its point of origin **(Figure 9)**. Three curved clamps are applied to the inferior mesenteric artery, and the vessel is divided and ligated with 00 silk. The inferior mesenteric vein should be ligated at this time, before the tumor has been palpated and compressed due to the manipulation required during resection.

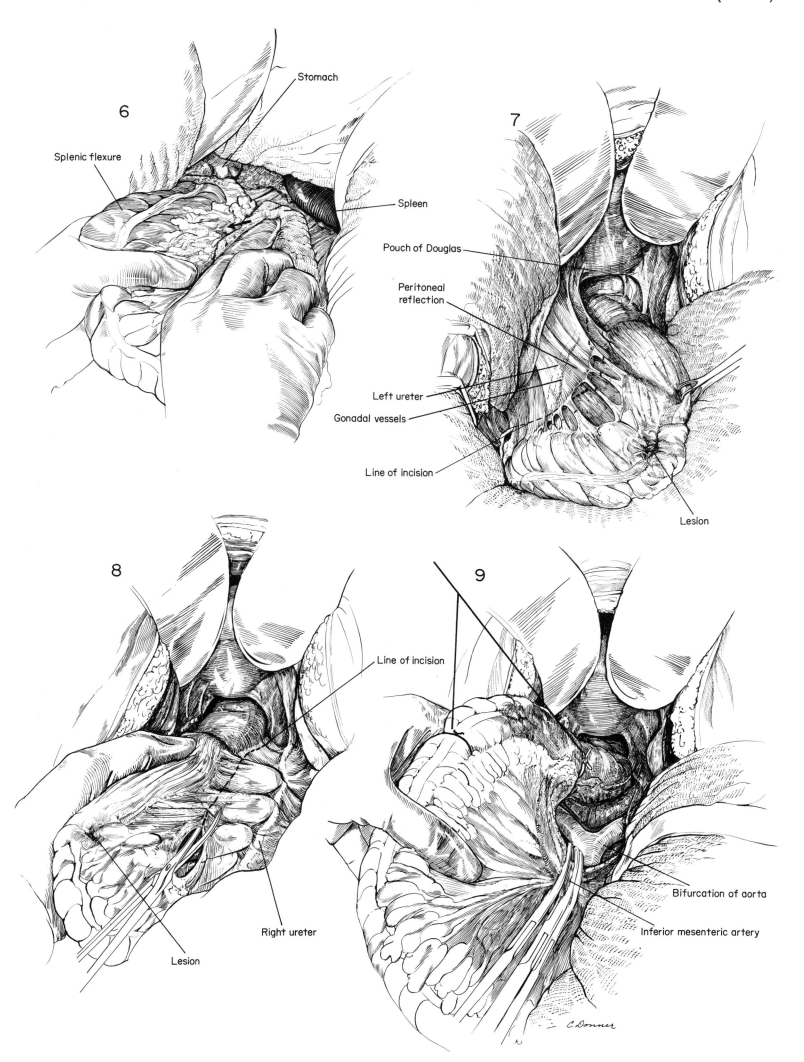

C Donner

PLATE LXIV · ANTERIOR RESECTION OF RECTOSIGMOID: SIDE-TO-END ANASTOMOSIS (BAKER)

DETAILS OF PROCEDURE (*Continued*). After the mesenteric vessels have been ligated and the rectum has been mobilized adequately, a Pace-Potts clamp is applied across the bowel at least 5 to 10 cm. below the tumor **(Figure 10A).** The position of both ureters should once again be identified before the clamp is applied. A straight clamp is applied 1 cm. proximal to the noncrushing clamp, and the bowel is divided **(Figure 10B).** As soon as possible the specimen is wrapped in a large pack held in place by encircling ties **(Figure 11).**

It is reassuring for the surgeon, especially in obese patients, to see active pulsations at the anastomotic site, and he should take the time to free the mobilized colon and to loosen any tension on the middle colic vessels. Procaine, 1 per cent, can be injected into the mesentery to strengthen pulsations in elderly patients or in the presence of large fat deposits in the mesentery **(Figure 11).** The small bowel should be returned to the abdomen from the plastic bag, since the base of the mesentery of the small intestine can compress the middle colic vessels, particularly if the small intestine is placed on the abdominal wall above and to the right of the umbilicus **(Figure 12).** The blood supply improves as the colon resection nears the middle colic vessels, since the descending colon is now dependent upon the marginal vessels of Drummond arising from the middle colic vessels **(Figure 12).** The entire transverse colon as well as the right colon may be mobilized by detaching the omentum and the peritoneal attachments as indicated by the dotted line **(Figure 12).**

The mesentery is divided up to the bowel wall **(Figure 13)** where active pulsations have been identified. The mesentery to the sigmoid is further mobilized and divided until a sufficient amount of bowel has been isolated proximal to the lesion.

The remaining colon must be sufficiently mobilized to then reach the rectal stump loosely and without tension. Extra mobility is mandatory, since postoperative distention of the bowel and subsequent tension on the suture line must be anticipated.

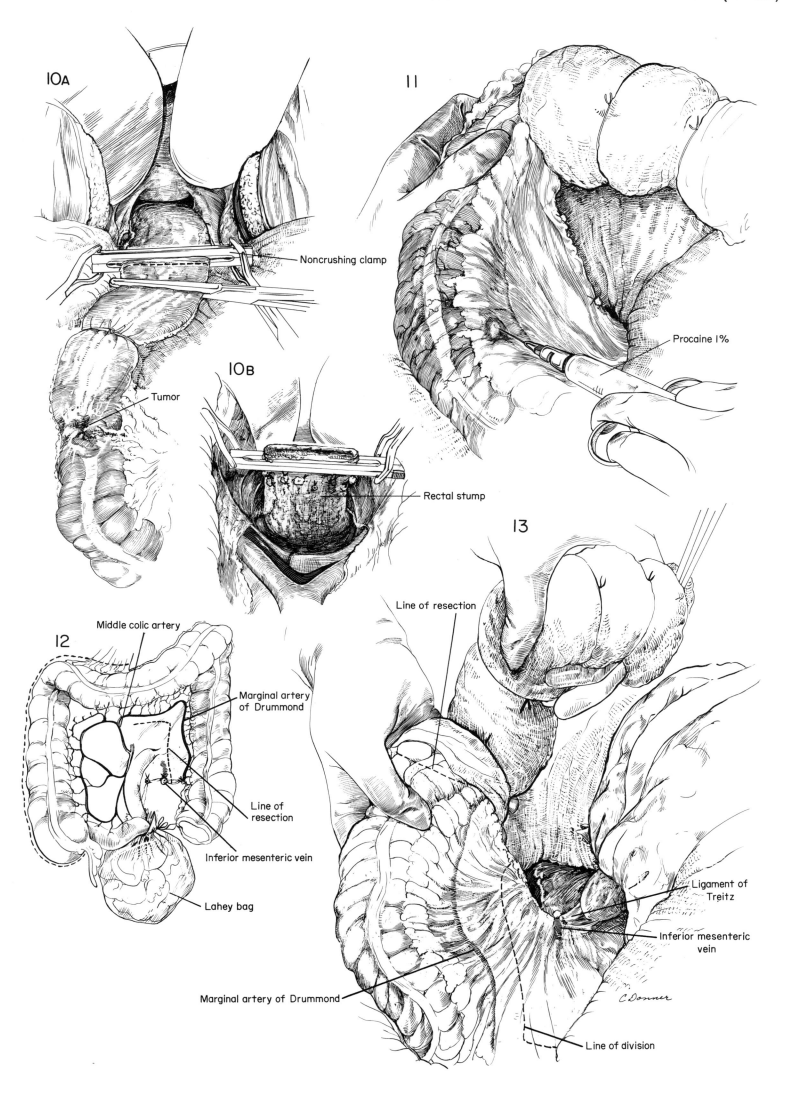

10A

Noncrushing clamp

Tumor

10B

Rectal stump

11

Procaine 1%

13

Line of resection

Middle colic artery

12

Marginal artery of Drummond

Line of resection

Inferior mesenteric vein

Lahey bag

Marginal artery of Drummond

Ligament of Treitz

Inferior mesenteric vein

Line of division

C Donner

PLATE LXV · ANTERIOR RESECTION OF RECTOSIGMOID: SIDE-TO-END ANASTOMOSIS (BAKER)

DETAILS OF PROCEDURE (*Continued*). The bowel is divided obliquely after the mesentery has been cleared off to about 1 cm. from the clamp **(Figure 14).** The mobility of this segment of bowel is tested by bringing it down to the region of the rectal stump to be absolutely certain that side-to-end anastomosis can be carried out without tension. If the initial segment is too tight, additional transverse colon may be mobilized. The hepatic flexure can be freed as well as the entire right colon. Any attachments constricting the mesentery of the descending colon can be divided. The presence of active arterial pulsations should be determined while the closed end of the colon is held deep in the pelvis. The end of the bowel is closed with two layers of 0000 silk sutures which may be left long for purposes of traction.

The taenia adjacent to the mesentery along the inferior surface of the mobilized segment is grasped with Babcock forceps, and traction sutures (A and B) are placed at either end of the proposed opening **(Figure 15).** These sutures keep the inferior taenia under traction during the subsequent placement of the posterior serosal row of interrupted 00 silk sutures **(Figure 16).** The traction suture (B) should be within 2 cm. of the closed end of the bowel, since it is undesirable to leave a long blind stump of colon beyond the site of the anastomosis. After this, the Pace-Potts clamp is removed. The margins of the rectal stump are protected by gauze pads to avoid gross spilling and contamination. It is advisable to excise the edge of the rectal stump if it has been damaged by the clamp. The color of the mucosa and viability of the rectal stump should be rechecked. Any bleeding points on the edge of the rectal stump are grasped and ligated with 0000 silk. It has been found useful for exposure to insert a traction suture (C) in the midportion of the anterior wall of the rectum. This keeps the bowel under modest traction and aids in subsequent placement of mucosal sutures. A noncrushing clamp may be applied across the colon to avoid the possibility of gross contamination. After the posterior suture row has been placed, an incision is made between the traction sutures (A and B) along the taenia, and the lumen of the proximal bowel is opened **(Figure 17).** All contamination is removed in both angles of the openings. The same type of traction suture (C) can be placed in the midportion of the wall of the sigmoid. The mucosa is approximated by interrupted 0000 silk sutures **(Figure 17).** These sutures are changed to an inverted Connell type as the angles are closed. The midline traction sutures remain, while the anterior mucosal row continues with interrupted Connell-type sutures **(Figure 18).**

This provides a large stoma. The patency of the stoma is determined by palpation. The anterior serosal row of interrupted parallel mattress sutures of 00 silk is placed to approximate the anterior rectal wall to the colon **(Figure 19).** After completion of the serosal row, traction sutures

can be removed. If the peritoneal reflection in the pouch of Douglas has been retained, and the anastomosis has been carried out near this level, the peritoneum may be anchored to the sigmoid for additional support **(Figure 20).**

To release tension from the suture line as the bowel becomes dilated in the early postoperative period, it is useful to anchor some fat pads to the peritoneal reflection in the iliac fossa. This seals off entrance into the pelvis as it anchors the bowel in this area. Likewise, the free medial edge of the mesentery should be approximated to the right peritoneal margin in order to cover all raw surfaces. As this peritoneum is closed, the course and location of both ureters must be identified repeatedly to avoid including them in a suture **(Figure 20).**

Just before the peritoneum is finally closed, the hollow of the sacrum should be irrigated with saline and emptied by suction of any collection of blood.

After completing the anastomosis, the surgeon should recheck the adequacy of the distal blood supply. The decision must now be made as to the necessity of providing decompression by a temporary cecostomy.

Cecostomy should be used in very obese patients when it is anticipated that the distended colon may not return to normal function quickly. Cecostomy is adequate, making prolonged nasogastric suction or temporary gastrostomy unnecessary. If the appendix is present, it can be removed and the base used for the introduction of a mushroom catheter. The catheter is inserted 10 to 12 cm. into the colon, and the opening inverted around it. The catheter is then brought out through a separate stab wound, and the tip of the cecum is anchored to the peritoneum. This avoids the possibility of leakage if the catheter is accidentally removed.

CLOSURE. The closure is made with interrupted mattress sutures of 00 silk to the peritoneum, figure-of-eight to the fascia, and fine silk to the fat and skin. Retention sutures may be used in the very obese patient and in patients with chronic coughing.

POSTOPERATIVE CARE. Blood volume should be restored as it is lost. The patient is continued on constant bladder drainage and the hourly output of urine maintained at 25 to 30 ml. The cecostomy tube is attached to a drainage bottle without suction. Electrolyte balance is maintained. Systemic antibiotics may or may not be given. Early on the first postoperative day the cecostomy catheter can be irrigated with saline to promote drainage and injected with an ounce of mineral oil. The cecostomy is then left open to provide decompression, and additional amounts of mineral oil can be added during subsequent days until normal bowel activity has been restored.

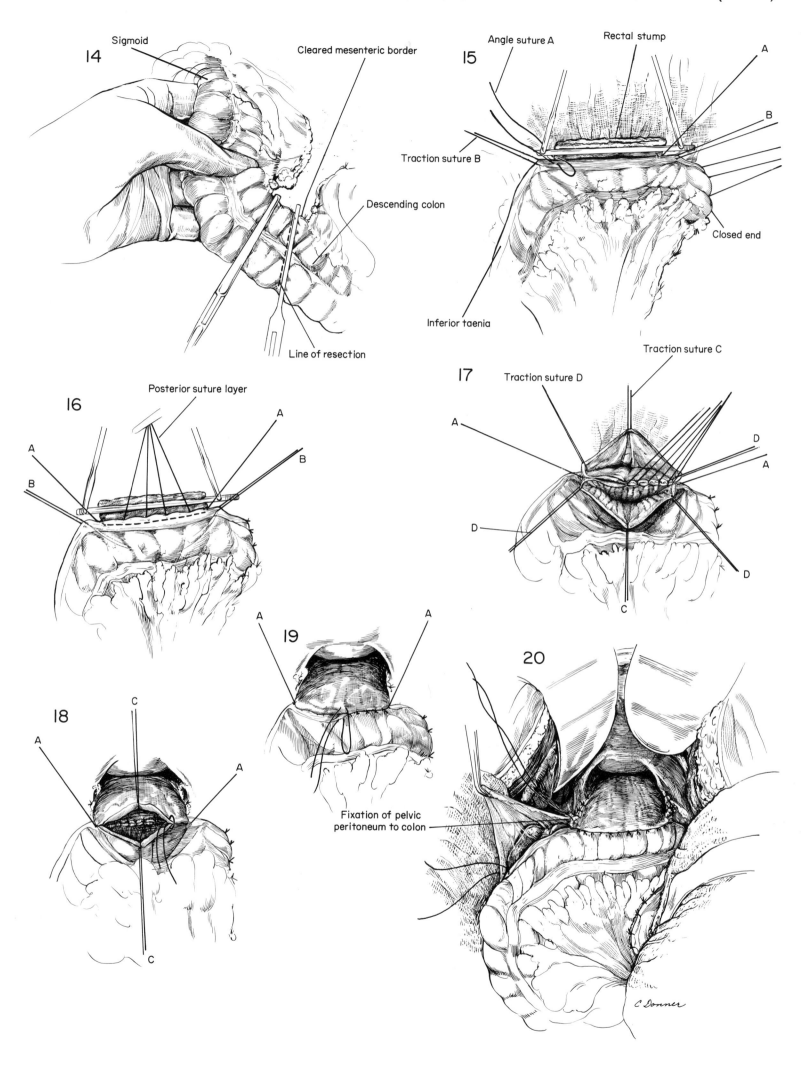

14   Sigmoid   Cleared mesenteric border

Descending colon

Line of resection

15   Angle suture A   Rectal stump   A

B

Traction suture B

Closed end

Inferior taenia

16   Posterior suture layer   A

A

B   B

17   Traction suture C   Traction suture D

A   D

A

D

D

C

18   C   19   A   A

A   A

C

Fixation of pelvic
peritoneum to colon

20

C. Donner

PLATE LXVI · COLOTOMY AND EXCISION OF POLYP

INDICATIONS. This operation is performed to diagnose and remove pedunculated lesions above the reach of the sigmoidoscope or not feasibly removed through the colonoscope. The principal indications for polypectomy are (1) size greater than 2 cm., (2) multiplicity, (3) a broad, sessile base, (4) progressive increase in size, and (5) appearance in a patient with previously documented bowel malignancy. These polyps should be visualized by preoperative barium enema with air contrast examination, and the remainder of the gastrointestinal tract must be evaluated.

PREOPERATIVE PREPARATION. The patient is prepared as for partial colectomy. During the preoperative evaluation it is imperative to correct any anemia that may be discovered and to correct hypokalemia if diarrhea has been a prominent part of the patient's symptomatology. Nonabsorbable intestinal antibiotics may be given for one to four days before surgery, along with a low-residue diet and vitamin K. A clear liquid diet is given on the day preceding the operation. A cathartic on the afternoon before surgery and enemas that evening complete the patient's preparation. The operator and assistant must carefully examine the barium studies to determine the location of the polyp relative to the pelvic brim and other landmarks. The assistant must determine that the sterile endoscopes and cautery are working satisfactorily before starting the skin preparation. A Foley catheter in the bladder and a rectal tube may facilitate exposure of sigmoid polyps.

ANESTHESIA. Either spinal or general anesthesia is satisfactory.

POSITION. The patient is placed in a comfortable supine position with the left side close to the edge of the table. A pillow is placed under the knees. Trendelenburg position may be advantageous, and it may be helpful to rotate the table slightly during colonoscopy.

OPERATIVE PREPARATION. The skin is prepared in the routine manner.

INCISION AND EXPOSURE. Since approximately 74 per cent of polyps of the large colon are located distal to the splenic flexure, the operator will most frequently use a low left paramedian incision **(Figure 1).** Polyps of the cecum and ascending colon may be visualized better through a right paramedian incision. It may be desirable to use an upper abdominal midline incision for lesions of the transverse colon. After opening the peritoneum, the operator carefully explores the abdomen, including the liver, to determine the presence of metastatic or unsuspected disease. The small bowel is held out of the operative field by packing. Attention is directed to the mesentery of the bowel where the polyp is thought to be located. If there is evidence of lymphadenopathy or induration of the adjacent bowel and base of the polyp suggestive of malignancy, partial colectomy is indicated. If no such findings are present, the operator then examines and palpates the colon in the affected region in order to locate the lesion. As the stalk is placed under gentle tension, the base of the lesion may be identified by invagination of the bowel wall **(Figure 3).** If necessary, the colon can be mobilized by incising its lateral peritoneal reflection and by taking down the splenic or hepatic flexures. In the presence of several widely separated polyps or recurrent polyps, the entire right, transverse, descending, and rectosigmoid colon should be mobilized to facilitate a thorough sigmoidoscopic examination. Increased mobility is provided if the greater omentum is detached from the transverse colon. Some prefer to insert a plastic wound protector to minimize the amount of possible wound contamination and potential wound infection.

DETAILS OF PROCEDURE. Common sites for introduction of the endoscope into the mobilized colon are shown in **Figure 1.** Sigmoid colotomy for colonoscopy should be performed as close as possible to the presumed level of the lesion. After the small bowel is packed away, the colon is brought into the wound, and the area is walled off with gauze pads. A purse-string suture of 0000 silk may be placed in the anterior taenia of the colon as an alternative to angle sutures. The surgeon incises the colon for a distance equal to one-half the circumference of the sigmoidoscope. The assistant facilitates introduction of the sigmoidoscope by grasping the edges of the colotomy with forceps or Babcock clamps **(Figure 2).** The endoscope is then passed distally, and a noncrushing intestinal clamp is applied below the level of the tip of this instrument. Another clamp is applied proximal to the instrument, and the purse-string or angle sutures are placed on tension. The operator may then distend the colon with air in order to slowly withdraw the endoscope to visualize any polyps present. When the lesion is identified, its level is marked by a loose suture through the epiploic appendix at this level or by application of a mosquito clamp to the appendix. Proximal colonoscopy may be performed by removing the proximal clamp and directing the instrument toward the splenic flexure.

After identification, the lesion may be removed by the use of a snare and cautery. As an alternative, it may be delivered into the operative wound by evagination of the colonic mucosa. If this cannot be achieved, the colotomy is closed, and a separate colotomy is performed along the presenting taenia at the level of the lesion.

After the area of the base of the polyp is brought into the operative wound, it is isolated by gauze pads. Angle sutures of 00 silk are placed at the lateral border of the presenting taenia. A longitudinal incision at the level of the base of the polyp is then made in the anterior taenia. The assistant is prepared to use suction while the bowel is opened **(Figure 3).** Noncrushing Babcock clamps are applied to the edges of the colotomy to effect hemostasis and facilitate exposure. The stalk of the polyp is then divided between straight mosquito clamps **(Figure 4),** and the specimen is sent for frozen-section pathologic examination. The base of the polyp is then transfixed with 0000 silk suture ligatures **(Figure 5).** After removing the clamp at the base of the polyp, the operator carefully inspects the stump to be sure that hemostasis is adequate. The stump of the polyp is then returned to the lumen of the bowel, and the adjacent area is inspected visually for other lesions **(Figure 6).** The assistant then places gentle tension on the angle sutures, and the colotomy is closed transversely in two layers. After closing the inner layer with interrupted inverting Connell stitches **(Figure 7),** the surgeon uses interrupted horizontal mattress stitches to approximate the seromuscular layer **(Figure 8).** The epiploic appendices are apposed over the closed colotomy wound, and the area is marked with a silver clip for subsequent identification of the site of the polyp during follow-up barium studies **(Figure 9).** The lumen is checked for adequacy with the thumb and forefinger. Contaminated pads and instruments are removed from the field.

If the stalk of the polyp is short, excision can be accomplished by removing a longitudinal elliptical wedge of mucosa with the specimen. In this event the mucosa is approximated in the transverse direction with interrupted 0000 silk sutures.

CLOSURE. The closure is made with interrupted mattress sutures of 00 silk to the peritoneum, figure-of-eight to the fascia, and fine silk to the fat and the skin.

POSTOPERATIVE CARE. Most patients are able to ambulate the evening of surgery and definitely should be walking on the day following surgery. Many will be able to take sips of water on the day after the operation. Intravenous fluids are used if necessary. No cathartics or enemas are given during the patient's convalescence. However, once oral intake is initiated, the patient should be given stool softeners. A low rectal tube may relieve gas. Following the patient's first postoperative bowel movement, he may be advanced to a soft and then a low-residue diet. Repeated sigmoidoscopic and air contrast studies should be scheduled for regular intervals.

PLATE LXVI   COLOTOMY AND EXCISION OF POLYP

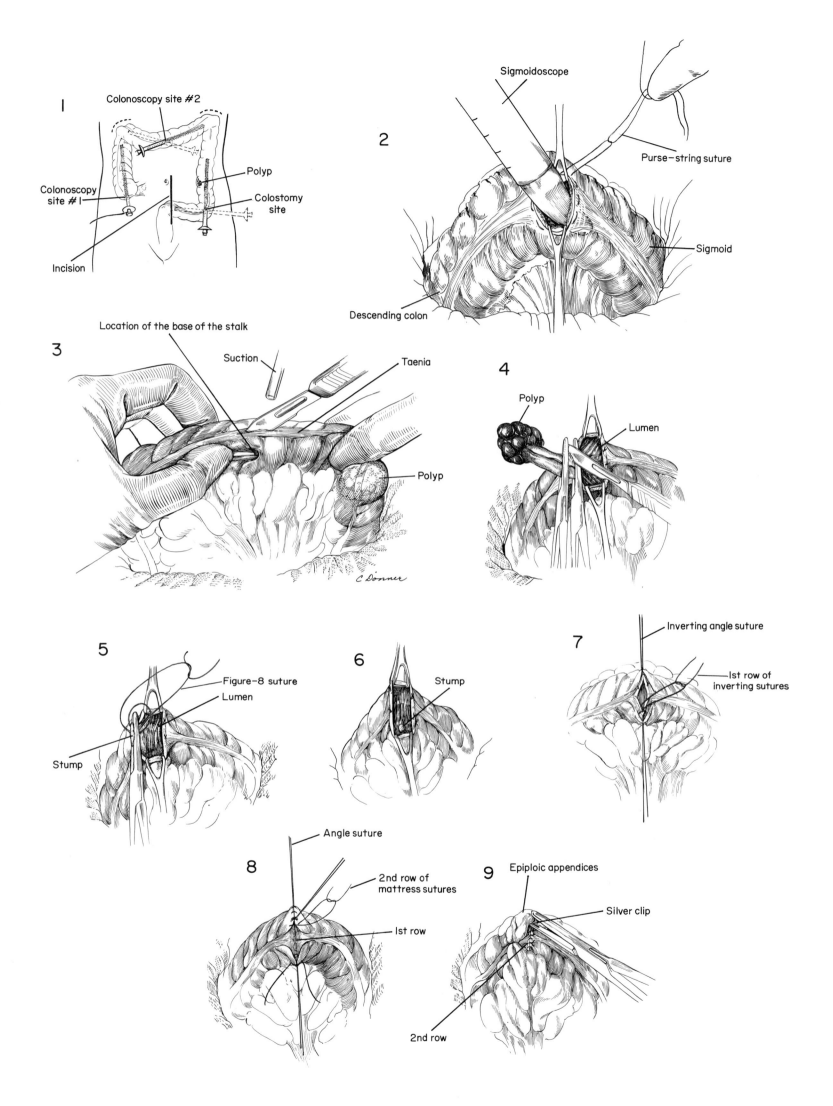

1
Colonoscopy site #2
Colonoscopy site #1
Incision
Polyp
Colostomy site

2
Sigmoidoscope
Purse-string suture
Sigmoid
Descending colon

3
Location of the base of the stalk
Suction
Taenia
Polyp

4
Polyp
Lumen

C Donner

5
Figure-8 suture
Lumen
Stump

6
Stump

7
Inverting angle suture
1st row of inverting sutures

8
Angle suture
2nd row of mattress sutures
1st row

9
Epiploic appendices
Silver clip
2nd row

PLATE LXVII · CHOLECYSTECTOMY, RETROGRADE METHOD

INDICATIONS. Cholecystectomy is indicated in patients with proven disease of the gallbladder that produces symptoms. The incidental finding of gallstones by X-ray or a history of vague indigestion is insufficient evidence for operation in itself, especially in the elderly, and does not justify the risk involved. On the other hand, it is doubtful whether gallstones ever can be considered harmless, because, if the patient lives long enough, complications are likely to develop.

PREOPERATIVE PREPARATION. A high-carbohydrate, high-protein, and high-fluid intake is advised. The patient should be free from respiratory infection. A roentgenogram of the chest is taken. Very obese patients should reduce their weight substantially by dieting, unless they are having recurrent attacks of colic. The entire gastrointestinal tract should be surveyed by barium studies for additional disorders, i.e., hiatus hernia, ulcer of the stomach or duodenum, and carcinoma or diverticulitis of the colon. Sigmoidoscopic examination is performed routinely.

ANESTHESIA. General anesthesia with endotracheal intubation is recommended. Deep anesthesia is avoided by the use of a suitable muscle relaxant. Spinal, either single-injection or continuous technic, may be used in preference to general anesthesia. In those patients suffering from extensive liver damage, minimal amounts of barbiturates and ether as well as other anesthetic agents suspected of hepatotoxicity should be avoided. In elderly or debilitated patients local infiltration anesthesia is satisfactory, although some type of analgesia is usually necessary as a supplement at certain stages of the procedure.

POSITION. The proper position of the patient on the operating table is essential to secure sufficient exposure. Arrangements should be made for an operative cholangiogram. An X-ray cassette is centered under the patient to ensure coverage of the liver, duodenum, and head of the pancreas. A sheet roll or sandbag should be placed under the left chest to ensure that the region of the lower end of the common duct rotates away from the spine. A preliminary roentgenogram is taken to ensure proper placement of the film as well as to permit correction of any exposure difficulties. While the cassette prevents the use of the gallbladder rest or break in the table at the costal margin, the exposure can be enhanced by tilting the table until the body as a whole is in a semierect position **(Figure 1)**. The weight of the liver then tends to lower the gallbladder below the costal margin. Retraction is also aided in this position, because the intestines have a tendency to fall away from the site of operation.

OPERATIVE PREPARATION. The skin is prepared in the routine manner.

INCISION AND EXPOSURE. Two incisions are commonly used: the vertical high rectus and the oblique subcostal **(Figure 2)**. A midline incision is used if other pathology, such as hiatus hernia or duodenal ulcer, requires surgical consideration. A transverse incision does not appear to be utilized as easily by junior surgeons as is the right rectus incision. This is true especially if the costal angles are high and narrow or if it is necessary to explore the common duct. Those favoring the subcostal incision believe the exposure is good, early postoperative wound discomfort minimal, and the incidence of late postoperative hernias much lower than that following the vertical incisions. After the incision is made, the details of the procedure are identical, irrespective of the type of incision employed.

A high right rectus incision is begun above the costal margin, to permit the skin incision to be a little longer than the peritoneal incision, and is carried to the level of the umbilicus. The costoxiphoid angle should be transected by the incision. The rectus sheath is then incised, and the muscle fibers are dissected free, medially, to permit lateral retraction of the entire rectus. Sharp dissection is required at each tendinous inscription where a small vessel usually requires ligation. All bleeding vessels are clamped and tied. If care is exercised, the majority of the underlying motor nerves can be preserved. The posterior rectus sheath and peritoneum are opened just to the right of the xiphoid; and the incision is continued to the umbilicus or below, depending upon the thickness of the abdominal wall and the distance between the xiphoid and the umbilicus. A properly made incision exposes the anterior surface of the liver which makes an easier presentation of liver and gallbladder. If the incision is started at the costal margin over the region of the gallbladder instead of near the midline adjacent to the xiphoid, the procedure is much more difficult.

After the peritoneal cavity has been opened, the gloved hand, moistened with warm saline solution, is used to explore the abdominal cavity, unless there is an acute suppurative infection involving the gallbladder. The stomach and particularly the duodenum are inspected and palpated, and a general abdominal exploration is carried out which includes careful evaluation of the size of the esophageal hiatus. Concomitant repair of a hiatus hernia usually can be carried out to ensure alleviation of gastrointestinal symptoms following the cholecystectomy. The surgeon next passes his right hand up over the dome of the liver, allowing air between the diaphragm and liver to aid in displacing the liver downward **(Figure 3)**.

When assistance is limited, a self-retaining retractor of the **Balfour** type may be used advantageously, or an ordinary retractor of the Halsted type may be used on the right side to retract the costal margin. A half-length clamp is applied to the round ligament and another to the fundus of the gallbladder **(Figure 4)**. Most surgeons prefer to divide the round ligament between half-length clamps, and both ends should be ligated; otherwise, active arterial bleeding will result. Downward traction is maintained by the clamps on the fundus of the gallbladder and on the round ligament. This traction is exaggerated with each inspiration as the liver is projected downward **(Figure 4)**. After the liver has been pulled downward as far as easy traction allows, the half-length clamps are pulled toward the costal margin to present the undersurfaces of the liver and gallbladder **(Figure 5)**. An assistant then holds these clamps while the surgeon prepares to wall off the field. If the gallbladder is acutely inflamed and distended, it is desirable to aspirate some of the contents through a trocar before the half-length clamp is applied to the fundus; otherwise, small stones may be forced into the cystic and common ducts. Adhesions between the undersurface of the gallbladder and adjacent structures are frequently found, drawing the duodenum or transverse colon up into the region of the ampulla. Adequate exposure is maintained by the assistant, who exerts downward traction with a warm moist sponge. The adhesions are divided with curved scissors until an avascular cleavage plane can be developed adjacent to the wall of the gallbladder **(Figure 6)**. After the initial incision is made, it is usually possible to brush these adhesions away with gauze sponges held in thumb forceps **(Figure 7)**. Once the gallbladder is freed of its adhesions, it can be lifted upward to afford better exposure. In order that the adjacent structures may be packed away with moist gauze pads, the surgeon inserts his left hand into the wound, palm down, to direct the gauze pads downward. The pads are introduced with long, smooth forceps. The stomach and transverse colon are packed away, and a final gauze pack is inserted into the region of the foramen of Winslow **(Figure 8)**. The gauze pads are held in position either by a large S retractor along the lower end of the field, or by the left hand of the first assistant, who, with fingers slightly flexed and spread apart, maintains moderate downward and slightly outward pressure, better defining the region of the gastrohepatic ligament.

PLATE LXVII   CHOLECYSTECTOMY, RETROGRADE METHOD

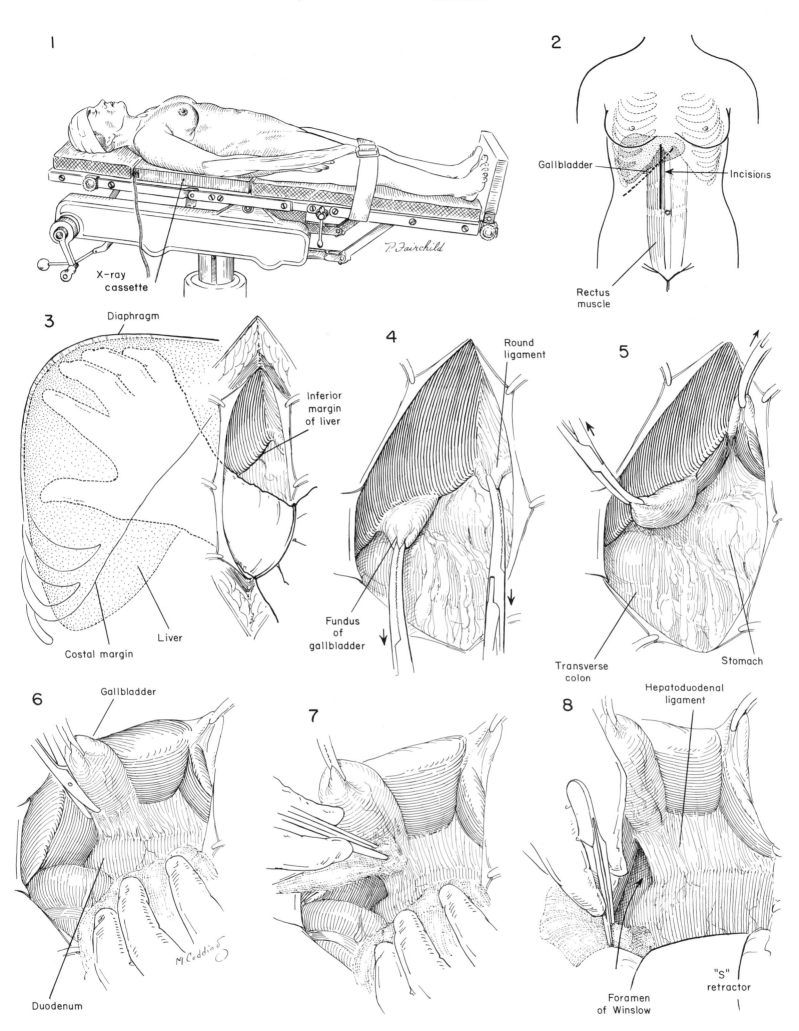

1

X-ray cassette

2

Gallbladder — Incisions

Rectus muscle

3

Diaphragm

Inferior margin of liver

Liver

Costal margin

4

Round ligament

Fundus of gallbladder

5

Transverse colon

Stomach

6

Gallbladder

Duodenum

7

8

Hepatoduodenal ligament

"S" retractor

Foramen of Winslow

PLATE LXVIII · CHOLECYSTECTOMY, RETROGRADE METHOD

DETAILS OF PROCEDURE (*Continued*). After the field has been adequately walled off, the surgeon introduces his left index finger into the foramen of Winslow and, with finger and thumb, thoroughly palpates the region for evidence of calculi in the common duct as well as for thickening of the head of the pancreas. A half-length clamp, with the concavity turned upward, is used to grasp the undersurface of the gallbladder to attain traction toward the operator **(Figure 9).** The early application of clamps in the region of the ampulla of the gallbladder is one of the frequent causes of accidental injury to the common duct. This is especially true when the gallbladder is acutely distended, because the ampulla of the gallbladder may run parallel to the common duct for a considerable distance. If the clamp is applied blindly where the neck of the gallbladder passes into the cystic duct, part or all of the common duct may be accidentally included in it **(Figure 10).** For this reason it is always advisable to apply the half-length clamp well up on the undersurface of the gallbladder before any attempt is made to visualize the region of the ampulla of the gallbladder. The enucleation of the gallbladder is started by dividing the peritoneum on the inferior aspect of the gallbladder and extending it downward to the region of the ampulla. The peritoneum usually is divided with a knife or long Metzenbaum dissecting scissors. The incision is carefully extended downward along the hepatoduodenal ligament **(Figures 11** and **12).** By means of blunt gauze dissection the region of the ampulla is freed down to the region of the cystic duct **(Figure 13).** After the ampulla of the gallbladder has been clearly defined, the clamp on the undersurface of the gallbladder is reapplied lower to the region of the ampulla.

With traction maintained on the ampulla, the cystic duct is defined by means of gauze dissection **(Figure 13).** A long right-angle clamp is then passed behind the cystic duct. The jaws of the clamp are separated cautiously as counterpressure is made on the upper side of the lower end of the gallbladder by the surgeon's index finger. Slowly and with great care, the cystic duct is isolated from the common duct **(Figure 14).** The cystic artery is likewise isolated with a long right-angle clamp. If the upward traction on the gallbladder is marked, and the common duct is quite flexible, it is not uncommon to have it angulate sharply upward, giving the appearance of a prolonged cystic duct. Under such circumstances injury to, or division of, the common duct may result when the right-angle clamp is applied to the supposed cystic duct **(Figure 15** and insert**).** Such a disaster may occur when the exposure appears too easy in a thin patient because of the extreme mobilization of the common duct.

After the cystic duct has been isolated, it is thoroughly palpated to ascertain that no calculi have been forced into it or the common duct by the application of clamps and that none will be overlooked in the stump of the cystic duct. The size of the cystic duct is carefully noted before the right-angle crushing clamp is applied. If the cystic duct is dilated, and if it seems from palpation that the gallbladder contains calculi so small that they could pass through it easily, it is advisable to perform a choledochostomy. Regardless, an operative cholangiogram is performed routinely through the cystic duct after it has been divided (Plate LXIX, **Figure 24).** Because it is more difficult to divide the cystic duct between two closely applied right-angle clamps, a curved half-length clamp is placed adjacent to the initial right-angle clamp. The curvature of the half-length clamp makes it ideally suited for directing the scissors downward during the division of the cystic duct **(Figure 16).** Whenever possible, unless occluded by severe inflammation, the cystic duct and cystic artery are isolated separately to permit individual ligation. Under no circumstances is a right-angle clamp applied to the supposed region of the cystic duct in the hope that both the cystic artery and cystic duct can be included in one mass ligature. It is surprising how much additional cystic duct can be developed many times by maintaining traction on the duct as blunt gauze dissection is carried out. After the cholangiogram, the cystic duct is ligated with a transfixing suture **(Figure 17).**

PLATE LXVIII   CHOLECYSTECTOMY, RETROGRADE METHOD

9

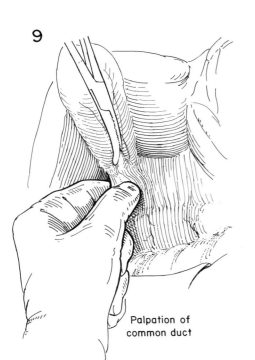

Palpation of
common duct

10

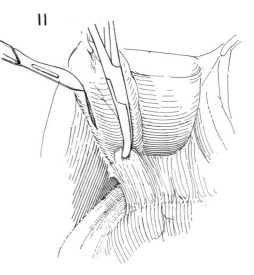

Danger
point

Common duct

11

Incision in hepatoduodenal
ligament

12

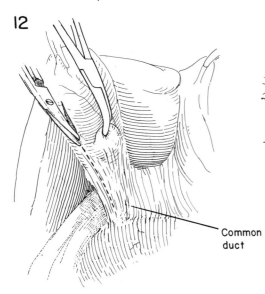

Common
duct

Point of reapplication
of clamp

13

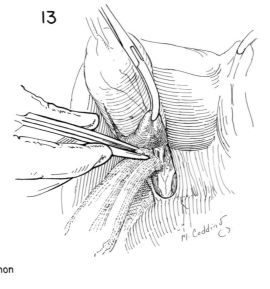

M. Codding

14

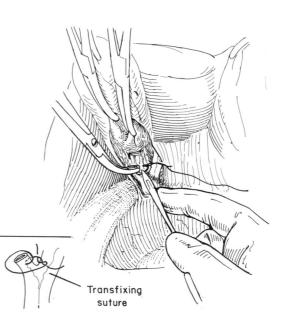

Cystic
duct

Common
duct

15

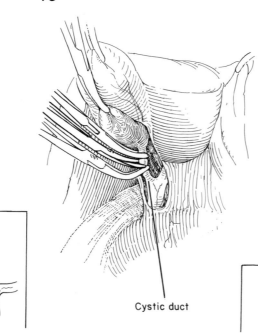

Danger
point

Angulation
of common duct

16

Cystic duct

17

Transfixing
suture

PLATE LXIX · CHOLECYSTECTOMY, RETROGRADE METHOD

DETAILS OF PROCEDURE (*Continued*). If the cystic artery was not divided before the cystic duct, it is now carefully isolated by a right-angle clamp similar to those used in isolating the cystic duct **(Figure 18)**. The cystic artery should be isolated as far away from the region of the hepatic duct as possible. A clamp is never applied blindly to this region, lest the hepatic artery lie in an anomalous location and be clamped and divided, resulting in a fatality **(Figure 19)**. Anomalies of the blood supply in this region are so common that this possibility must be considered in every case. The cystic artery is divided between clamps similar to those utilized in the division of the cystic duct **(Figure 20)**. The cystic artery should be tied as soon as it has been divided to avoid possible difficulties while the gallbladder is being removed **(Figure 21)**. If desired, the ligation of the cystic duct can be delayed until after the cystic artery has been ligated. Some prefer to ligate the cystic artery routinely and leave the cystic duct intact until the gallbladder is completely freed from the liver bed. This approach minimizes possible injury to the ductal system as complete exposure is obtained before the cystic duct is divided. If the clamp or tie on the cystic artery slips off, resulting in vigorous bleeding, the hepatic artery may be compressed in the gastrohepatic ligament by the thumb and index finger of the left hand, temporarily controlling the bleeding **(Figure 22)**. The field can be dried with suction by the assistant, and, as the surgeon releases his compression of the hepatic artery, a hemostat may be applied safely and exactly to the bleeding point. The stumps of the cystic artery and cystic duct are each thoroughly inspected and, before the operation proceeds, the common duct is again visualized to make certain that it is not angulated or otherwise disturbed. Blind clamping in a blood field is all too frequently responsible for injury to the ducts, producing the dreaded complication of stricture. Classic anatomic relationships in this area should never be taken for granted since normal variations are more common in this critical zone than anywhere else in the body.

After the cystic duct and artery have been tied, removal of the gallbladder is begun. The incision initially made on the inferior surface of the gallbladder about 1 cm. from the liver edge is extended upward around the fundus **(Figure 23)**. An edematous cleavage plane can be developed easily by injecting a few milliliters of saline between the serosa and the seromuscular layer, utilizing this cleavage plane for dissection. It is important that the serosa be divided with a scalpel or scissors along both the lateral and medial margins of the gallbladder, so that the gallbladder is not torn from the liver bed by traction. If this occurs, raw liver surface results, and it may be impossible to peritonealize the liver bed. With his left hand the surgeon holds the clamps that have been applied to the gallbladder and, by careful scissors dissection, divides the loose areolar tissue between the gallbladder and the liver. This allows the gallbladder to be dissected from its bed without dividing any sizable vessels. Before the fundus of the gallbladder is finally removed from its cleft in the liver, advantage may be taken of the traction that can be exerted upon it to keep the liver edge everted, thereby preserving the exposure of the deeper parts of the field. Fine 0000 interrupted silk sutures are placed to close the open bed of the gallbladder on the undersurface of the liver **(Figure 25)**. These sutures are tied from below upward as tension on the gallbladder is released while it is being peeled away from the liver. The final peritoneal attachment between gallbladder and liver is severed.

When facilities permit, an operative cholangiogram **(Figure 24)** should be made routinely to ensure complete clearance of the ductal system. When this procedure is planned, the cystic duct is not ligated before the gallbladder has been removed and the liver bed approximated. An extra length of cystic duct should be retained initially to facilitate the procedure. Small mosquito clamps grasp the end of the divided cystic duct as the

right-angle clamp is removed. Since the valves of Heister tend to block the introduction of the small polyethylene tube into the cystic duct, the channel should be cleared by the introduction of a small metal probe. A syringe of saline as well as diluted contrast media should be connected by a two-way adapter in a closed system to avoid the introduction of air into the ducts. The polyethylene tube, size 190, is filled with saline as it is introduced a short distance into the common duct. The tube is secured in the cystic duct by one tied suture utilizing a surgeon's knot. All gauze packs, clamps, and retractors are removed as the table is returned to a level position by the anesthetist. Five milliliters of contrast media, 20 to 25 per cent concentration, are injected and the X-ray immediately taken. Limited amounts of a dilute solution prevent the obliteration of any small calculi within the ducts. A second injection of 15 to 20 ml. is made to outline the ductal system completely and ensure patency of the ampulla of Vater. The tube should be displaced laterally and the duodenum gently pushed to the right to ensure a clear roentgenogram without interference from the skeletal system or the tube filled with contrast media. Two roentgenograms are taken to provide a comparison in case doubtful shadows are noted. If the appendix is present, it is removed during the interval required to develop the roentgenogram. If no further studies are warranted, the tube is removed and the cystic duct ligated near the common duct.

If the round ligament has been divided, it is reapproximated, and the rent in the falciform ligament is likewise repaired. A warm, moist gauze sponge is then laid along the suture line to make certain there is no oozing and the field is absolutely dry. Some type of coagulant may be placed over the repair in the liver bed. As a further aid in walling off this area, the omentum may be tucked against the gallbladder bed.

CLOSURE. The table is leveled, and any sandbags or pillows used for elevation of the costal margin are removed before attempting closure to avoid unnecessary tension on the structures of the abdominal wall. The closure may follow each operator's accustomed method. When the transverse incision or the oblique Kocher incision is used, tension sutures are not necessary; but when the usual right paramedian incision is utilized, particularly in the case of the elderly and obese patient or in the presence of anticipated cardiorespiratory difficulties, it is wise to use retention sutures.

A small soft rubber drain is left along the cleft in the liver from which the gallbladder has been removed. This drain passes by the foramen of Winslow and is positioned into Morrison's pouch above the kidney and lateral to the spinal column. It is preferable to bring the drain out through a separate stab wound so placed as to ensure an oblique tract without angulation around the liver margin. The drain is anchored to the skin with a silk suture and a safety pin.

POSTOPERATIVE CARE. The patient is placed in a semi-Fowler's position and is moved from side to side frequently. The fluid balance is maintained by the intravenous injection of 5 or 10 per cent glucose in water and/or isotonic saline. Constant gastric suction is optional for 24 to 48 hours. The diet is rapidly increased as soon as the tube is withdrawn. The patient is permitted out of bed on the first postoperative day. Careful daily examination should be made of the lower extremities to rule out the presence of deep venous thrombosis because of the susceptibility of these patients to pulmonary embolus. The rubber drain is removed within 24 to 48 hours unless there is bile leakage. In this instance the drain is not removed until a sinus tract forms, which ordinarily takes three to seven days. The patient should gradually add those items to the diet that precipitated discomfort previous to cholecystectomy.

PLATE LXIX   CHOLECYSTECTOMY, RETROGRADE METHOD

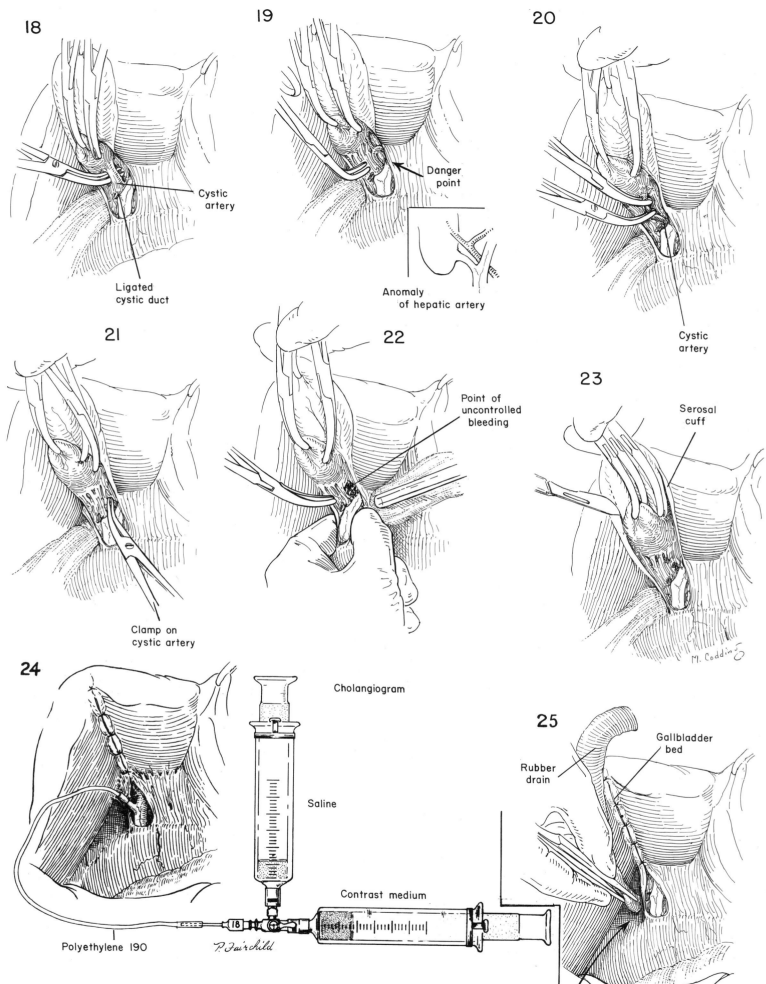

18

Cystic
artery

Ligated
cystic duct

19

Danger
point

Anomaly
of hepatic artery

20

Cystic
artery

21

Clamp on
cystic artery

22

Point of
uncontrolled
bleeding

23

Serosal
cuff

M. Coddin

24

Cholangiogram

Saline

Contrast medium

Polyethylene 190

P. Fairchild

25

Rubber
drain

Gallbladder
bed

Foramen of Winslow

PLATE LXX · CHOLEDOCHOSTOMY

INDICATIONS. The decision to explore the common duct depends not only on the patient's preoperative history and laboratory examination but also upon the anatomic findings by palpation and inspection at the time of operation. The presence of jaundice or a recent history of jaundice is a strong indication for exploration of the common duct. The common duct is explored: if there is, on palpation, a suspicion of a stone; if the common duct is thickened or dilated; if the cystic duct is sufficiently dilated to permit stones to pass into the common duct; if the head of the pancreas is thickened, suggesting a chronic pancreatitis; or if there are one or more very small stones in the gallbladder or cystic duct, which, because of their size, could easily pass into the common duct. Over 40 per cent of patients with cholelithiasis present indications for exploration of the common duct unless a routine cholangiogram through the cystic duct is clearly negative. In approximately one-third of the common ducts explored, one or more stones will be recovered. **Figure 1** depicts schematically the more common locations of calculi.

PREOPERATIVE PREPARATION. In the presence of deep jaundice it is desirable to delay operation for a few days to effect general improvement. During this time all of the clinical and laboratory data are gathered together on a so-called jaundice balance sheet. The evidence for and against an obstructive jaundice amenable to surgery or a medical jaundice caused by hepatitis or drug reaction must be carefully assessed. The blood prothrombin level is determined. In the presence of jaundice and low prothrombin levels, vitamin K and whole blood transfusions are administered before operation. Surgery is further delayed if the prothrombin levels do not show a good response to vitamin administration. A diet high in proteins, carbohydrates, and vitamins is given either orally or parenterally in preparing for operation. Appropriate antibiotic or chemotherapy is begun if infection is suspected. In order to avoid hypotension, the blood volume should be restored before surgery, and whole blood should be available at the time of operation to replace losses as they occur. At no time during the operation or in the early postoperative period must the patient be permitted to have a period of hypotension because of the threat of renal shut-down.

ANESTHESIA. General anesthesia with endotracheal intubation is recommended. Spinal, either single injection or continuous technic, may be used in preference to general anesthesia. In those patients suffering from extensive liver damage, barbiturates, ether, as well as other anesthetic agents suspected of hepatotoxicity, should be avoided. Blood is promptly replaced as it is lost to avoid the development of hypotension.

OPERATIVE PREPARATION. The skin is prepared in the routine manner.

INCISION AND EXPOSURE. The incision and exposure are carried out as described for cholecystectomy (Plate LXVII). The peritoneal reflection of the ampulla of the gallbladder, which is continuous with the structures about the common duct, is visualized and incised with long, curved scissors. This liberates the ampulla from its position against the common duct and cystic duct **(Figure 2)**. When this is done carefully, it is usually unnecessary to ligate any vessels. In the presence of jaundice the cystic duct is not clamped or divided, nor is the gallbladder removed until it is certain that any obstruction in the region of the papilla can be relieved, since the gallbladder may be needed for a short-circuiting procedure.

The size of the common duct, the thickness of the wall, the presence of inflammation, and any other pathologic findings are noted, together with the factors mentioned previously, to determine whether exploration of the common duct is necessary. Routine cholangiography through the cystic duct will decrease the number of choledochostomies. In doubtful situations the common duct is identified by its position in the hepatoduodenal ligament, by its direct relation to the cystic duct, by the presence of a vein running over its wall, and by the aspiration of bile from it through a fine needle **(Figure 3)**. Anomalies of the structures in this location occur so frequently that careful and accurate identification of the duct is mandatory.

DETAILS OF PROCEDURE. In order to explore the common duct, two fine 0000 silk sutures are placed a few millimeters apart in its wall just below the entrance of the cystic duct into the common duct **(Figure 4)**. Traction on these sutures and tension on the gallbladder and cystic duct, unsevered from the biliary system until after the common duct procedures are completed, provide excellent exposure of the field **(Figure 5)**. If the field is obscured by a distended gallbladder, however, adequate exposure is obtained by aspiration or removal of the gallbladder and closure of the liver bed. The liver margin is returned into the peritoneal cavity and retracted upward by a Richardson retractor. When the exposure is difficult, removal of the gallbladder from the fundus downward should be considered. Safer identification and ligation of the cystic artery and cystic

duct may result. The common duct can be explored after removal of the gallbladder and fixation of the cystic duct by a right-angle clamp **(Figure 6)**. The field is entirely walled off with moist gauze packs, and a suction tube is placed down to the foramen of Winslow to remove the bile that escapes while opening the duct. The common duct is opened between these sutures with a sharp scalpel for about 1 cm. The opening is made parallel to the long axis of the duct, avoiding a blood vessel commonly found in its anterior wall. This opening is large enough to admit a small scoop without traumatizing or tearing the duct **(Figure 5)**. The colon and consistency of the bile are noted.

Should the cystic duct be sufficiently large to permit exploration of the common duct through it, it is opened between sutures placed just above its point of junction with the common duct.

The duct is held open and explored with a metal probe, such as a uterine sound, which is directed downward to Vater's papilla and into the duodenum if possible. The patency of the papilla is determined at this time. With a finger inserted into the foramen of Winslow to give counterresistance as the metal probe passes, a grating of metal against stone may be sensed, and a calculus may be found that otherwise might be overlooked. If a probe passes into the duodenum, it does not assure that a calculus either is not impinged at the ampulla of the common duct or is not resting in a sacculation of the duct. A small, pliant metal scoop, such as a Cushing pituitary curet, is then repeatedly directed into the region of the papilla of the common bile duct, and any stones are removed **(Figure 5)**. A scoop, 8 by 15 mm., with an easily molded handle is entirely adequate; large scoops with rigid handles should not be used. If a stone is impacted in a diverticulum to one side of the ampulla of the bile duct, the left forefinger and thumb may fix the stone so that it is fragmented by the scoop and can be removed piecemeal or by irrigation. The scoop is directed upward into both hepatic ducts, for small calculi may lodge in the larger intrahepatic bile ducts **(Figure 1)**. Also, a Fogarty balloon catheter may be useful in extracting stones and verifying patency of the ampulla. After stone removal, a silk woven catheter, No. 8 or 10F, is inserted toward the liver, and warm saline (less than 110° F.) is injected as the catheter is withdrawn. The catheter is then directed downward. A sudden increase in resistance will be encountered when it passes through Vater's papilla into the duodenum **(Figure 6)**. Saline is gently injected, and if the tip of the catheter is in the duodenum, the duodenum will balloon out **(Figure 7)**. As the catheter is withdrawn slowly, saline is again injected gently to dislodge any calculi. The scooping is then repeated. Once its patency has been established, no attempt is made to dilate the papilla beyond the gentle passage of a No. 12 or 14F silk woven catheter.

After manipulations upon the common duct have been completed, a small T-tube common-duct catheter, No. 14 or 16, is inserted through the opening in the duct. The larger size may permit secondary mechanical removal of overlooked calculi. The arms of the T-tube are usually shortened, and a wedge is excised opposite the main stem of the catheter to facilitate its subsequent removal **(Figure 8)**. The opening in the duct about the catheter is closed securely with fine 0000 silk sutures on French needles **(Figure 9)**. The suture line is tested by injecting saline through the T-tube **(Figure 10)**. The gallbladder is then removed as described for cholecystectomy (Plate LXIX).

CLOSURE. A rubber drain is introduced down past the foramen of Winslow into Morrison's pouch **(Figure 11)**. The catheter and drain are brought out through a stab wound lateral to the incision at a level that avoids acute angulation of the catheter and T-tube (see Plate LXIX, **Figure 20**). The catheter is attached to the skin of the abdomen with a skin suture and adhesive tape.

POSTOPERATIVE CARE. Hypotension must be avoided to decrease the possibility of uremia. If the bile loss is excessive, sodium lactate or bicarbonate should be added to compensate for the excessive sodium loss. The fluid balance is maintained by daily administration of approximately 2,000 to 3,000 ml. of 5 to 10 per cent dextrose in water or isotonic saline. The catheter is connected to a drainage bottle, and the amount of drainage over a 24-hour period is recorded. In the presence of jaundice with a bleeding tendency, whole blood and vitamin K are given. The drain is removed in 24 to 48 hours, and the patient may be out of bed on the first postoperative day. The common-duct catheter is removed in seven to ten days. A cholangiogram is advisable before the catheter is removed if this was not done at the time of surgery. If a T-tube has been used, the catheter may be clamped off during the day and allowed to drain during the night. If there is no reaction to these procedures, the catheter is removed by gentle, sustained traction. In some instances of prolonged biliary drainage, it may be useful to refeed the bile back to the patient in a mixture of grape juice or through a gastric or enterostomy tube. Loss of bile through external drainage often results in poor appetite, and the patient's nutrition becomes a problem.

PLATE LXX   CHOLEDOCHOSTOMY

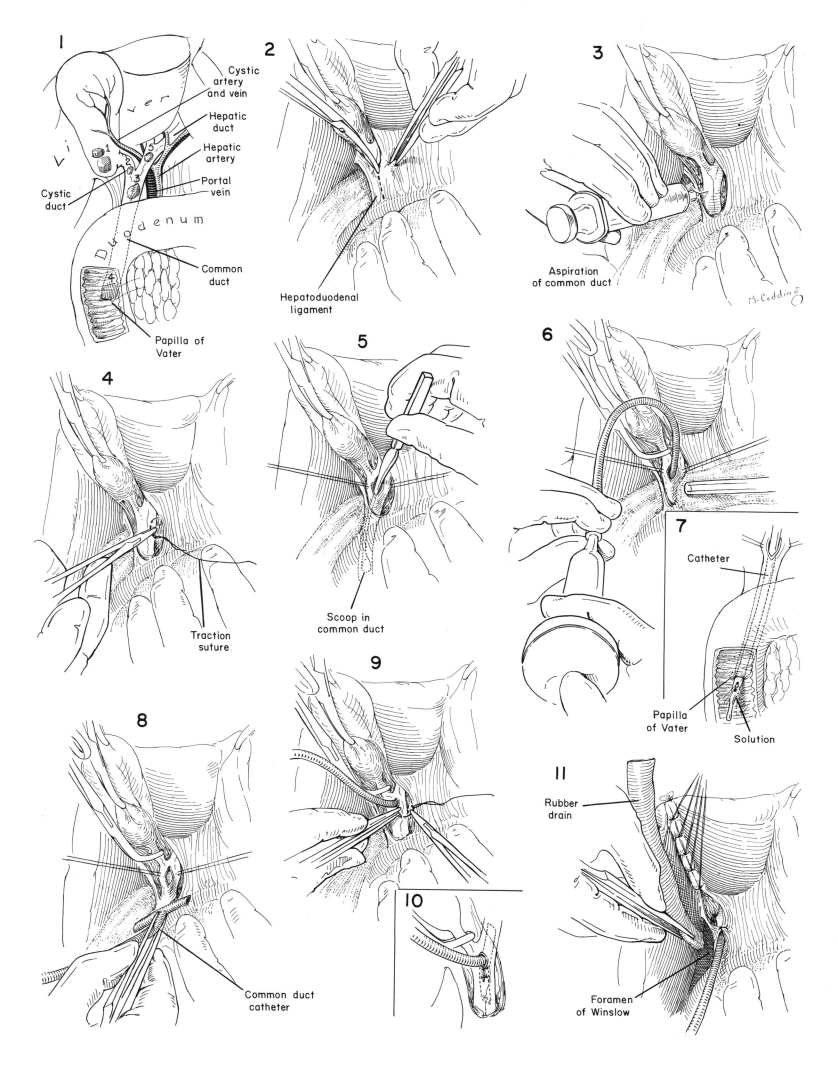

1
Cystic
artery
and vein
Hepatic
duct
Hepatic
artery
Portal
vein
Common
duct
Cystic
duct
Liver
Duodenum
Papilla of
Vater

2
Hepatoduodenal
ligament

3
Aspiration
of common duct

M. Codding

4
Traction
suture

5
Scoop in
common duct

6

7
Catheter
Papilla
of Vater
Solution

8
Common duct
catheter

9

10

11
Rubber
drain
Foramen
of Winslow

PLATE LXXI · CHOLEDOCHOSTOMY, TRANSDUODENAL APPROACH

DETAILS OF PROCEDURE (*Continued*). Sometimes it is impossible to dislodge a calculus from the region of Vater's papilla by careful and repeated manipulation, and a more radical procedure is followed. Under such circumstances the duodenum is mobilized by the Kocher maneuver, and the common duct is exposed throughout its course down to the duodenal wall. An incision is made in the lateral part of the peritoneal attachment of the duodenum, making it possible to mobilize the second portion of the duodenum **(Figure 12).** After the peritoneal attachment has been incised with long, curved scissors, blunt gauze dissection is used to sweep the duodenum medially. Occasionally, this will expose the retroduodenal portion of the common duct and will allow more direct palpation **(Figure 13).** A blunt metal probe is introduced downward to the point of the obstruction, and the location of the stone is more accurately determined by palpation. A scoop is passed down to the region of the ampulla of the common bile duct, and its course is directed carefully with the index finger and thumb of the surgeon's left hand **(Figure 14).** With the tissues being held firmly by the thumb and index finger, it is usually possible to break up the impacted calculus with the scoop. Should this prove unsuccessful, it is necessary to open the anterior duodenal wall and to expose Vater's papilla **(Figure 15).** Since opening the duodenum tends to increase the risk of complications, it should not be considered until all indirect methods have been tried.

By exerting gentle pressure on a uterine sound inserted to the common duct, the surgeon can determine the exact location of the papilla by palpation over the anterior wall of the duodenum. With the duodenal wall held taut in Babcock forceps or by silk sutures, an incision 3 to 4 cm. long is made over this area, parallel to the long axis of the bowel. The field must be completely walled off by gauze sponges, and constant suction must be maintained to avoid contamination by bile and pancreatic juice. Small gauze sponges are then introduced upward and downward within the lumen of the duodenum to prevent further soiling. Long silk sutures are attached to each of these gauze sponges to ensure their subsequent removal **(Figure 15).** Even at this point the calculus may be dislodged by direct palpation. If this is still impossible, the probe is reintroduced and directed firmly against the region of the papilla to determine the direction of the duct, so that a small incision may be made directly parallel to it **(Figure 15).** This incision enlarges the papilla so that a calculus can either be expressed or be removed with fenestrated stone forceps **(Figure 16).** Following this, the patency of the common duct is ascertained by introducing a silk woven bougie into the opening of the common duct and downward through the papilla **(Figure 17).** Any bleeding points from the incision into the papilla are controlled by fine 0000 interrupted silk sutures **(Figure 18).** The pancreatic duct must not be occluded by these sutures. No effort is made to reconstruct the papilla to its natural size, the opening being allowed to remain enlarged as a result of the incision.

The small gauze sponges that plugged the duodenum are withdrawn, and the intestine is closed. The bowel is closed in the opposite direction from that in which the incision was made. This avoids constricting the lumen of the bowel **(Figure 19).** The duodenal wall is sutured with interrupted 0000 silk sutures, starting at the angle adjacent to one of the Babcock clamps. The serosa is reinforced with a layer of interrupted Halsted mattress sutures of 00 silk **(Figure 19).** This closure must be watertight and secure to avoid the complication of duodenal fistula. A catheter is introduced into the common duct, and the duodenum is distended with normal saline to make certain that there is no leakage. A small T-tube is then directed into the initial opening of the common duct, and the technic from this point on is observed as described in Plate LXX. A rubber drain is inserted down past the foramen of Winslow into Morrison's pouch in all cases and remains there until there is no danger of duodenal fistula. It is advisable to bring the common-duct catheter and rubber drain out through a stab wound lateral to the incision **(Figure 20).** It is safest to avoid clamping the common-duct catheter, permitting it to drain into a sterile gauze sponge until it is attached to a drainage bottle. The bile is cultured for bacterial content and antimicrobial sensitivities.

CLOSURE. The closure is made in the routine manner (see Plates VII and VIII).

POSTOPERATIVE CARE. Constant gastric suction is employed for 24 to 48 hours. The fluid balance is maintained by the administration of 5 to 10 per cent dextrose in water or isotonic saline in daily amounts of approximately 3,000 ml. In the case of elderly patients with known cardiac weakness, the amount is decreased appropriately. The common-duct catheter is connected to a sterile drainage bottle. Every effort is made to avoid pulmonary complications and pulmonary embolism. The patient is placed in a semi-Fowler's position and moved from side to side frequently; likewise, exercise of the legs is instituted. In the presence of jaundice with a bleeding tendency, whole blood and vitamin K should be given. The rubber drain is removed in 24 to 48 hours, and the patient may be out of bed on the first postoperative day. Liquids and food are permitted as tolerated. The common-duct catheter, which usually drains up to 500 ml. of bile in 24 hours, is removed in seven to ten days. If the bile drainage is excessive, perfusion pressures should be taken to make certain the ampulla is patent. The excessive loss of sodium must be replaced by the addition of sodium lactate or bicarbonate solutions. The appetite is often poor during the loss of bile. Attention to the caloric intake and the refeeding of bile is essential, especially in the elderly poor-risk patient. A cholangiogram is advisable before the catheter is removed, even if this has been done at the time of surgery. Retained stones may be lysed with chemical irrigations or extracted with a basket catheter under fluoroscopic control. The sinus tract should heal promptly after the common-duct catheter has been removed.

PLATE LXXI   CHOLEDOCHOSTOMY, TRANSDUODENAL APPROACH

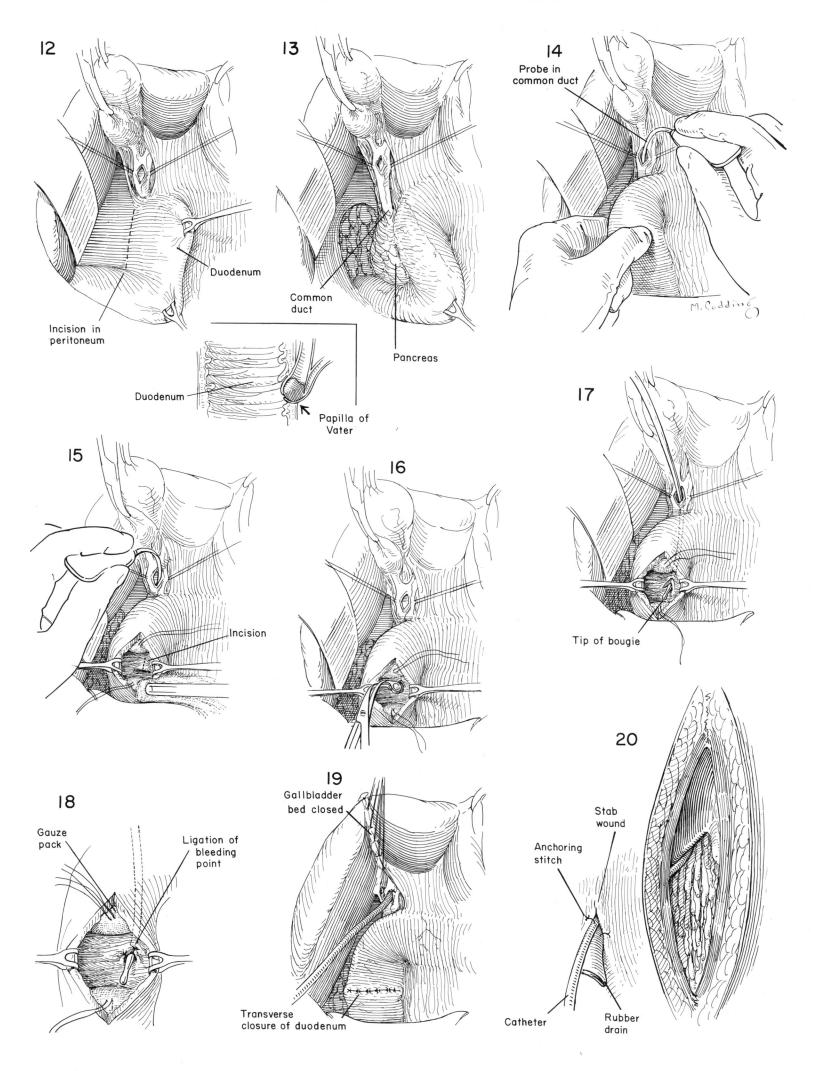

12

Incision in
peritoneum

Duodenum

13

Common
duct

Pancreas

Duodenum

Papilla of
Vater

14

Probe in
common duct

M. Codding

15

Incision

16

17

Tip of bougie

18

Gauze
pack

Ligation of
bleeding
point

19

Gallbladder
bed closed

Transverse
closure of duodenum

20

Stab
wound

Anchoring
stitch

Catheter

Rubber
drain

PLATE LXXII · CHOLECYSTECTOMY—PARTIAL CHOLECYSTECTOMY

A. Cholecystectomy from Fundus Downward

INDICATIONS. Cholecystectomy from the fundus downward is the desirable method in many cases of acute cholecystitis where exposure of the cystic duct is difficult and hazardous. Extensive adhesions, a large, thick-walled, acutely inflamed gallbladder, or a large calculus impacted in the ampulla of the gallbladder make this the safer and wiser procedure. Better definition of the cystic duct and cystic artery is ensured with far less chance of injury to the common duct. Some prefer this method of cholecystectomy as a routine procedure.

PREOPERATIVE PREPARATION. In the presence of acute cholecystitis the preoperative treatment depends upon the severity and the duration of the attack. Early operation is indicated in patients seen within 48 hours after the onset, as soon as fluid balance has been established. Frequent clinical and laboratory evaluation over a 24-hour period is necessary. The patient is placed in the semi-Fowler's position, and fluid balance is maintained. Constant gastric suction may be advisable. The value of chemotherapy is questionable. Regardless of the duration of the acute manifestations, surgical intervention is indicated if there is recurrence of pain, a mounting white cell count, or an increase in the signs and symptoms suggesting a perforation. The gallbladder may show advanced acute inflammation despite a normal temperature, white count, and negative physical findings. Blood must be available for transfusion. About 75 per cent of the patients will respond to conservative treatment, and surgery in this group can be delayed a few days until fluid and caloric intake returns to normal. Approximately one patient in five with acute cholecystitis will not progressively improve and may worsen. Such patients require operation as an "off-schedule" urgent procedure.

ANESTHESIA. See Plate LXVII.

POSITION. The patient is placed in the usual position for gallbladder surgery. If local anesthesia is used, the position may be modified slightly to make the patient more comfortable.

OPERATIVE PREPARATION. The skin is prepared in the usual manner.

INCISION AND EXPOSURE. Incision and exposure are carried out as shown in Plate LXVII. The omentum must be separated carefully by either sharp or blunt dissection from the fundus of the gallbladder, care being taken to tie all bleeding points. An oblique incision below the costal margin should be considered, especially if the mass presents rather far laterally.

DETAILS OF PROCEDURE. The appearance of the fundus and the patient's general condition determine whether it is safer to drain the gallbladder or to remove it from the fundus downward, or to proceed with the retrograde cholecystectomy. Blunt dissection only is utilized to free the omentum and other structures from the gallbladder wall. It is safer to empty the contents immediately to decrease the bulk and to give more exposure. A short incision is made through the serosa of the fundus, a trocar is introduced, and the liquid contents are removed by suction. Cultures are taken. A fenestrated forceps is introduced deep into the gallbladder to remove any calculi in the ampulla. The opening is closed with hemostats, which prevents further soiling and serves as traction.

An incision is made into the serosa of the gallbladder with a scalpel along both sides about 1 cm. from the liver substance **(Figure 1)**; otherwise, excessive traction will result in avulsion of the gallbladder from the liver bed. Separation is accomplished by blunt or scissors dissection, especially since the loose tissue beneath the serosa is edematous in the presence of acute cholecystitis **(Figure 2).** The cuff of gallbladder wall in the region of the fundus is held with forceps, while the gallbladder is further freed by scissors dissection **(Figure 3).**

As an alternate method, since the contents have been aspirated and are frequently sterile, the opening in the fundus is enlarged, permitting the index finger or a gauze sponge to be inserted to give counterresistance and to aid in dissecting within the developed cleavage plane.

The serosa is incised on each side down to the ampulla of the gallbladder. Since there may be difficulty from oozing because the cystic artery is intact, all bleeding points should be meticulously clamped. As the cuff at the margin of the liver is held by a curved, half-length clamp, a relatively dry field is obtained if the cuff is closed with interrupted sutures as the dissection progresses down to the ampulla **(Figure 4).** Great care must be taken in isolating the ampulla from the common duct. It may be possible by finger compression to dislodge a calculus impinged in the ampulla and to separate the distorted ampulla from the adjacent structures. Alternate sharp and gauze dissection is advisable until the majority of adhesions have been separated. The gallbladder is retracted medially and outward to assist in identifying the cystic duct and cystic artery. After the ampulla is defined, the cystic duct is isolated with a right-angle clamp cautiously introduced from the lateral side to avoid injury to the common duct and to the right hepatic artery **(Figure 4).** The cystic artery is isolated with any accompanying indurated tissue. The artery may be much larger than normal, and the right hepatic artery may be in an anomalous position. It is safer to isolate the cystic artery as near the gallbladder wall as possible. The cystic artery and adjacent tissues are divided between a half-length and a right-angle clamp **(Figure 5)** and ligated with a transfixing suture.

The cystic duct is palpated carefully, especially if acute cholecystitis is present, to ensure that a stone has not been overlooked. The common duct is palpated carefully, and exploration is avoided unless the cholangiogram showed clear-cut evidence of a calculus there. If choledochostomy is not indicated, the cystic duct is divided between right-angle and half-length clamps **(Figure 6)** and tied with a transfixing suture, unless a cholangiogram is planned through the cystic duct. After thorough inspection of the area for oozing, the clamp is removed from the liver margin, and a final suture is taken to close the gallbladder bed. Since inflammation and technical difficulties have made this procedure necessary, a rubber drain is inserted down to the region of the cystic duct. Because of bile leakage, if raw liver surface has been exposed, drainage is always indicated. A coagulant may be applied to the liver bed. The bile is cultured for bacterial growth and antimicrobial sensitivities.

B. Partial Cholecystectomy

Fewer cholecystostomies are necessary if the principle of partial cholecystectomy is utilized occasionally. If a classic cholecystectomy appears hazardous because of advanced inflammation, or if the gallbladder is partially buried in the liver, or if structures in the cystic duct region cannot be safely identified, the full thickness of the gallbladder is left within the liver bed. The gallbladder is aspirated, and traction is exerted on the fundus. The inferior surface is divided cautiously down to the ampulla, which may be densely adherent to the adjacent structures **(Figure 7).** Calculi impacted in the ampulla or cystic duct are removed with fenestrated forceps **(Figure 8).** The gallbladder wall beyond the liver margin is excised, and any bleeding points are controlled by interrupted sutures of fine silk **(Figure 9).** The mucosa is removed from the retained portion of the gallbladder bed by sharp and blunt dissection, or it is destroyed by electrocoagulation. When the cystic duct is not ligated, its patency is ascertained, and it is drained with a small catheter **(Figure 9).** A cholangiogram may be made at this time. Several rubber drains are introduced down to the region of the cystic duct, and the omentum is brought up around these drains.

CLOSURE. The customary closure is made. The catheter and drains may be brought out through a separate stab wound.

POSTOPERATIVE CARE. The care described in Plate LXXI is observed. Bile drainage is expected from the tube or about the drain. After systemic and local signs of inflammation have disappeared and drainage has subsided, a cholangiogram should be considered before the catheter is removed, unless one was made at the time of surgery. The rubber drains are withdrawn several inches daily, beginning several days after operation.

PLATE LXXII   CHOLECYSTECTOMY—PARTIAL CHOLECYSTECTOMY

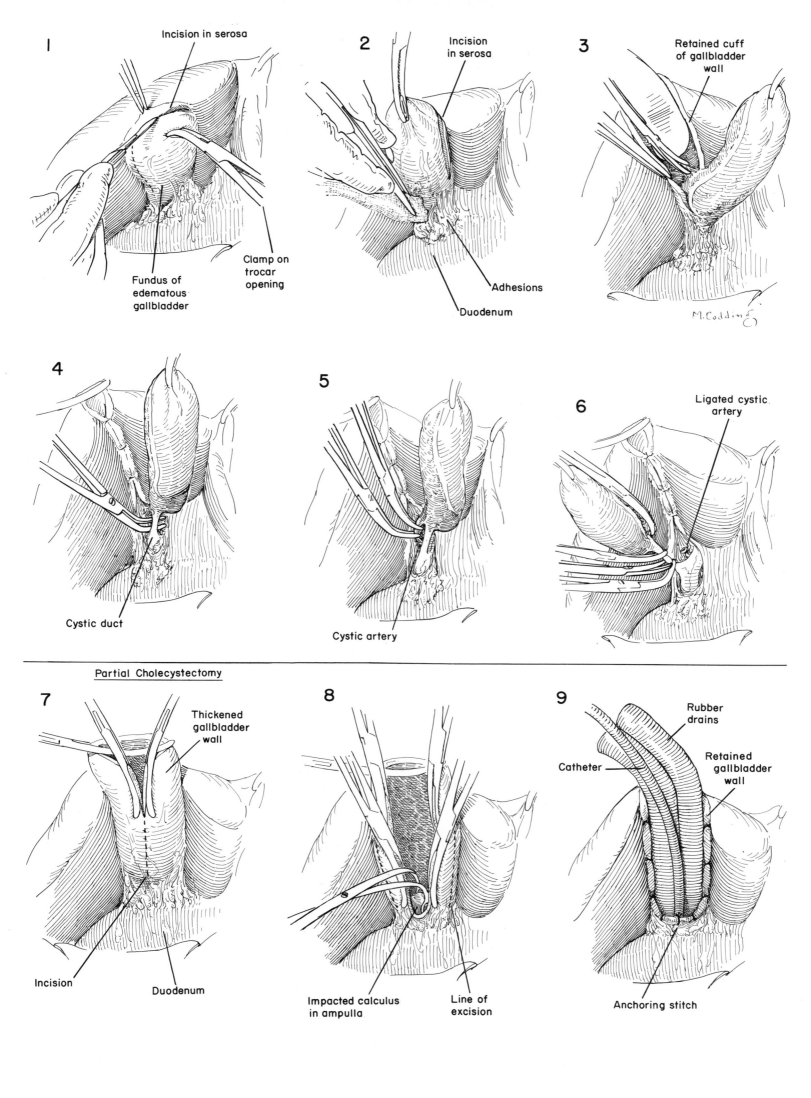

1 Incision in serosa
Fundus of edematous gallbladder
Clamp on trocar opening

2 Incision in serosa
Adhesions
Duodenum

3 Retained cuff of gallbladder wall
M. Codding

4 Cystic duct

5 Cystic artery

6 Ligated cystic artery

Partial Cholecystectomy

7 Thickened gallbladder wall
Incision
Duodenum

8 Impacted calculus in ampulla
Line of excision

9 Rubber drains
Retained gallbladder wall
Catheter
Anchoring stitch

PLATE LXXIII · CHOLECYSTOSTOMY—CHOLEDOCHOPLASTY

A. Cholecystostomy

INDICATIONS. Cholecystostomy, while not recognized as routine treatment for cholelithiasis, may be a life-saving procedure. It is the operation of choice in some elderly patients with acute cholecystitis, in poor surgical risks who present a well-defined mass, in seriously ill patients in whom minimal surgery is desirable when a large abscess surrounds the gallbladder, and when technical difficulties make cholecystectomy hazardous. If there is obstruction of the common duct with longstanding jaundice and a tendency toward hemorrhage which cannot be controlled by vitamin K and transfusions, preliminary cholecystostomy for decompression may be the procedure of choice.

PREOPERATIVE PREPARATION. See Plate LXVII.

ANESTHESIA. See Plate LXVII.

POSITION. The position for a gallbladder operation as described in Plate LXVII is used. With local anesthesia this is modified if the patient is uncomfortable.

OPERATIVE PREPARATION. The skin is prepared in the routine manner.

INCISION AND EXPOSURE. A small incision is made with its midportion directly over the maximum point of tenderness in the right upper quadrant. Occasionally, when unsuspected technical difficulties or inflammation more severe than anticipated are encountered, the procedure is carried out through the usual upper right rectus or infracostal incision. The adhesions are not dissected from the undersurface of the gallbladder, unless it is thought that cholecystectomy might be feasible **(Figure 1).**

DETAILS OF PROCEDURE. The fundus is walled off with gauze before the evacuation of its contents. An incision is made just through the serosa of the bulging fundus **(Figure 2).** A trocar is inserted to remove the liquid contents **(Figure 3).** Suction is maintained adjacent to the incision in the fundus as the trocar is withdrawn. A culture is taken routinely. The edematous wall is then grasped with Babcock forceps, and the opening is extended **(Figure 4).** A purse-string suture of fine catgut is placed about the opening in the fundus to control oozing and to close the fundus about the drainage tube. Any liquid or grumose material remaining in the lumen of the gallbladder is removed by suction. Since there is usually an impacted stone in the ampulla of the cystic duct, a determined effort is made to remove it to permit the escape of bile from the biliary ducts. A small, flexible scoop, such as a Cushing pituitary curet, is directed down to the ampulla **(Figure 5).** If the scoop cannot dislodge the stones, a fenestrated forceps is used. The lumen of the gallbladder is repeatedly flooded with saline. A small rubber catheter is inserted and anchored with an interrupted silk suture **(Figures 6 and 7),** or a Foley catheter may be used. The previously placed purse-string suture is tied snugly about the drainage tube **(Figure 7).** If the inflammation is severe, or if an abscess was encountered, or if there has been soiling about the wall, a rubber tissue drain is inserted along the wall of the gallbladder.

CLOSURE. Stitches are taken to anchor the fundus to the overlying peritoneum to prevent the soiling of the peritoneal cavity before the area is sealed off **(Figure 8).** A routine closure is made. After a sterile dressing has been applied, the drainage tube is anchored to the skin with a suture or adhesive tape and is connected to a drainage bottle.

POSTOPERATIVE CARE. See Plate LXXI. While the drainage tube is in place, a radiopaque substance may be injected and a cholangiogram taken for evidence of overlooked calculi. If the patient is in good condition, and the postoperative recovery is uncomplicated, a subsequent cholecystectomy may be performed through the original wound within several weeks. A secondary operation after cholecystostomy is not recommended in the extremely poor-risk patient.

B. Choledochoplasty

INDICATIONS. Plastic repair of the extrahepatic bile ducts is usually required as a result of stenosis or stricture following technical difficulties or errors, such as a fatty exposure or excessive bleeding that occurred during a previous cholecystectomy. The surgeon may hurriedly clamp and ligate blindly to control bleeding and include part or all of an extrahepatic bile duct. The ampulla of the gallbladder often lies parallel and adjacent to the common duct, so that the clamps applied roughly to the ampulla may also include a portion of the common duct.

During operation if the extrahepatic ducts have been injured or divided accidentally, they should be repaired immediately.

PREOPERATIVE PREPARATION. See Plate LXVII.

ANESTHESIA. See Plate LXVII.

POSITION. See Plate LXVII.

OPERATIVE PREPARATION. The skin is prepared in the routine manner.

INCISION AND EXPOSURE. The incision may be made through the old scar and may be extended if necessary. If there is an external biliary fistula, a small probe is introduced to facilitate the dissection of the sinus down to its origin. Sharp dissection may be necessary to divide the adhesions between the anterior surface of the liver and the overlying peritoneum. Because of the previous cholecystectomy, the duodenum or hepatic flexure of the colon may be drawn up toward the hilus of the liver, and meticulous dissection is required to separate these structures from the old gallbladder bed until the region of the hepatoduodenal ligament is visualized. The dissection may be started far out laterally, progressing toward the midline until the foramen of Winslow can be identified. The remainder of the abdomen is packed off with warm, moist gauze.

DETAILS OF PROCEDURE. The lateral margin of the hepatoduodenal ligament should be searched carefully for the common duct. The hepatoduodenal ligament is incised along its lateral margin. Usually, it is easier if the dilated upper end of the common duct can be located. This may require searching well up toward the hilus of the liver. The second portion of the duodenum should be mobilized to permit visualization of the common duct by incising the peritoneal reflection along its lateral border **(Figure 9).** The duodenum is retracted medially by blunt dissection to expose the head of the pancreas and the lower portion of the common duct **(Figure 10).** Traction sutures are placed in either side of the isolated duct, and an opening is made either above or below the stricture, depending upon the space available **(Figure 10).** An attempt is made to pass a probe past the constriction, and an incision is made on the probe up and down along the constricted area **(Figure 11).** Additional traction sutures are placed in the cut edges of the duct. Saline is injected through a catheter that is directed downward through Vater's papilla to prove the patency of the lower end of the duct. A rubber T-tube, No. 12 or 14F, is then passed through the opening that was made below the stricture **(Figure 12).** One arm is directed beyond the stricture and the other downward **(Figures 13 and 14).** Before the area of stricture is repaired, the duodenum is well mobilized to ensure that there will be no tension on the suture line. The distance gained must be more than the length of the vertical incision made through the strictured portion of the duct. The duodenum is pulled upward to the hilus of the liver, and its superior margin is anchored to the thickened hepatoduodenal ligament with interrupted sutures **(Figures 14 and 15).**

The vertical opening through the stricture is closed horizontally **(Figure 13).** The lateral traction sutures are gently manipulated so that the upper and lower lips of the opening approximate **(Figure 13).** Interrupted sutures are taken, including just the margin of the cut duct, and tied with the knot on the inside **(Figure 13).** A reinforcing layer of sutures is added if the tension is not too great and the tissue included does not encroach upon the lumen of the duct **(Figure 14).** The suture line is tested by injecting saline through the catheter, and a cholangiogram is made. If the ductal system is clear and contrast medium enters the duodenum freely, a final inspection to ensure that there is no tension on the suture line is made. The area is covered with omentum, and a rubber drain is inserted.

CLOSURE. Closure is routine.

POSTOPERATIVE CARE. Postoperative care is carried out as described in Plate LXXI. The common-duct catheter should not be removed for two or three weeks. The status of the extrahepatic biliary ducts should be determined by a cholangiogram before the catheter is removed. Accurate blood volume replacement is essential both during operation and postoperatively to avoid any prolonged period of hypotension. Hypotension in the jaundiced patient predisposes to uremia and should be carefully avoided by maintenance of a normal blood volume. Bile losses must be measured accurately. Sodium deficits are corrected by the administration of sodium lactate or sodium bicarbonate, depending upon the extent of the loss.

PLATE LXXIII   CHOLECYSTOSTOMY—CHOLEDOCHOPLASTY

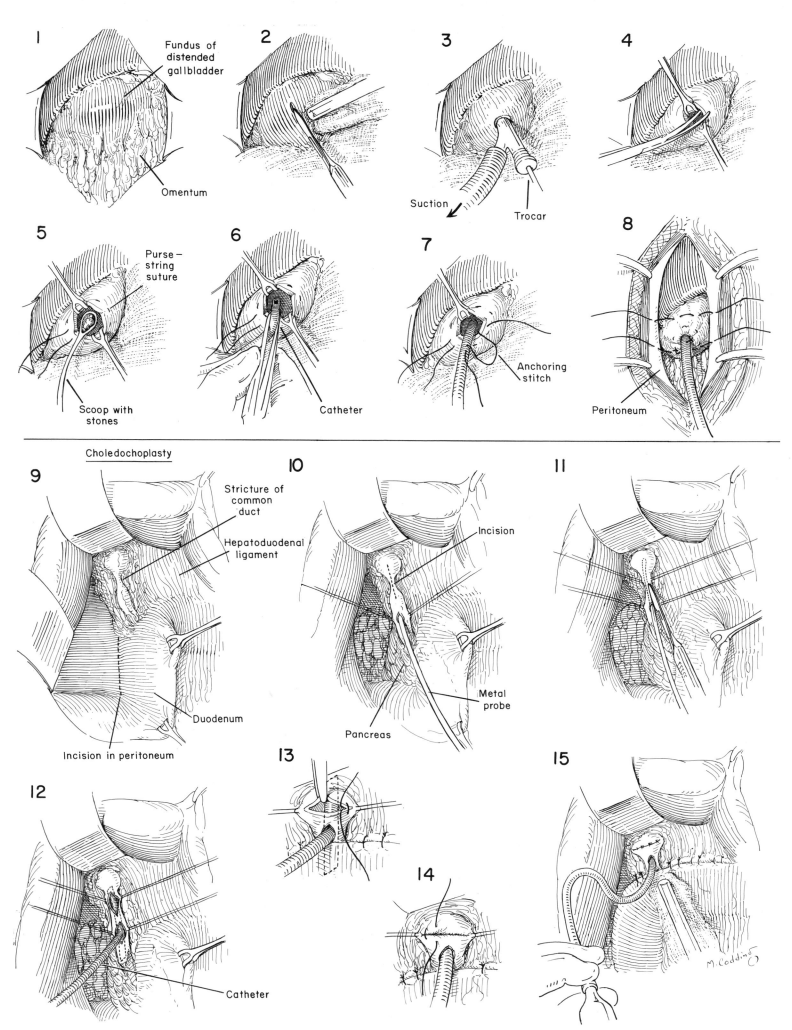

1

Fundus of distended gallbladder

Omentum

2

3

Suction

Trocar

4

5

Purse-string suture

Scoop with stones

6

Catheter

7

Anchoring stitch

8

Peritoneum

Choledochoplasty

9

Stricture of common duct

Hepatoduodenal ligament

Duodenum

Incision in peritoneum

10

Incision

Metal probe

Pancreas

11

12

Catheter

13

14

15

M. Codding

PLATE LXXIV · CHOLEDOCHOJEJUNOSTOMY—END-TO-END ANASTOMOSIS

A. Choledochojejunostomy (Mucosal Graft, Rodney Smith)

DETAILS OF PROCEDURE. The surgeon is occasionally faced with the difficult problem of finding the strictured area or blind end of the hepatic duct. The adhesions between the duodenum and hilus of the liver are carefully divided by sharp and blunt dissection **(Figure 1)**. Great care must be exercised to avoid unnecessary bleeding and possible injury to the underlying structures. Usually, it is easier to start the dissection quite far laterally and to free up the superior surface of the right lobe of the liver from the adherent duodenum, hepatic flexure of the colon, and omentum. Sharp dissection is used along the liver margins to avoid tearing the liver capsule, which results in a troublesome ooze. After the edge of the adhesion has been incised, blunt dissection will be more effective and safer in freeing up the undersurface of the liver. The exposure should be directed toward identifying and exposing the foramen of Winslow. The stomach may or may not have to be dissected away from the liver. Usually, the duodenum is drawn up into the old gallbladder bed and fixed by dense adhesions. The second portion of the duodenum is mobilized medially, following division of the peritoneum along its lateral margin **(Figure 2)**. As the duodenum is reflected downward and the undersurface of the liver is retracted upward, the upper portion of the dilated duct may be verified by aspiration of bile through a fine hypodermic needle **(Figure 3)**, and a cholangiogram may be performed. The needle may be left in place, and an incision is made alongside the needle until a free flow of bile is obtained. A blunt-nosed, curved clamp is inserted upward into the dilated duct and the opening gradually enlarged by dilatation, which may include an additional incision to enlarge the opening. No effort is made to free up the entire circumference of the ductal system, since the mucosal graft will be eventually intussuscepted well up into the duct without a direct end-to-end anastomosis **(Figure 6)**.

Following the opening of the dilated common hepatic duct, a long curved clamp is inserted, usually toward the left side, and extended up through the liver substance. A rubber tube (14-16F) is pulled down through the liver and partially out through the duct opening **(Figure 4)**. Following this, a Roux-en-Y arm of jejunum is prepared in the usual way. The end of the mobilized jejunal arm is closed with two layers of interrupted silk. On the antimesenteric border of the jejunum a 5-cm. segment of the seromuscular coat is excised approximately 5 cm. from the closed end **(Figure 4)**. Care should be taken to avoid making any additional openings in the mucosa except in the very apex of the protruding mucosal pocket. The tube which was pulled down through the liver is now directed through the small opening made in the apex of the mucosal pocket and directed down into the arm of jejunum for 10 or more centimeters. A purse-string suture of catgut is placed in the mucosa about the tube and tied. After the tube has been passed the desired distance down the Roux-en-Y limb, a No. 2 chromic catgut suture is passed completely through the jejunal walls and around the tube to fix it in position when tied just distal to the mucosal outpocketing. A centimeter or two distally a similar suture of catgut is taken to ensure further fixation **(Figure 6, A and B)**. These are the only sutures utilized to fix the tube to the wall of the jejunum. These sutures ensure fixation of the jejunal mucosa to the tube as it is withdrawn. Several holes are cut around the tube just above the mucosal graft to ensure drainage of the right as well as the left hepatic duct. Traction then is placed on the end of the tube coming out of the dome of the liver in order to pull the mucosal graft carefully and firmly up into place inside the common hepatic duct. This provides an intussusception of the jejunal mucosa up into the dilated common hepatic duct and ensures direct mucosa-to-mucosa approximation **(Figure 6)**. In very high strictures it may be necessary to use a tube into the left as well as the right hepatic radical. Special tubes have been devised for very high strictures that sparate the right from the left hepatic ducts. The Roux-en-Y loop is securely anchored in place beneath the liver by several catgut sutures placed through the seromuscular coat and the scar tissue around the opening into the duct system **(Figure 5)**.

CLOSURE. The tube is brought out through a separate stab wound to one side or the other of the incision and anchored securely in place with nonabsorbable suture material. The wound is closed in layers after suction drainage is instituted to the undersurface of the liver by a plastic tube with many perforations.

POSTOPERATIVE CARE. The tube going to the anastomosis is placed on low-grade constant suction to divert bile until the newly made junction is healed. The appropriate antibiotic therapy should be adjusted following culture and sensitivity studies of the bile. The tube may be irrigated with saline intermittently to wash out all debris or small calculi. In addition, the tube provides a means of taking postoperative transhepatic cholangiograms from time to time to evaluate the security of the anastomosis and the evidence of regression in the size of the formerly obstructed ducts. Ordinarily, the tube is left in place for a minimum of four months. A complete evaluation with liver function studies and several cultures of the bile should be made, as well as a cholangiogram, before it is advisable to remove the tube.

B. End-to-End Anastomosis

In rare instances the common duct may be accidentally divided and the injury fortunately discovered at once. This is likely to occur just below the junction of the hepatic and cystic ducts as a result of technical errors. The surgeon should always inspect the common and hepatic ducts at the completion of cholecystectomy to make certain that they are not angulated or otherwise injured. If there is any question, sufficient time should be spent to make certain that the extrahepatic biliary system has not been damaged. The surgeon should be alert for any error at the time of operation and take steps to remedy it. If the common duct has been completely divided, a direct end-to-end anastomosis may be performed.

The peritoneum on the lateral wall of the duodenum should be divided, and the duodenum should be mobilized to relieve any possible tension on the suture line. Clamps are not applied to the severed ends of the ducts. Irregular or frayed edges are excised. Both ends of the duct are held in position with guide sutures of fine 0000 silk **(Figure 7)**. A posterior layer of interrupted sutures is placed without entering the lumen to approximate the posterior duct walls **(Figure 8)**. Upon completion of the posterior layer all of the sutures are divided except one at either angle to serve for purposes of traction **(Figure 9)**. The posterior layers of mucous membrane are closed with very fine interrupted silk sutures. Following this the common duct is exposed for a short distance, preferably downward, to permit the opening of the duct, as in choledochostomy, and the introduction of a T-tube catheter **(Figure 10)**. One arm of the tube is passed up beyond the suture line to ensure an adequate lumen for the duct when the anterior layer of sutures is placed, and the other is directed downward. If the duct has been divided quite low, the opening may be made above the suture line with one arm of the tube directed downward. The mucous membrane of the common duct is closed over the T-tube with interrupted 0000 silk sutures with the knots on the inside **(Figure 11)**. The second layer of sutures is placed close to the original layer to reinforce the line of anastomosis **(Figure 12)**.

All the sutures taken in the duct must be accurately placed with small needles and fine 0000 silk and must include only a very small bite of tissue to avoid stenosis. After the anastomosis has been completed, saline is injected into the catheter to make certain that there is no leakage about the suture line, and a cholangiogram is made. A final inspection verifies the absence of undue tension on the suture line. A rubber drain is inserted past the foramen of Winslow into Morrison's pouch.

CLOSURE. The rubber drain and common-duct catheter are brought out through a stab wound lateral to the incision. The wound is closed in the routine manner. The catheter is anchored to the skin with a silk suture and adhesive tape. Sterile dressings are applied.

POSTOPERATIVE CARE. See Plate LXXI.

PLATE LXXIV   CHOLEDOCHOJEJUNOSTOMY—END-TO-END ANASTOMOSIS

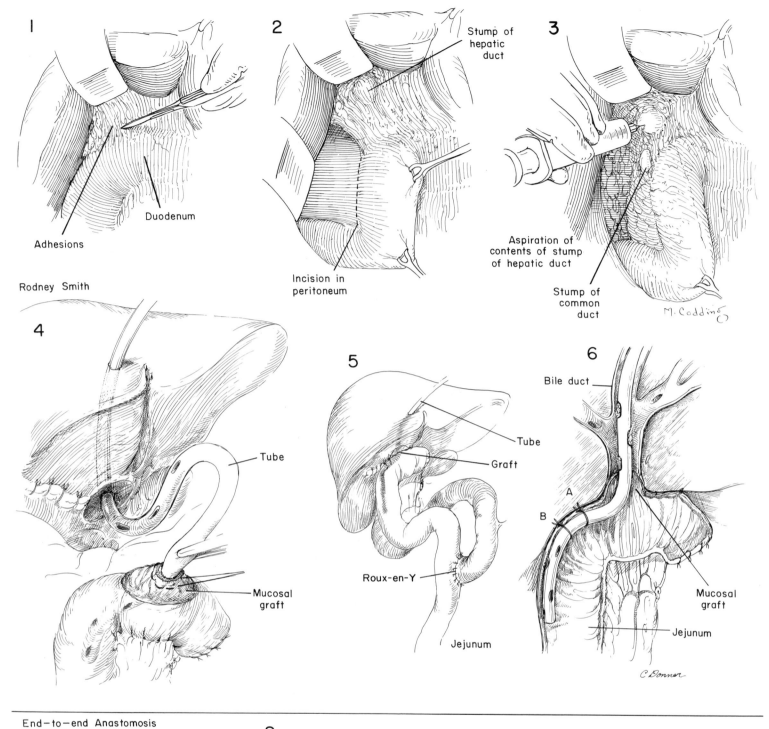

1

Adhesions

Duodenum

2

Stump of
hepatic
duct

Incision in
peritoneum

3

Aspiration of
contents of stump
of hepatic duct

Stump of
common
duct

M. Codding

Rodney Smith

4

Tube

Mucosal
graft

5

Tube

Graft

Roux-en-Y

Jejunum

6

Bile duct

A

B

Mucosal
graft

Jejunum

C. Donner

End-to-end Anastomosis

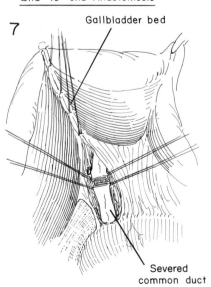

7

Gallbladder bed

Severed
common duct

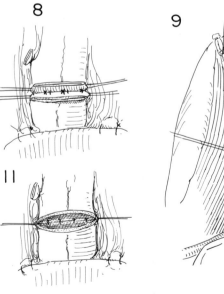

8

11

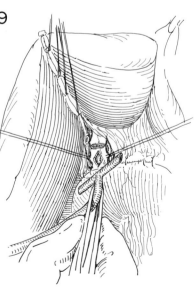

9

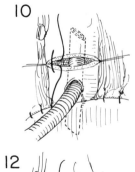

10

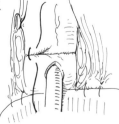

12

PLATE LXXV · CHOLECYSTOGASTROSTOMY—BIOPSY OF LIVER

A. Cholecystogastrostomy

INDICATIONS. This procedure may be utilized in poor-risk patients having a limited life expectancy because of inoperable malignant disease obstructing the common duct. Occasionally, it is used as a first-stage procedure in a poor-risk patient in order to relieve the jaundice and improve the patient's general condition preliminary to a radical resection of the head of the pancreas. In making this short-circuiting anastomosis, it is preferable to utilize the nearest portion of the upper gastrointestinal tract that can easily be approximated to the gallbladder without tension. The gallbladder should not be utilized in an attempt to relieve obstructive jaundice if the cystic duct is obstructed or if the lower end of the common duct is to be removed in a radical resection. In such instances it is desirable to anastomose the open end of the retained common duct to the jejunum, lest leakage develop at the site of the common duct closure. Visualization of the gallbladder and ducts by contrast media may be worth while to prove beyond any doubt the site of obstruction.

PREOPERATIVE PREPARATION. Although the operation is a simple one, the patients are such poor risks that they require careful preparation to avoid a fatality. A high-carbohydrate, high-vitamin, and high-protein diet is given, or hyperalimentation may be needed. As a rule, the patient is deeply jaundiced, and there is already serious liver damage. Whole blood transfusions and large doses of vitamin K are indicated until the prothrombin level returns to a normal range. If the blood volume is not restored, hypotension may occur with a greatly increased tendency toward uremia. At no time should a period of hypotension be permitted in the presence of severe jaundice because of the threat of a renal shutdown.

ANESTHESIA. See Plate LXVII.

POSITION. The position of the patient is adjusted as described for cholecystectomy (Plate LXVII); if local anesthesia is used, this position may be modified for the patient's comfort.

OPERATIVE PREPARATION. The skin is prepared in the usual manner.

INCISION AND EXPOSURE. Usually, a right paramedian incision about 2 or 3 cm. lateral to the midline and reaching from the xiphocostal junction almost to the umbilicus is made, opening the rectus sheath anteriorly and posteriorly. However, either a transverse or a Kocher oblique incision is satisfactory for those familiar with these approaches to the gallbladder. Bleeding and oozing points in the wound or within the peritoneal cavity are meticulously ligated. Exploration is carried out to determine the nature of the disease causing the obstruction, i.e., whether there is a tumor located in or about the common duct or in the head of the pancreas, whether the tumor is primary or metastatic, or whether there is a common duct stone. In the presence of malignant disease obstructing the common duct without distant metastasis, the duodenum should be mobilized and the operability of the lesion determined. Involvement about the portal vein contraindicates surgery. If extensive involvement or dislocation of the duodenum by tumor is apparent, a posterior gastroenterostomy should also be planned to avoid possible late obstruction. A determined attempt should be made to prove the suspicion of tumor, even though extra effort may be required to obtain the biopsy. For biopsy purposes, mobilization of the duodenum may be indicated to expose the posterior side of the head of the pancreas, if the tumor seems more superficial there.

DETAILS OF PROCEDURE. If the lesion is inoperable and the life expectancy short, the surgeon must determine whether it is easier to anastomose the distended gallbladder to the stomach, the duodenum, or the jejunum as a palliative measure. The same type of anastomosis is used whichever viscus is chosen. The more complicated but efficient types of anastomosis, such as a Roux-en-Y anastomosis, are not necessary unless they are part of a radical extirpation of a malignant lesion with a reasonable chance of prolonged life expectancy.

As a rule, it is easy to perform the anastomosis to the stomach, preferably 2 to 4 cm. above the pylorus and near the greater curvature. Should such an anastomosis be likely to leave the gallbladder under tension when the patient is erect, the anastomosis should be made to the duodenum or upper jejunum.

A portion of the bowel is held up to the gallbladder on its medial side about 2 to 3 cm. below the fundus (**Figure 1**). If the gallbladder is greatly distended, it may be emptied through a trocar before the anastomosis is started; if not, a posterior row of interrupted fine silk sutures is placed to bring the two viscera in apposition without opening either of them (**Figure 2**). These sutures should not enter the lumen. The interrupted sutures (S_1) on either end of the posterior serosal layer are left long, and the others are cut to expose the field where the incisions into the gallbladder and stomach are to be made (**Figure 3**). The incisions are then made with the scalpel paralleling the suture line, with suction used to control the spread of any contents from either viscus (**Figure 3**). With scissors, the incisions are then lengthened to give a stoma of 1 to 2 cm. (**Figure 4**). To avoid contamination some surgeons prefer to carry out this procedure with enterostomy clamps applied to the gallbladder and stomach. The bleeding from the mucosa of the stomach, which is the only bothersome element, can be controlled easily by placing a mosquito snap on each of the major vessels. The clamps should be loosened and all bleeding points ligated before closure of the anterior layer.

When the field is dry, the operator places a series of interrupted 0000 fine silk sutures in the mucosal layers (**Figure 5**). The anterior mucosal layer is closed with interrupted sutures with the knots on the inside (**Figure 6**). After the mucosal sutures are laid, an anterior row of interrupted sutures is placed between the serosal coats to complete the anastomosis (**Figures 7** and **8**). The patency of the stoma is tested by palpation between the thumb and index finger, and as a precaution several sutures may be inserted at either angle. The field must be free of oozing points.

CLOSURE. After the table is leveled, the omentum is brought up about the anastomosis. A temporary gastrostomy may be made, since gastric emptying will be delayed. The incision is closed without drainage in a routine fashion.

POSTOPERATIVE CARE. The patient is placed in a semi-Fowler's position. Special attention is given to combating hemorrhagic tendencies with vitamin K therapy and whole blood transfusions. The administration of fluids and food by mouth is restricted for a few days, as in other intestinal anastomoses. The appearance of bile in the stools and a decreasing icteric index indicate that the anastomosis is functioning. A high-vitamin, high-protein, and high-carbohydrate diet is resumed as soon as tolerated. The gastrostomy tube is removed within ten days or when gastric emptying is assured and the oral caloric intake is adequate. In elderly, poor-risk patients who refuse to eat, the gastrostomy tube can be used for the refeeding of bile mixed with milk and other liquids in order to hasten their recovery.

B. Biopsy of Liver

INDICATIONS. It is not uncommon during an exploratory laparotomy to remove a small fragment of the liver for histologic study. Biopsy of the liver is indicated in most patients who have a history of splenic or liver disease, or in the presence of a metastatic nodule. The specimen should not be taken from an area near the gallbladder, since the vascular and lymphatic connections between the liver and gallbladder are such that a pathologic process involving the gallbladder may have spread to the neighboring liver, and, as a result, the biopsy would not give a true picture of the liver as a whole.

DETAILS OF PROCEDURE. Two deep 00 silk sutures, a and b, are placed about 2 cm. apart at the liver border (**Figure 1**). If a silk suture is placed, a fine needle is used; if catgut, an atraumatic type of needle. The suture is passed through the edge of the liver and back through again to include about one-half the original distance (**Figure 1A**). This prevents the suture from slipping off the biopsy margin with resultant bleeding. These sutures are tied with a surgeon's knot, which will not slip between the tying of the first and second parts (**Figure 1A**). The thread should be pulled as tightly as possible without cutting into the liver, for the tension under which these knots are tied is the important factor in the procedure. Such sutures control the blood supply to the intervening liver substance. The two sutures are placed not more than 2 cm. apart, deep in the liver substance; yet as they are tied, at least 2 cm. of liver are included at the free margin to increase the size of the biopsy by making it triangular in shape. An additional mattress suture, c, may be taken at the tip of the triangular wound (**Figure 2**). After the biopsy is removed with a scalpel (**Figure 3**), the wound is closed by tying together the sutures, a and b, or by placing an additional mattress suture, d, beyond the limits of the original sutures (**Figures 4** and **5**). The area of biopsy is covered with some type of coagulant.

PLATE LXXV   CHOLECYSTOGASTROSTOMY—BIOPSY OF LIVER

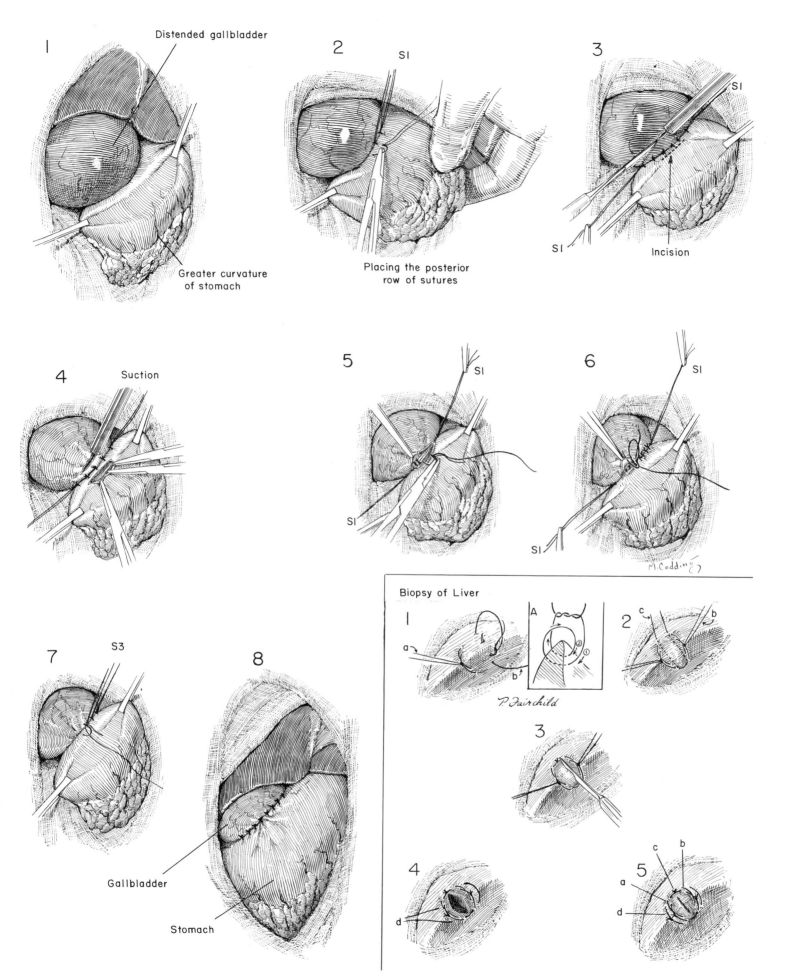

1 — Distended gallbladder / Greater curvature of stomach

2 — SI / Placing the posterior row of sutures

3 — SI / SI / Incision

4 — Suction

5 — SI / SI

6 — SI / SI

7 — S3

8 — Gallbladder / Stomach

M. Codding

Biopsy of Liver

1 — a / b' / A / P. Fairchild

2 — c / b

3

4 — d

5 — c / b / a / d

PLATE LXXVI · ANATOMY AND RESECTIONS OF THE LIVER

SURGICAL ANATOMY OF LIVER. The liver is divided into eight major subsegments or areas (excluding the caudate lobe), with the principal line of division between the right and left sides extending cephalad and obliquely from the middle of the gallbladder fossa to the center of the inferior vena cava between the right and left main hepatic veins **(Figure 1, A-A¹).** The true anatomic left lobe thus defined is divided into medial and lateral segments approximately along the line of the falciform or round ligament, and each of these segments is then subdivided into a superior (cephalad) area and an inferior (caudad) area **(Figure 2).** In contrast, the right lobe is divided into anterior and posterior segments by a plane from the anteroinferior edge of the liver that extends both superiorly and posteriorly. This cleavage is similar to the oblique fissure above the right lower lobe of the lung, and it is roughly parallel to it. These segments of the right hepatic lobe are then split into superior and inferior areas similar to those on the left **(Figure 2).**

Although the segmentation of the liver appears straightforward, successful segmentectomy or lobectomy depends upon a thorough understanding of the difference between the portal vein, biliary duct, and hepatic artery distribution as opposed to the hepatic vein drainage. In general, the portal triad structures bifurcate in a serial manner and ultimately lead directly into each of the eight areas. The specific exception to this rule is the parumbilicalis of the left hepatic branch of the portal vein, as this structure straddles the division between the left inferior medial and lateral segments. Thus it lies roughly under the round ligament **(Figure 1, 7).** The superior and inferior areas of the left lateral lobe have a portal venous supply from either end of the parumbilicalis **(Figure 1, 9 and 10);** however, special note should be made of the paired medial supply to the superior and inferior areas of the medial segment **(Figure 1, 8 and 12).** It is equally important at this point to examine the biliary and arterial supply of this area **(Figure 7).** The main left hepatic duct and artery proceed with the expected bifurcations out through the superior and inferior divisions of the left lateral segment; however, the left medial segment duct and artery **(Figure 7, 13)** do not divide and send a large branch to the superior and inferior areas, but rather send long paired structures out in each direction from the junction of the two areas **(Figure 7, 12 and 13).**

In contrast, the portal triad distribution to the right hepatic lobe is by a straightforward arborization with major divisions first into anterior and posterior segments followed by secondary divisions into superior and inferior subsegmental vessels **(Figure 1, 2 through 5).** Interestingly, the caudate lobe straddles the major right and left cleavage plane and simply receives its portal supply directly from the right and left main branches of the portal vein, hepatic arteries, and biliary ducts. Its venous return, however, is usually a single caudate lobe hepatic vein that enters the inferior vena cava on its left side just distal to the main hepatic veins **(Figure 1, 11).**

The hepatic veins, in general, run between the hepatic segments in a manner analogous to the pulmonary veins. The right hepatic vein lies in the major cleft between the anterior and posterior segments on that side **(Figure 1, 14).** The left hepatic vein **(Figure 1, 15)** drains predominantly the lateral segment, while the middle hepatic vein **(Figure 1, 16)** crosses between the left medial segment and the right lobe. It is imperative to know that this middle vein usually joins the main left hepatic vein within a few centimeters of the junction with the vena cava and that this vein has two major tributaries that cross over into the right anterior inferior and the left medial inferior areas **(Figure 1, 17).** Appropriate preservation of these channels is, of course, all-important in specific segmental resections, as hepatic venous occlusion results in necrosis of the entire area(s) involved.

The remaining figures demonstrate the four most common hepatic resections, whose specific details are covered in the operative text (Plates LXXVII through LXXX). Of specific note are the "danger points" along the parumbilicalis of the left branch of the portal vein **(Figures 4, 5, and 6).** It is in these areas that the surgeon must be certain of the integrity of the hepatic venous drainage before dividing any major venous branches. Also shown is the use of interlocking full-thickness mattress sutures for hemostasis in the partial and total left lateral segmentectomies, a common technic **(Figures 3 and 4),** as is the finger fracture technic.

PLATE LXXVI   ANATOMY AND RESECTIONS OF THE LIVER

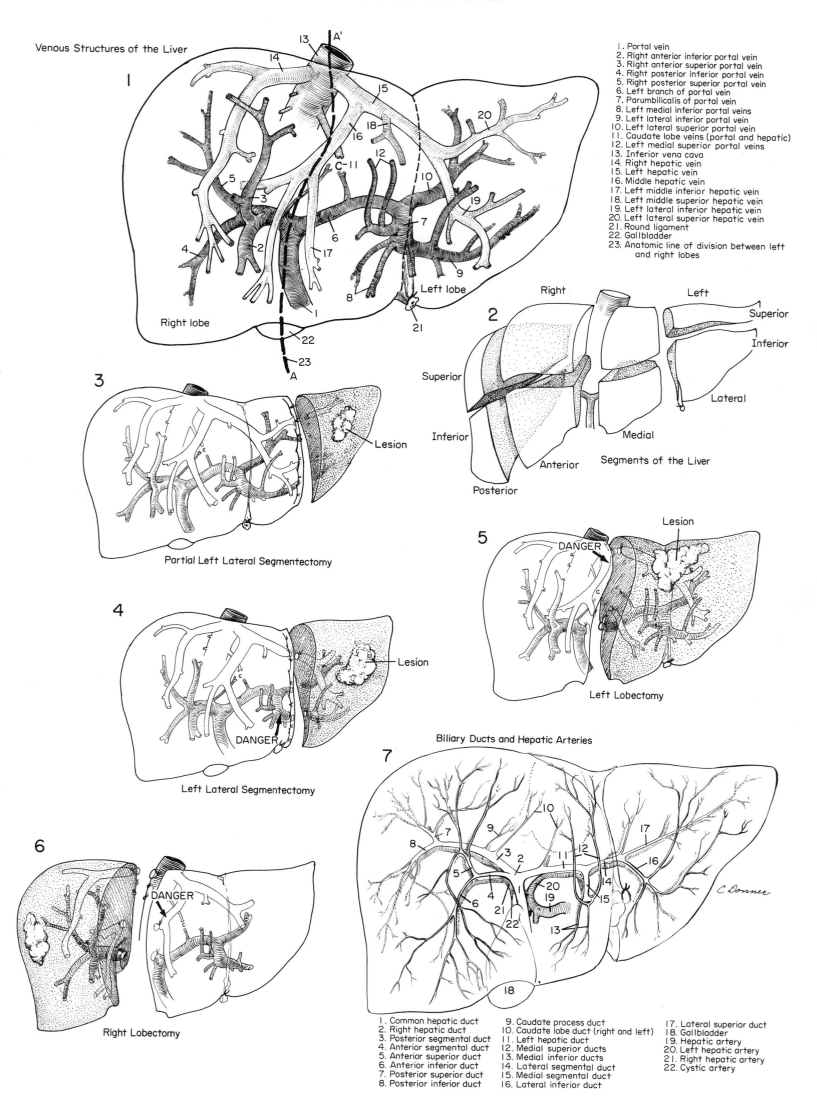

Venous Structures of the Liver

1. Portal vein
2. Right anterior inferior portal vein
3. Right anterior superior portal vein
4. Right posterior inferior portal vein
5. Right posterior superior portal vein
6. Left branch of portal vein
7. Parumbilicalis of portal vein
8. Left medial inferior portal veins
9. Left lateral inferior portal vein
10. Left lateral superior portal vein
11. Caudate lobe veins (portal and hepatic)
12. Left medial superior portal veins
13. Inferior vena cava
14. Right hepatic vein
15. Left hepatic vein
16. Middle hepatic vein
17. Left middle inferior hepatic vein
18. Left middle superior hepatic vein
19. Left lateral inferior hepatic vein
20. Left lateral superior hepatic vein
21. Round ligament
22. Gallbladder
23. Anatomic line of division between left and right lobes

Partial Left Lateral Segmentectomy

Segments of the Liver

Left Lateral Segmentectomy

Left Lobectomy

Right Lobectomy

Biliary Ducts and Hepatic Arteries

1. Common hepatic duct
2. Right hepatic duct
3. Posterior segmental duct
4. Anterior segmental duct
5. Anterior superior duct
6. Anterior inferior duct
7. Posterior superior duct
8. Posterior inferior duct
9. Caudate process duct
10. Caudate lobe duct (right and left)
11. Left hepatic duct
12. Medial superior ducts
13. Medial inferior ducts
14. Lateral segmental duct
15. Medial segmental duct
16. Lateral inferior duct
17. Lateral superior duct
18. Gallbladder
19. Hepatic artery
20. Left hepatic artery
21. Right hepatic artery
22. Cystic artery

C. Donner

PLATE LXXVII · RIGHT HEPATIC LOBECTOMY

INDICATIONS. Massive hepatic resection may be indicated for hepatic carcinomas, cysts, and liver-cell adenomas, gallbladder or bowel carcinomas in continuity, hemangiomas, or traumatic rupture of liver parenchyma. Metastatic malignancy within the liver is not ordinarily an indication for resection, unless it presents a technically easy resection, as a solitary metastasis, and its primary origin, preferably the colon, has been removed. Possible hemorrhage associated with the giant hemangiomas and the probability of malignant degeneration in liver-cell adenomas are the major reasons for vigorous pursuit of these lesions. Lastly, resection for massive traumatic rupture confined to an anatomic lobe is usually preferred if multiple mattress sutures or hepatic artery ligations are inadequate in controlling loss of blood and bile.

PREOPERATIVE PREPARATION. In patients with liver trauma the primary preoperative considerations, of course, are concerned with the maintenance of an adequate blood volume and assessment and treatment of associated injuries. The majority of patients undergoing elective hepatic resection have normal liver function. In these no specific preparation is indicated other than hepatic angiography, which should be done in all patients before elective resection to provide information regarding the arterial blood supply. In about one-fourth of the patients, in whom liver function is altered preoperatively, assessment should be made similar to that recommended for patients undergoing portacaval anastomosis. In general, patients with severe degrees of sodium sulfobromophthalein retention, hypoalbuminemia, and hypoprothrombinemia should not be considered for massive resection. Large doses of antibiotics that have a high concentration in bile may be given.

ANESTHESIA. Careful preoperative preparation, control of blood volume and blood pressure, and avoidance of anoxia are more important than the choice of an anesthetic agent. However, because of the possible relationship between liver damage and the use of halogenated anesthetics, these agents or any potentially hepatotoxic drugs should not be used in patients undergoing massive liver resection.

POSITION. The patient should be placed on the operating table with the right side elevated about 30 degrees. Rotation of the shoulder somewhat more than the hips by the use of appropriately placed pads will facilitate the thoracic extension of the incision. The right arm should be placed in a position that will not cause undue pressure or traction. Suspending the arm from a soft sling attached to the ether screen is satisfactory.

OPERATIVE PREPARATION. In patients with abnormal liver function the preoperative measures outlined should be continued up to the time of operation. In addition, in these patients as well as those with normal liver function, ambulation should be encouraged up to the day of operation. Blood volume deficits should be replaced, and the patient should stop smoking. In anticipation of possible hepatic insufficiency, chemical and mechanical preparation of the bowel should be accomplished in the period immediately before operation. The prophylactic administration of vitamin K despite normal prothrombin activity may be useful. It is also wise to assure the availability of four units of fresh whole blood, fresh frozen plasma, and other agents that may prove useful for the management of postoperative complications. Appropriate intraoperative monitoring should include arterial and central venous pressure measurement.

INCISION AND EXPOSURE. Of several suitable incisions a long right subcostal incision extending across the left rectus muscle and then extended in a T fashion into the chest through the seventh or eighth right intercostal space provides adequate exposure **(Figure 1).** A midline abdominal incision, extended up as a median sternotomy, provides good exposure.

DETAILS OF PROCEDURE. Figure 2 shows the plan of the resection. The hepatoduodenal structures are divided in the order the numbers suggest. The line of resection of liver extends from the gallbladder bed to the vena cava **(Figure 2).** The diaphragm is radially incised between clamps to the orifice of the inferior vena cava **(Figure 3).** By carefully avoiding the main trunk of the phrenic nerve, postoperative diaphragmatic paralysis may be minimized. Suture ligation of the cut surface of the diaphragm is recommended.

Dissection is begun in the hilar region, where the structures of the hepatoduodenal ligament are dissected free and identified. The gallbladder is removed after division of the cystic artery and duct **(Figure 4).** The right primary branches of the hepatic artery, portal vein, and bile ducts must be exposed and identified with great care to avoid injury to the structures serving the remaining left lobe of the liver. The right hepatic duct and artery are ligated and divided in order **(Figures 5** and **6).** If doubt exists, trial occlusion of the vessels by a noncrushing clamp may be helpful. If both the arterial and portal venous supply to the right lobe are occluded, a line of color demarcation can be detected corresponding to the anatomic division between the right and left lobes, extending from the midpoint of the gallbladder fossa to the midpoint of the inferior vena cava.

PLATE LXXVII   RIGHT HEPATIC LOBECTOMY

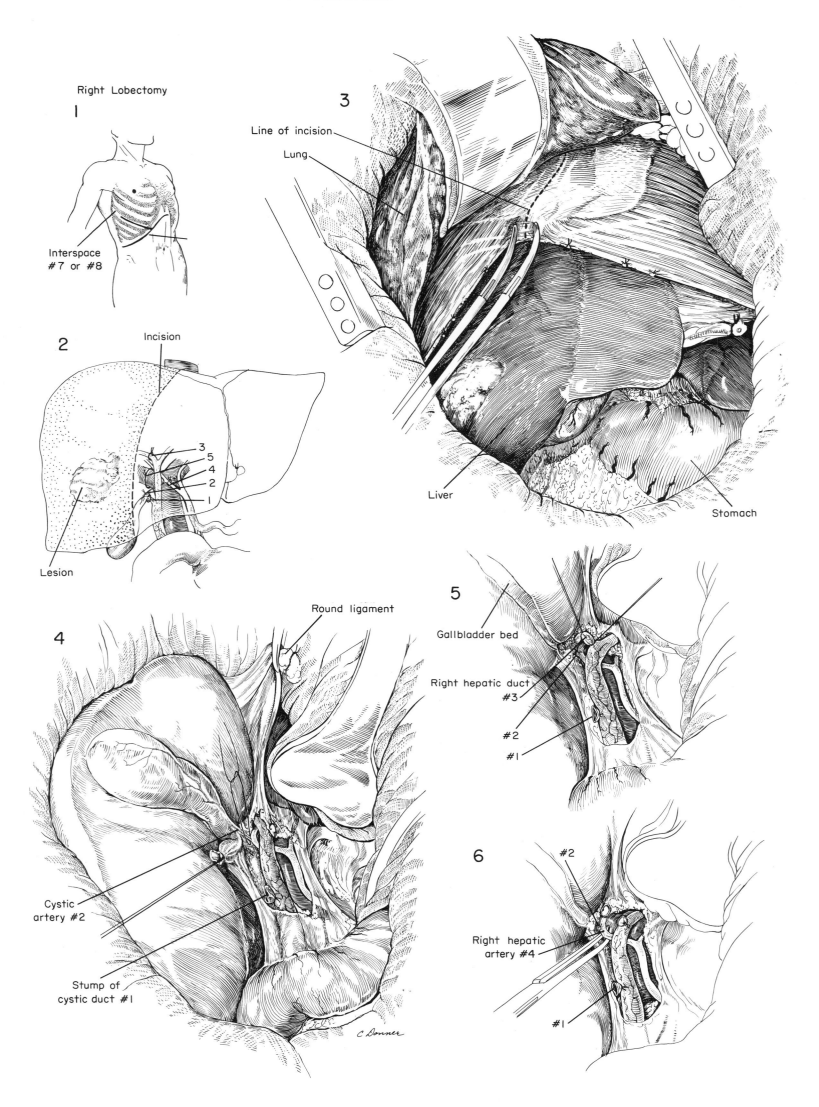

Right Lobectomy

1

Interspace #7 or #8

2

Incision

3
5
4
2
1

Lesion

3

Line of incision

Lung

Liver

Stomach

4

Round ligament

Cystic artery #2

Stump of cystic duct #1

5

Gallbladder bed

Right hepatic duct #3

#2

#1

6

#2

Right hepatic artery #4

#1

C Donner

PLATE LXXVIII · RIGHT HEPATIC LOBECTOMY

DETAILS OF PROCEDURE (*Continued*). The right branch of the portal vein supplying the right lobe is sufficiently isolated to ensure a double ligation of the proximal stump which includes a distal stick tie **(Figure 7).** Further mobilization of the liver is obtained by dividing the relatively avascular right triangular ligament **(Figure 8).** It is preferable now to ligate the right hepatic vein and the right accessory veins which enter the inferior vena cava at the diaphragm. This may be done by rotating the liver down and to the left, exposing first the right hepatic vein as it enters the vena cava. It must be borne in mind that because these veins are extremely short and easily torn, this dissection must be carried out with extreme care, and vascular clamps should be readily available **(Figure 9).** The method of dividing the liver substance involves placing interlocking mattress sutures of heavy catgut along the line of proposed resection. A variety of methods is available to assist in the placement of these sutures, which include large circular needles or long straight ligature carriers designed for this purpose. Care is taken to leave behind a margin of the demarked area, thus avoiding tying the middle hepatic vein with the mattress sutures **(Figure 10).** After a shallow incision is made between the rows of sutures, fluid losses may be reduced by dividing the parenchyma bluntly with the finger or a blunt instrument, such as the handle of the scalpel, individually securing and ligating the vessels and bile ducts as they are encountered **(Figure 10).** Dissection is begun just to the right of the center of the gallbladder fossa. By beginning at this point and continuing the dissection at a slight angle toward the left, one can ordinarily follow the main trunk of the middle hepatic vein in the interlobar fissure **(Figure 10).**

PLATE LXXVIII   RIGHT HEPATIC LOBECTOMY

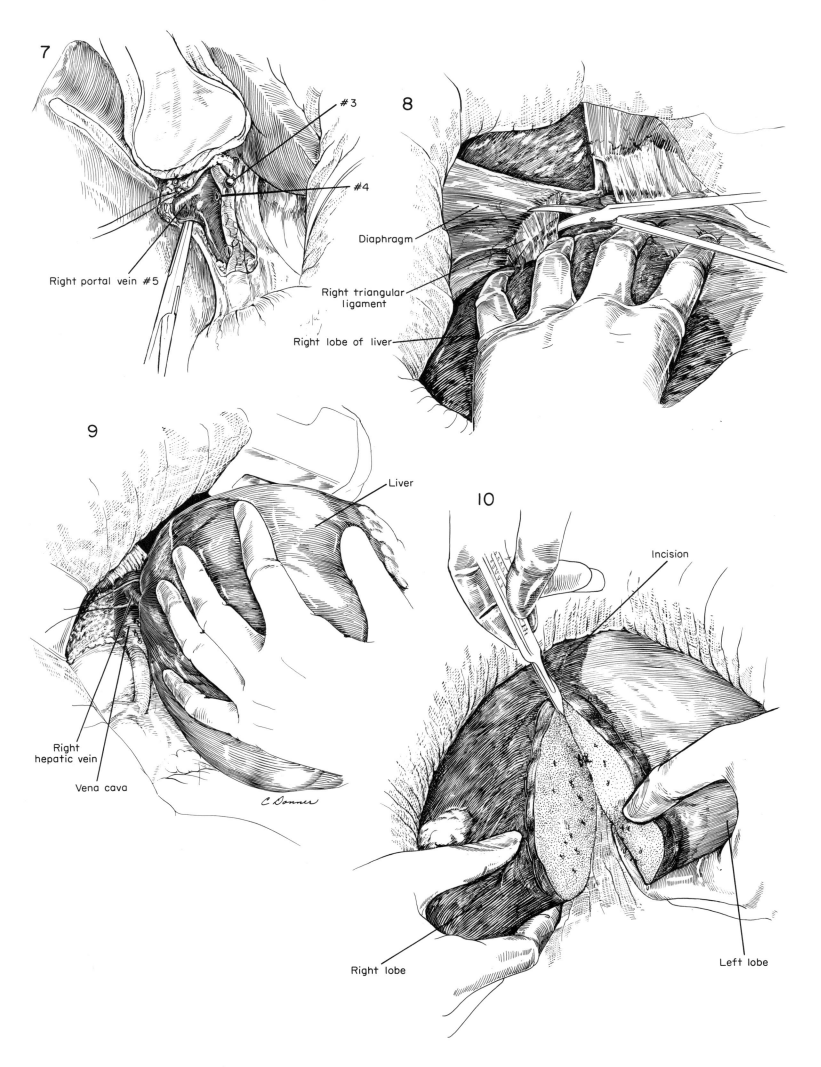

7

Right portal vein #5

#3

#4

8

Diaphragm

Right triangular
ligament

Right lobe of liver

9

Liver

Right
hepatic vein

Vena cava

C Donner

10

Incision

Right lobe

Left lobe

PLATE LXXIX · RIGHT HEPATIC LOBECTOMY

DETAILS OF PROCEDURE (*Continued*). The line of color demarcation in the liver following ligation of the hilar structures corresponds to the interlobar fissure. Using the darkened area as a guide, dissection is continued more deeply into the liver substance, controlling the tributaries of the hepatic veins from the right lobe individually, as schematically outlined in **Figure 11.** This dissection is then carried down to the vena cava **(Figure 12).** This technic will leave a small amount of devitalized liver tissue along the margin, since the dissection should be slightly to the right of the fissure. If mattress sutures are used, they must be placed in the left lobe, leaving a sufficient cuff of tissue of the right hepatic lobe to ensure against injury of the middle hepatic vein, which should be preserved. After the vena cava is reached, the right lobe is freed of any remaining attachments and removed **(Figure 12).** A flap of peritoneum or omentum is

useful but not necessary in sealing the raw surface of the liver after removal of the excised lobe **(Figure 13).** Before closure, injection of methylene blue into the biliary system will reveal any open biliary ducts that may have escaped detection, but this step is not necessary. Following major hepatic resection, especially for trauma, decompression of the biliary tree with a T-tube may be advisable. The edges of the diaphragm as well as the sternum are reapproximated as indicated.

CLOSURE. Two catheter-type sump drains are placed in the wound, one inserted through the lateral end of the wound and the other placed more medially near the intersection of the T incision. These can be used for cross-flushing the tremendous cavity remaining after the right hepatectomy. The incision is closed in layers.

PLATE LXXIX   RIGHT HEPATIC LOBECTOMY

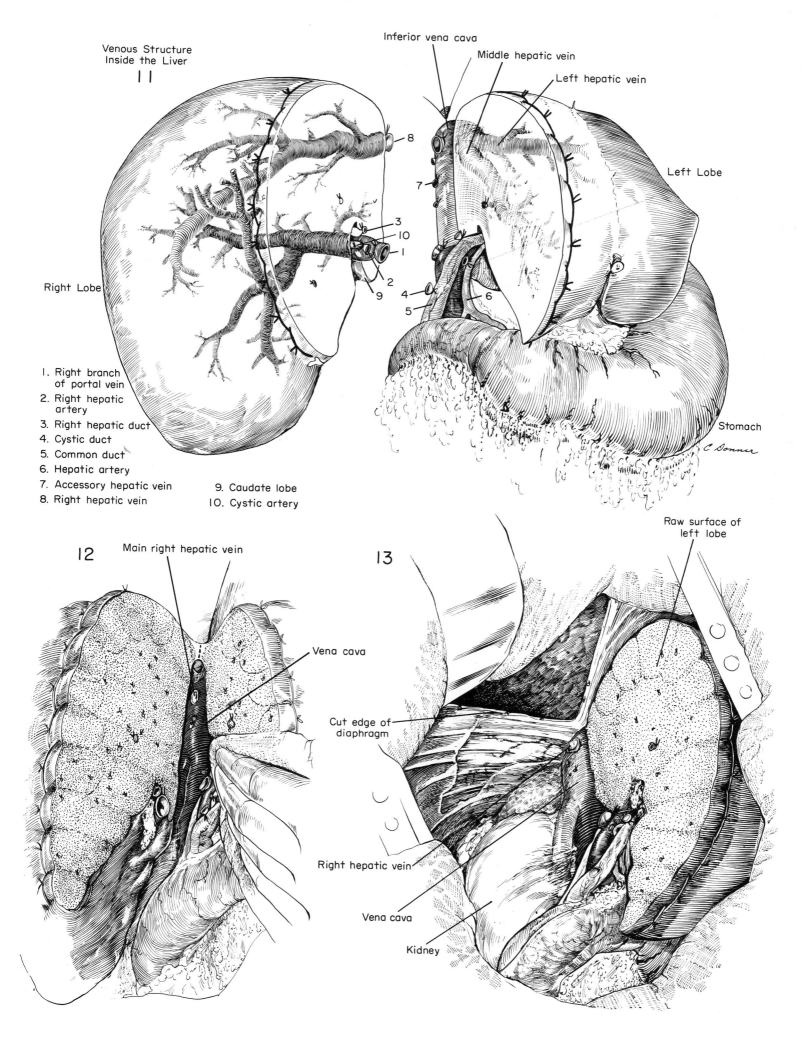

Venous Structure
Inside the Liver
11

Inferior vena cava

Middle hepatic vein

Left hepatic vein

Left Lobe

8

3
10
1

2

9

Right Lobe

7

4
5

6

Stomach

C Donner

1. Right branch
   of portal vein
2. Right hepatic
   artery
3. Right hepatic duct
4. Cystic duct
5. Common duct
6. Hepatic artery
7. Accessory hepatic vein
8. Right hepatic vein
9. Caudate lobe
10. Cystic artery

12   Main right hepatic vein

Vena cava

13

Raw surface of
left lobe

Cut edge of
diaphragm

Right hepatic vein

Vena cava

Kidney

PLATE LXXX · LEFT HEPATIC LOBECTOMY

INDICATIONS. The same basic considerations apply here as for the right lobectomy. This operation is a true anatomic left lobectomy and not a resection of the left lateral segment, which is only that liver substance lateral to the falciform ligament.

PREOPERATIVE PREPARATION. See Plate LXXVII.

ANESTHESIA. See Plate LXXVII.

POSITION. See Plate LXXVII.

OPERATIVE PREPARATION. See Plate LXXVII.

INCISION AND EXPOSURE. The same incision is used as for the right hepatic lobectomy **(Figure 14)**.

DETAILS OF PROCEDURE. The middle hepatic vein is the guideline for dissection within the hepatic parenchyma, and it should be preserved. The middle hepatic vein may drain into the right hepatic vein or independently into the vena cava, but frequently it joins the left hepatic vein in the liver parenchyma just prior to its entrance into the vena cava **(Figure 15)**. Mobilization of the ductal structures proceeds in the same order as for the right lobectomy **(Figure 16)**. Again, it is convenient to remove the gallbladder immediately. The left triangular ligament is divided to mobilize the superior surface of the left lobe **(Figure 17)**. By gentle medial and downward traction on the liver, the hepatic veins can be exposed. The left hepatic vein should be dissected carefully up into the liver substance to locate and isolate the entrance of the middle hepatic vein into it. The left hepatic vein only is carefully ligated and divided **(Figure 18)**. A double row of overlapping heavy catgut sutures is placed and tied to control the bleeding preliminary to division of the liver substance. Sharp and blunt dissections are used to divide the liver substance, beginning just to the left of the gallbladder fossa and proceeding to the vena cava, again leaving behind a border of the left lobe. The left lobe is freed of its remaining attachments and removed **(Figure 19)**.

CLOSURE. The wound is closed in layers after the drains are placed.

Left Lateral Segmental Resection

This is perhaps the most commonly employed hepatic resection.

INCISION AND EXPOSURE. The same incision previously described is used, but the left branches of the portal triad *must not be ligated* or divided. This will result in devitalization of the medial segment of the left lobe. The plane of dissection should be approximately 1 cm. to the left of the falciform ligament to avoid damaging the structures of the medial segment of the left lobe and the parumbilicalis of the left branch of the portal vein (Plate LXXVI, **Figure 1,** 7). Interlocking mattress sutures may be used to control blood and bile losses but are not essential. In this resection such sutures may obviate the need for blunt dissection through the liver, with individual vessel control; but the latter method still appears to be the preferable procedure. The falciform ligament provides a convenient peritoneal surface for covering the raw area of the liver after this procedure.

CLOSURE. Adequate drainage with several Penrose drains through a lateral stab wound is provided. The wound is closed in layers.

POSTOPERATIVE CARE. Careful attention should be given to postoperative blood volume maintenance, and the use of arterial and central venous pressure catheters can be quite useful. To avoid hepatic anoxia, ventilation should be adjusted using arterial blood gases as a guideline. In addition, the arterial blood sample can be used in following the patient's acid-base status. Serial hematocrits and coagulation profiles should be obtained. Copious drainage may be encountered from the operative site, and therefore scrupulous attention should be paid to the drain sites to be sure that they are draining freely. The drains may be enclosed in a plastic bag to lessen the chance of infection, permit inspection of the drainage, and accurately measure the losses. Despite careful technic, there is still a chance of delayed hemorrhage, which, of course, must be watched for and treated according to its severity. An occasional patient will develop a hemorrhagic diathesis after major hepatic resection. Expert hematologic advice should be sought, and, in general, the use of fresh whole blood and/or its components will prove to be the most useful means of combating this problem.

Each patient having undergone a massive liver resection should be treated postoperatively as if hepatic insufficiency existed. Albumin (50 to 75 Gm. daily) should be given and vitamin K administered daily. Hyperalimentation may be necessary to ensure adequate calories and intake of amino acids, vitamins, and minerals. It is ordinarily useful to administer antibiotics that have a high concentration in bile. Serial blood sugars should be obtained to detect early the onset of postresection hypoglycemia. Serial determinations of SGOT, SGPT, LDH, alkaline phosphatase, and total bilirubin should be obtained to detect early signs of hepatic decompensation, in which event vigorous treatment must be instituted. Large doses of analgesics and sedatives that are metabolized by the liver should be avoided.

Following major hepatic resection significant enlargement of both spleen and hepatic remnant may occur secondary to a reduction in hepatic outflow tracts. Although splenomegaly may be demonstrated radiographically for six to eight weeks, clinically apparent hypersplenism does not develop.

PLATE LXXX   LEFT HEPATIC LOBECTOMY

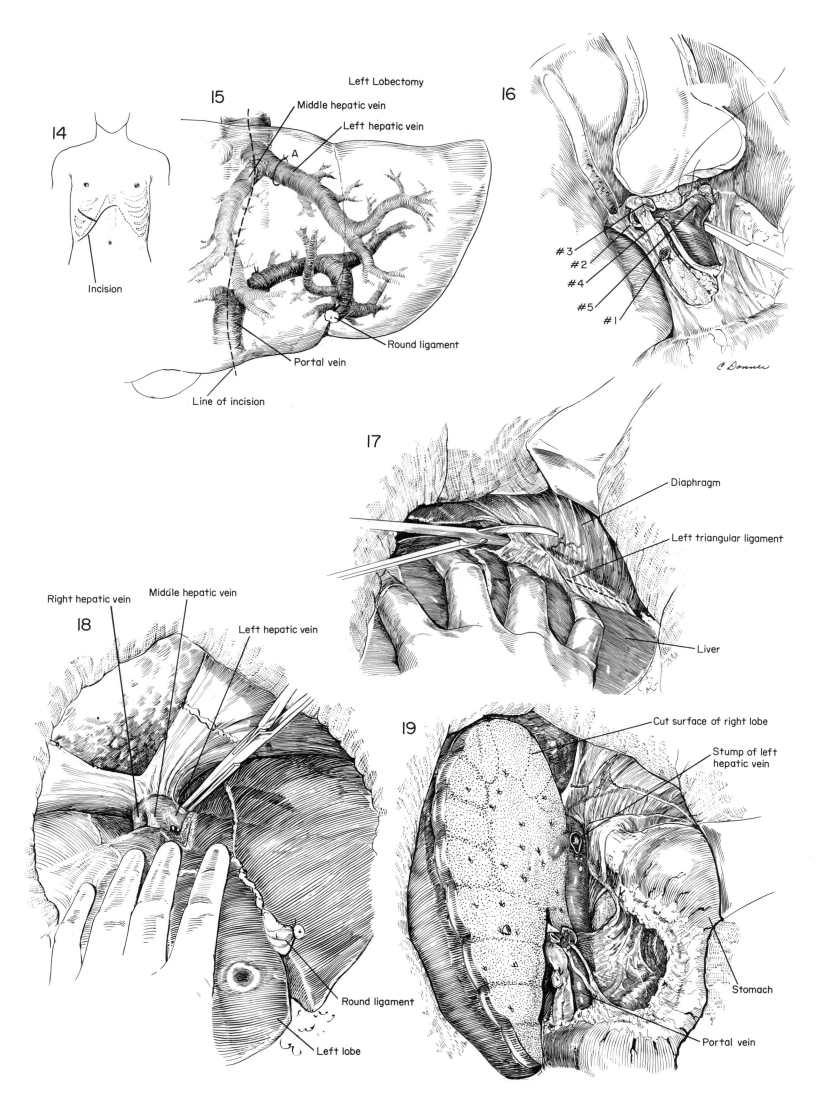

Left Lobectomy

14

Incision

15

Middle hepatic vein

Left hepatic vein

A

Round ligament

Portal vein

Line of incision

16

#3
#2
#4
#5
#1

C Donner

17

Diaphragm

Left triangular ligament

Liver

18

Right hepatic vein   Middle hepatic vein

Left hepatic vein

Round ligament

Left lobe

19

Cut surface of right lobe

Stump of left hepatic vein

Stomach

Portal vein

PLATE LXXXI · DRAINAGE OF CYST OR PSEUDOCYST OF THE PANCREAS

INDICATIONS. Pseudocysts of the pancreas are not an uncommon sequela of acute pancreatitis, chronic pancreatitis, and blunt abdominal trauma with resultant traumatic pancreatitis. Pancreatic pseudocysts should be suspected when the serum amylase remains elevated after apparently satisfactory response to treatment of the acute episode. However, the serum amylase may be normal, and quantitative urinary amylases may establish the diagnosis. Blood calcium levels should be followed during severe episodes. A palpable mass can usually be detected in the upper abdomen, most frequently in the midepigastrium or the left upper quadrant. These cysts do not have an epithelial lining as do the true pancreatic cysts. They are most commonly found in the body and tail of the pancreas but also may be found in the neck and head of the pancreas. Gastrointestinal barium studies confirm the diagnosis and can demonstrate a large, round filling defect in the posterior wall of the stomach with lateral displacement, depression of the transverse colon and/or splenic flexure, widening of the duodenal C-loop, or deformity of the gastric antrum. Films of the chest and abdomen may demonstrate elevation of the left hemidiaphragm with or without basilar atelectasis or pleural effusion. Treatment of cysts that do not regress spontaneously consists most commonly of internal drainage via the stomach, duodenum, or jejunum, although external tube drainage with subsequent fistula may be rarely indicated.

The ideal time to drain these pseudocysts internally is six to eight weeks after their appearance, when the cyst is intimately attached to the surrounding structures, and the surrounding inflammatory reaction is quiescent. At this time the cyst wall is strong enough for the technical anastomosis. External tube drainage of the cyst may be necessary if the cyst wall is friable or if the patient is septic or has a rapidly expanding pseudocyst. In all cases the interior of the cyst should be thoroughly examined and the cyst wall biopsied. Externally drained cysts usually close spontaneously, but pancreatic fistulas can occur and tend to condemn the procedure. Cysts may resolve gradually, particularly those associated with stones in the common duct and acute pancreatitis.

PREOPERATIVE PREPARATION. It is most important that these patients be in satisfactory metabolic condition before surgery. Accordingly, deficiencies in electrolytes, red cell mass, serum protein, or prothrombin levels are corrected preoperatively, and hyperalimentation should be considered. A clear liquid diet is given on the day before surgery, and the colon is emptied by the use of oral cathartics and enemas.

ANESTHESIA. General anesthesia with intratracheal intubation is satisfactory.

POSITION. The patient is placed in a comfortable supine position as near the operator's side as possible. The knees are flexed on a pillow. Moderate elevation of the head of the table facilitates exposure. Facilities for operative pancreatic cystogram as well as cholangiogram should be available.

OPERATIVE PREPARATION. The lower thorax and abdomen are prepared in the usual manner.

INCISION AND EXPOSURE. An epigastric midline incision or paramedian incision on the side of the cyst can be used for this procedure. Resection of the xiphoid process will give an additional 5 to 7.5 cm. of exposure if necessary.

DETAILS OF PROCEDURE. After the peritoneal cavity is entered, thorough exploration is carried out with particular emphasis on the gallbladder and common duct. Fat necrosis in the omentum or transverse mesocolon is commonly found. The cysts of the pancreas are best drained into that portion of the upper gastrointestinal tract most intimately adherent to the cyst, as shown in **Figure 1A.** Cystoantrostomy or cystoduodenostomy is quite satisfactory when it can be performed easily. In addition, the cystoduodenostomy affords the opportunity for sphincterotomy. Loop cystojejunostomy or Roux-en-Y cystojejunostomy may be performed also **(Figure 1B).** The latter is the preferred method, unless the cyst is intimately attached to the posterior gastric wall, and has the added advantage of preventing reflux of intestinal contents into the cyst, with less chance of leakage about the suture line.

After the field is walled off by gauze pads, the omentum overlying the cyst is opened and all bleeding points ligated **(Figure 2).** The diagnosis of a cyst is confirmed by needle aspiration of the suspected area. The cyst is then partly aspirated, permitting the operator to determine the thickness of the cyst wall and confirm the diagnosis **(Figure 3).** Specimens of the cyst contents are sent for culture and sensitivity, amylase and electrolyte determination. At this time operative cystography can be performed. Since the cyst fluid will dilute the contrast medium, it is better to inject 5 to 10 ml. of an undiluted contrast medium into the cyst.

Guide sutures A and B are placed into the wall of the cyst, and a 2- to 3-cm. opening is made at the desired level for drainage **(Figure 4).** Suction should be available for aspirating the cyst contents. The full thickness of cyst wall is biopsied **(Figure 4).**

The surgeon should explore the interior of the cyst with the index finger, carefully checking for coexistent neoplasm and pocketing within the cystic cavity **(Figure 5).** To prevent tension on the cystoduodenostomy, it is advisable to perform a Kocher maneuver to mobilize the duodenum.

PLATE LXXXI   DRAINAGE OF CYST OR PSEUDOCYST OF THE PANCREAS

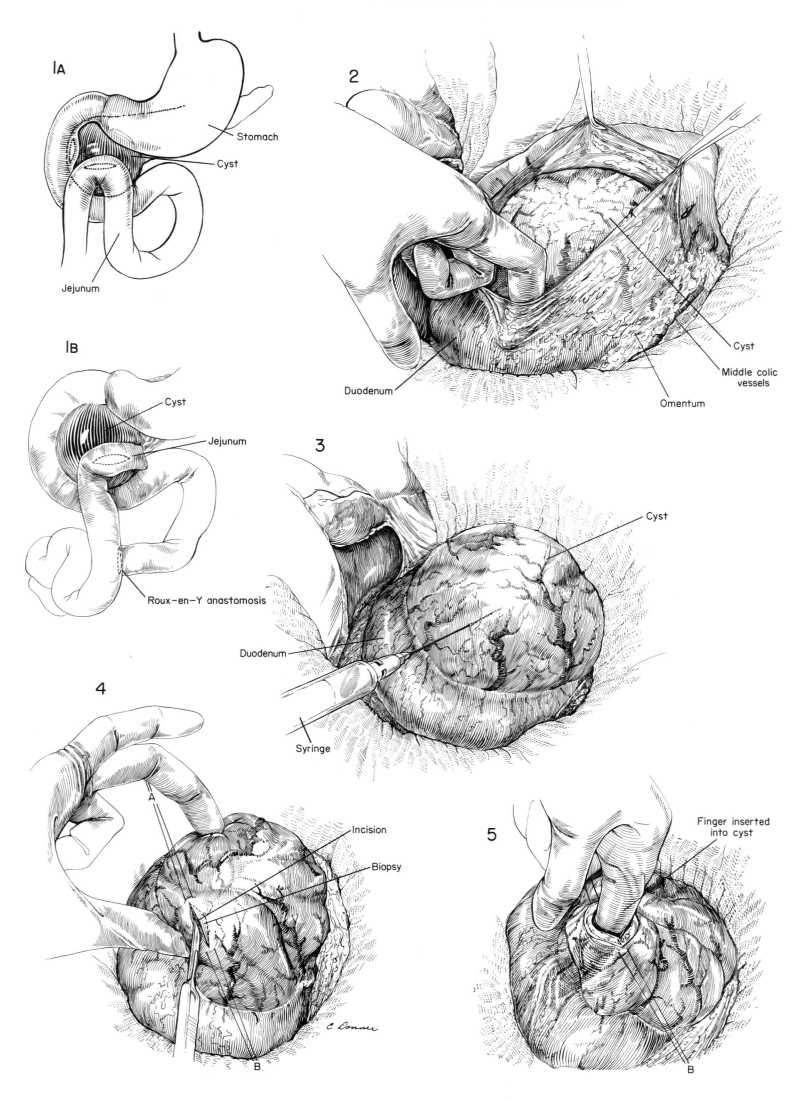

1A

Stomach

Cyst

Jejunum

1B

Cyst

Jejunum

Roux-en-Y anastomosis

2

Duodenum

Cyst

Middle colic vessels

Omentum

3

Cyst

Duodenum

Syringe

4

Incision

Biopsy

A

B

C Donner

5

Finger inserted into cyst

B

PLATE LXXXII · DRAINAGE OF CYST OR PSEUDOCYST OF THE PANCREAS

DETAILS OF PROCEDURE (*Continued*). Gentle tension is put on the duodenum with noncrushing clamps, and a posterior row of 00 interrupted silk horizontal mattress sutures is placed **(Figure 6).**

Traction angle sutures are placed at the angles of the proposed opening in the duodenum. The incision into the duodenum is made slightly smaller than that in the cyst. All bleeding points are meticulously ligated with 0000 silk **(Figure 6).** The full thickness of the cyst wall is approximated to the full thickness of the duodenal incision, using interrupted 0000 silk sutures **(Figure 7).** Through the duodenal incision, adequate exposure of the ampulla of Vater can be obtained. If a sphincterotomy is considered, a small probe or French woven whistletip catheter, No. 10 or No. 12, is passed through the papilla of Vater into the duct **(Figure 8).** The superior margins of the ampulla are grasped by straight mosquito forceps **(Figure 9).** The sphincter is incised superiorly **(Figure 9),** and a full-thickness biopsy is taken before the ductal mucosa is approximated to the duodenal mucosa by interrupted fine silk sutures on the lateral edge only **(Figure 10).** After hemostasis has been obtained and an adequate flow of bile observed upon compressing the gallbladder, the pancreatic duct is likewise probed. After the patency of the ducts has been determined, the full thickness of the cyst wall and the full thickness of the duodenum are approximated with interrupted 0000 silk inverting sutures **(Figure 11).** The seromuscular layer of the duodenum is approximated to the cyst wall in order to provide the outer layer of the two-layer anastomosis **(Figure 12).** This layer is carried well beyond the margins of the interior anastomosis in order to prevent tension on the anastomosis. .

PLATE LXXXII   DRAINAGE OF CYST OR PSEUDOCYST OF THE PANCREAS

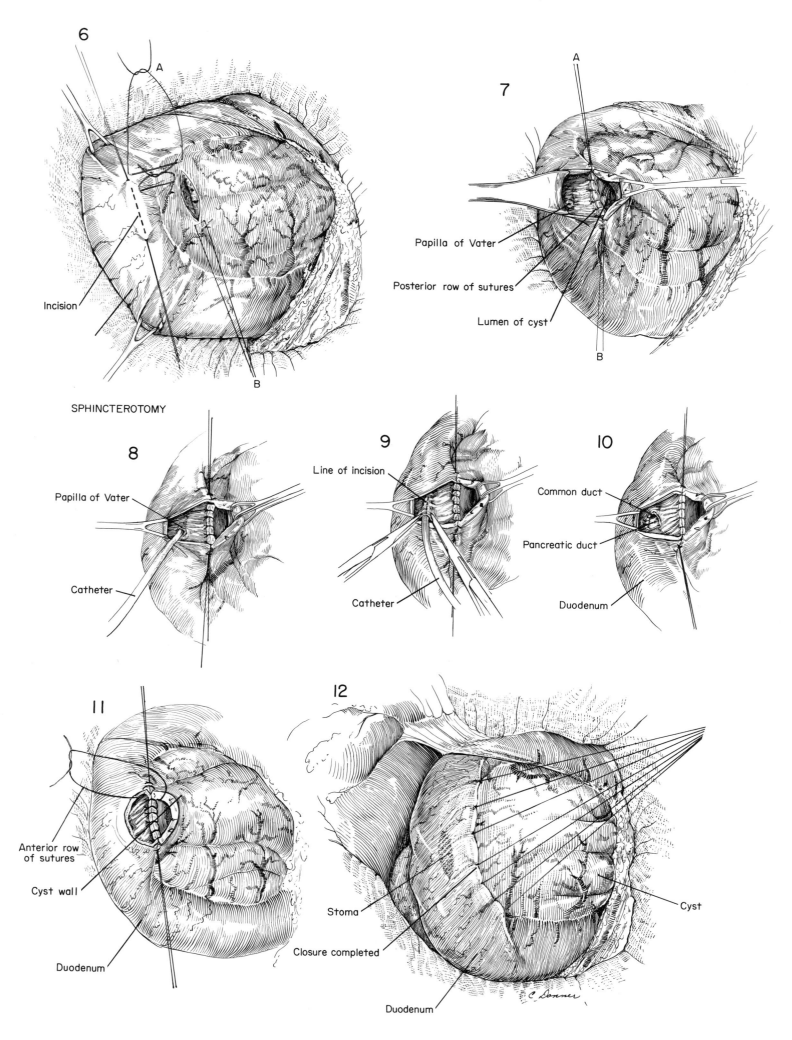

6

A

Incision

B

7

A

Papilla of Vater

Posterior row of sutures

Lumen of cyst

B

SPHINCTEROTOMY

8

Papilla of Vater

Catheter

9

Line of incision

Catheter

10

Common duct

Pancreatic duct

Duodenum

11

Anterior row
of sutures

Cyst wall

Duodenum

12

Stoma

Closure completed

Duodenum

Cyst

C. Donner

PLATE LXXXIII · DRAINAGE OF CYST OR PSEUDOCYST OF THE PANCREAS

DETAILS OF PROCEDURE (*Continued*). Pseudocysts of the body and tail of the pancreas are usually drained most easily by transgastric cystogastrostomy **(Figure 13).** The lesser sac is carefully explored to determine where the posterior stomach wall is adherent to the pancreas. This can be done either above the lesser curvature or by separating the greater omentum from the midtransverse colon for a short distance. As shown in **Figure 14,** the field is walled off with gauze pads, and guide sutures are placed in the anterior wall of the stomach over the most prominent portion of the palpated cyst and where the cyst is most adherent to the stomach. An incision is made in the anterior gastric wall parallel to the blood supply. The margins of the gastrotomy are grasped with noncrushing clamps for exposure as well as hemostasis.

The cyst is localized by partial aspiration through the posterior wall of the stomach at the point where the cyst and stomach are intimately attached. Aspiration confirms the diagnosis and provides a specimen of the cyst fluid for culture as well as amylase and electrolyte determination **(Figure 15).** At this point operative cystography can be performed to determine the size and extent of the cyst. The mucosa of the posterior wall of the stomach is gently grasped with fine-toothed forceps by the surgeon and the assistant, and the full thickness of the posterior wall of the stomach and the full thickness of the cyst wall are then incised **(Figure 16).** The contents of the cyst cavity are then aspirated with suction. The interior of the cyst is explored with the index finger, and biopsy of the cyst wall performed. All bleeding points are ligated with 0000 silk sutures. Firm attachment between the cyst wall and stomach is essential rather than dependence upon suture approximation. All bleeding points should be suture ligated. A one-layer anastomosis using interrupted 00 silk sutures is

performed **(Figure 17A).** It is imperative that the full thickness of the stomach as well as the full thickness of the cyst wall be included in each suture **(Figure 17B).**

When all bleeding has been controlled and the cyst completely evacuated, drainage into the cavity may be carried out. A soft rubber tissue drain may be securely anchored with several silk sutures to the end of the nasogastric or gastrostomy tube and the other end introduced into the cyst cavity. This drain comes out with removal of the tube. Upon completion of the cystogastrostomy anastomosis, the gastrotomy is closed in two layers, using an inner layer of interrupted 0000 inverting silk sutures and an outer layer of interrupted 00 horizontal mattress sutures **(Figure 18).** The advantages of temporary tube gastrostomy should be considered. The stomach wall may be anchored to the round ligament to provide fixation of the stomach if gastrostomy is not performed. Cholecystectomy may be performed in good-risk patients with calculi, as may operative cholangiography.

CLOSURE. The abdomen is then closed in the usual manner.

POSTOPERATIVE CARE. Nasogastric suction or gastrostomy drainage is maintained until the gastrointestinal tract begins to function again. This is most easily ascertained by the appearance of carmine red in the stool and the absence of symptoms of pancreatitis. Daily blood amylase determinations are made. Stimulation of the pancreas is decreased initially by intramuscular atropine and nasogastric suction or gastrostomy drainage, and later by antacids and a bland diet consisting of six feedings per day without caffeine-containing hot or cold liquids.

PLATE LXXXIII   DRAINAGE OF CYST OR PSEUDOCYST OF THE PANCREAS

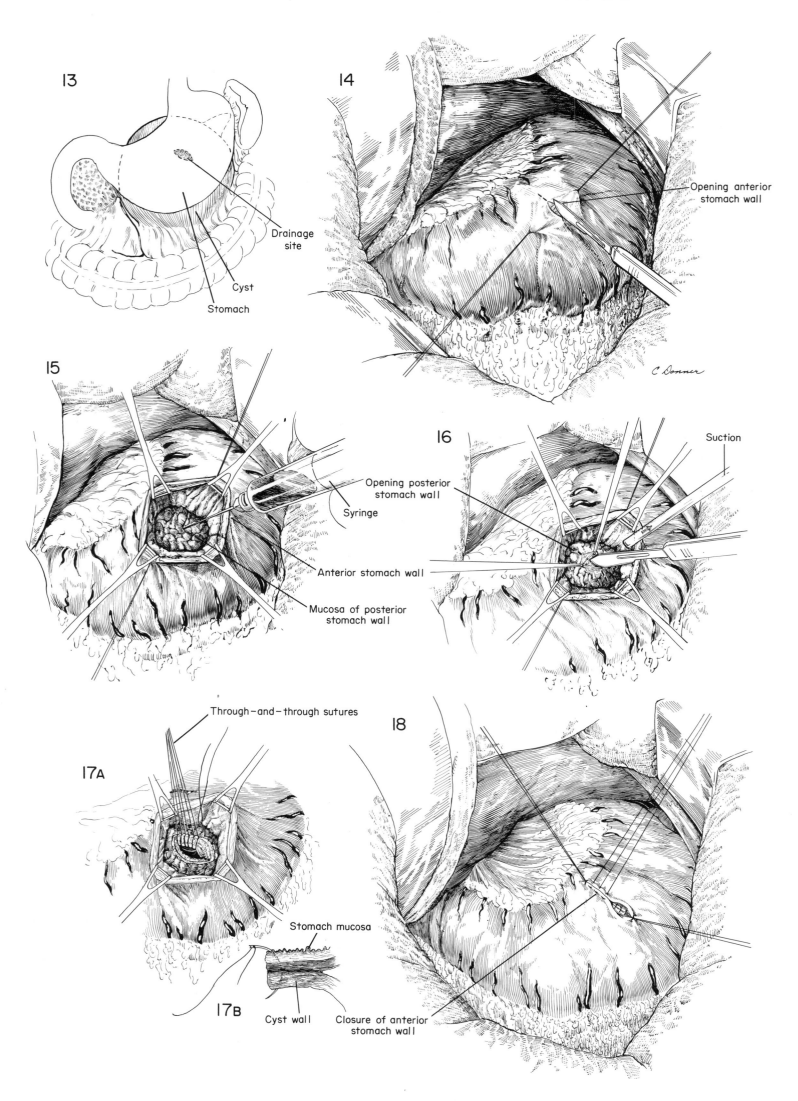

13

Drainage site

Cyst

Stomach

14

Opening anterior stomach wall

C. Donner

15

Opening posterior stomach wall

Syringe

Anterior stomach wall

Mucosa of posterior stomach wall

16

Suction

17A

Through—and—through sutures

Stomach mucosa

17B

Cyst wall

Closure of anterior stomach wall

18

PLATE LXXXIV · PANCREATICOJEJUNOSTOMY
(PUESTOW-GILLESBY PROCEDURE)

INDICATIONS. Drainage of the pancreatic duct by anastomosis to the jejunum may be indicated in the treatment of symptomatic chronic recurrent calcific pancreatitis. Before this procedure is carried out, all stones from the biliary tract should be removed by cholecystectomy and choledochostomy. There should be evidence of free drainage of bile through the papilla of Vater into the duodenum. Decompression of the obstructed pancreatic duct should be considered because of recurrent or persistent pain and evidence of progressive destruction of the pancreas.

PREOPERATIVE PREPARATION. All too often these patients are addicted to alcohol and/or narcotics because of persistent pain. Evidence of advanced pancreatic disease may be diabetes, steatorrhea, and poor nutrition. The entire gastrointestinal tract should be surveyed by barium studies and the biliary system evaluated by oral as well as intravenous methods. Stones in the gallbladder or the common duct should be suspected, and ulceration of the duodenum is not uncommon. Evidence for or against gastric hypersecretion should be determined by overnight 12-hour secretion studies. The stools should be examined to determine the degree of pancreatic insufficiency, insofar as fats are concerned. Particular attention should be given to restoring the blood volume and controlling existing diabetes. Blood calcium and phosphorus levels should be determined to rule out a parathyroid adenoma.

ANESTHESIA. General anesthesia is used.

POSITION. The patient is placed supine on the table with a Potter-Bucky tray available for a cholangiogram or pancreatogram.

OPERATIVE PREPARATION. The upper abdomen is prepared in the usual manner.

INCISION AND EXPOSURE. A curved incision following the costal margin on the left and extending across the midline around to the right or a long midline incision, which may extend below the umbilicus on the left side, may be used.

DETAILS OF PROCEDURE. The stomach and duodenum should be thoroughly evaluated for evidence of an ulcer. Likewise, the gallbladder should be carefully palpated for evidence of stones, and the size of the common duct determined. In the presence of stones the gallbladder is removed and a cholangiogram is taken through the cystic duct. A small amount of contrast medium (5 ml.) is first injected to avoid a dense shadow, which may hide small calculi in the common duct. Sufficient contrast medium should be subsequently injected to determine the patency of the papilla of Vater by visualization of the duodenum. It is advisable to carry out a Kocher maneuver to palpate the head of the pancreas, especially if there is radiographic evidence of an enlarged C-loop. Under such circumstances, needle aspiration may be carried out to search for evidence of a pancreatic cyst. The omentum, which is often quite vascular, is freed in the usual fashion from the transverse colon across to the region of the splenic flexure. The lesser sac may be obliterated, and sharp dissection may be required to separate the adhesions between the stomach and the pancreas which may be due to chronic pancreatitis. The stomach should be freed until the entire length of the fibrotic and lobulated pancreas can be easily explored **(Figure 1)**. The transverse colon is returned to the peritoneal cavity, while the stomach is retracted upward with a large S retractor. The posterior wall of the antrum should be freed from the pancreas so that the pancreatic duct can be palpated and opened as far to the right as possible to remove any calculi that might be impacted in the duodenal end **(Figure 2)**. After the lobulated fibrotic pancreas has been clearly exposed, an effort is made to identify the location of the pancreatic duct by needle aspiration **(Figure 1)**. Occasionally, it is desirable to aspirate pancreatic juice from the dilated pancreatic duct and then to inject a limited amount of contrast medium to ensure X-ray visualization of the pancreatic duct. Evidence of calculi in the duct is obtained as well as evidence to indicate whether the papilla of Vater is blocked or patent.

If there is evidence of a large and obstructed pancreatic duct, decompression is performed by anastomosing it to the jejunum. The capsule of the pancreas is incised directly over the needle **(Figure 3)**. This is done with a small scalpel or with an electrocautery unit. Some prefer the electrocautery unit to control the bleeding; otherwise, the bleeding points need to be grasped with fine forceps and ligated as the fibrotic pancreas overlying the duct is divided.

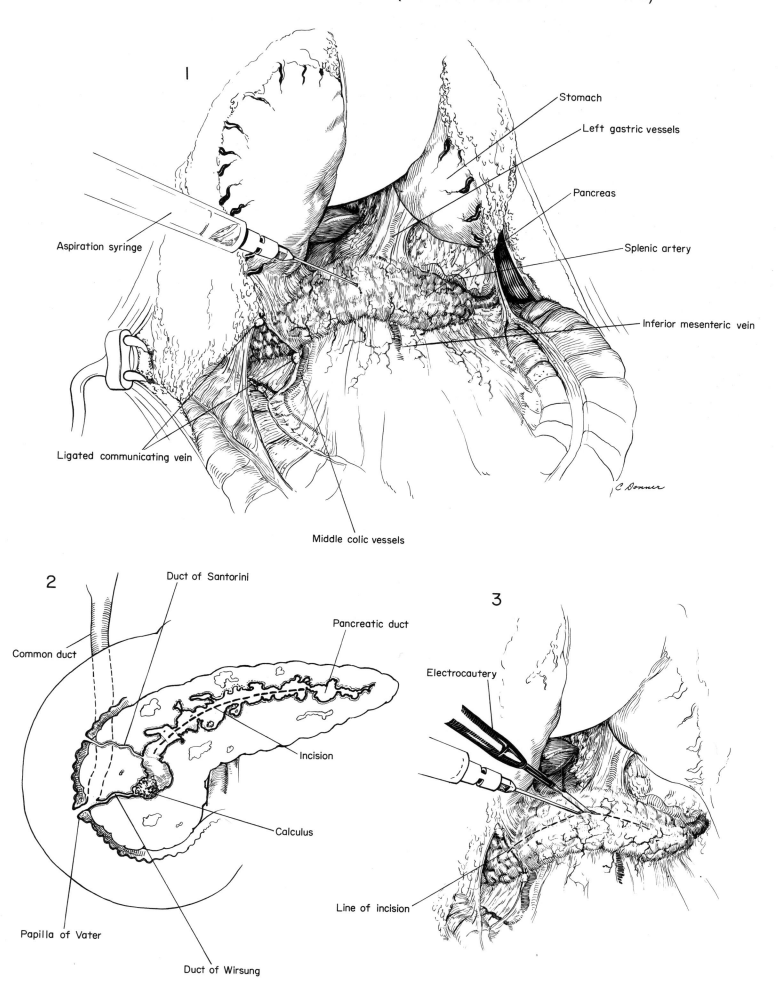

1

Stomach

Left gastric vessels

Pancreas

Splenic artery

Inferior mesenteric vein

Aspiration syringe

Ligated communicating vein

Middle colic vessels

C. Donner

2

Duct of Santorini

Pancreatic duct

Common duct

Incision

Calculus

Papilla of Vater

Duct of Wirsung

3

Electrocautery

Line of incision

PLATE LXXXV · PANCREATICOJEJUNOSTOMY (PUESTOW-GILLESBY PROCEDURE)

DETAILS OF PROCEDURE (*Continued*). A rather liberal incision is made in the pancreatic duct and carried over toward the right side but not up against the posterior wall of the duodenum, lest the pancreaticoduodenal vessels be divided and massive hemorrhage occur. A dilated pancreatic duct is usually encountered, and intermittent lakes or segmental dilatations may be found **(Figure 4)**. As the pancreatic duct is divided, the fibrotic margins are grasped by Allis forceps, and all bleeding points are controlled **(Figure 4)**. An effort can be made to establish the patency between the remaining segment of the pancreatic duct in the head of the pancreas and the lumen of the duodenum through the papilla of Vater. Frequently one or more calculi may need to be dislodged with a gallbladder type of scoop or small, fenestrated type of forceps commonly used to remove ureteral calculi **(Figure 4)**. Considerable time may be consumed in clearing the major pancreatic duct of calculi. A French woven catheter can be directed into the pancreatic duct to determine the patency of the papilla of Vater **(Figure 5)**. Patency can be proved by distention of the duodenum after an injection of saline. If in doubt, it may be advisable to inject contrast medium followed by a roentgenogram to visualize the remaining short segment of the pancreatic duct.

Ordinarily, the pancreatic duct is opened for 6 to 8 cm., and a decision must then be made as to the type of anastomosis that will be carried out: the Roux-en-Y arm as in a jejunal "fishmouth" lateral anastomosis, full-width side-to-side anastomosis, or implantation of the mobilized pancreas into the lumen of the jejunal segment. The jejunum is prepared for the Roux-en-Y anastomosis by dividing it 10 to 15 cm. below the ligament of Treitz (Plate XXIX). The vessels in the mesentery of the upper jejunum are visualized, and several vascular arcades are divided some distance from the mesenteric border. This permits mobilization of a sufficient length of jejunum to allow it to reach up into the region of the pancreas. An opening is made in the mesocolon to the left of the middle colic vessels in an avascular portion near the base of the mesentery. The arm of the jejunum is then tested for length and is turned with the open end to the right as well as to the left to determine which position of the mobilized jejunum produces the least interference with the blood supply. Many procedures can be followed in accomplishing the pancreaticojejunostomy.

First Technic—Lateral Fishmouth Anastomosis. One procedure that may be followed is to crush the open end of the jejunum along its antimesenteric border with a Payr clamp **(Figure 6)**. The distance crushed should be greater than the opening that has been made in the pancreas **(Figure 6)**. The crushed area is divided with scissors for the necessary distance, and any active bleeding is controlled with interrupted sutures of fine silk **(Figure 7)**.

The pancreas is anchored to the opened jejunum with one layer of interrupted sutures of 00 silk **(Figure 8)**. These sutures go through the entire wall of the jejunum but through only the capsule of the pancreas. The full thickness of the fibrotic pancreatic wall down to the opened pancreatic duct should not be sutured because there are numerous intramural smaller ducts that would be blocked and then would deliver pancreatic secretions into the peripancreatic tissue instead of to the intestinal lumen.

PLATE LXXXV   PANCREATICOJEJUNOSTOMY (PUESTOW-GILLESBY PROCEDURE)

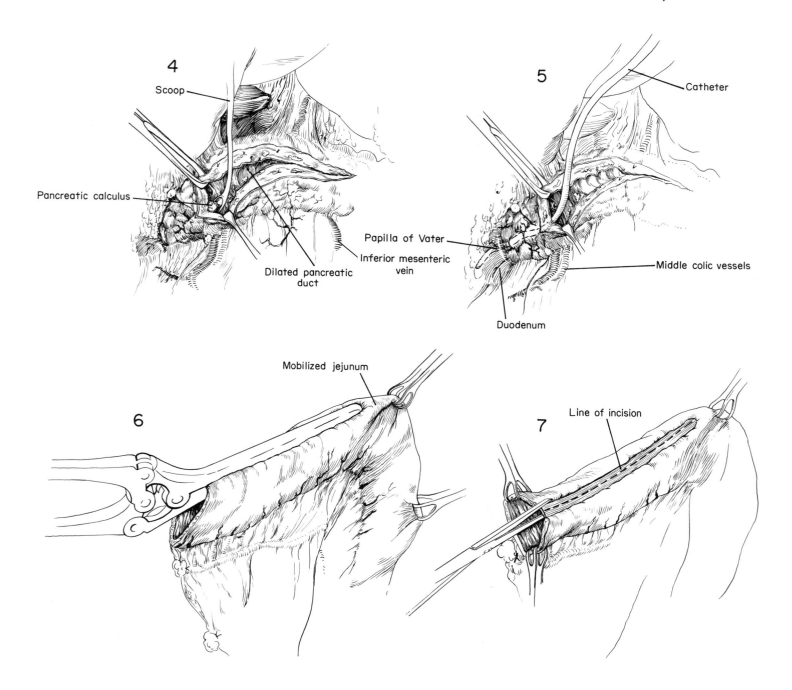

4

Scoop

Pancreatic calculus

Dilated pancreatic duct

Inferior mesenteric vein

Papilla of Vater

5

Catheter

Middle colic vessels

Duodenum

6

Mobilized jejunum

7

Line of incision

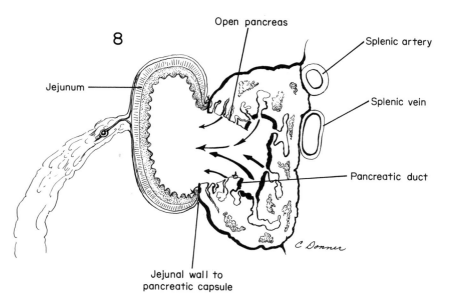

8

Open pancreas

Splenic artery

Splenic vein

Jejunum

Pancreatic duct

Jejunal wall to pancreatic capsule

C Donner

PLATE LXXXVI · PANCREATICOJEJUNOSTOMY (PUESTOW-GILLESBY PROCEDURE)

DETAILS OF PROCEDURE. Lateral Fishmouth Anastomosis (*Continued*). The open end of the jejunal arm is anastomosed over the opened pancreatic duct **(Figure 9).** The jejunum is anchored to the capsule of the tail of the fibrotic pancreas just beyond the end of the incision into the duct, and the full thickness of the jejunal wall is anchored to the cut margins of the capsule of the pancreas throughout the full length of the opened pancreatic duct. The open (fishmouth) end of the jejunum may need to be tailored from time to time, as outlined by the dotted lines **(Figure 9),** to ensure a sealed anastomosis around the duct. Again, only the capsule is included in these sutures, and the fibrotic wall of the pancreas is left free to promote drainage of the fine ducts, many of which are filled with small calculi. The anterior layer is also made with interrupted sutures, and the free end of the jejunum is anchored to the capsule with three or four additional sutures toward the tail of the pancreas **(Figure 10).** When the pancreas is shortened and thickened, a splenectomy may be necessary to adequately mobilize the pancreas and facilitate this anastomosis.

Second Technic—Full-Width Side-to-Side Anastomosis. Some prefer to close the end of the Roux-en-Y arm of jejunum with two layers of interrupted silk sutures (Plate XXIX) and anastomose the jejunum to the pancreas in a manner similar to a lateral anastomosis of small intestine **(Figures 11** and **12).** Only one layer of sutures is used, but they must be placed accurately and close enough together to prevent subsequent leakage.

When the Roux-en-Y principle is used, the jejunum near the ligament of Treitz is anastomosed to the arm of the jejunum going to the pancreas by an end-to-side anastomosis **(Figure 13).** The free margin of the mesentery should be secured by interrupted sutures (A) to the ascending jejunum to obliterate any opening for the subsequent development of an internal hernia **(Figure 13).** The opening in the mesocolon is closed about the jejunal arm.

PLATE LXXXVI   PANCREATICOJEJUNOSTOMY (PUESTOW-GILLESBY PROCEDURE)

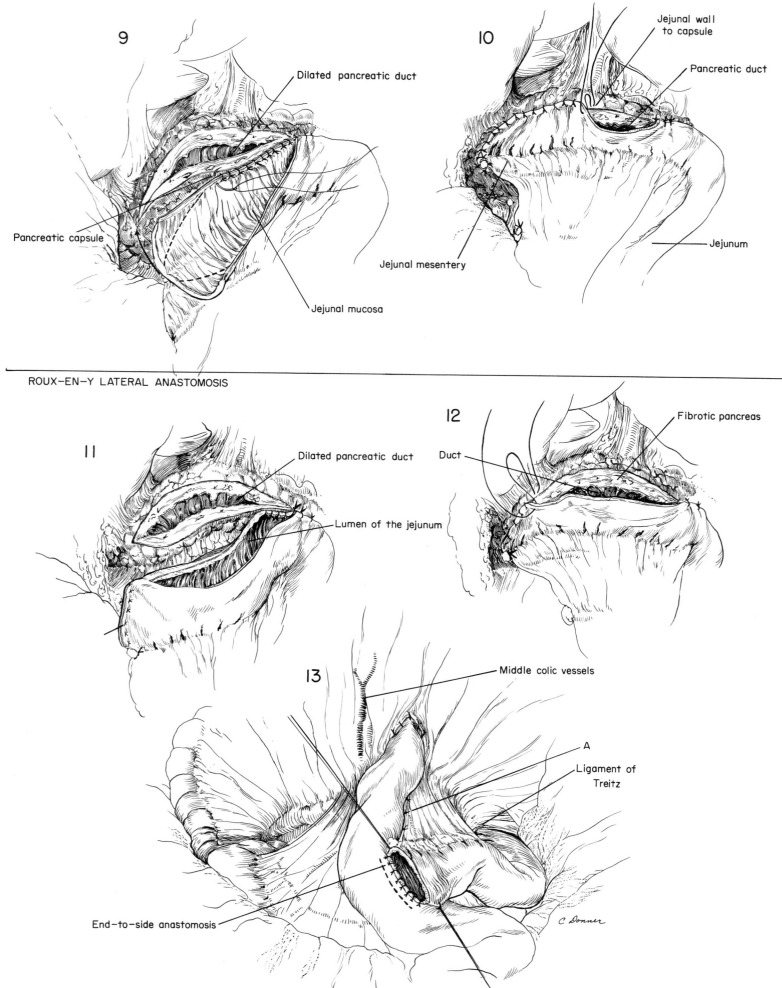

9

Dilated pancreatic duct

Pancreatic capsule

Jejunal mucosa

10

Jejunal wall to capsule

Pancreatic duct

Jejunal mesentery

Jejunum

ROUX—EN—Y LATERAL ANASTOMOSIS

11

Dilated pancreatic duct

Lumen of the jejunum

12

Duct

Fibrotic pancreas

13

Middle colic vessels

A

Ligament of Treitz

End-to-side anastomosis

C Donner

PLATE LXXXVII · PANCREATICOJEJUNOSTOMY
(PUESTOW-GILLESBY PROCEDURE)

DETAILS OF PROCEDURE (*Continued*). **Third Technic—Pancreatic Implantation Within Jejunum.** In addition to the previous procedures described, drainage of the body and tail of the pancreas may be accomplished by implanting the left end of the pancreas into the open end of the arm of jejunum which has been brought up for a Roux-en-Y type of anastomosis.

When the pancreas is severely inflamed, small, and contracted, it may be advisable to mobilize as much of the tail and body as possible and to remove the spleen in anticipation of implantation into the jejunum. Once the presence or absence of a dilated duct is confirmed by needle aspiration and palpation **(Figure 14)**, the peritoneum is incised superior and inferior to the body and tail of the pancreas, care being taken not to injure the inferior mesenteric vein **(Figure 14)**. After the peritoneum has been incised, the surgeon inserts his index finger behind the pancreas and can very easily, by a backward and forward motion, free the posterior wall of the body and tail of the pancreas from adjacent tissues. The finger is inserted completely around the pancreas, including the splenic artery and vein, which run along the superior surface of the pancreas **(Figure 15)**. A rubber drain is passed through this opening in order to provide gentle traction on the pancreas for the dissection of the tail and exposure during the freeing of the remainder of the pancreas and the splenectomy **(Figure 16)**. The gastrosplenic ligament is divided, and the blood supply along the greater curvature of the stomach is transfixed to the gastric wall with interrupted sutures of 00 silk. Any attachments between the superior pole of the spleen and the diaphragm are divided, and the spleen is mobilized well into the wound. The pedicle of the attachments between the inferior surface of the spleen and the colon is likewise divided. The blood supply to the spleen is divided and ligated. The vessels are then doubly ligated with 00 silk ligatures **(Figure 17)**.

PLATE LXXXVII   PANCREATICOJEJUNOSTOMY (PUESTOW-GILLESBY PROCEDURE)

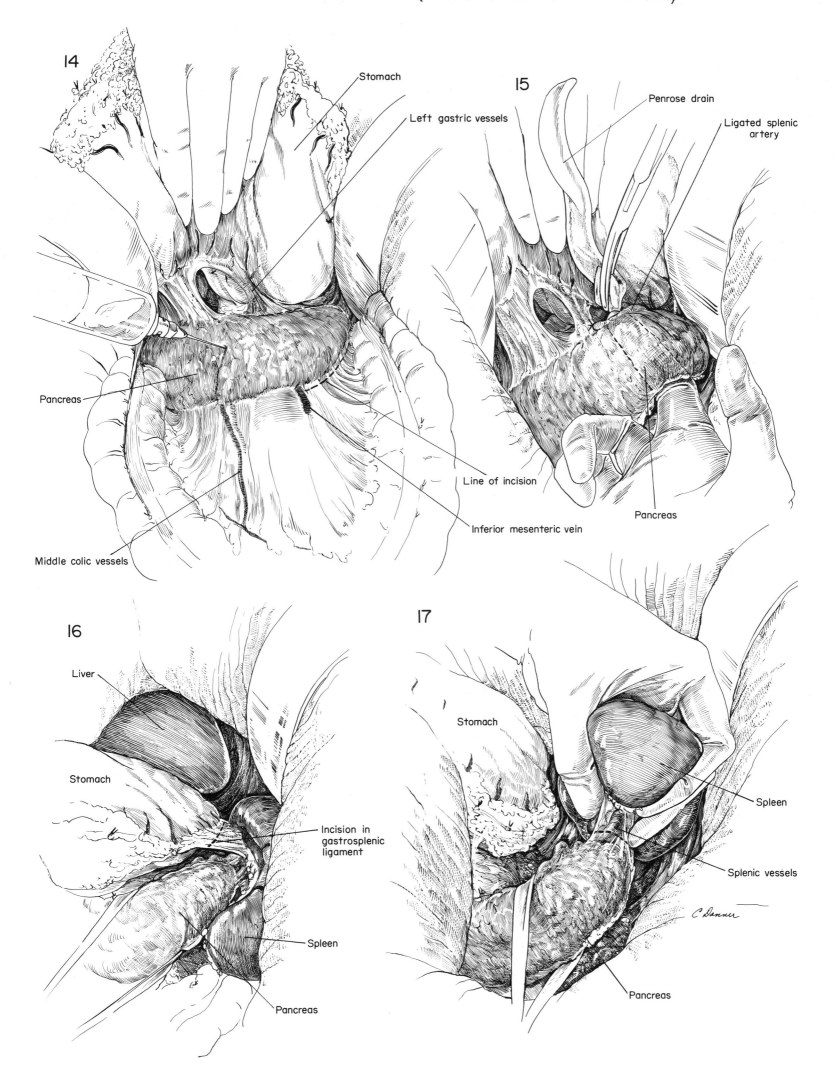

14

Stomach

Left gastric vessels

Pancreas

Line of incision

Inferior mesenteric vein

Middle colic vessels

15

Penrose drain

Ligated splenic artery

Pancreas

16

Liver

Stomach

Incision in gastrosplenic ligament

Spleen

Pancreas

17

Stomach

Spleen

Splenic vessels

Pancreas

C. Danner

PLATE LXXXVIII · PANCREATICOJEJUNOSTOMY (PUESTOW-GILLESBY PROCEDURE)

DETAILS OF PROCEDURE. Pancreatic Implantation Within Jejunum (*Continued*). The tail and body of the pancreas, now freely mobilized, are rotated toward the midline so that the courses of the splenic artery and vein are clearly visualized **(Figure 18).** The splenic artery should be doubly ligated and divided near its point of origin. It is advisable to remove the artery from this point of ligature out to the tip of the pancreas. Likewise, the splenic vein should be carefully dissected free of the adjacent pancreas and doubly ligated very near its junction with the inferior mesenteric vein **(Figure 18).** After the artery and vein have been removed from the distal half of the pancreas, the tail of the pancreas is stabilized with a suture or Allis forceps, and the end of the pancreas is carefully transected until the pancreatic duct is identified **(Figure 19).** The small amount of bleeding that occurs can be easily controlled by compressing the pancreas between the thumb and index finger, clamping the individual bleeding points, and then ligating them with 0000 silk **(Figure 19).** As soon as the pancreatic duct is located, a probe is inserted into the duct **(Figure 20).** The duct is usually a little nearer the superior than the inferior margin of the pancreas. The surgeon then grasps the pancreas with his thumb and index finger and makes an incision directly down onto the probe, completely exteriorizing the major pancreatic duct **(Figure 21).** The incision should be carried medially, and soon the pancreatic duct will greatly enlarge. With intermittent strictures and dilatations, there is a tendency of the duct to form a chain of individual lakes. Multiple calculi may be encountered and small calcifications noted in many small ducts within the wall of the fibrosed pancreas. The incision is carried from the tail of the pancreas downward as near as possible to the medial border of the duodenum **(Figure 22).** This is accomplished by stabilizing the pancreas with the left hand and inserting scissors into the lumen of the duct and carrying the dissection medially **(Figure 22).** The finger is inserted into the enlarged proximal portion of the dilated duct, and any calculi are removed. A small probe may be introduced into this area to determine whether or not there is free communication between the pancreatic duct and the duodenum through the ampulla, but this is not absolutely necessary **(Figure 23).** During the dissection the fibrotic wall of the pancreas is grasped with multiple Allis forceps, usually at the points of active bleeding. When these clamps are removed, the individual points are carefully ligated with interrupted silk sutures. No effort is made to approximate the wall of the duct and the fibrous capsule so that free drainage from the smaller ducts will be possible.

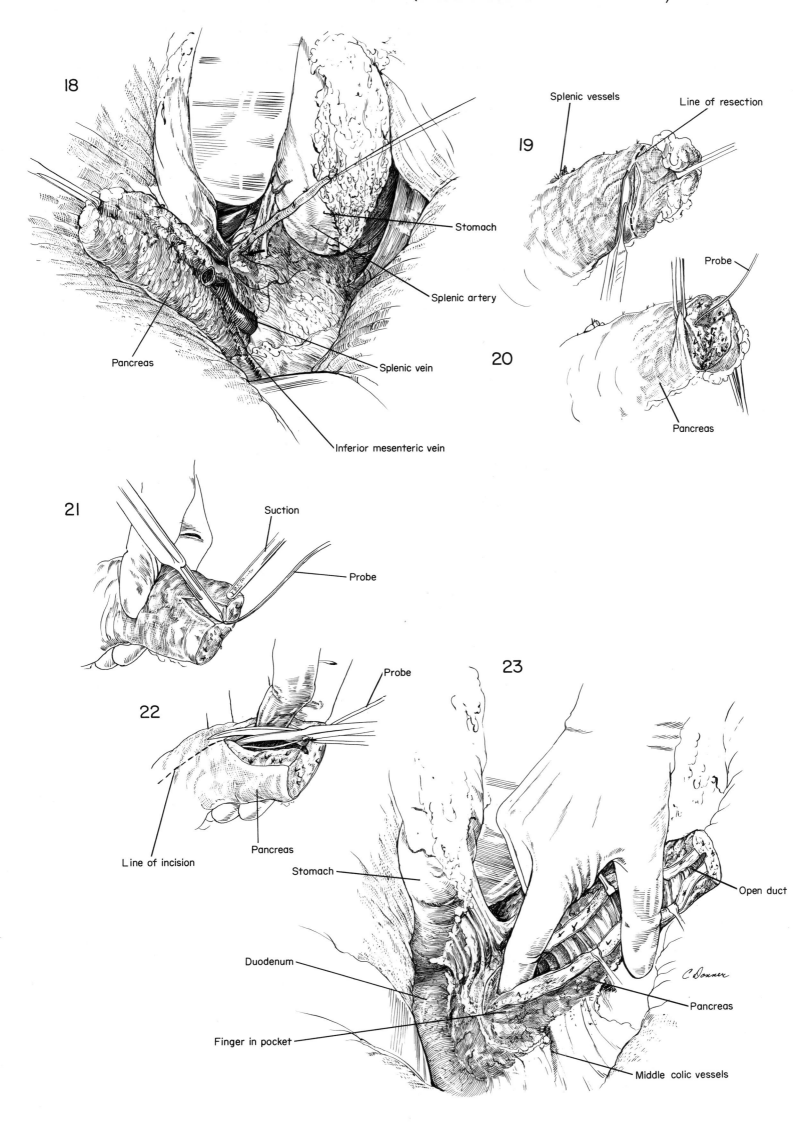

18

Stomach

Splenic artery

Pancreas

Splenic vein

Inferior mesenteric vein

19   Splenic vessels   Line of resection

20   Probe

Pancreas

21   Suction

Probe

22   Probe

Line of incision   Pancreas

23   Open duct

Stomach

Duodenum

Pancreas

Finger in pocket

Middle colic vessels

PLATE LXXXIX · PANCREATICOJEJUNOSTOMY (PUESTOW-GILLESBY PROCEDURE)

DETAILS OF PROCEDURE. Pancreatic Implantation Within Jejunum (*Continued*). The jejunum is held up out of the wound. By transillumination the surgeon can study the vascular arcades to select more accurately the blood vessels to be divided for mobilizing the arm of the jejunum to be brought up to the pancreas (Plate XXIX). The jejunum is divided at a point 10 to 15 cm. beyond the ligament of Treitz. A small opening is made in the mesocolon to the left of the middle colic vessels, just over the ligament of Treitz. The jejunum is pulled through this opening and measured along the full length of the pancreas **(Figure 24).** The length of the pancreas from just beyond the end of the opened duct to the end of its tail is marked, point X, on the jejunum, by Babcock forceps placed on its antimesenteric border **(Figure 24).** The tail of the pancreas will be drawn into the bowel lumen and approximated to point X. Here the surgeon must be certain that there is adequate jejunal length and that the mesenteric vascular pedicle will reach easily without angulation. Traction sutures (A and B) of 00 silk are placed on the superior and inferior borders of the capsule of the pancreas **(Figure 25)** to aid in pulling the tail to point X. The Potts forceps are removed from the open end of the jejunum and replaced by Babcock forceps at the antimesenteric border. The jejunum is gently stretched between the two Babcock forceps as the needles, with attached traction sutures A and B, are introduced into the lumen of the bowel. During insertion the needles are held parallel to the long axis of the holder with points backward so that the bowel wall is not punctured **(Figure 26A).** At point X, the needle is sharply retracted to puncture the wall and carry the suture externally **(Figure 26B).** Gentle traction is maintained upon these sutures to aid in pulling the pancreas up into the jejunum. When the pancreas is completely encased inside the bowel, sutures A and B are tied together, bringing the tail to point X **(Figure 27).** The opened end of the jejunum is then circumferentially tracked down to the capsule with interrupted silk sutures. The posterior row is placed first, beginning at the mesenteric border and proceeding superiorly to the antimesenteric surface. The anterior row is also begun at the mesenteric border of the jejunum. If the jejunal circumference is too small, the bowel may be longitudinally incised to accommodate the girth of the pancreas **(Figure 27).**

The adequacy of the blood supply of the jejunum is repeatedly checked. Intestinal continuity is established through a Roux-en-Y jejunojejunostomy, beyond the ligament of Treitz, using two layers of fine silk sutures **(Figure 28).** All free edges of the mesentery should be closed with interrupted 0000 silk sutures, care being taken that the marginal blood supply within the mesentery is not compromised. Before closure the blood supply of the jejunum should be carefully rechecked. A few sutures are taken to anchor the vascular margin of the mesentery to adjacent structures to prevent its rotation and the formation of an internal hernia. The window in the mesocolon is also secured to the pancreatic arm of the Roux-en-Y.

CLOSURE. If biliary tract surgery has simultaneously been performed, a cigarette drain is inserted in the foramen of Winslow. If T-tube drainage of the common duct has been instituted, the tube is brought out through a separate stab wound on the right side. Drainage is unnecessary for the pancreaticojejunostomy itself. The wound is closed in layers with fine silk. In the presence of impaired nutrition it may be advisable to supplement the closure with retention sutures.

POSTOPERATIVE CARE. Although varying degrees of pancreatitis can be anticipated following this procedure, the postoperative course is surprisingly mild. Blood amylase and sugar levels are determined and attention given to the narcotic requirements. These patients tend to be addicted to narcotics and may be difficult to sedate because of chronic alcoholism. Pancreatic enzyme therapy should be instituted, the diabetic tendency should be regulated, and any previous addiction should be corrected, if possible, before the patient is discharged from the hospital. A rigid ulcer type of dietary program should be followed with a gradual return to a more liberal diet.

PLATE LXXXIX   PANCREATICOJEJUNOSTOMY (PUESTOW-GILLESBY PROCEDURE)

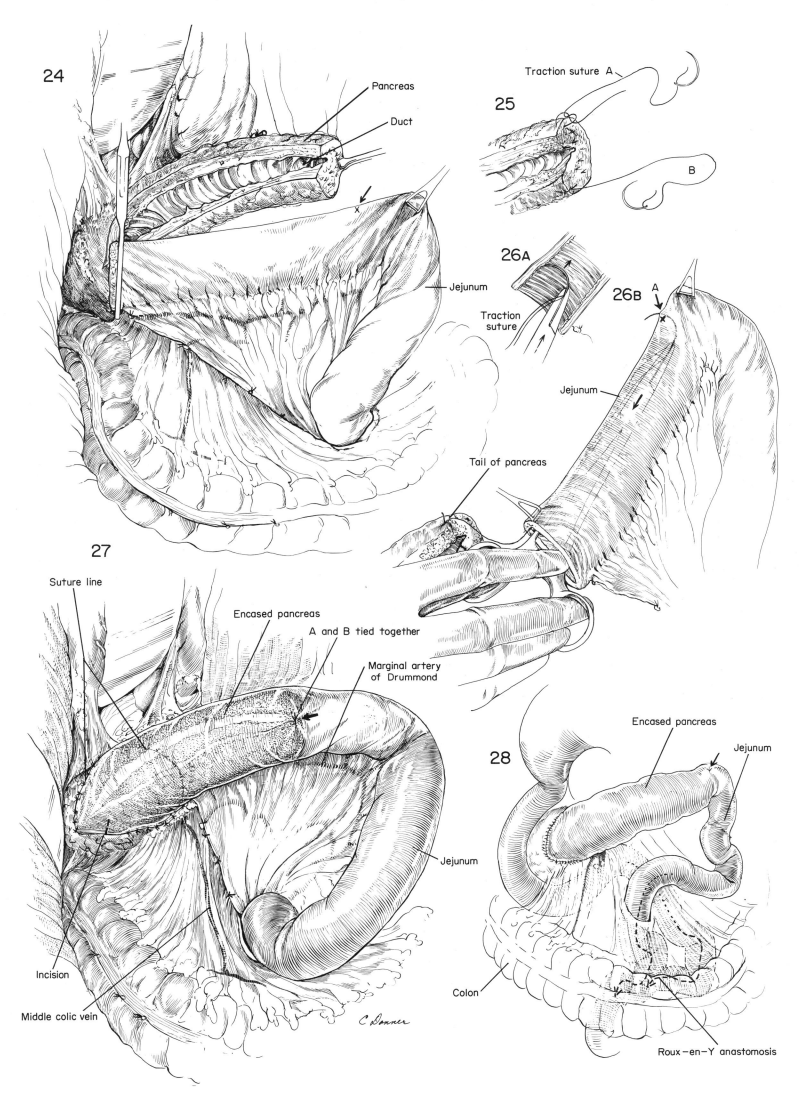

24

Pancreas

Duct

Jejunum

25

Traction suture A

B

26A

Traction suture

26B

A

Jejunum

Tail of pancreas

27

Suture line

Encased pancreas

A and B tied together

Marginal artery of Drummond

Jejunum

Incision

Middle colic vein

C Donner

28

Encased pancreas

Jejunum

Colon

Roux—en—Y anastomosis

PLATE XC · RESECTION OF THE TAIL OF THE PANCREAS

INDICATIONS. The more common indications for resecting the body and tail of the pancreas include localized adenocarcinoma in this area, islet cell adenomas of the beta cell and non-beta cell type, cysts, and chronic calcific pancreatitis.

PREOPERATIVE PREPARATION. The preparation is related to the preoperative diagnosis. The blood volume should be restored.

The patient with a beta cell adenoma, suggested by repeated fasting blood sugars of below 50 mg. per cent, requires supplementary glucose by mouth or intravenously at regular intervals for 24 hours preceding surgery and intravenously during surgery. Steroids in moderate dosage are sometimes given.

When an ulcerogenic tumor is suspected, the fluid and electrolyte balance should be corrected, particularly if there have been large losses of gastric secretion or losses from enteritis. Serum gastrin levels may establish the diagnosis, so that the patient should be prepared for a total gastrectomy by a thorough discussion of the postoperative dietary problems and vitamin requirements that follow this procedure.

ANESTHESIA. General anesthesia with endotracheal intubation.

POSITION. Supine position with the feet lower than the head.

OPERATIVE PREPARATION. The skin is shaved from the level of the nipples well out over the chest wall and down over the abdomen, including the flanks.

INCISION AND EXPOSURE. Either a long vertical midline or an extensive curved incision parallel to the costal margins, as described for pancreaticoduodenectomy (Plate XCIII).

DETAILS OF PROCEDURE. When the procedure is carried out for an inflammatory lesion of the body and tail of the pancreas, a direct exploration of this region is performed. When the procedure is carried out for tumor, a thorough exploration of the abdomen, with particular reference to the liver and the gastrohepatic ligament in the region of the celiac plexus, should be made for evidence of metastasis. Since the adenomas of either the beta cell or non-beta cell type can be distributed throughout the pancreas, the head of the pancreas must be thoroughly explored by visualization and palpation preliminary to a definitive type of procedure on the left half of the pancreas. Evidence of gastric hypersecretion, as indicated by increased vascularity and thickening of the gastric wall, along with a hyperemic and hypertrophic duodenum and an ulcer in the duodenum or beyond the ligament of Treitz, adds support to the potential diagnosis of non-beta islet cell tumor of the pancreas. Likewise, the inner wall of the duodenum should be carefully palpated in the search for small adenomas extending into the lumen of the duodenum from the pancreatic side. After the abdomen has been explored and the region of the head of the pancreas evaluated, the greater omentum is reflected upward, and downward traction is maintained on the transverse colon as the omentum is separated by sharp dissection and the lesser sac entered **(Figure 1).** Usually, the stomach is easily separated from the pancreas, but sharp dissection may be required to separate it from the capsule of the pancreas, especially if there have been repeated bouts of acute inflammation. Sharp as well as blunt dissection is used to sweep the posterior gastric wall away from the pancreas, particularly in the region of the antrum, to make certain the middle colic vessels have not been angulated upward and attached to the posterior gastric wall. A clear view must be assured of the entire pancreas and first part of the duodenum all the way over to the hilus of the spleen **(Figure 1).** To avoid troublesome bleeding, it is usually desirable to divide the communicating vein between the right gastroepiploic vessels and the middle colic vein inferior to the pylorus. This permits better mobilization in the region of the antrum. Large S retractors can be used to retract the stomach upward as the transverse colon is either pulled downward outside the wound or returned to the abdomen and packed away. The pancreas should be thoroughly inspected and palpated to verify the pathology. It is safer and far easier to mobilize and remove the spleen rather than attempt to separate the pancreas from the splenic artery and vein running along the superior surface of the body and tail of this organ.

In carcinoma the tumor's mobility and the presence or absence of regional metastasis must be determined before a radical resection is planned. In beta cell adenoma it is more common to find only one tumor, and this may be enucleated without removing a large segment of the pancreas, depending on the adenoma's location and relationship to the major pancreatic duct and vessels. In contrast, the tendency of the non-beta cell adenomas to be multiple, combined with an over-all 50 per cent incidence of malignancy, makes removal of all acid-bearing tissue of the stomach by a total gastrectomy a concomitant surgical procedure. Finding a solitary non-beta cell adenoma of considerable size may tempt the surgeon to do a local excision for proof of diagnosis despite an anticipated ulcer recurrence rate of well over 50 per cent.

When the lesion cannot be seen or palpated by digital examination of the anterior surface of the gland, the body and tail must be mobilized for direct palpation with the thumb and index finger and for visualization of the underside of the pancreas. This is accomplished by incising the peritoneum along the inferior surface of the pancreas **(Figure 2).** Only a few small blood vessels are encountered. The inferior mesenteric vein should be identified, and the incision should avoid it as well as the middle colic vessels. After the inferior surface of the peritoneum has been incised, a finger can be rather easily introduced underneath the pancreas, and the substance of the gland can be palpated quite easily between the thumb and index finger **(Figure 3).** As a matter of fact, the finger can be inserted completely around the pancreas following the incision in the peritoneum just above the splenic artery and vein.

PLATE XC   RESECTION OF THE TAIL OF THE PANCREAS

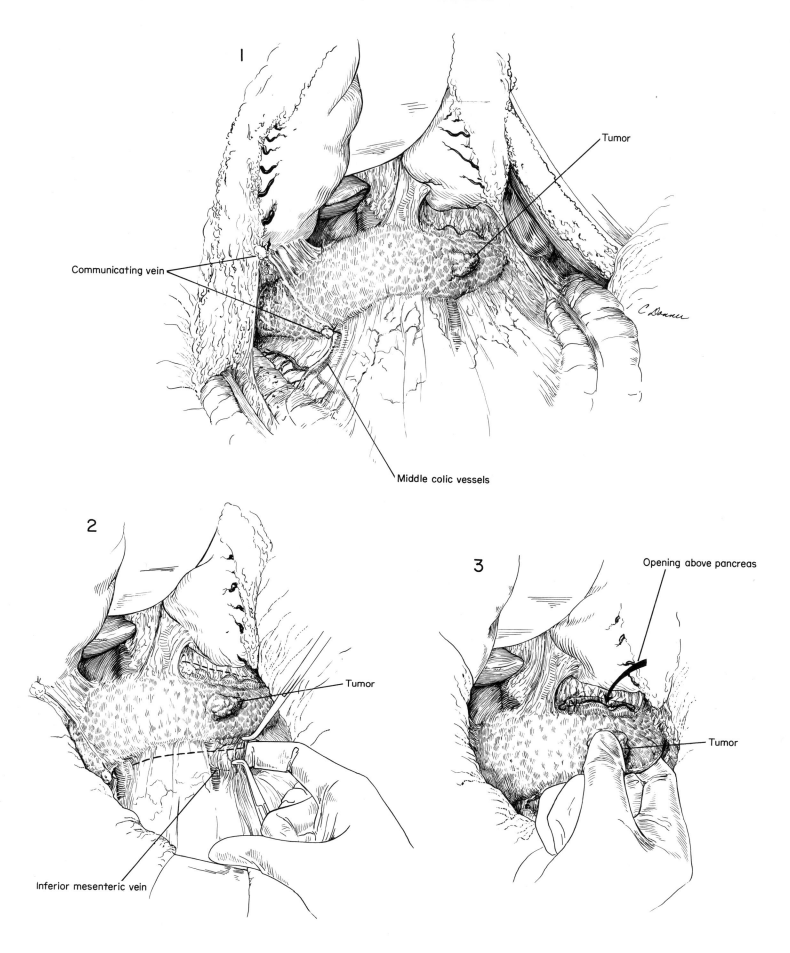

PLATE XCI · RESECTION OF THE TAIL OF THE PANCREAS

DETAILS OF PROCEDURE (*Continued*). In the presence of a tumor that necessitates removal of the left half of the pancreas, steps should be taken to mobilize and remove the spleen. The splenic artery is doubly ligated with 00 silk near its point of origin. This tends to decrease the blood loss following manipulation of the spleen and permits blood to drain from this organ into the systemic circulation during the subsequent steps of its removal. The left gastroepiploic vessel is doubly clamped and ligated, and the short gastric vessels are then divided all the way up to the diaphragm. The blood supply on the greater curvature should be ligated by transfixing sutures that incorporate a bite of the gastric wall to prevent hemorrhage if gastric distention should occur and the ligature slip off the gastric side **(Figure 4).** The splenorenal ligament is divided as the surgeon pulls the spleen medially with his left hand **(Figure 5).** Blunt and sharp dissection may be carried out to free the tail of the pancreas, but this is rather easily done by finger dissection as the organ is reflected medially **(Figure 6).** The left adrenal and kidney are clearly visualized as well as a segment of the left renal vein. The inferior mesenteric vein is ligated at the inferior border of the pancreas. The splenic artery is divided near its point of origin and ligated and then transfixed distally with double ties of 00 silk. The splenic vein is cleared and separated from the posterior surface of the pancreas and is followed over to the point where it joins the superior mesenteric vein to form the portal vein **(Figure 7).** The splenic vein is gently freed from the pancreas, using blunt-nosed right-angle clamps **(Figure 7).** The vessel is ligated and is transfixed proximally to this tie to avoid any possible late hemorrhage. The spleen and body of the pancreas can then be sufficiently mobilized to be brought outside the peritoneal cavity.

PLATE XCI   RESECTION OF THE TAIL OF THE PANCREAS

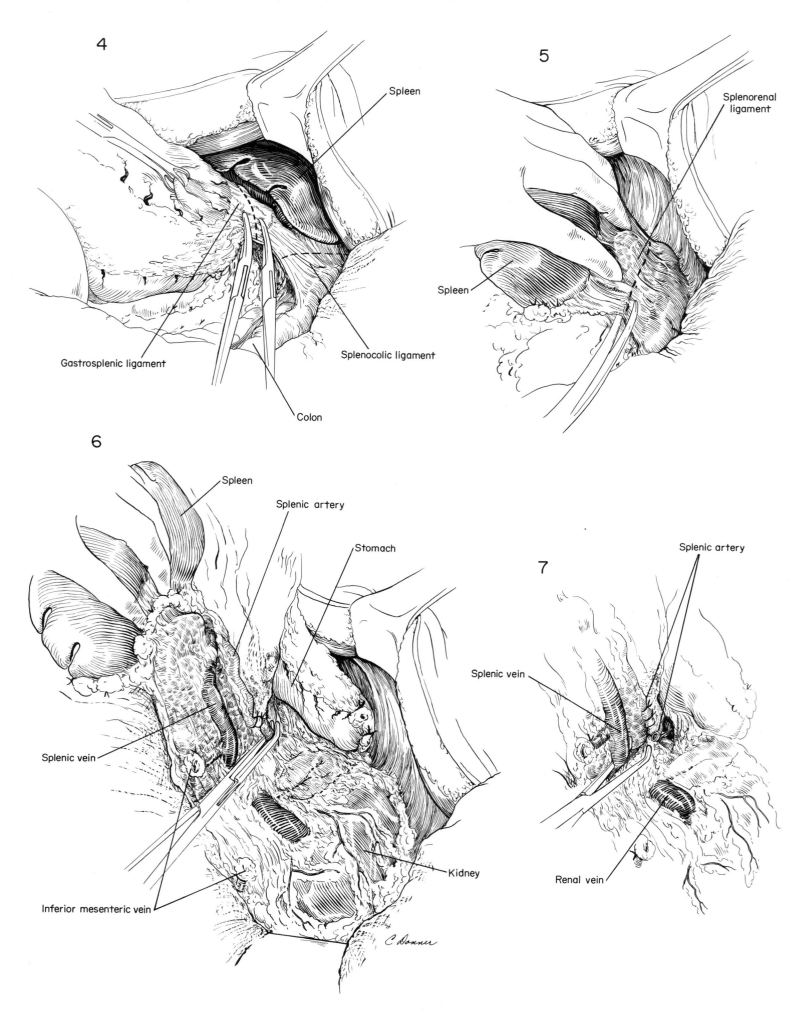

4

Spleen

Gastrosplenic ligament

Splenocolic ligament

Colon

5

Splenorenal
ligament

Spleen

6

Spleen

Splenic artery

Stomach

Splenic vein

Inferior mesenteric vein

Kidney

7

Splenic artery

Splenic vein

Renal vein

PLATE XCII · RESECTION OF THE TAIL OF THE PANCREAS

DETAILS OF PROCEDURE (*Continued*). After the spleen and the tail of the pancreas have been mobilized outside the peritoneal cavity, the entire pancreas is palpated once again for evidence of tumor involvement. The pancreas can be divided to the left of the portal vein or, if need be, even to the right side of the portal vein, provided that a finger has been introduced between the vein and the pancreas to free its anterior margin. Noncrushing specially constructed forceps are applied in pairs in the region of the pancreas, and the pancreatic tissue is divided **(Figure 8).**

The surgeon usually finds it advisable to make multiple serial sections of the pancreas in searching for additional adenomas and in determining whether his line of incision is free of tumor. Frozen-section consultations may be obtained, although pancreatic tissue is difficult to evaluate under these circumstances, and the final diagnosis may have to be delayed until the permanent sections have been made.

Before removing the noncrushing forceps, a row of interrupted overlapping 00 silk sutures of the mattress type is placed entirely through the pancreas and tied **(Figure 9).** After the clamp has been removed, additional sutures are taken, particularly where there is persistent bleeding in the area where the major pancreatic duct has been visualized **(Figure 10).**

CLOSURE. Rubber tissue drainage from the stump of the pancreas may be instituted. The drain is brought out either directly through a stab wound in the midportion of the abdomen or to either side through a separate stab wound incision. The wound is closed in layers with silk.

POSTOPERATIVE CARE. The postoperative care is routine except for repeated laboratory checks on the blood sugar and amylase levels. A mild degree of pancreatitis may occur, and colloids and other solutions should be given in adequate amounts to maintain a slow pulse. A transient diabetic tendency may occur; on the other hand, it is difficult to determine in the immediate postoperative period what effect the surgical procedure will have on total pancreatic function.

PLATE XCII   RESECTION OF THE TAIL OF THE PANCREAS

8

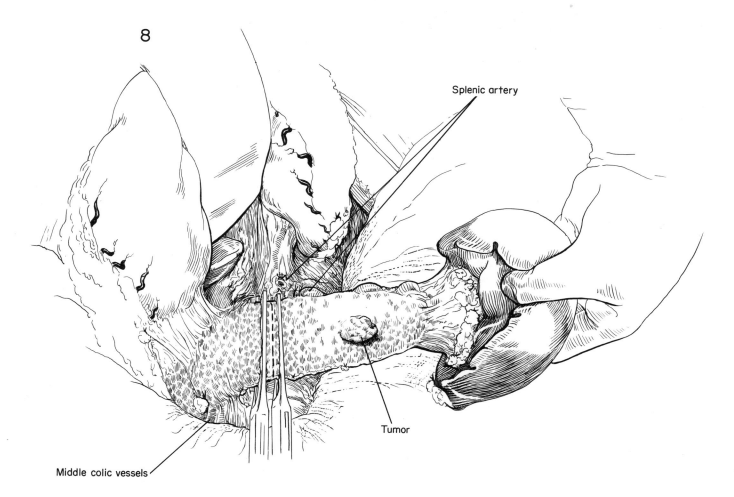

Splenic artery

Tumor

Middle colic vessels

9

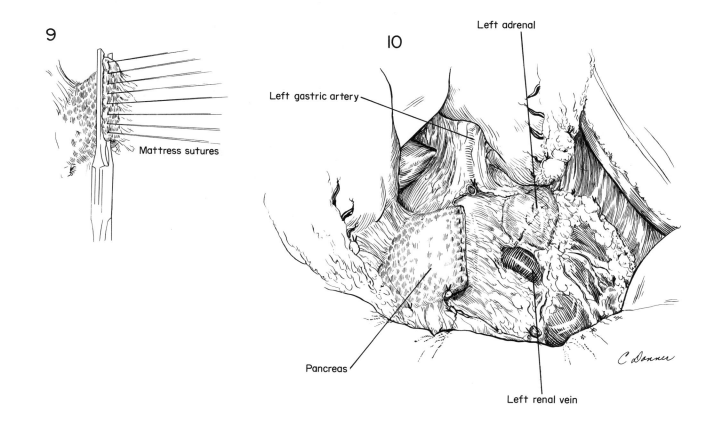

Mattress sutures

10

Left adrenal

Left gastric artery

Pancreas

Left renal vein

C Donner

PLATE XCIII · PANCREATICODUODENECTOMY (WHIPPLE PROCEDURE)

INDICATIONS. The head of the pancreas is usually removed for malignancy involving the ampulla of Vater, the lower end of the common duct, the head of the pancreas, or the duodenum. Far less frequently, the procedure is carried out to manage intractable pain associated with a chronic calcific pancreatitis. In the presence of malignancy the resection is indicated in the absence of proven metastases and if the tumor is of such a limited size that the portal vein is not involved. In a poor-risk patient with deep jaundice it may be advisable to carry out a two-stage procedure: the obstruction of the common duct is relieved by cholecystoenterostomy, and later the head of the pancreas and the duodenum are resected. The patient should be made aware of the possibility of diabetes mellitus after operation as well as the need for daily pancreatic enzyme replacement.

PREOPERATIVE PREPARATION. Three or four units of blood may be required preoperatively to restore the blood volume and decrease the tendency to hypotension and eventual renal shutdown after operation. The electrolyte levels should be returned to normal, and particular care should be taken that the prothrombin level is well above 50 per cent of normal and that the kidney function is not impaired, as shown by creatinine and blood urea nitrogen levels. Whole blood should be available, since the systolic blood pressure levels in the jaundiced patient must be sustained above 100 mm. of mercury at all times, including the period of induction of anesthesia, during the surgical procedure, and in the early postoperative period, to minimize the possibility of renal failure. The measured blood loss should be replaced as lost during the operative procedure, preferably via a central venous catheter. It is advisable to have a catheter in the bladder in order to follow the postoperative hourly output of urine. Prophylactic antibiotic therapy starting 24 hours before operation should be considered because of the possibility of compromising the blood supply to the liver.

ANESTHESIA. A nasogastric tube is inserted. General anesthesia with endotracheal intubation is recommended. Hepatotoxic agents should be avoided.

POSITION. The patient is placed supine on the table with the feet slightly lower than the head. Facilities should be available for performing a cholangiogram or pancreaticogram.

OPERATIVE PREPARATION. The skin should be shaved from the level of the nipples well out over the chest wall and down over the abdomen, including the flanks.

INCISION AND EXPOSURE. A type of incision should be selected that will ensure the extensive and free visualization of the upper abdomen, especially on the right side. While an upper midline **(Figure 1, A)** or right paramedian incision that may extend below the umbilicus is useful, many prefer an oblique or curved incision that parallels the costal margins **(Figure 1, B).** When the xiphoid is long and the xiphocostal angle narrow, further exposure may be obtained by excision of the xiphoid process. On the other hand, very good exposure can usually be obtained by the oblique or curved incision, first carried out over the right upper quadrant and then extended across the midline and as far to the left as the surgeon believes

necessary to ensure a liberal exposure. All bleeding points must be carefully clamped and tied to keep blood loss at a minimum, especially in jaundiced patients. Regardless of the type of incision used, the round ligament is divided **(Figure 2).** The contents of the curved clamps must be securely ligated to avoid bleeding from a vessel in the round ligament. Further mobility of the liver can be obtained if the falciform ligament is divided well up over the dome of the liver **(Figure 2).** Occasionally, small blood vessels are present in it which should be ligated. After the round ligament has been divided, a self-retaining retractor can be inserted and the margins of the wound freed of all clamps after the ligation of their contents.

DETAILS OF PROCEDURE. The type, location, and extent of the pathologic process must now be determined by thorough exploration. Evidence of metastatic spread to the liver, the lymph nodes around the celiac axis, and the region above the pancreas, as well as in the hepatoduodenal ligaments, should be sought by careful exploration.

When a very large gallbladder and common duct are encountered in the presence of an obstructive jaundice, it may be helpful to aspirate the contents of the gallbladder to enhance the exposure and at the same time to accurately localize the site of obstruction by injecting radiopaque contrast material into the biliary system. A point for the needle aspiration should be selected on the underside of the fundus, since this area may be required for a cholecystoenterostomy if resection is found to be contraindicated. Since the bile is often thick and inspissated, a rather large-bore needle, such as an 18- or 20-gauge, is useful, and as much bile as possible is aspirated. The needle is left in place, 50 to 150 ml. of 35 per cent iodinated contrast medium is injected, and the patient is made ready for a cholangiogram. A purse-string suture is placed in the wall of the gallbladder around the needle so that the opening in the gallbladder can be closed as the needle is withdrawn.

While the surgeon is waiting for the return of the cholangiograms for his inspection, he can proceed with mobilization of the duodenum and head of the pancreas by the Kocher maneuver **(Figure 3).** The duodenum is grasped with one or more Babcock forceps and retracted medially as the peritoneum along the lateral wall of the duodenum is incised. Usually, it is not necessary to ligate vessels in this area, but in the presence of jaundice it is advisable to carry out a meticulous hemostasis. Finger or gauze dissection is used to push the posterior wall of the pancreas from the underlying vena cava and right kidney. An avascular cleavage plane can easily be developed **(Figure 4).** A column of peritoneum remains which forms the lower boundary of the foramen of Winslow **(Figure 5).** The surgeon can place this column of peritoneum under tension by inserting his index and middle fingers on either side of the peritoneum and should incise it very carefully, avoiding injury to the underlying vena cava. In the presence of recurrent ulceration in the region of the second part of the duodenum, considerable scarring and fixation in this area may be encountered.

After the posterior wall of the duodenum and head of the pancreas have been carefully inspected for evidence of tumor or metastatic involvement, further freeing of the second or third part of the duodenum is indicated to determine whether the lesion is operable. Care should be exercised in sweeping away the middle colic vessels which, surprisingly enough, frequently cross to the hepatic flexure of the colon high up over the second part of the duodenum **(Figure 6).**

PLATE XCIII   PANCREATICODUODENECTOMY (WHIPPLE PROCEDURE)

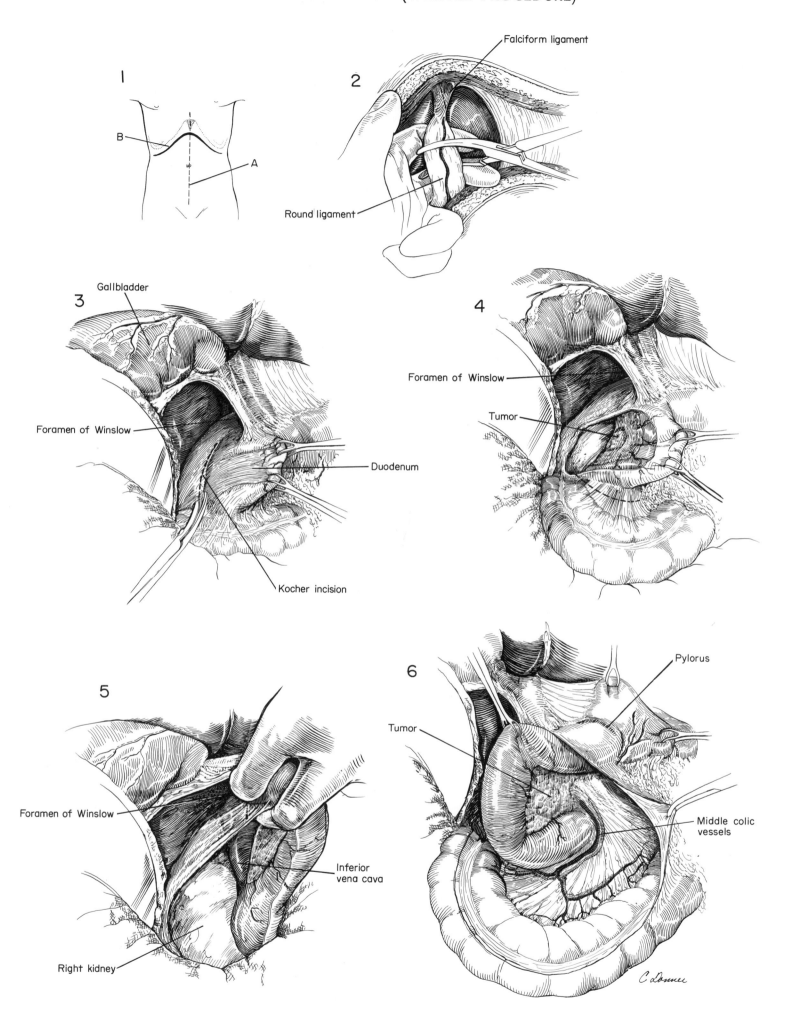

1

2

Falciform ligament

Round ligament

3

Gallbladder

Foramen of Winslow

Duodenum

Kocher incision

4

Foramen of Winslow

Tumor

5

Foramen of Winslow

Inferior vena cava

Right kidney

6

Tumor

Pylorus

Middle colic vessels

C. Donner

PLATE XCIV · PANCREATICODUODENECTOMY (WHIPPLE PROCEDURE)

DETAILS OF PROCEDURE (*Continued*). The gallbladder, antrum of the stomach, head of the pancreas, and duodenum have been separated to call attention to the various relationships, including the blood vessels that must be ligated in this procedure. These structures are numbered for convenient identification. The gallbladder is removed since there is a tendency for gallstone formation in case of long survival. To facilitate the anastomosis, as much of the common duct as possible should be saved below the junction of the cystic duct. The common hepatic artery and its branches must be carefully identified. The right gastric and the pancreaticoduodenal vessels are identified and ligated in order to gain access to the region of the portal vein. Since no vessels enter at the anterior surface of the portal vein, this is the logical point for dividing the head of the pancreas from the body and tail. A number of pancreatic veins enter at the lateral border of the portal vein opposite the point where the splenic vein joins the superior mesenteric to form the portal vein. The middle colic artery and vein should be preserved.

Before the blood supply of the head of the pancreas is compromised, the antrum of the stomach is resected, using the landmarks for hemigastrectomy (see Plate XVII). The division of the first part of the duodenum or the adjacent stomach provides a direct approach to the pancreas in the region of the portal vein.

The pancreatic duct varies in size, depending upon the amount of obstruction that may have occurred as a result of a prolonged block by calculi or tumor formation. If it is quite small, direct implantation of the duct is impossible, and direct implantation of the tail of the pancreas into the lumen of the jejunum can be carried out. The pancreatic duct may be ligated, rather than implanted, providing pancreatic enzyme replacement is carried out indefinitely to avoid subsequent gastric hypersecretion. Usually, there is one blood vessel that needs to be ligated above the pancreatic duct in the substance of the gland and two below.

Since marginal peptic ulceration may occur in a prolonged survival, the ability of the stomach to produce acid must be controlled insofar as possible by vagotomy and by removing the entire antrum of the stomach. The latter can be accomplished by hemigastrectomy, selecting as the point of division the stomach at the level of the third vein on the lesser curvature and the point on the greater curvature where the epiploic vessels are nearest the gastric wall (see Plate XVII).

One of the most difficult parts of the procedure is the freeing of the third part of the duodenum, because of the short mesentery in this area. A portion of the upper jejunum should be resected along with the duodenum to ensure free mobilization of the upper jejunum which is to be brought through the opening in the mesentery to the right of the middle colic vessel.

1. Tumor
2. Duodenum
3. Pancreaticoduodenal artery and vein: (a) Superior (b) Inferior
4. Right gastroepiploic artery and vein
5. Right gastric artery
6. Right gastric vein
7. Gastroduodenal artery

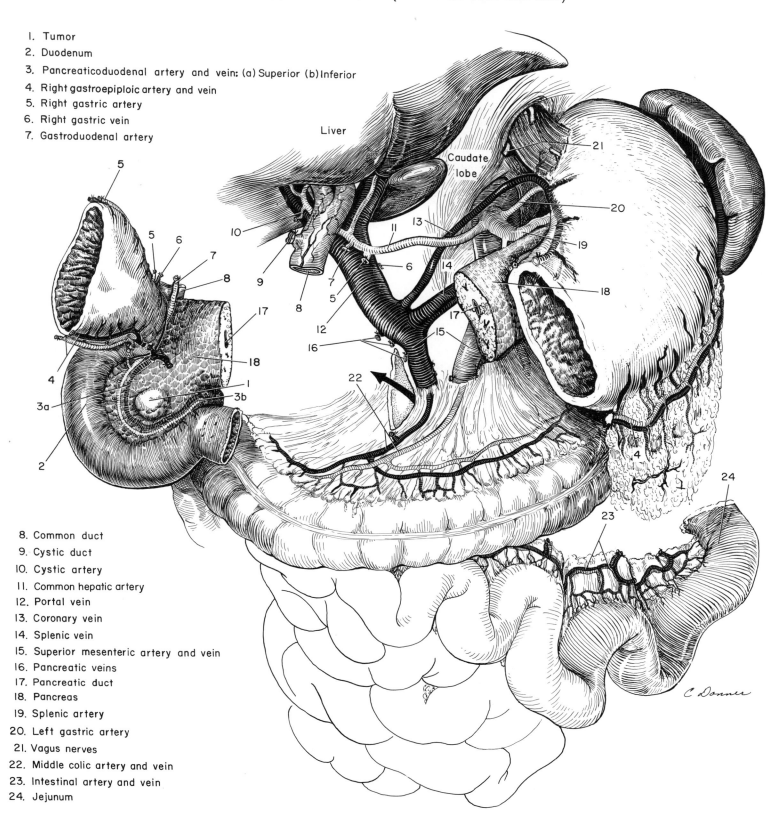

8. Common duct
9. Cystic duct
10. Cystic artery
11. Common hepatic artery
12. Portal vein
13. Coronary vein
14. Splenic vein
15. Superior mesenteric artery and vein
16. Pancreatic veins
17. Pancreatic duct
18. Pancreas
19. Splenic artery
20. Left gastric artery
21. Vagus nerves
22. Middle colic artery and vein
23. Intestinal artery and vein
24. Jejunum

PLATE XCV · PANCREATICODUODENECTOMY (WHIPPLE PROCEDURE)

DETAILS OF PROCEDURE (*Continued*). When the second and third parts of the duodenum are well mobilized, the surgeon may or may not have proved the presence and the extent of a tumor. He can obtain additional information by palpating the head of the pancreas between his thumb and index finger **(Figure 7).** It should be remembered that occasionally pancreatic adenomas are found extending into the wall of the duodenum on the inner curvature side. The presence of a tumor involving the lower end of the common duct, and particularly ulceration with tumor involvement in the region of the ampulla of Vater, may be verified by palpation. A major concern when a tumor is felt or visualized is to determine whether it is a benign or malignant lesion and whether the portal vein is involved. There should be good evidence that the tumor does not extend into or about the portal vein before deciding to proceed with the radical extirpation of the head of the pancreas.

It is not unusual to have considerable difficulty in proving the presence or absence of a malignant tumor deep in the head of the pancreas producing an obstructive jaundice. A surgeon is often reluctant to adequately mobilize the head of the pancreas and to carry out a biopsy to prove the presence of tumor because of the fear of complications such as hemorrhage or a pancreatic fistula. Hence, a transduodenal needle biopsy is utilized by some surgeons. For a number of reasons, however, it is advisable to make a special effort to obtain sufficient material for frozen-section diagnosis. Proof of the diagnosis should be obtained if at all possible before proceeding with such an extensive procedure as extirpation of the head of the pancreas. The risks involved in establishing a diagnosis are far less than those which may follow a radical procedure for a benign lesion. Even though the lesion is not resectable and palliation is to be provided by such surgical procedures as cholecystoenterostomy and gastroenterostomy, chemotherapy may be advisable. Microscopic proof is needed to decide upon the type of chemotherapy and to evaluate its effectiveness. And last, microscopic proof of malignancy is essential for an accurate prognosis. It permits a more rational plan for the patient's care, which may extend over a long period. The surgeon must decide whether the best approach for the biopsy of the tumor is anteriorly or posteriorly **(Figure 8).** A biopsy needle, such as the Vim-Silverman type, can be inserted into a deep-seated tumor and biopsies taken. If the pathologist is hesitant to provide a diagnosis from the minimal amount of tissue available, the surgeon must consider the possibility of proceeding with a wedge biopsy using a small knife blade **(Figure 9).**

A small blade can be used to remove a wedge of tumor and the adjacent tissue compressed together with a transfixing suture of 00 silk on French needles. All bleeding must be controlled. This is not believed to be particularly dangerous, provided the sutures are not so deeply placed as to obstruct the major pancreatic duct. While awaiting the pathologist's report of the biopsies taken, the surgeon should proceed with further mobilization of the pancreas by entering the lesser sac **(Figure 10).** The omentum is retracted upward and the incision made into the lesser sac for more thorough evaluation of potential metastases above the pancreas and about the region of the celiac axis. Since some tumors of the pancreas are multiple, it is important that the entire pancreas be visualized and palpated, especially if a diagnosis of islet cell tumor has been considered. It is usually advisable to open the lesser sac completely by freeing the omentum from the underlying transverse colon all the way over to and including the region of the splenic flexure of the colon **(Figure 11).** It should be kept in mind that the blood vessels to the colon may be angulated upward and attached for several centimeters to the undersurface of the mesocolon. The incision should therefore be made several centimeters away from the visualized bowel wall, as shown in **Figure 11.** It may be necessary to free the spleen, especially during the exploration of the pancreas for islet cell adenomas. If the diagnosis of a localized malignancy involving the region of the head of the pancreas is proved without gross evidence of distant metastases, the surgeon proceeds to reevaluate the patient as a surgical risk. The blood pressure must be sustained and blood replaced as lost while he proceeds to identify and further explore the structures above the first part of the duodenum **(Figure 12).** The contents of the enlarged gallbladder can be aspirated if exposure is limited. The peritoneum is incised over the superior border of the duodenum, which is an initial step in isolating the common duct from the adjacent vascular structures.

PLATE XCV   PANCREATICODUODENECTOMY (WHIPPLE PROCEDURE)

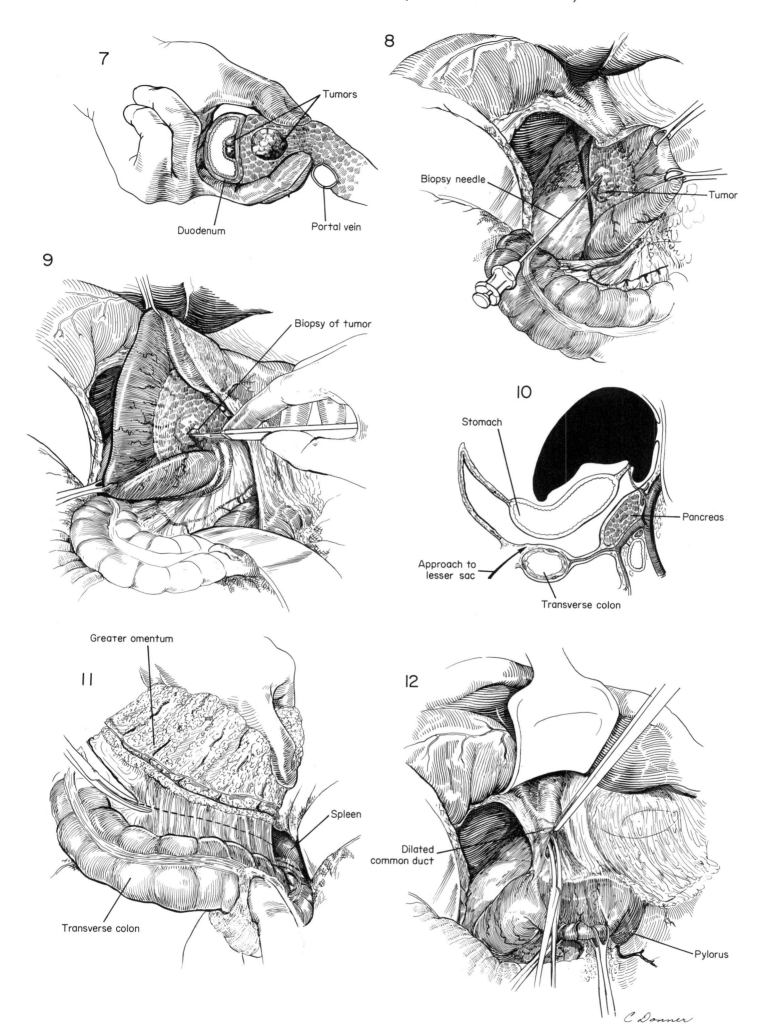

7

Tumors

Duodenum

Portal vein

8

Biopsy needle

Tumor

9

Biopsy of tumor

10

Stomach

Pancreas

Approach to
lesser sac

Transverse colon

11

Greater omentum

Spleen

Transverse colon

12

Dilated
common duct

Pylorus

C Donner

PLATE XCVI · PANCREATICODUODENECTOMY (WHIPPLE PROCEDURE)

DETAILS OF PROCEDURE (*Continued*). Mobilization of the superior part of the duodenum is continued in an effort to isolate as long a segment of the common duct as possible. This can be accomplished by gently spreading a right-angle clamp about the dilated common duct and meticulously controlling all bleeding **(Figure 13).**

An effort should be made to completely free this portion of the common duct; the surgeon can then palpate behind the duodenum with his index finger in an effort to develop a cleavage plane between the duodenum and portal vein, and at the same time he can determine more accurately whether there is fixation by the tumor to this vein. Once he has assured himself that resection is safe without injury to the portal vein, he proceeds to ligate the blood supply necessary for antrectomy. The right gastroepiploic vessels should be ligated and tied **(Figure 14).** Following this, the antrum can be encircled with tape, gentle medial and downward traction applied to the stomach, and the right gastric vessels identified **(Figure 15).**

It is helpful to insert a straight clamp above the duodenum and spread the clamp parallel to the small right gastric vessels in order to better define the vascular pedicle to be doubly ligated **(Figure 15).** Crushing clamps can be used across the duodenum, as shown in **Figure 16,** since these tissues are to be sacrificed. The duodenum is divided. Since peptic ulceration is one of the late complications following radical amputation of the head of the pancreas and duodenum, it is essential to control the acid-producing ability of the remaining stomach. This can be accomplished by hemigastrectomy, which ensures complete removal of the antrum. This is accomplished if the resection includes all of the stomach distal to the third vein on the lesser curvature and the area on the greater curvature where the gastroepiploic vessels are nearest the gastric wall. Some prefer to add vagotomy to the hemigastrectomy. An area the width of the index finger should be cleared on either curvature to prepare for the anastomosis after the blood supply has been doubly ligated **(Figure 17).** A crushing clamp is applied adjacent to the traction sutures, which are left in place to define the areas prepared for anastomosis **(Figure 17).** The removal of the antrum greatly assists in the subsequent exposure of the more difficult portion of the resection.

PLATE XCVI   PANCREATICODUODENECTOMY (WHIPPLE PROCEDURE)

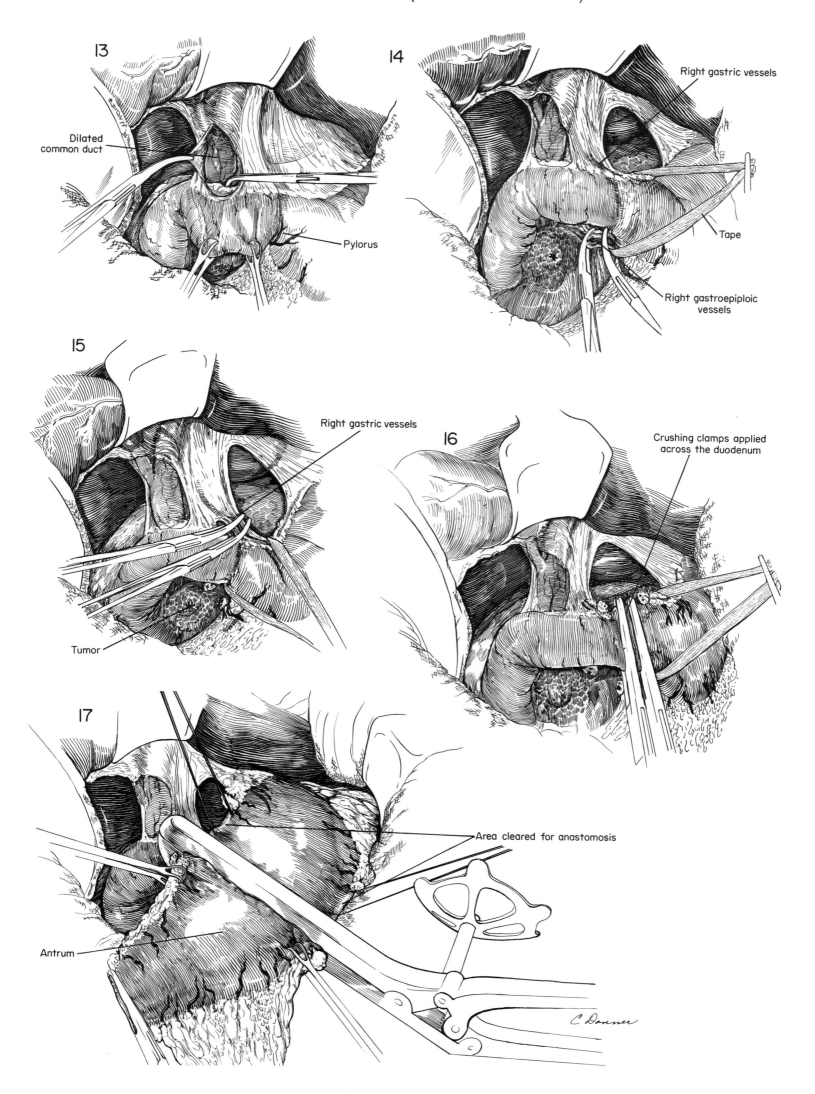

13

Dilated
common duct

Pylorus

14

Right gastric vessels

Tape

Right gastroepiploic
vessels

15

Right gastric vessels

Tumor

16

Crushing clamps applied
across the duodenum

17

Area cleared for anastomosis

Antrum

C Donner

PLATE XCVII · PANCREATICODUODENECTOMY (WHIPPLE PROCEDURE)

DETAILS OF PROCEDURE (*Continued*). If there is oozing between the clips applied by the sewing clamp, it is controlled by interrupted sutures of 0000 silk. The upper half of the approximated gastric outlet is inverted by a layer of interrupted 00 silk mattress sutures **(Figure 18).** A sufficient length of the gastric outlet near the greater curvature is retained to provide a stoma approximately two to three fingers wide. This portion of the gastric wall should not be excised until the final steps of the anastomosis, although it may be necessary to apply several sutures along the line of the clips to control oozing.

A very critical point now involves the identification of the common hepatic artery and the gastroduodenal artery, which runs downward over the pancreas behind the duodenum **(Figure 19A).** The common hepatic artery may be located by palpation just above the pancreas. The peritoneum over it is carefully incised and this major artery clearly visualized to avoid its injury. By blunt dissection the surrounding tissue is separated until the origin of the gastroduodenal artery is visualized. This vessel must be clearly identified and doubly ligated **(Figure 19B).** The lumen of the common hepatic artery must not be encroached upon. The tissues about the right gastric artery also must be gently freed and separated upward, as shown by the dotted line **(Figure 19B).** Following the ligation of these two vessels, blunt dissection with a long right-angle clamp may be undertaken to further free the region of the common duct and portal vein **(Figure 20).** Since these patients are often rather emaciated, there is relatively little tissue to be separated away from the portal vein. Great care should be taken to develop gently a cleavage plane over the portal vein, which will permit the surgeon to introduce carefully a blunt-nosed hemostat, such as a right-angle clamp, behind the pancreas and to open and close the clamp as the tissues are separated from the underlying portal vein. It may be safer and easier for the surgeon to introduce his index finger directly behind the pancreas and over the portal vein. Considerable time should be spent in manipulating the pancreas off the portal vein. This can be done since no vessels enter from the anterior surface of the portal vein. The tissues about the inferior surface of the pancreas may need to be incised so that the finger can be introduced completely underneath the pancreas and come out inferiorly near the region of the middle colic vein **(Figure 21).**

The subsequent technical details of the procedure can be enhanced if the pancreas is divided at this point. A crushing clamp of the Kocher type can be applied across the pancreas on the common duct side, while a modified noncrushing vascular-type clamp may be applied across the pancreas to control the bleeding as the pancreas is divided with the scalpel **(Figure 22).** There is usually one sizable bleeding point above the pancreatic duct, and it is divided with a scalpel **(Figure 23).** The duodenum and head of the pancreas to be excised are grasped primarily with the surgeon's left hand as he proceeds to identify gently the friable vessels entering the head of the pancreas from the right side of the portal vein.

PLATE XCVII   PANCREATICODUODENECTOMY (WHIPPLE PROCEDURE)

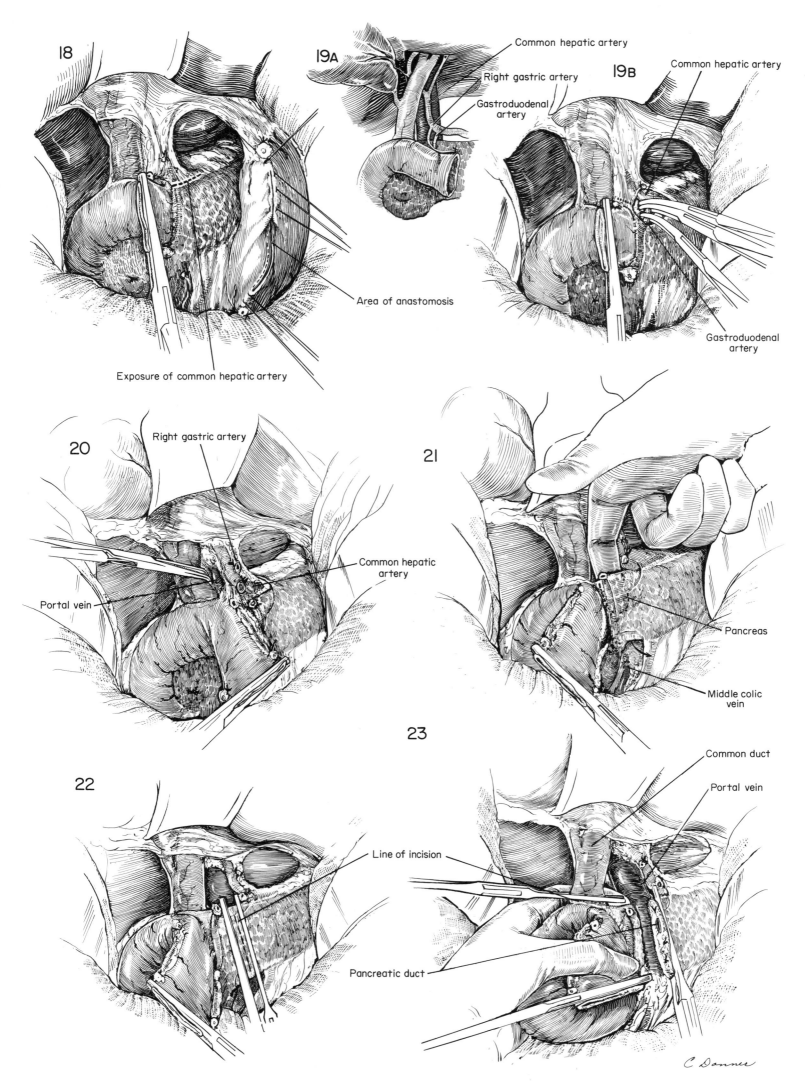

18

Exposure of common hepatic artery

19A
Common hepatic artery
Right gastric artery
Gastroduodenal artery

19B
Common hepatic artery
Gastroduodenal artery

Area of anastomosis

20
Right gastric artery
Common hepatic artery
Portal vein

21
Pancreas
Middle colic vein

22

23
Common duct
Portal vein
Line of incision
Pancreatic duct

C Donner

PLATE XCVIII · PANCREATICODUODENECTOMY (WHIPPLE PROCEDURE)

DETAILS OF PROCEDURE (*Continued*). With the index finger of the left hand above and the thumb below compressing the specimen to be excised, the surgeon applies right-angle clamps in pairs to the strand of tissue that extends from the portal vein into the pancreas **(Figure 24).** Within this strand of tissue there are a number of small veins that must be very carefully ligated lest troublesome bleeding occur. All areas should be ligated to keep the specimen as free of clamps as possible while the third portion of the duodenum is free from the region of the ligament of Treitz and the superior mesenteric vein and artery **(Figure 25).** This can be one of the most difficult steps in the procedure. An incision into the peritoneum about the third portion of the duodenum produces an opening directly into the general peritoneal cavity, through which the upper jejunum will eventually be pulled for the anastomosis **(Figure 25).** The blood supply in the mesentery to the third part of the duodenum and adjacent jejunum is very short, and it is often difficult to mobilize the area about the ligament of Treitz with a minimal loss of blood. Small bits of the mesentery near the duodenal wall are incorporated between pairs of small curved clamps, and the contents are ligated as this area of the duodenum is further freed **(Figure 26).** The attachment of the duodenum that tends to fix the duodenum beneath the inferior mesenteric vein may be more easily identified and clamped if a portion of the upper jejunum is pulled through the opening made in the transverse mesocolon in the region of the ligament of Treitz **(Figure 27).** The remaining short mesenteric attachments, including arterial branches going into the inferior mesenteric artery, can then be carefully clamped with curved clamps and the contents ligated **(Figure 28).** This completely frees the head of the pancreas. A pair of Kocher clamps may be applied to the upper jejunum adjacent to the third part of the duodenum, and the upper jejunum may be divided in this area to dispose of the specimen and provide more room for subsequent mobilization of the upper jejunum and removal of the gallbladder.

PLATE XCVIII   PANCREATICODUODENECTOMY (WHIPPLE PROCEDURE)

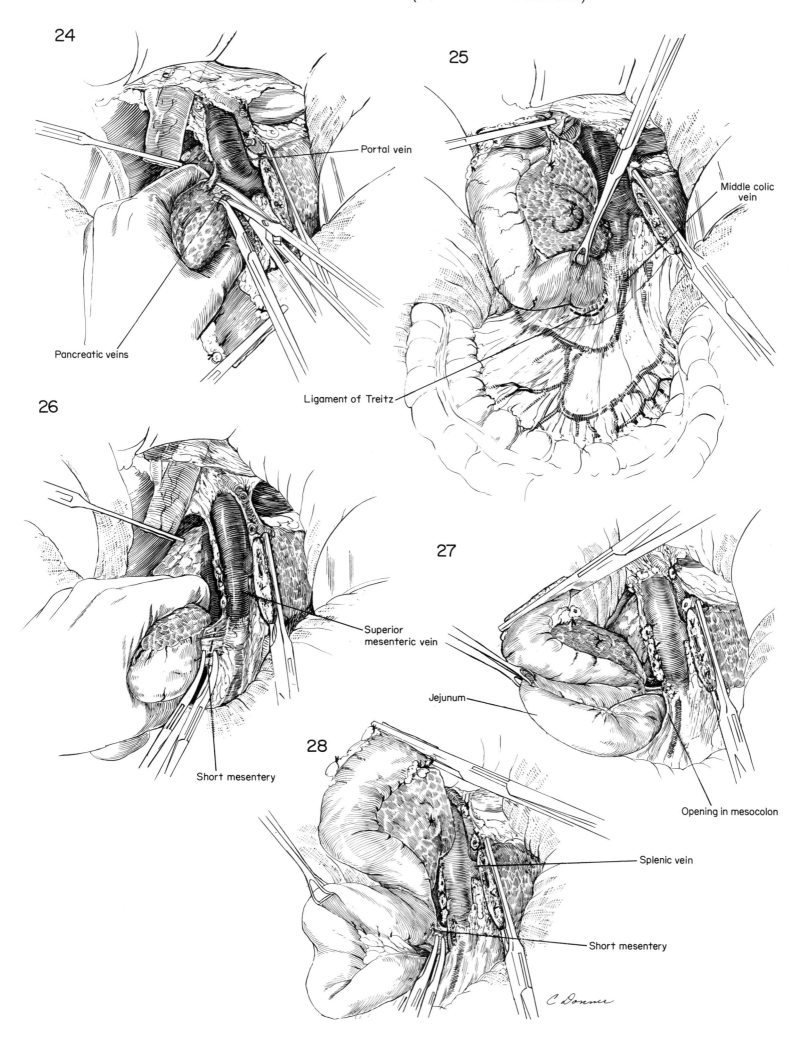

24

Portal vein

Pancreatic veins

25

Middle colic vein

Ligament of Treitz

26

Superior mesenteric vein

Short mesentery

27

Jejunum

Opening in mesocolon

28

Splenic vein

Short mesentery

PLATE XCIX · PANCREATICODUODENECTOMY (WHIPPLE PROCEDURE)

DETAILS OF PROCEDURE (*Continued*). Since the gallbladder is often quite large and distended, it should be removed to provide additional room and to prevent late complication from gallstone formation **(Figure 29)**. The liver bed is very carefully closed after the gallbladder has been removed, and the cystic duct is doubly ligated. Attention is now directed toward further mobilization of the upper jejunum in the region of the ligament of Treitz **(Figure 30)**. Usually, the peritoneum has been opened from above the colon, just about where the dotted line is shown. The upper jejunum is grasped with Babcock forceps and the bowel held up in order to enhance the visualization of the arcades providing the rich blood supply to the jejunum. Incisions are made through the avascular portion of these arcades so that two or three of the basic arcades can be divided and doubly ligated to enhance the mobilization of the upper jejunum **(Figure 31)**. The identification of the arcade to be divided must be done very carefully, and no vessels should be ligated in the mesentery near the mesenteric border of the bowel, since the blood supply to that segment may be compromised. When a segment of the mesentery of the upper jejunum has been divided, the jejunum is brought up through the opening in the mesocolon underneath the superior mesenteric vein **(Figure 31)**. If crushing clamps have been applied to the jejunum originally, it is frequently necessary to reapply noncrushing clamps of the modified vascular type on the oblique, after selecting a point where the mesenteric blood supply is obviously good **(Figure 31)**. About a centimeter of the mesenteric border is freed of blood supply, since this end of the bowel usually will be closed and then invaginated. The loop brought up through the opening in the mesocolon must be long enough to reach well up into the gallbladder fossa without undue tension or compromise of the blood supply. If there appears to be considerable tension, the bowel should be returned back below the colon and additional mesentery divided.

PLATE XCIX   PANCREATICODUODENECTOMY (WHIPPLE PROCEDURE)

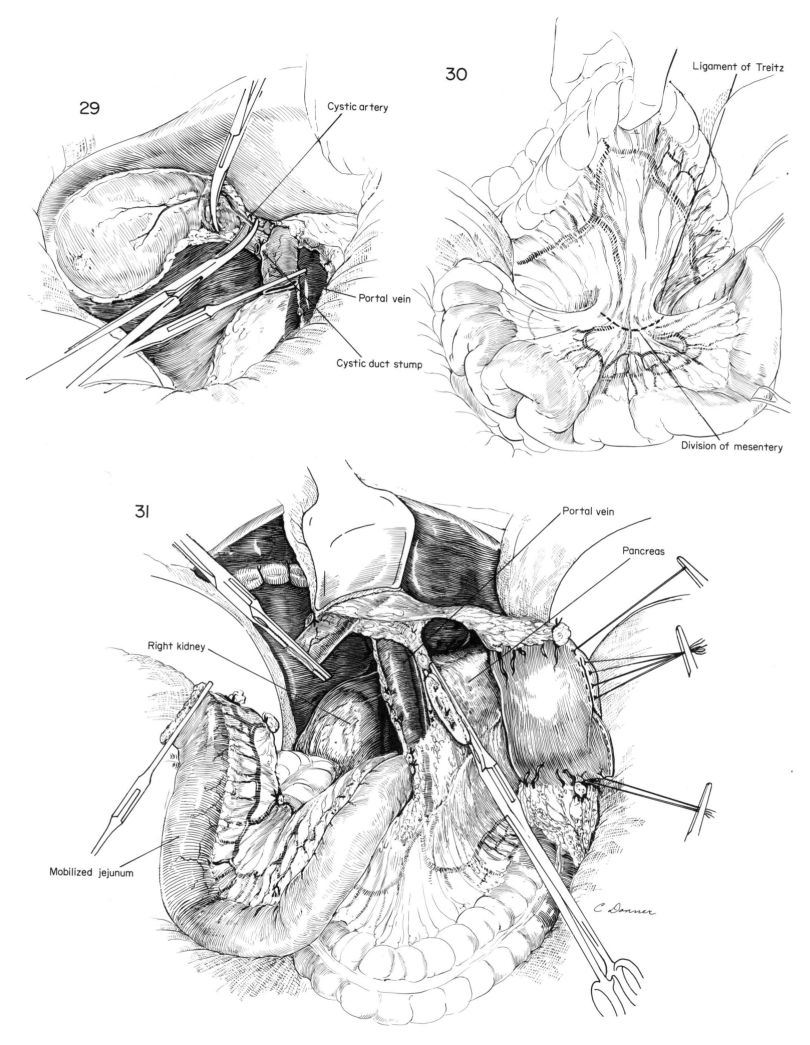

29

Cystic artery

Portal vein

Cystic duct stump

30

Ligament of Treitz

Division of mesentery

31

Portal vein

Pancreas

Right kidney

Mobilized jejunum

C. Donner

PLATE C · PANCREATICODUODENECTOMY (WHIPPLE PROCEDURE)

DETAILS OF PROCEDURE (*Continued*). The diagrams in **Figures 32A** and **32B** outline two of the many variations of reconstruction after removal of the duodenum and head of the pancreas that have been developed. The bile and pancreatic ducts are arranged to empty their alkaline juices into the jejunum before the acid gastric juice as a measure of protection against peptic ulceration. The mobilized jejunum can be used safely in a variety of ways for the several anastomoses required. The end of the jejunum can be closed and anchored up into the region of the gallbladder bed, followed by direct anastomosis with the dilated common duct and pancreatic duct within a very short distance of the closed end of the jejunum. The jejunum is then anastomosed to the partly closed end of the gastric pouch **(Figure 32A)**. Some prefer to ligate the pancreatic duct, since it tends to simplify the procedure and does not appear to increase the incidence of pancreatic fistula. This may be done if pancreatic enzymes are given immediately during the postoperative period and thereafter to prevent the development of gastric hypersecretion. Many prefer not to close the end of the jejunum but rather to implant the open end of the pancreas directly into the open end of the jejunum **(Figure 32B)**. This is perhaps a simpler procedure than that in **Figure 32A**, unless the pancreatic duct is quite large. The common duct is then anastomosed to the jejunum and at an easy point of approximation to the stomach. **Figures 33** and **34** demonstrate details of the technic as shown in **Figure 32A.** The end of the jejunum should then be anchored to the tissues medial to the common duct or even up into the lower portion of the closed liver bed. Great care should be taken, however, that sutures do not include the right hepatic artery, which may curve upward into this area. The end of the common duct is then anchored with interrupted 0000 silk sutures to the serosa of the jejunum. Silk sutures of 0000 size are used to fix either side of the end of the common duct to maintain the wall under slight tension as a row of interrupted sutures is placed to anchor it to the serosa of the jejunum. The fixed angle sutures are allowed to remain for traction **(Figure 33),** while an incision is made into the adjacent jejunal wall a little shorter than the diameter of the lumen of the common duct **(Figure 33)**. A series of interrupted 0000 silk sutures is used to accurately approximate the mucosa of the jejunum to the common duct. A large rubber catheter of a size that almost fills the common duct is introduced up into the common duct, and the lower end is inserted into the lumen of the jejunum. This catheter, which will be subsequently removed at the time of the gastrojejunal anastomosis, tends to facilitate the accurate placement of the interrupted sutures in the closure of the anterior layer **(Figure 34)**. The catheter also ensures a sizable stoma. A second layer of interrupted sutures reinforces the mucosal closure. The peritoneum, which tends to be thickened over the region of the common duct, is then anchored with interrupted sutures to the serosa of the jejunum, starting beyond the angles of the anastomosis and extending anteriorly parallel with the anastomosis **(Figures 35 and 36)**. The jejunum is then rotated laterally alongside the noncrushing clamp which holds the divided end of the pancreas **(Figure 36)**. The clamp may be released, and at least three major vessels, one above the pancreatic duct and two below, will require ligation with 0000 silk sutures. With the clamp in place the posterior capsule of the pancreas is anchored with interrupted 00 silk sutures to the serosa of the jejunum **(Figure 37)**. There should be no tension and preferably some redundancy of the jejunum between the several sites of anastomosis. The patency and size of the pancreatic duct are determined by inserting a soft rubber catheter. With the catheter in place to serve as a stent, the margins of the duct are freed for a short distance to facilitate an accurate anastomosis to the jejunal mucosa **(Figure 38)**.

PLATE C   PANCREATICODUODENECTOMY (WHIPPLE PROCEDURE)

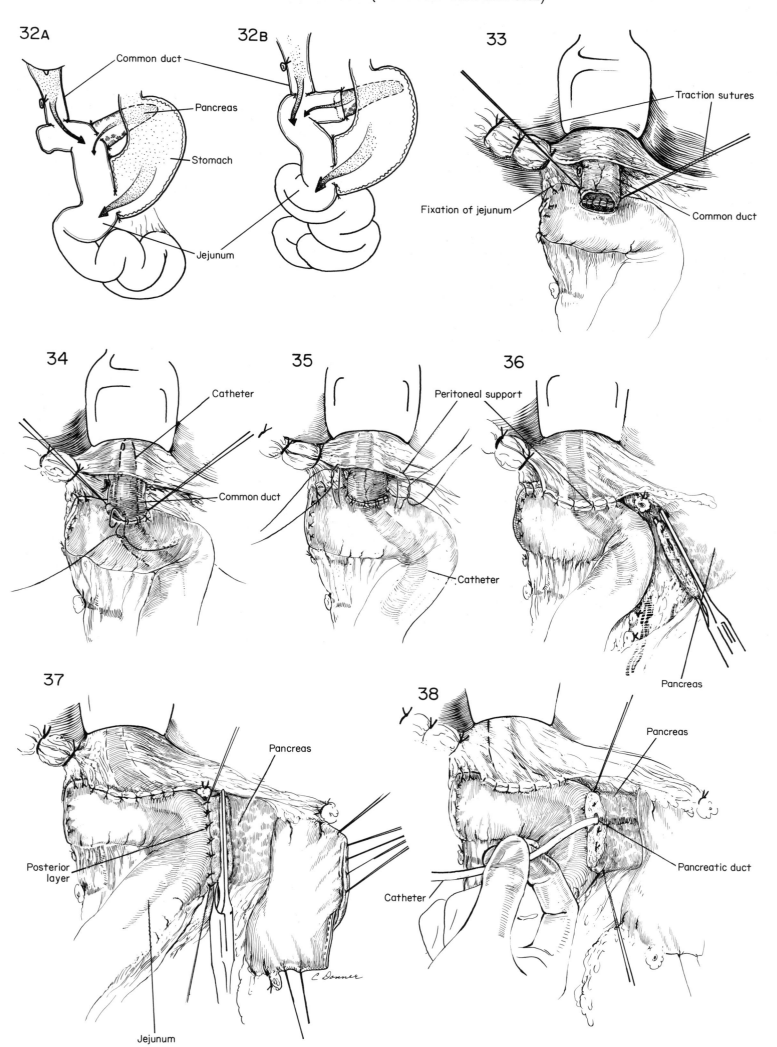

32A

Common duct

Pancreas

Stomach

Jejunum

32B

33

Traction sutures

Fixation of jejunum

Common duct

34

Catheter

Common duct

35

Peritoneal support

Catheter

36

Pancreas

37

Pancreas

Posterior layer

Jejunum

38

Catheter

Pancreas

Pancreatic duct

C Donner

PLATE CI · PANCREATICODUODENECTOMY
(WHIPPLE PROCEDURE)

DETAILS OF PROCEDURE (*Continued*). A very small opening related to the size of the pancreatic duct is made into the lumen of the jejunum, and interrupted 0000 silk sutures are placed at both angles **(Figure 39).** The catheter is rotated to the left while the posterior layer of sutures is placed, and it is then inserted into the lumen of the bowel as the anterior layer of sutures is finally completed. The catheter serves as a stent and makes it easier to place the sutures more accurately through the mucosa of the jejunum as well as the pancreatic duct. When this anastomosis has been completed, the capsule of the pancreas is anchored to the serosa to seal off the raw end of the gland against the wall of the jejunum **(Figure 40).**

Some prefer to insert the open end of the pancreas into the open end of the jejunum, especially when the pancreatic duct is quite small **(Figure 41A).** The margins near the cut end of the pancreas should be freed for several centimeters in preparation for telescoping the end of the jejunum over it, and all bleeding points should be carefully ligated. The end of the jejunum is usually large enough to admit the end of the pancreas. If not, it may be necessary to incise the full thickness of the jejunum along the antimesenteric border to make the opening large enough to easily match the size of the end of the pancreas. After all bleeding is controlled, the mucosa of the jejunum is sewed to the capsule of the pancreas in a manner similar to an end-to-end anastomosis. A small soft rubber catheter can be inserted into the lumen of the pancreatic duct to ensure its patency during the completion of the anastomosis. It is subsequently removed before closure of the gastrojejunostomy. An additional one or two layers of interrupted sutures of 00 silk are placed to pull the jejunal wall up over the capsule of the pancreas for approximately 1 cm. **(Figure 41B).** The common duct and gastric anastomosis to the jejunum are not altered.

The gastrojejunal anastomosis may be made over the entire length of the gastric outlet, or the outlet may be partly closed and the stoma limited in size. After withdrawal of the nasogastric tube, a gastric clamp, such as a Scudder, may be applied across the stomach to prevent soiling and control the bleeding. The full thickness of the gastric wall, including the clips, is excised to provide a stoma two to three fingers wide **(Figure 42).** The noncrushing clamp is relaxed, any retained gastric contents are aspirated, and all bleeding points in the mucosa of the gastric wall are controlled by transfixing sutures of 0000 silk. The serosa of the jejunum near the mesenteric border is then anchored to the posterior wall of the stomach from one curvature to the other with 00 silk **(Figure 43).** The jejunum should be approximated loosely so that there is some laxity between the anastomosis of the pancreas and the gastric wall in the region of the lesser curvature. An opening about two fingers wide is made in the jejunum, and the gastrojejunal mucosa is approximated with interrupted 0000 silk sutures **(Figure 43).** At this point the catheters that were introduced into the common duct and the pancreatic duct are removed **(Figure 43).** The gastrojejunal anastomosis is then completed with a layer of interrupted 0000 silk sutures, with the knots buried on the inside. The second layer of the gastrojejunal anastomosis is then completed with a layer of interrupted 00 sutures from one curvature to the other **(Figure 44).** The opening about the region of the ligament of Treitz and the peritoneum about the ligament of Treitz should be approximated to the jejunal wall **(Figure 44)** to prevent prolapse of small bowel up through this opening. A temporary tube gastrostomy may be used.

CLOSURE. The abdominal wall is closed in layers with interrupted sutures of 00 silk with 0000 silk to the fat and skin. In the presence of malignancy, jaundice or emaciation, and in the older age group, it may be advisable to close the fascia with a so-called four-pound-figure-of-eight stitch or by the addition of numerous retention sutures.

POSTOPERATIVE CARE. It is of paramount importance, especially in the jaundiced patient, to make certain that the blood volume is restored at all times and that a period of hypotension does not occur. A period of hypotension in a jaundiced patient tends to be associated with eventual renal failure. Fluid balance is sustained by administration of 5 per cent glucose in water, with vitamins C and K added, daily. Blood sugar and amylase levels are obtained. The hourly urine output should be watched carefully and should be maintained at 30 to 40 ml. per hour. The administration of intravenous fluids should be balanced through the 24-hour period rather than given all at one time, such as early in the morning. Urinary output of about 1,000 ml. and the replacement of gastric drainage will determine the amount of fluids required.

A 12-hour gastric secretion test should be done before removing the gastrostomy tube or the inlying nasal catheter as a baseline for subsequent treatment should symptoms of marginal ulceration occur. If the pancreatic duct has been ligated, it is important to give adequate daily dosage of pancreatic enzymes, starting early in the postoperative period and continuing for an indefinite period; this is the best insurance against gastric hypersecretion and subsequent marginal ulceration. The patient's weight must be watched carefully, and an adequate daily caloric and vitamin intake assured. Blood sugar levels should be determined at regular intervals and the stools examined for evidence of pancreatic insufficiency.

PLATE CI   PANCREATICODUODENECTOMY (WHIPPLE PROCEDURE)

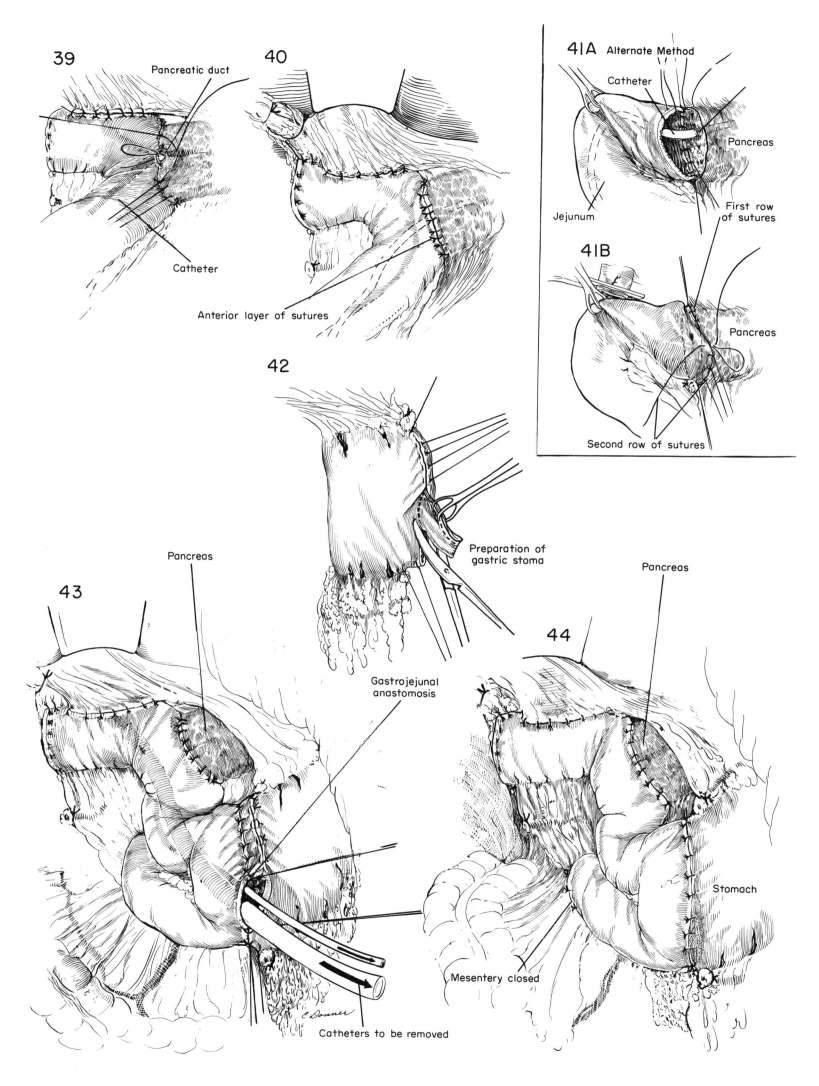

39

Pancreatic duct

Catheter

40

Anterior layer of sutures

41A Alternate Method

Catheter

Jejunum

Pancreas

First row
of sutures

41B

Pancreas

Second row of sutures

42

Preparation of
gastric stoma

43

Pancreas

Gastrojejunal
anastomosis

Catheters to be removed

44

Pancreas

Stomach

Mesentery closed

C. Donner

MISCELLANEOUS ABDOMINAL PROCEDURES

PLATE CII · SPLENECTOMY

INDICATIONS. The most common indications for splenectomy are traumatic rupture; blood dyscrasias, such as congenital hemolytic icterus, essential thrombocytopenic purpura, primary splenic neutropenia, splenic panhematopenia; staging of Hodgkin's disease; and cysts and tumors of the spleen. Symptomatic benefit may follow splenectomy in certain other conditions, such as secondary hypersplenism, Felty's syndrome, Banti's syndrome, Boeck's sarcoid, or Gaucher's disease. Thorough clinical studies are essential, including evaluation by a competent hematologist of the bone marrow and ferrokinetics. Emergency splenectomy may be indicated if the patient with a low platelet count shows signs of intracranial hemorrhage, or evidence of a rapid downhill course despite steroid therapy. Elective splenectomy should be delayed until after the age of two years because of the possibility of immunologic deficiency.

PREOPERATIVE PREPARATION. It is necessary to consider the nature of the disease for which splenectomy is indicated to give the proper preoperative treatment. In congenital hemolytic icterus, preoperative transfusion is contraindicated, even in the presence of the most severe anemia, because of the likelihood of precipitating a hemolytic crisis. In cases of thrombocytopenic purpura, platelet transfusions may be given the night before and the morning of operation if indicated. The patient with primary splenic neutropenia, panhematopenia, or other types of hypersplenism is transfused as indicated by his general condition and the information gained from the clinical studies. Antibiotic therapy is given in the presence of neutropenia. Large amounts of whole blood should be available in cases of suspected traumatic rupture of the spleen, and the patient should be operated upon as soon as his condition permits. Prompt splenectomy may be a lifesaving procedure in some patients with a blood dyscrasia, especially those with primary thrombocytopenic purpura. Previous steroid therapy should be continued preoperatively and during the early postoperative period.

ANESTHESIA. General anesthesia is usually satisfactory and may be supplemented with depolarizing or nondepolarizing muscle relaxants. Patients who have severe anemia should receive little premedication, and ample oxygen should be administered with the anesthetic. In the presence of a low platelet count great care is taken to avoid trauma to the mouth and upper respiratory passages, since hemorrhage may occur.

POSITION. The patient is placed in a supine position. The spleen is made more accessible by tilting the table to lower the feet.

OPERATIVE PREPARATION. The skin is prepared in the routine manner. Gastric intubation is avoided in portal hypertension or in the presence of a low platelet count, i.e., thrombocytopenic purpura, in order to avoid initiating hemorrhage. However, in other indications it can be used to ensure a collapsed stomach and an improved exposure.

INCISION AND EXPOSURE. Two types of incision are commonly used —a liberal vertical incision through the middle of the left rectus sheath extending over the costal margin adjacent to the xiphoid and down to the level of the umbilicus **(Figure 1,** A), or a left oblique subcostal incision **(Figure 1,** B). The vertical incision is usually employed. In the presence of proven gallstones the incision is placed in the midline to facilitate removal of the diseased gallbladder, if the splenectomy has progressed satisfactorily and was uneventful.

If a bleeding tendency exists in the presence of blood dyscrasias, it is necessary to exercise rigid control of all bleeding points. In the very ill and anemic patient the general oozing may be controlled by pressure with warm, moist gauze pads, so that the abdomen may be opened and the splenic artery ligated as soon as possible. This will often effect a marked decrease in the bleeding tendency as soon as the artery is clamped. In the absence of acute intra-abdominal hemorrhage or an acute hemolytic blood crisis, the abdomen is explored. The gallbladder should be carefully palpated if the splenectomy has been indicated for hemolytic jaundice, since gallstones frequently occur in such patients. The pelvic organs in the female are carefully palpated for evidence of other pathology that might be responsible for excessive blood loss from the reproductive system. Enlarged lymph nodes should be biopsied.

The colon is packed downward out of the field of operation by warm, moist gauze, and the first assistant maintains downward traction with a large S retractor. A Babcock forceps is applied to the stomach, and a retractor is placed under the rib margin on the left to facilitate the exposure of the spleen.

DETAILS OF PROCEDURE. The exact procedure depends upon many factors: the size and mobility of the spleen, the presence of extensive adhesions between the spleen and the parietal peritoneum, the length of the

splenic pedicle, the presence of active bleeding from a ruptured spleen, or the patient's poor general condition as a result of blood dyscrasia. The approach to the immobilization and control of the blood supply of the spleen must be individualized in each case. A thorough understanding of the attachments and blood supply of the spleen is essential **(Figure 2).**

When splenectomy is indicated for blood dyscrasias, a careful search should be made for an accessory spleen both before and after the spleen is removed and hemostasis is effected **(Figure 2).** A routine search is made in the following order: the hilar region, A; the splenorenal ligament, B; the greater omentum, C; the retroperitoneal region surrounding the tail of the pancreas, D; the splenocolic ligament, E; and the mesentery of the large and small intestines, F **(Figure 2).** If accessory spleens are found in two or more locations, one is usually in the hilus. In some cases of blood dyscrasias the clinical course of the patient may suggest recurrence of the disease because of a retained accessory spleen. In such instances not only should the above-mentioned sites be searched, but the search should also be extended to the adnexa in the pelvis. The spleen must not be lacerated, nor should remnants be left within the abdomen because of the danger of seeding which may result in splenosis.

The diagram in **Figure 2** illustrates the anatomic relationships of the spleen. As traction is exerted on the stomach medially, an avascular area in the gastrosplenic ligament may be incised, giving direct entrance to the lesser sac. Several blood vessels in the gastrosplenic ligament are divided and ligated to provide adequate exposure of the splenic artery. Along the upper margin of the pancreas, the tortuous course of the splenic artery can be palpated. The peritoneum over the vessel is carefully incised, and a long right-angle clamp is introduced beneath the artery to isolate it and to facilitate its ligation. The splenic vein is immediately beneath the artery. One or more 00 silk sutures are drawn beneath the artery and carefully tied **(Figure 3).** Preliminary ligation of the splenic artery has many advantages. It allows blood to drain from the spleen, providing an autotransfusion. The spleen tends to shrink, making its removal easier and with less blood loss. Finally, blood transfusions can be given immediately to the patient with hemolytic anemia. This preliminary step does not prolong the procedure and tends to ensure a safer splenectomy with minimal blood loss.

After the splenic artery has been secured, the remainder of the gastrosplenic ligament is divided between small curved clamps **(Figure 4).** Great care is exercised, especially toward the upper margin of the spleen, to avoid injuring the gastric wall during the application of clamps, for in this area the gastrosplenic ligament is sometimes extremely short. This is especially true when the spleen is very large or in the presence of portal hypertension. Failure to secure the uppermost vein in the gastrosplenic ligament can result in serious blood loss. Because of the danger of postoperative bleeding following gastric dilatation, the vessels along the greater curvature should be ligated with a transfixing suture that includes a bite of the gastric wall. In addition, in this area several vessels commonly extend from the hilus of the spleen over to the posterior wall near the greater curvature high on the fundus. At the inferior margin of the spleen, fairly sizable vessels, the left gastroepiploic artery and vein, will commonly be encountered in the gastrosplenic ligament **(Figure 4).** The contents of the clamps are ligated on both the gastric and splenic sides, since the division of the gastrosplenic ligament will leave a large opening directly into the lesser sac.

The preliminary ligation of the major splenic artery makes mobilization of the spleen easier and safer. The surgeon passes the left hand over the spleen in an effort to deliver it into the wound **(Figure 5).** Dense adhesions may be present between the spleen and the peritoneum of the abdominal wall; however, the spleen usually can be mobilized after a few avascular adhesions and the gastrosplenic ligament have been divided.

As the spleen is mobilized, the surgeon passes his fingers over its margin to expose the splenorenal ligament, which should be carefully incised **(Figure 6).** The peritoneal reflection in this area is usually rather avascular; however, it is necessary to ligate many bleeding points in the presence of portal hypertension. Usually, the index finger can be inserted into the peritoneal opening, and by blunt dissection with the index finger of the left hand, which extends over the surface of the spleen, the margin of the spleen can be freed easily **(Figure 7).** This must be done gently since the capsule may be torn, resulting in troublesome bleeding or seeding of splenic tissue.

After the posterior margin of the spleen has been mobilized, the spleen may be brought well outside the abdomen; however, if dense adhesions between the spleen and the parietal peritoneum are encountered, it is easier to incise the overlying peritonum and carry out a subperitoneal resection which leaves a large, raw space. This may be safer than attempting to free the spleen with sharp dissection. Warm, moist packs may be introduced into the splenic bed to control oozing. Active bleeding points should be ligated by transfixion.

PLATE CII   SPLENECTOMY

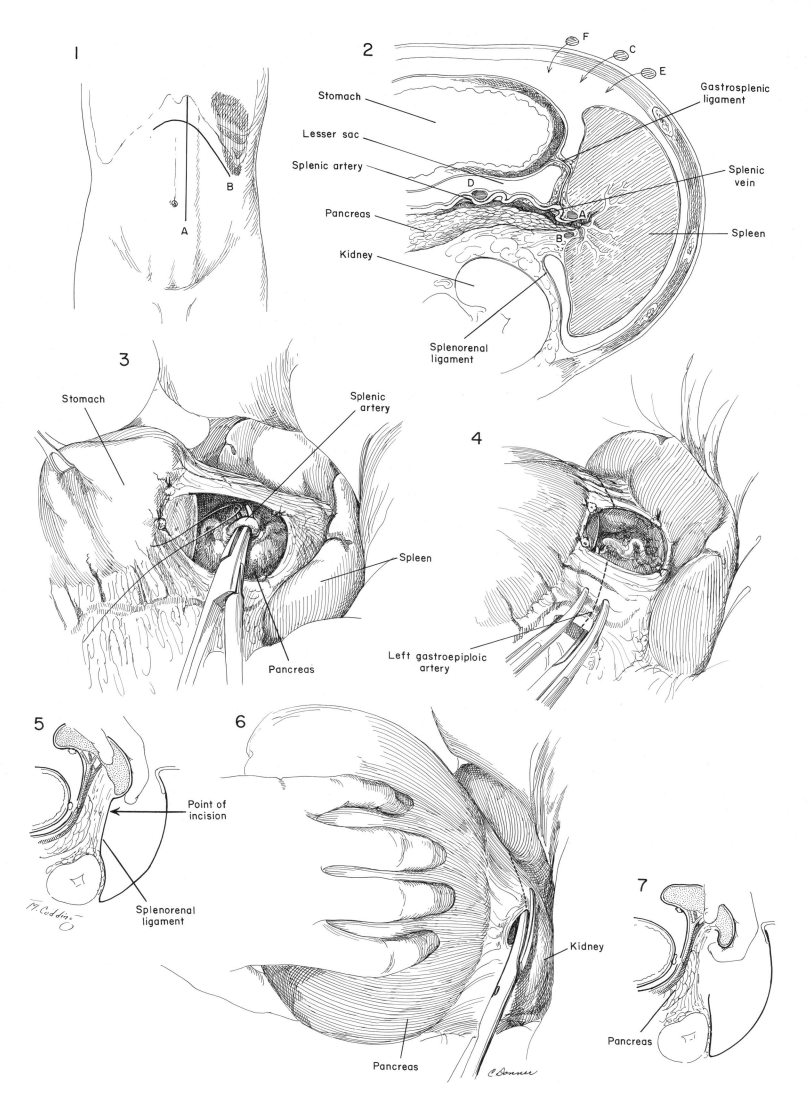

1

2

Stomach

Lesser sac

Splenic artery

Pancreas

Kidney

Splenorenal
ligament

F

C

E

Gastrosplenic
ligament

Splenic
vein

Spleen

D

A

B

3

Stomach

Splenic
artery

Spleen

Pancreas

4

Left gastroepiploic
artery

5

Point of
incision

Splenorenal
ligament

M. Codding

6

Kidney

Pancreas

C Donner

7

Pancreas

PLATE CIII · SPLENECTOMY

DETAILS OF PROCEDURE (*Continued*). When the spleen is mobilized outside the wound, the splenocolic ligament is divided between curved clamps **(Figure 8)**. This procedure is carried out carefully in order to avoid any possibility of damage to the colon. The contents of these clamps are ligated with a transfixing suture of 00 silk. In the presence of portal hypertension many large veins may be present in this area. The spleen is then retracted medially by the surgeon's left hand, while the tail of the pancreas, if it extends up to the splenic hilus, is separated by blunt dissection from the splenic vessels in order to avoid damage to it by the subsequent ligation of the pedicle **(Figures 9 and 10)**. The surgeon should keep in mind the possibility of accessory spleens in this location. The spleen is held upward and laterally by an assistant, while the large vessels in the pedicle are separated from the adjacent tissues to permit the application of several curved clamps to the individual vessels **(Figure 11)**. These vessels should be ligated at the base of the pedicle proximal to the bifurcation of the splenic vessels. Despite the fact that the splenic artery has been previously ligated, it is tied again proximally and transfixed distally **(Figure 12)**. The same principle of double ligature for the splenic vein is also carried out. In those instances where preoperative transfusions have been contraindicated, they may be started as soon as the splenic artery has been divided. The operative site is searched for evidence of persistent oozing. Warm, moist packs or a coagulant may be introduced to control the small bleeding points. Following this, a final careful search is made for any existing accessory spleens. Reperitonealization of the splenic bed may be useful in controlling persistent oozing. Interrupted sutures are used.

Alternate Method

When the spleen is quite mobile and the pedicle is long, which is apt to be the case in the presence of splenomegaly of long standing, splenectomy may be facilitated if the splenorenal ligament is first incised without an attempt to divide the gastrosplenic ligament **(Figure 13)**. The spleen is gently pulled upward and medially, providing exposure of the vessels in the pedicle from the lateral side **(Figure 14)**. It may be necessary to divide the splenocolic ligament first in order to better expose the contents of the splenic pedicle. In the presence of a ruptured spleen the urgency of the situation may require mass clamping of the splenic pedicle; however, individual ligation of the major vessels is safer and more desirable. This may be accomplished by ascertaining the position of the splenic artery by palpation followed by blunt dissection, in an effort to isolate the splenic artery **(Figure 14)**. When the splenic artery has been divided, the spleen should be compressed to ensure an autotransfusion through the intact splenic vein. Since the gastrosplenic ligament has not been previously divided, it may be included in the clamps applied to the splenic pedicle, thereby sealing off the lesser omental sac **(Figure 15)**. If the gastrosplenic ligament is to be included in these clamps, great care is necessary to avoid including a portion of the greater curvature of the stomach, especially when the gastrosplenic ligament is very short. This is more apt to occur high in the region of the fundus of the stomach. The inclusion of the gastrosplenic ligament in the clamps applied to the splenic pedicle should not be attempted unless the pedicle is long and all structures may be easily and clearly identified **(Figure 16)**. The contents of the clamps applied to the splenic pedicle are doubly ligated. The most superficial of these ligatures should be of the transfixing type. Deep transfixing sutures should not be taken, since troublesome hemorrhage may result, especially from the splenic vein.

Except in cases of traumatic rupture of the spleen, the surgeon should consider the advisability of routine liver biopsy to provide additional microscopic evaluation of the reticuloendothelial system (Plate LXXV). It is not uncommon to convert a diagnosis of so-called primary to secondary hypersplenism because of the finding of a primary disease, such as lymphosarcoma, in the biopsy.

In good-risk patients cholecystectomy is performed if gallstones are found, especially in association with congenital hemolytic anemia. A routine cholangiogram is also carried out. In the younger age groups with primary hypersplenism the appendix is removed if the cecum is easily mobilized.

Staging of Hodgkin's Disease

Splenectomy may be indicated as part of the procedure of "staging" to determine the extent of Hodgkin's disease. Patients have usually had the diagnosis proved by a peripheral lymph node biopsy. In addition to an extensive hematological evaluation, these patients should have had extensive liver function studies as well as lymphangiograms in search of retroperitoneal lymph node involvement.

The abdominal incision may need to be extended below the level of the umbilicus if the preoperative studies indicate the need to biopsy the periaortic lymph nodes. The liver and spleen should be carefully palpated for evidence of tumor involvement. Lymph nodes about the hilus of the spleen should be removed for microscopic study. The splenic pedicle should be marked with several Cushing metal clips. A liberal biopsy of the liver should be taken and lymph nodes about the pancreas excised for microscopic examination. Proof of retroperitoneal involvement often requires exploration along the aorta, starting beneath the mobilized body of the pancreas. A silver clip or clips should be applied to all biopsy sites. They may serve as a guide to radiation therapy, and their subsequent displacement may suggest the extent of any recurrences.

CLOSURE. The wound edges can be more easily approximated by returning the table to its original horizontal position, thus facilitating return of the abdominal contents to their anatomical location. A routine silk closure is done without drainage.

POSTOPERATIVE CARE. This will vary, depending upon the requirement for whole blood replacement. Within a short time after splenectomy for a blood dyscrasia involving a bleeding tendency, it is usually noted that the platelet count rises rapidly; thus, transfusion may be unnecessary for this purpose. It is good practice to monitor platelet counts postoperatively, even in elective procedures, because of the marked thrombocytosis that is occasionally seen. In patients with markedly elevated platelet counts or abnormal platelet function, anticoagulants, such as acetylsalicylic acid and dipyridamole, may be indicated. Anticoagulants are rarely necessary in routine splenectomy. A marked leucocytosis commonly follows splenectomy and should not be interpreted as indicative of infection. Constant gastric suction for several days is often advisable. The patient is permitted out of bed on the first postoperative day. Fluid balance is carefully maintained according to the patient's general condition. Any steroid therapy given preoperatively is continued during the postoperative period. Further steroid therapy will be regulated by the hematologist, who will be guided by the patient's blood picture response to splenectomy. In patients with secondary hypersplenism, their primary disease will not be altered, although the patient's life has been saved or prolonged by removal of the overactive spleen.

PLATE CIII   SPLENECTOMY

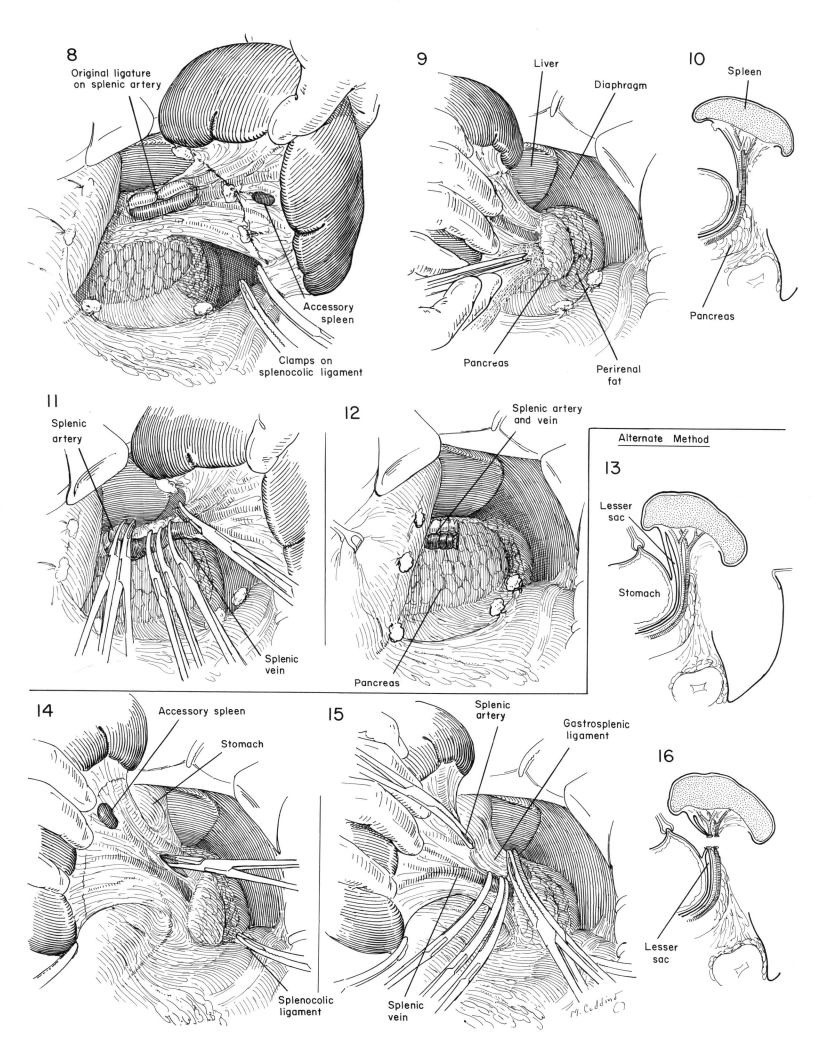

8 Original ligature on splenic artery
Accessory spleen
Clamps on splenocolic ligament

9 Liver
Diaphragm
Pancreas
Perirenal fat

10 Spleen
Pancreas

11 Splenic artery
Splenic vein

12 Splenic artery and vein
Pancreas

Alternate Method
13 Lesser sac
Stomach

14 Accessory spleen
Stomach
Splenocolic ligament

15 Splenic artery
Gastrosplenic ligament
Splenic vein

16 Lesser sac

M. Codding

PLATE CIV · BILATERAL ADRENALECTOMY

INDICATIONS. The presence of cortical or medullary tumors of either malignant or benign adenomatous nature is a well-established indication for unilateral adrenalectomy. In recent years, however, the number of indications for bilateral adrenalectomy has gradually increased. It is occasionally performed to control complex endocrine states after partial or unilateral adrenalectomy has failed to alleviate hyperaldosteronism or hypercorticism, as in Cushing's syndrome. Some also recommend bilateral adrenalectomy in cases of advanced carcinoma of the breast or prostate to decrease circulating sexual hormones when the metastatic tumors are hormone-dependent.

PREOPERATIVE PREPARATION. The most important preoperative procedure is to establish a firm diagnosis. Clinical findings often indicate the altered pathophysiology, but extensive endocrine studies are usually necessary, not only to establish the disorder within the adrenals but also to rule out associated disorders in other endocrine glands. Tumors are seldom large enough to be identified by pyelography, tomography, retroperitoneal gas injection, or aortography. Accordingly, the reader should refer to current texts on diagnostic endocrinology for the required procedures. When adrenalectomy is decided upon, the surgeon should investigate and, if possible, correct many of the secondary systemic and metabolic effects that are the direct result of the altered functional activity of the adrenal. The management of the hypertension and its cardiovascular sequelae is a major problem with pheochromocytomas. Problems associated with hypercorticism include hypokalemia with alkalosis, hypertension, polycythemia, musculoskeletal depletion with osteoporosis and hypercalcemia, abnormal glucose tolerance, multiple areas of skin furunculosis, and finally, poor wound healing. Thus, the surgeon must be aware that many organ systems and their response to surgery are profoundly affected by adrenal malfunction.

ANESTHESIA. Preoperative consultation and communication among endocrinologist, surgeon, and anesthetist are necessary. The anesthetist must be prepared for adequate blood and endocrine replacement and occasionally for a prolonged procedure that may be extended into the chest. Electrolytes should be in optimum condition and the patient prepared with parenteral cortisone the evening before and on the morning of surgery for hypercorticism or bilateral adrenalectomy. Adequate blood must be available, as hypertension plus increased vascularity and fragile veins about the adrenals all tend to increase blood losses.

General anesthesia with endotracheal intubation is preferred. Hypotensive agents such as Regitine (phentolamine methane sulfonate) may be used for several days in preparation for surgery upon pheochromocytomas. However, during operation both Regitine and norepinephrine (Levophed) must be set up as drips into a *secure* intravenous line to combat possible rapid and violent changes in blood pressure. Once the tumor is out, norepinephrine is run continuously for one to two days with a gradual taper as tolerated. The use of antihypertensive drugs preoperatively, however, should be made known to all the physicians, as anesthesia frequently potentiates their hypotensive effect.

POSITION. The patient is placed supine with the foot of the table slightly down, so that moderate hyperextension can be obtained if necessary. A posterior approach to the adrenals can be used but is not described here.

OPERATIVE PREPARATION. The patient's hair should be completely removed, with minimal trauma to the skin. In the anterior approach the skin of the lower chest and abdomen well into the flanks should be included in the preparation, since in a transverse incision it may be necessary to go far into the flanks in obese patients.

INCISION AND EXPOSURE. The surgeon stands on the patient's right side and outlines an incision about two to three fingerbreadths below the costal margin with its apex about two fingers below the tip of the xiphoid process **(Figure 1).** Increased vascularity in the subcutaneous tissue is common in these cases, particularly in Cushing's syndrome. Thus, meticulous ligation with 0000 silk of all bleeding points should be carried out before the peritoneal cavity is opened. Both recti muscles are divided, and then the transversus muscle and peritoneum are incised through a liberal incision. This is necessary since many of these patients tend to be obese. Additional exposure may be obtained by dividing the internal oblique muscles in the direction of their fibers out into the flanks. The round ligament to the liver is divided between curved hemostats and then ligated with 00 silk.

DETAILS OF PROCEDURE. The surgeon must first be aware of the anatomic differences of the two adrenal glands **(Figure 2).** The right adrenal is close to the superior pole of the kidney, the vena cava medially, and the right lobe of the liver superiorly. Its main arterial supply comes directly to its medial edge from the aorta **(Figure 2, 11),** and the main right adrenal vein (5) comes directly from the inferior vena cava in a parallel manner. In contrast, the left adrenal is in proximity to the aorta medially, the renal vein inferiorly, and the superior pole of the left kidney. Its main arterial supply comes directly from the aorta (12), but the main left adrenal vein (6) usually comes from the left renal vein (8). Both adrenal glands, however, have many arterial twigs from both the inferior phrenic arteries (9 and 10) and both renal arteries.

The operative exposure of the right adrenal is shown first **(Figure 3);** it is begun with a classic Kocher maneuver, after the transverse colon and omentum have been carefully packed away and the right lobe of the liver has been gently retracted. After the peritoneum lateral to the duodenum has been incised, it is mobilized in the usual manner by blunt dissection with the surgeon's index finger under the head of the pancreas. The inferior vena cava is exposed in its position directly posterior to the second portion of the duodenum **(Figure 4)** and then cleared to show the right renal vein. The superior pole of the right kidney is located and exposed with further blunt finger dissection. The adrenal is identified by its characteristic yellowish color, lobulated appearance, and clearly definable blunt lateral edge. This generally avascular area is then incised **(Figure 5),** and additional exposure and mobility of the adrenal gland may be obtained by gentle blunt finger dissection directly posterior to the gland. The surgeon should bear in mind that the vascular attachments are usually on or near the medial and superior edges of the gland rather than on its broad surfaces.

PLATE CIV   BILATERAL ADRENALECTOMY

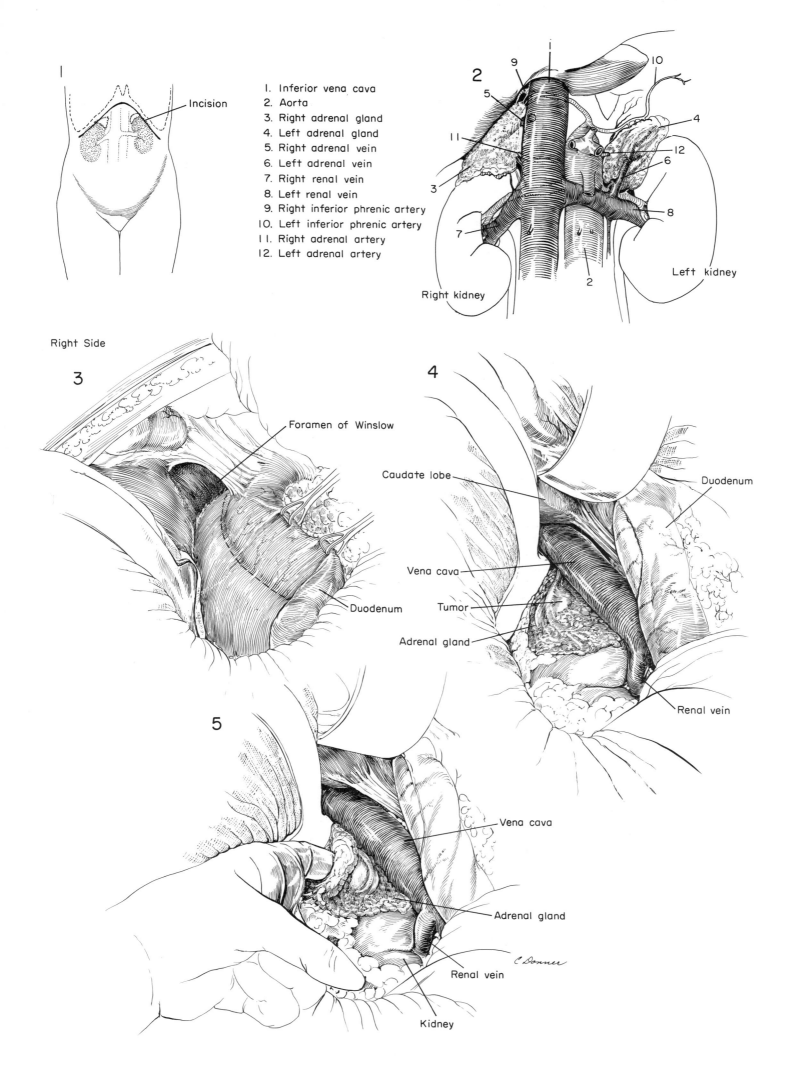

Incision

1. Inferior vena cava
2. Aorta
3. Right adrenal gland
4. Left adrenal gland
5. Right adrenal vein
6. Left adrenal vein
7. Right renal vein
8. Left renal vein
9. Right inferior phrenic artery
10. Left inferior phrenic artery
11. Right adrenal artery
12. Left adrenal artery

Right kidney

Left kidney

Right Side

3

Foramen of Winslow

Duodenum

4

Caudate lobe

Duodenum

Vena cava

Tumor

Adrenal gland

Renal vein

5

Vena cava

Adrenal gland

Renal vein

Kidney

C Donner

PLATE CV · BILATERAL ADRENALECTOMY

DETAILS OF PROCEDURE (*Continued*). Usually, the principal adrenal vein is first identified and then doubly ligated with 00 silk **(Figure 6).** The surgeon then cautiously works his way about the medial and inferior edges of the gland and ligates the principal artery or accessory arteries in a similar manner. He must also either carefully ligate or secure with clips the many minor vessels encountered.

The approach to the left adrenal via the transabdominal route may take either of two courses, as demonstrated in **Figures 7** through **10.** The usual approach is shown in cross section in **Figures 7** and **8.** The surgeon carefully packs the abdominal contents toward himself and then, carefully grasping the spleen, divides the avascular splenorenal ligament so that the spleen is mobilized somewhat toward himself. With blunt dissection it is then possible to dissect above Gerota's fascia but beneath the pancreas and primary splenic artery and vein. This dissection may be carried medially as far as the superior mesenteric vein, which will give a degree of mobilization as shown in **Figure 11.** The surgeon then incises the Gerota's fascia over the left kidney **(Figure 8),** and with blunt dissection clears the superior pole of the left kidney and comes upon the adrenal, which is shown here in a somewhat medial and inferior location. The left lobe of the liver is also identifiable, but it is usually not necessary to mobilize or retract it. The same general principles of exposure apply to the left adrenal gland, except that the prominent adrenal vein **(Figure 11)** is shown being secured first. The surgeon then works his way about the periphery of the gland, ligating all prominent vessels. This is often slow, meticulous work, but if in doubt it is safer to ligate with 000 silk each suspicious vascular area.

Many surgeons have found it useful to approach the left adrenal through the transverse mesocolon, after mobilizing the inferior border of the body and tail of the pancreas **(Figure 9).** This is accomplished by first removing most of the greater omentum from its attachment along the transverse mesocolon and carefully securing any bleeding points with 000 silk in this generally avascular area. Care must be taken to preserve the middle colic vessels, since the omentum is sometimes closely blended with the mesocolon, and these vessels are therefore liable to damage during the procedure. An incision is then made along the distal or inferior margin of the pancreas from the tip of its tail back along the body to the region of the inferior mesenteric vein (Danger Point, **Figure 9).** This allows the surgeon to mobilize the distal pancreas with blunt finger dissection so that it may be elevated in a cephalad manner and to expose the Gerota's fascia directly over the left kidney, whose midportion is usually directly exposed by this approach. This fascia is then incised and the dissection carried about the superior pole of the kidney, where the adrenal can be identified **(Figure 12).** Its lateral edge is then approached and its removal performed as in the procedure described above.

CLOSURE. The closure may follow each surgeon's accustomed method. However, retention sutures are recommended in hypercorticism, as poor wound healing is a known complication.

POSTOPERATIVE CARE. Blood losses must be carefully replaced, and patient observation and blood pressure monitoring must be unfailingly frequent. Should blood pressure continue to fall in the recovery area or during closure despite adequate endocrine replacement, retroperitoneal hemorrhage from an unsecured vessel must be strongly suspected. In patients who have had a pheochromocytoma removed, a postoperative vasopressor in the form of norepinephrine is usually necessary for 24 to 36 hours, after which time it is gradually tapered as tolerated.

Patients will experience a drop in the level of circulating corticosteroids after removal of an hyperfunctioning tumor or after subtotal or total adrenalectomy. Therefore, they must have cortisone support before, during, and after surgery. Cortisone acetate in the dose of 100 mg. is given intramuscularly the evening before and on the morning of surgery. Supplemental intravenous hydrocortisone is given during the operation as needed. A final dose of 100 mg. cortisone acetate is given intramuscularly in the evening after surgery, with a total dose of approximately 300 mg. being given the day of surgery. This is gradually tapered down over the next seven to ten days to approximately 50 mg. per day, which may be given in divided doses. It is felt that 30 to 50 mg. per day of oral cortisone represents reasonable maintenance therapy. However, it may be necessary to add an active mineralocorticoid to this if maintaining sodium and potassium balance is difficult. In the immediate postoperative period, however, the major problem is to ensure adequate cortisone replacement, as it is easy to undertreat but almost impossible to overtreat with cortisone.

The postoperative ileus and return to alimentation should be handled the same as for any laparotomy. Wound healing, however, will be impaired in patients with hypercorticism, and infection is a possibility, as many of these patients also have extensive furunculosis. Lastly, it is important that the patient's long-term medical management and his follow-up and endocrine replacement be clearly defined.

PLATE CV   BILATERAL ADRENALECTOMY

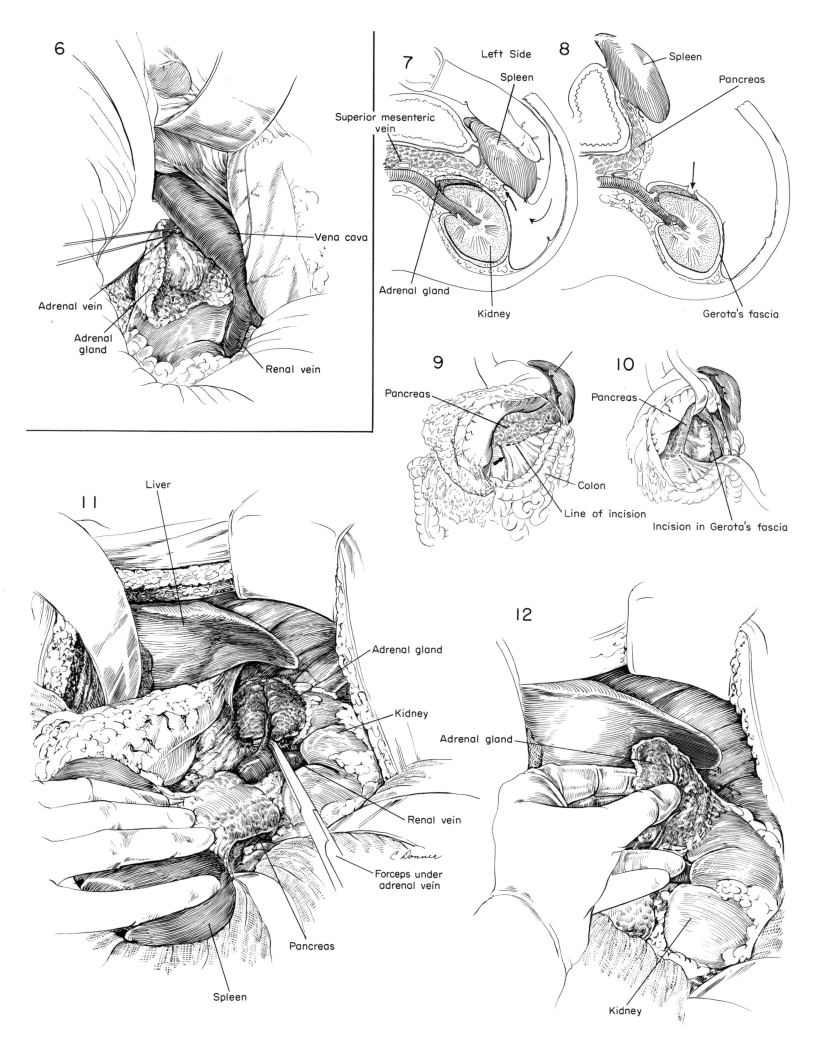

VASCULAR PROCEDURES

PLATE CVI · RESECTION OF ABDOMINAL AORTIC ANEURYSM

INDICATIONS. Aneurysms of the abdominal aorta occurring below the renal vessels should, in general, be replaced. This is particularly true if they are enlarging, if they are producing pain, or if there is evidence of impending or actual perforation. In poor-risk patients with small aneurysms less than 5 cm. in diameter, observation may be the better course. Although the operation is of considerable magnitude, anticipated mortality associated with spontaneous rupture and exsanguination from an aneurysm is such as to warrant the risk of surgery in the great majority of patients. Emergency operations may be the only chance of patient survival if there is evidence of leakage or perforation of the aneurysm. A past history of coronary occlusion is not a contraindication to surgery.

PREOPERATIVE PREPARATION. Aortography is carried out if there is a question about the extent of the aneurysm, if distal occlusive disease is present, and when renal vascular disease or mesenteric insufficiency is suspected. An electrocardiogram is performed, and extensive laboratory evaluation of renal and pulmonary function is carried out by appropriate studies.

In elective resection of an aneurysm the preoperative preparation consists of emptying the large intestine by a mild cathartic. The intravenous antibiotic coverage is started the night before surgery, and a fluid load of "crystaloid" is given, approximately 100 to 150 ml. per hour, beginning the evening before operation. A nasogastric tube is inserted, and constant bladder drainage is initiated to accurately follow the hourly output of urine, especially during the immediate postoperative period. Catheters are placed for central venous and arterial monitoring.

ANESTHESIA. General anesthesia with endotracheal intubation is routine. The arterial line permits instantaneous evaluation of blood pressure changes, and blood gas sampling can be done when required. Several large-bore (15-gauge) polyethelene catheters should be placed intravenously for adequate control of fluid and blood replacement.

POSITION. The patient is placed in a slight head-down position to aid in natural retraction of the small intestine from the region of the lower abdomen. The needles are secured in place in both arms and adequately protected from dislodgment. The urethral catheter is connected to a constant bladder drainage bottle. Since the presence of pulsations of the dorsalis pedis must be verified after the prosthesis has been inserted, some type of low support should be provided over the feet and lower third of the legs to assist in evaluating the presence of arterial pulsations.

DETAILS OF PROCEDURE. After rapid palpation and visualization of the aorta and confirmation of the diagnosis of aneurysm, steps are taken to empty the abdominal cavity of small intestine. Unless the abdominal wall is quite thick, the greater portion of the small intestine can be retracted upward and to the right and inserted into a plastic bag, the mouth of which can be partly constricted by a tape **(Figure 2)**. Saline is added to the plastic bag to keep the intestine moist. A sterile gauze pad is inserted into the neck of the plastic bag to avoid undue constriction and prevent the escape of the small intestine from the bag. It may be advisable (if the aneurysm is sizable and involves the right common iliac) to mobilize the appendix, terminal ileum, and cecum, and to retract the right colon upward. A large S retractor over a sterile gauze pad adequately retracts the intestine and readily exposes the aneurysm. Additional exposure can be gained by dividing the peritoneum about the ligament of Treitz to permit further retraction of the small intestine upward and to the right **(Figure 2)**. What at first may appear to be an inoperable aneurysm may eventually prove to be rather easily resectable, since the aneurysm tends to bulge anteriorly and seems to extend up so high as to suggest involvement of the renal vessels **(Figure 3)**. The bulk of the aneurysm tends to come forward from under the left renal vein. The incised peritoneum over the anterior surface of the aneurysm is reflected by blunt and sharp dissection until the left renal vein is visualized. Blunt and sharp dissection frees the left renal vein from the underlying aorta **(Figure 4)**. The renal vein is retracted upward with a retractor **(Figure 5)** to gain additional space for the application of the occluding clamp to the aorta above the aneurysm.

PLATE CVI   RESECTION OF ABDOMINAL AORTIC ANEURYSM

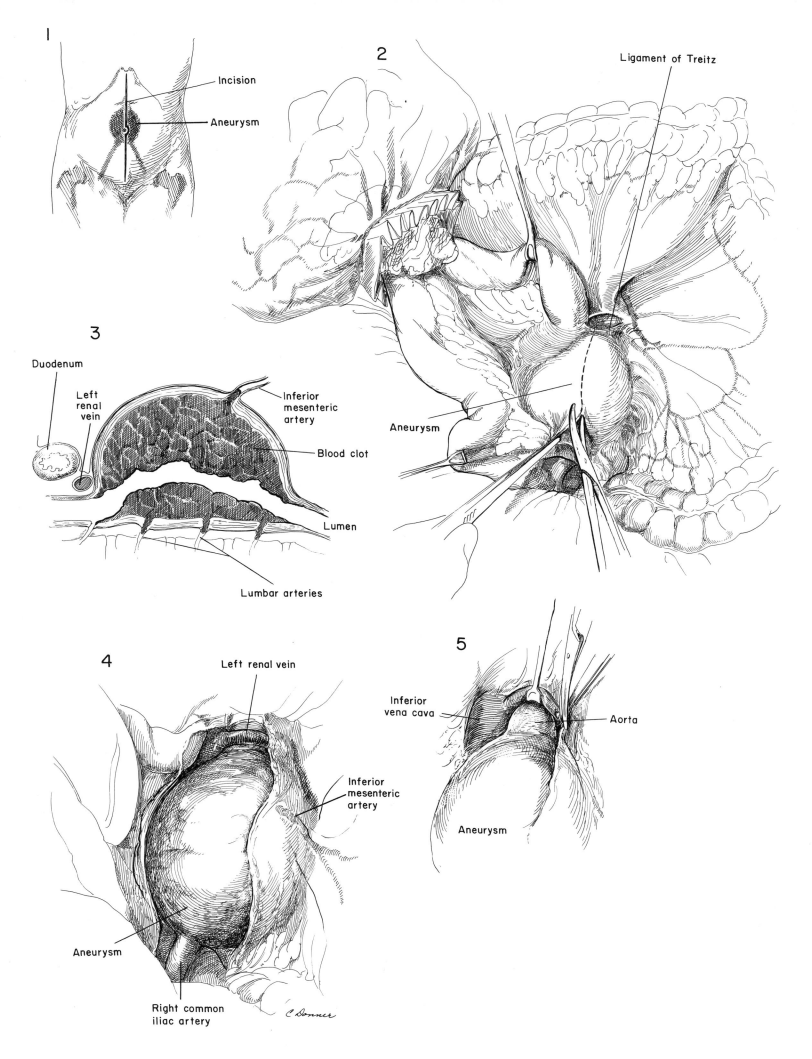

1

Incision

Aneurysm

2

Ligament of Treitz

Aneurysm

3

Duodenum

Left renal vein

Inferior mesenteric artery

Blood clot

Lumen

Lumbar arteries

4

Left renal vein

Inferior mesenteric artery

Aneurysm

Right common iliac artery

5

Inferior vena cava

Aorta

Aneurysm

C Donner

PLATE CVII · RESECTION OF ABDOMINAL AORTIC ANEURYSM

DETAILS OF PROCEDURE (*Continued*). The inferior mesenteric artery is identified, clamped, and divided **(Figure 6).** The mesenteric side is controlled with a suture ligature. Usually, this vessel is small and sclerotic, in which case sacrifice is of little consequence. In rare instances, it is large and serves as a major contributor to the left colon blood supply, especially if internal iliac and mesenteric occlusive disease is present. In such a case reimplantation of this vessel into the aortic graft may be required to protect the colon.

The common iliac arteries are then exposed on their anterior, lateral, and medial surfaces in preparation for clamp placement. It is not necessary to encircle these vessels completely, and dissection posteriorly can result in troublesome hemorrhage from the underlying iliac veins. During the iliac artery exposure the ureters are identified and protected from injury throughout the procedure **(Figure 6).**

Blood is now aspirated from the aneurysm and used for preclotting of the graft. This markedly reduces bleeding from the interstices of the graft if carried out carefully.

Heparin is then injected directly into the aneurysm to provide protective anticoagulation for the extremities during aortic clamping.

An aortic clamp is used to occlude the aorta proximal to the aneurysm and distal to the renal arteries. A careful identification of the position of the renal arteries is mandatory before clamp application. Angled vascular clamps are applied to the distal common iliac arteries. The aneurysm is then opened through a linear arteriotomy **(Figure 7).** The mural thrombus is extracted **(Figure 8).** Bleeding from the paired lumbar arteries is controlled with suture ligatures **(Figure 9).** The aortic cuff is next prepared by dividing all but the posterior wall. Leaving this portion attached prevents troublesome bleeding from lumbar veins often found in this area **(Figure 10).** The iliac arteries are prepared in similar fashion; the posterior wall is undisturbed to protect the iliac veins **(Figure 10).**

PLATE CVII   RESECTION OF ABDOMINAL AORTIC ANEURYSM

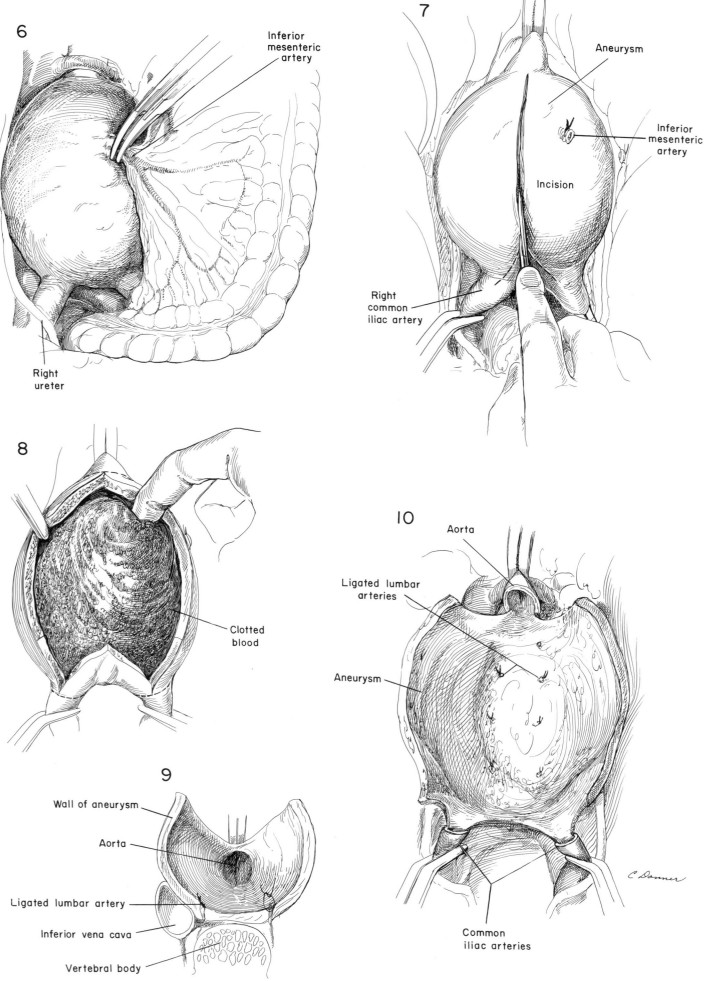

6

Inferior
mesenteric
artery

Right
ureter

7

Aneurysm

Inferior
mesenteric
artery

Incision

Right
common
iliac artery

8

Clotted
blood

10

Aorta

Ligated lumbar
arteries

Aneurysm

Common
iliac arteries

9

Wall of aneurysm

Aorta

Ligated lumbar artery

Inferior vena cava

Vertebral body

C Donner

PLATE CVIII · RESECTION OF ABDOMINAL AORTIC ANEURYSM

DETAILS OF PROCEDURE (*Continued*). The clotted knitted dacron graft of appropriate size is then stretched and tailored to fit the aortic defect **(Figure 11)**. Suturing of the graft begins in the midline posteriorly with a double-arm swaged-on 00 suture. The initial stitch begins by passing both needles from outside inward on the graft and from inside outward on the aorta. This suture is then tied **(Figure 12)**. Over-and-over suturing is then carried from the midline position, proceeding from outside the graft to inside the aorta **(Figure 12)**. At the midline anteriorly, this suture is again tied.

Vascular clamps are temporarily applied to the iliac limbs of the graft, and the aortic clamp is momentarily released to check the proximal suture line for hemostasis and the preclotting of the graft. Should leaks be noted in the anastomosis, they can be controlled by individual mattress sutures.

The iliac anastomoses are done in the same manner as that of the aorta **(Figure 14)**. Just before completion of the anastomosis, the aortic clamp is opened momentarily to flush any clots that may have accumulated in the aorta or graft **(Figure 15)**. This flushing-out greatly lessens the incidence of subsequent thrombosis in either extremity and justifies a considerable loss of blood.

PLATE CVIII   RESECTION OF ABDOMINAL AORTIC ANEURYSM

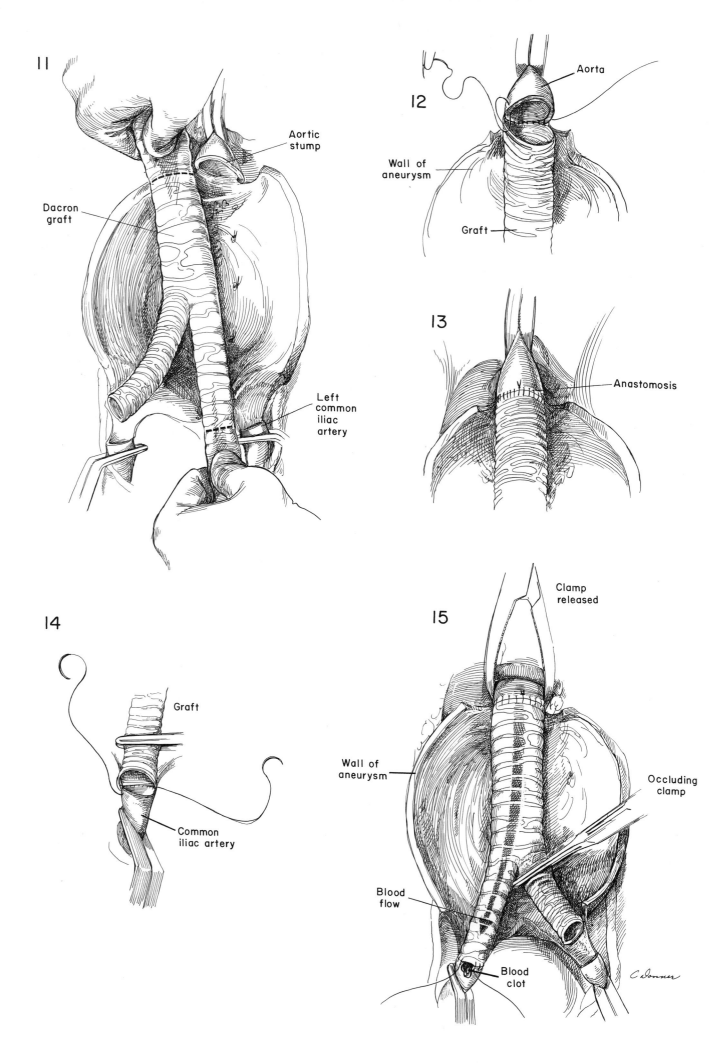

11

Aortic stump

Dacron graft

Left common iliac artery

12

Aorta

Wall of aneurysm

Graft

13

Anastomosis

14

Graft

Common iliac artery

15

Clamp released

Wall of aneurysm

Occluding clamp

Blood flow

Blood clot

PLATE CIX · RESECTION OF ABDOMINAL AORTIC ANEURYSM

DETAILS OF PROCEDURE (*Continued*). The clamp is closed and the suture line completed and tied. The completed limb is occluded by finger control, and the aortic clamp is slowly removed. Blood flow is gradually reestablished to the limb to prevent hypotension **(Figure 16).** Close coordination between surgeon and anesthesiologist is required at this point so that the rate of opening the graft is compensated by fluids and blood administration with maintenance of stable blood pressure.

The other iliac anastomosis is carried out in similar fashion **(Figure 17).** The aneurysm sac, if adequate, is closed over the graft with a running suture **(Figure 18).** The posterior peritoneum is reapproximated, with care taken not to injure the ureters.

In the presence of occlusive disease of the common iliac in addition to the aneurysm, the common iliac may be divided and oversewn with a continuous suture **(Figure 19)** on both sides following removal of the aneurysm. The preclotted knitted dacron graft is tailored to permit anastomosis of the aorta above the aneurysm with end-to-end anastomosis to the external iliacs beyond the points of stenosis. This bypass procedure makes extensive endarterectomy unnecessary and prevents sacrifice of the hypogastric arteries.

CLOSURE. The small intestine is returned to the peritoneal cavity from the plastic bag, and the peritoneal cavity is cleared of blood clots and sponges. Some prefer to insert a temporary gastrostomy tube to combat an anticipated paralytic ileus, especially in elderly and poor-risk patients. Before closure particular attention is given to the adequacy of the blood supply to the sigmoid. Ordinarily, the blood supply is adequate after ligation of the inferior mesenteric artery. Evidence of bleeding from the prosthesis or at the site of anastomosis is thoroughly searched for before the closure is finally completed. The femoral vessels should be palpated from time to time to ensure that thrombosis has not occurred and that a good flow of blood is going through to the lower extremities. In case of doubt it may be necessary to reexplore one or both sides and remove any blood clots that are found. Routine abdominal closure is done.

POSTOPERATIVE CARE. Postoperative care is usually provided in an intensive care unit for the first 24 to 48 hours. In the postoperative period it is particularly important to ensure that there is a good blood supply to the lower extremities and a good hourly output of urine. Blood should be given until all major blood loss has been replaced, and the blood pressure is satisfactory. Intravenous fluids are slowly administered during the first 24 hours to ensure a steady output of urine from the indwelling catheter. The presence or absence of pulsation in the dorsalis pedis arteries should be recorded. Confirmation may be difficult at first, but the pulsations usually become more apparent later in the postoperative period. If pulsations are absent and there is a cold extremity, thrombosis may have occurred, and reexploration and removal of the blood clot should be considered.

An electrocardiogram is taken in the early postoperative period. Laboratory studies to evaluate the blood volume and kidney function are performed daily until the convalescence is uneventful. A tendency to paralytic ileus should be combatted by gastric suction until there is evidence that peristalsis has returned. Renal failure should be suspected if there has been preoperative evidence of impaired renal function or if there has been a prolonged period of hypotension.

If adequate hourly output of urine is not maintained, despite an adequate intake, anuria should be suspected and appropriate therapy instituted.

PLATE CIX   RESECTION OF ABDOMINAL AORTIC ANEURYSM

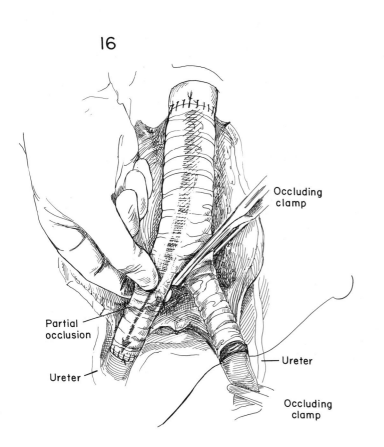

16

Occluding
clamp

Partial
occlusion

Ureter

Ureter

Occluding
clamp

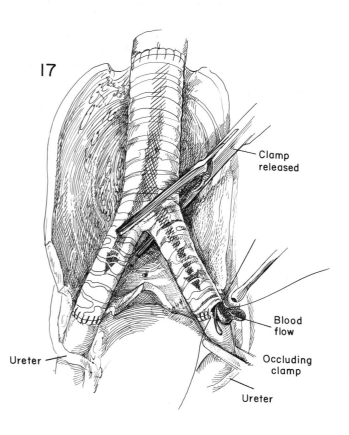

17

Clamp
released

Blood
flow

Occluding
clamp

Ureter

Ureter

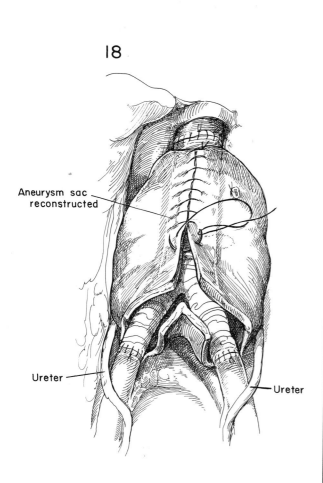

18

Aneurysm sac
reconstructed

Ureter

Ureter

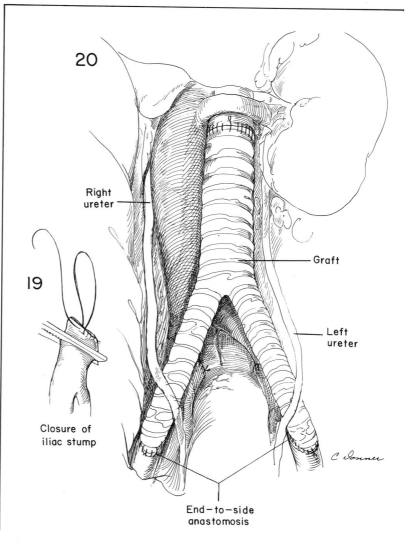

20

19

Right
ureter

Graft

Left
ureter

Closure of
iliac stump

End-to-side
anastomosis

C Donner

PLATE CX · AORTOFEMORAL BYPASS

INDICATIONS. Only patients with severe and debilitating occlusive disease of the aortoiliac segment should be considered for surgery. In general, these patients will have claudication that is progressing or disabling. Patients with rest pain, ulceration, or gangrene who fall in the limb salvage group may require surgery to preserve limb function. These patients are generally elderly and have associated generalized arteriosclerosis with a high incidence of coronary disease and hypertension. In addition, the majority are long-time smokers, and it is not unusual for limitation of pulmonary function to be present. The risks associated with these factors must be carefully weighed against the benefits expected from a successful surgical procedure. The careful selection of patients is of the utmost importance.

PREOPERATIVE PREPARATION. See Plate CVI.

ANESTHESIA. See Plate CVI.

POSITION. See Plate CVI.

OPERATIVE PREPARATION. See Plate CVI.

INCISION AND EXPOSURE. A midline incision is made from the xiphoid to the pubis to afford maximum exposure **(Figure 1).** The abdomen is explored for the presence of other pathology, and the intra-abdominal arterial tree is carefully assessed. **Figure 2** demonstrates typical aortoiliac occlusive disease. The aorta is freed by entering the retroperitoneal space. The posterior peritoneum is divided, and the duodenum is mobilized until the renal vein is identified. Sharp and blunt dissection is then used to clear the aorta on its anterior, lateral, and medial surfaces **(Figure 3).** It is not necessary usually to encircle the aorta or to free it completely; this oftentimes leads to troublesome bleeding from lumbar arteries and veins. Blood is obtained for preclotting the graft, and heparin is injected intra-arterially to protect the distal extremities from thrombosis, as outlined for resection of abdominal aortic aneurysm (Plate CVII).

DETAILS OF PROCEDURE. An aortic clamp is then used to clamp the aorta proximally just below the renal arteries **(Figure 4).** A second aortic clamp is placed horizontally to occlude the iliac vessels and the lumbar arteries, as depicted in **Figures 4** and **5.** A small vascular clamp should be applied to the inferior mesenteric artery. It is important to have the distal aorta freed sufficiently so that this clamp can be placed far posteriorly to avoid interference with the arteriotomy and the anastomosis. A linear arteriotomy is made in the aorta to a point just above the inferior mesentery artery take-off **(Figure 5).** An attempt is made to preserve that vessel if at all possible. The graft is beveled **(Figure 6A),** and an end-to-end anastomosis is then created **(Figures 6B, 7, 8,** and **9)** with a running 000 vascular suture, beginning at the inferior margin of the arteriotomy with a mattress suture, much as described in Plate CVIII. The running suture is then carried up each side of the arteriotomy, and finally the anastomosis is completed in the middle of the arteriotomy on the operator's side.

PLATE CX   AORTOFEMORAL BYPASS

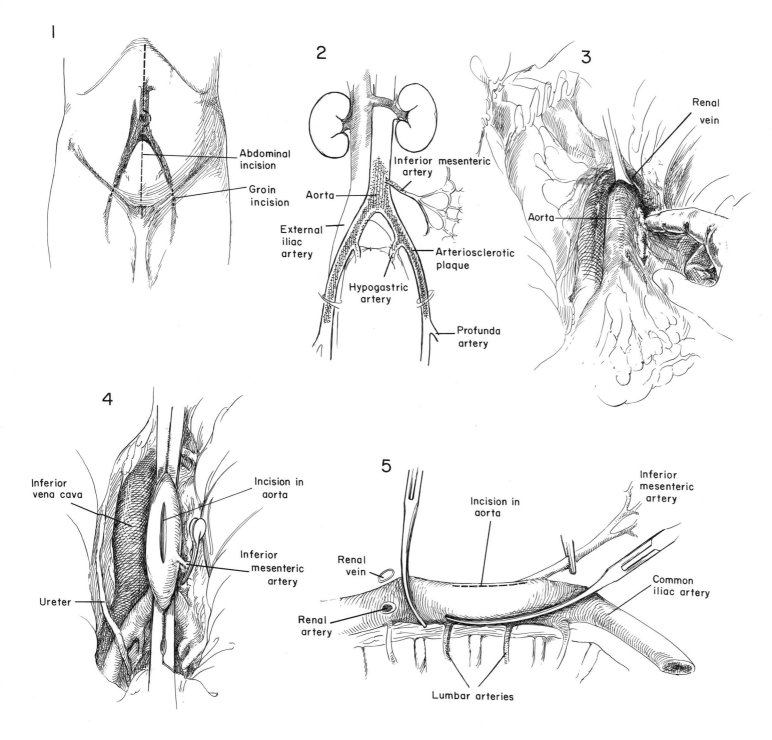

1

2

Abdominal
incision

Groin
incision

Inferior mesenteric
artery

Aorta

External
iliac
artery

Arteriosclerotic
plaque

Hypogastric
artery

Profunda
artery

3

Renal
vein

Aorta

4

Inferior
vena cava

Ureter

Incision in
aorta

Inferior
mesenteric
artery

5

Incision in
aorta

Inferior
mesenteric
artery

Renal
vein

Renal
artery

Common
iliac artery

Lumbar arteries

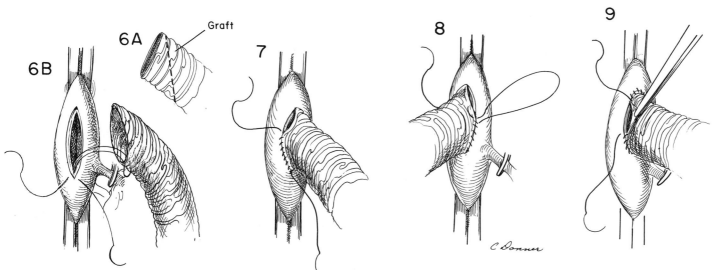

Graft

6A

6B

7

8

9

C Donner

PLATE CXI · AORTOFEMORAL BYPASS

DETAILS OF PROCEDURE (*Continued*). A linear incision is made in the groin over the femoral artery **(Figure 10),** and the common femoral, the profunda femoris, and the superficial femoral artery are carefully isolated. It is important to dissect at least several centimeters of the profunda femoris to evaluate the presence of disease in this vessel. If it is significantly involved, profunda endarterectomy should be considered, because this procedure appears to increase the longevity of graft function. A retroperitoneal tunnel is then made overlying the iliac artery and extending into the femoral incision **(Figure 10)** by blunt finger dissection from above as well as from below the inguinal ligament. It is important to make this tunnel on the artery so that the ureter does not become entrapped. Care should be given to anterior displacement of the ureter so that after the procedure it will overlie the prosthetic graft.

The graft is pulled into the groin incision **(Figure 11)** and the end beveled **(Figure 12).** Vascular clamps have been placed on the common femoral, the profunda femoris, and the superficial femoral arteries **(Figure 13),** and the linear arterotomy is made. It is not necessary to excise a button of artery wall. The anastomosis is carried out in the same manner as the upper end-to-side anastomosis of the graft to the aorta **(Figures 14 and 15).** Just before completion of the femoral anastomosis, a clamp is placed on the opposite iliac limb of the graft and across the right common iliac beyond the bifurcation. The aortic clamp is opened momentarily to allow any potentially clotted material to be flushed out from the graft **(Figure 16).** The clamp is replaced and the anastomosis is completed. Then the aortic clamp is removed, with secure digital compression of the graft in order to ensure a gradually increased flow to the limb **(Figure 17).** This limb is slowly allowed to fill so that hypotension does not occur, much as was outlined in the aortic aneurysm procedure. A similar procedure is followed in completing the anastomosis of the graft to the left common femoral artery.

CLOSURE. All wounds are closed with interrupted sutures. See Chapter I.

POSTOPERATIVE CARE. See Plate CIX. Acute flexion of the thighs should be avoided for seven to ten days.

PLATE CXI   AORTOFEMORAL BYPASS

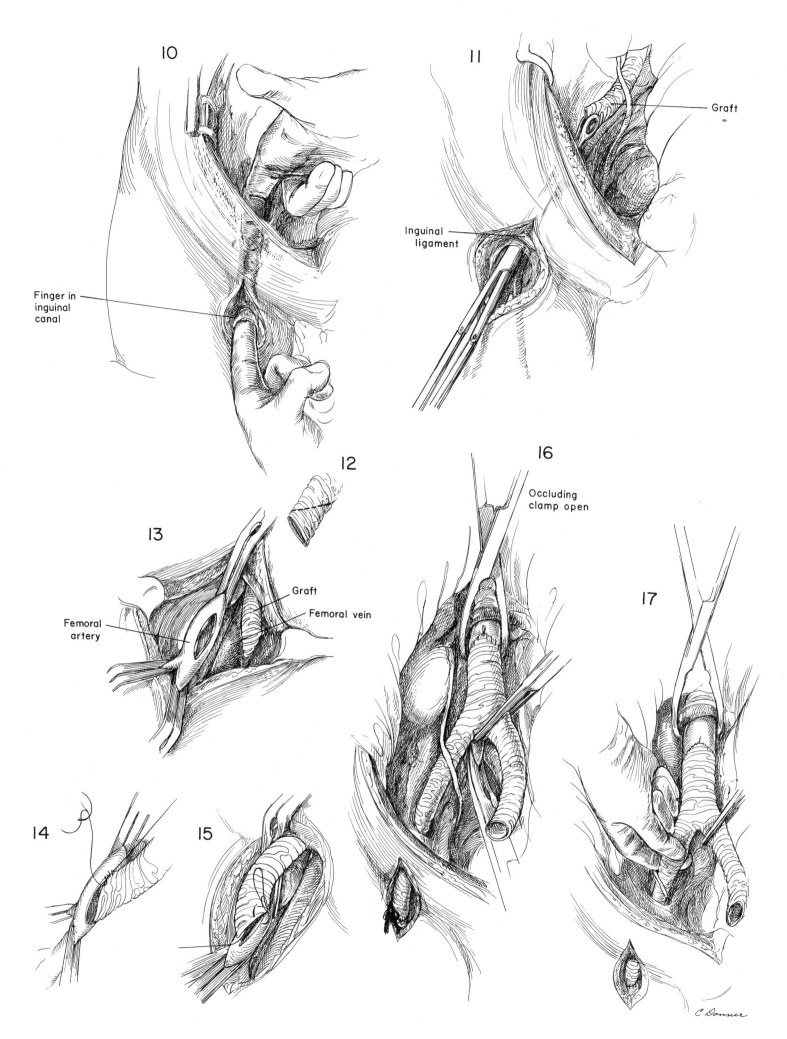

10

Finger in
inguinal
canal

11

Graft

Inguinal
ligament

12

13

Femoral
artery

Graft

Femoral vein

16

Occluding
clamp open

17

14

15

C Donner

PLATE CXII · HIGH LIGATION AND STRIPPING OF THE SAPHENOUS VEINS

INDICATIONS. High ligation and stripping of the greater saphenous trunk and its major varicose tributaries are indicated in patients who have valvular incompetence or incompetent communicating veins. Such patients should have a complete peripheral vascular examination to (1) determine whether varicosities are primary or secondary, (2) evaluate the status of the deep venous system, and (3) assess the arterial circulation. Stigmata, history or suspicion of deep venous incompetence, or obstruction implying that the varicosities may be secondary are indications for a venogram to ascertain the status of the deep system as well as to demonstrate the possible role of the superficial venous system in return collateral flow.

Contraindications. (1) The presence of severe incompetence or obstruction of the deep venous system demonstrated by venogram, to an extent that the superficial venous system is the predominant route of return flow, or a positive Perthes' test contraindicates complete saphenous system stripping. However, limited stripping below knee level may be safe after careful assessment and use of critical judgment by the surgeon. (2) Cutaneous infections or stasis ulcers that are not surgically clean may lead to postoperative infection. (3) Pregnancy, advanced age, and serious systemic diseases are relative contraindications except in unusual circumstances.

PREOPERATIVE PREPARATION. Healing of varicose ulcers and elimination of stasis eczema can almost always be achieved by use of local treatment, compression dressings, and elevation when at rest. If such lesions are healed at least four weeks before operation, the incidence of postoperative infections will be minimized and wound healing will be accelerated.

The patient is instructed to take two cleansing showers within 12 hours before operation. After the groin and extremity have been shaved, the involved saphenous trunks, major varicose tributaries, and location of suspected incompetent communicating veins, which can be detected by walking with a tourniquet applied at various levels, are then marked with indelible skin dye (Bonnie's blue or brilliant cresyl green) while the patient is standing. It is imperative that the surgeon understand that incompetent communicating veins often connect with major varicose tributaries, which must also be stripped to ensure a good result and to minimize necessary postoperative injections with sclerosing solutions.

ANESTHESIA. General anesthesia is usually preferred.

POSITION. The patient is supine with the thigh and knee in slight external rotation and flexion. After the high ligation, division of the primary tributaries below the medial malleolus, and passage of the stripper through the entire length of the greater saphenous vein, moderate Trendelenburg position is used during segmental resection of the varicose tributaries and before the stripping. This lowers venous pressure and decreases bleeding during and after the procedure.

OPERATIVE PREPARATION. The skin of the foot, lower extremity, and groin is prepared in the usual manner. The forefoot is covered by a rubber glove, and usual draping is used **(Figure 1).** Specially designed holders may be used to suspend the leg at 30 to 40 degrees to facilitate skin preparation. The holder is adjustable and, as an alternative, may be used for positioning throughout the procedure.

INCISION AND EXPOSURE. A 6-cm. oblique incision is made in the femoral skin crease with its lateral end over the femoral pulse **(Figure 1).** After the superficial fascia is incised, the proximal part of the saphenous trunk, one or more of its tributaries, and occasionally an accessory saphenous vein will be exposed at the center of the incision. The saphenofemoral junction is located two fingerbreadths laterally and below the pubic tubercle.

DETAILS OF PROCEDURE. The adventitial sheath of the saphenous trunk is incised longitudinally, and circumferentially separated from the vein. This greatly facilitates dissection proximally to the saphenofemoral junction as well as exposure of various tributaries. The vein is transected between hemostats, and the proximal segment is mobilized to its junction with the common femoral vein. During this dissection the medial and lateral superficial circumflex iliac **(Figure 2,** a and b**),** the superficial epigastric (c), the superficial external pudendal (d), the medial superficial femoral cutaneous (e), and occasional deep muscular venous branches (f) must be meticulously divided and ligated to avoid later development of collaterals that would result in recurrences of the varices. The medial circumflex iliac artery lies at the lower margin of the fossa ovalis and consequently is a reliable anatomic reference to the saphenofemoral junction, which is just above it **(Figure 3).** The proximal stump of the saphenous trunk is doubly ligated with a proximal free tie and then a transfixing suture ligature of 0000 silk **(Figure 3).** The other end of the saphenous trunk is dissected distally till a large medial tributary, the medial superficial femoral cutaneous, is exposed, divided, and ligated **(Figure 4).** This avoids postoperative hematomas and excessive extravasation and ecchymosis of the medial thigh.

A 2-cm. transverse incision, placed one fingerbreadth below and just anterior to the tip of the medial malleolus, and downward retraction will expose the trifurcated origin of the saphenous vein **(Figure 5).** Each of the three primary tributaries is divided and ligated. The saphenous vein is then dissected proximally above the malleolus for 4 cm. Sizable anterior and posterior tributaries are usually exposed, divided, and ligated **(Figure 6).** The edges of the transected lower end of the saphenous trunk are grasped between two mosquito hemostats and slit 1 cm. to enhance the insertion of the probe end of the stripper **(Figure 7).** The instrument is then gently passed proximally with guidance by palpating, advancing fingers. The stripper can usually be passed through the entire length of the vein but may be arrested by large varices, tributaries, communicating veins, or by stenosis resulting from previous phlebitis. At these points an additional small transverse incision may be made to expose the vein and the tip of the stripper. The tip may then be manually guided proximally, or the vein may be transected to allow introduction of an additional stripper through the proximal end. Alternatively, a second stripper may be inserted into the proximal end of the divided saphenous trunk through the femoral incision and passed distally till it contacts the instrument inserted from the ankle. The end of the saphenous trunk is then securely tied to the stripper with two encircling ligatures of 00 silk, about 2 cm. apart, to prevent inversion of the vein over the stripper **(Figure 8).**

At this point the surgeon may choose to strip the lesser saphenous vein, if indicated. Approximately 20 per cent of patients with varicose veins have involvement of one or both lesser saphenous systems which should also be stripped. Adequate positioning can be achieved by flexing the knee 90 degrees, placing the sole of the foot flat on the operating table, and slightly internally rotating the hip **(Figure 9).** The primary tributaries converging on the lateral side of the ankle to form the lesser saphenous trunk can be exposed through a 2-cm. transverse incision between the posterior tip of the lateral malleolus and the lateral edge of the Achilles tendon. Careful attention is given to avoid damage to the sural nerve **(Figure 9).** The branches are divided and ligated, and a short stripper is inserted and passed proximally in the lesser saphenous trunk up to the popliteal skin crease. A small transverse incision is made over the palpable stripper probe, and the vein is isolated, divided, and the proximal end is ligated. Major varicose tributaries identified and marked before operation are segmentally stripped, as described below for the greater saphenous stripping. A large varicose tributary connecting the greater and lesser saphenous trunks is often present at the level of the upper medial bulge of the calf and requires similar resection.

PLATE CXII   HIGH LIGATION AND STRIPPING OF THE SAPHENOUS VEINS

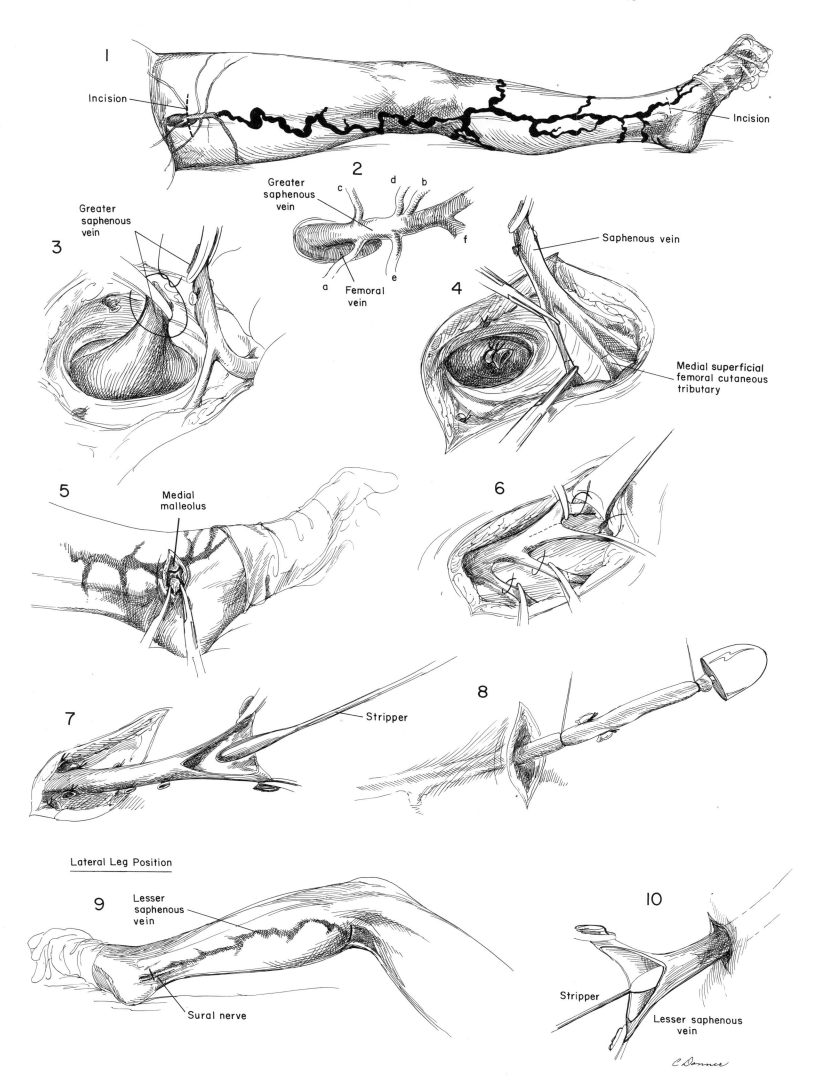

1

Incision

Incision

2

Greater
saphenous
vein

c   d   b

f

a   Femoral
vein

e

3

Greater
saphenous
vein

4

Saphenous vein

Medial superficial
femoral cutaneous
tributary

5

Medial
malleolus

6

7

Stripper

8

Lateral Leg Position

9

Lesser
saphenous
vein

Sural nerve

10

Stripper

Lesser saphenous
vein

C. Donner

DETAILS OF PROCEDURE (*Continued*). With the greater and perhaps the lesser saphenous trunks traversed by strippers, attention is then turned to the varicose tributaries and suspected sites of incompetent communicating veins of the greater saphenous system **(Figure 11)**. The latter most often occur adjacent to the saphenous trunk, at the junction of the middle third with the lower and upper thirds of the leg below the knee. Small 1- to 2-cm. transverse incisions are made at 4- to 6-cm. intervals along the involved major varicose tributaries which were marked with skin dye preoperatively **(Figure 11)**. The veins are exposed, doubly clamped, and divided between hemostats. Subcutaneous dissection with tonsil hemostats in the plane between the vein and skin will mobilize and permit segmental stripping of these tributaries **(Figure 12)**. During this dissection communicating veins may be encountered, divided, and ligated. Other suspected sites of incompetent communicating veins located by a preoperative walking tourniquet test or venogram should be explored to allow appropriate ligation.

The distal end of the stripper is pulled upward about 6 cm. to a subcutaneous position, and all the distal incisions are carefully and accurately closed with vertical mattress sutures of 0000 silk **(Figure 13)**. The greater saphenous trunk is then removed by pulling the stripper from distally out through the femoral incision. The lesser saphenous vein may be similarly stripped. Stripping in this direction is more effective in removing longer segments of undivided tributaries and is less likely to result in tearing the saphenous trunk and avulsing it from the stripper. Free blood is then milked and extruded from the saphenous channel. The femoral incision is approximated in two layers with 0000 interrupted silk sutures. The operated extremities are snugly wrapped with a layer of elastic cotton gauze and compression elastic bandages from the base of the toes to the groin.

POSTOPERATIVE CARE. The extremities are elevated 10 to 15 degrees until the patient becomes ambulatory, which should be as early as possible. Once ambulatory, the patient should not stand still for long periods or sit in a chair without elevating the legs. After 48 hours the original dressings are removed, and hospital elastic stockings are applied up to the knee. The patient may begin showering. Except at night, the stockings are worn for two or three weeks until all discoloration, edema, and tenderness have disappeared. The patient should be reexamined at four- to six-month intervals, at which time any residual or recurrent varicosities can be obliterated by injection with sodium tetradecyl sulfate.

Vena Caval Interruption

INDICATIONS. Life-threatening pulmonary embolism is a frequent complication of many medical illnesses and surgical procedures when antecedent venous thrombosis is associated with low flow states, venous injuries, obesity, prolonged immobilization, hypercoagulability, and the poorly understood effects of certain malignant tumors.

Anticoagulants and heparin in particular are generally accepted as the primary therapy for thromboembolic disease. Venous interruption, proximal to the site of venous thrombosis, is usually reserved for patients who have recurrent, documented pulmonary emboli despite well-controlled heparinization, who have a large life-threatening embolus such that an additional one might be fatal, who cannot be anticoagulated because of bleeding problems, or who are developing progressive pulmonary hypertension from repeated emboli.

Superficial femoral ligation has largely been abandoned because of the inability to precisely localize the proximal extent of the process and the likelihood of undetected thrombus in the opposite extremity or deep pelvic veins. Inferior vena caval ligation avoids these uncertainties and is primarily indicated for recurrent small septic emboli usually associated with pelvic infections.

Vena caval interruption by partially occlusive serrated clips has the advantage of maintaining caval flow with a minimal increase in downstream venous pressure, arresting all but the smallest thrombi, and minimizing the resultant edema of the lower extremities. The cava remains intact, the new channels are uniform in size, and there are no intraluminal sutures for potential thrombosis as in the sieve technic.

PREOPERATIVE PREPARATION. Most patients are heparinized when the decision for vena caval interruption is made. Since heparin is usually administered intravenously and its duration of anticoagulation effect is limited, there should be little delay beyond six to eight hours after the last injection. Protamine sulfate should be available during the procedure for heparin reversal, but this is rarely needed. These patients may have impaired cardiac function and abnormal ventilation/perfusion of the lung, such that vigorous cardiac and pulmonary support must be given.

ANESTHESIA. Epidural or general anesthesia is favored. Airway maintenance for increased oxygenation must be anticipated, and a secure cutaneous catheter for medications or transfusions is essential.

POSITION. The patient is supine with the right flank slightly elevated with a pillow or pads under the hips and lateral chest/shoulder. The operative site should be at the break level of the operating table, as hyperextension may improve the operative exposure. If the patient has been receiving heparin, a Lee-White coagulation time should be obtained immediately before operation to ensure that it is not unduly prolonged. Both lower extremities should be firmly wrapped with elastic bandages from ankles to groins, and electrodes should be placed to allow electrocardiographic monitoring. The operative site is widely prepped and draped as usual.

INCISION AND EXPOSURE. The transperitoneal approach is used when simultaneous ligation of the ovarian veins is indicated, as in pelvic thrombophlebitis; otherwise, the extraperitoneal method is preferred. This approach is tolerated better and is more easily performed. A transverse incision is made just above the level of the umbilicus **(Figure 1)**. It is carried from the lateral border of the right rectus muscle to midway between the costal margin and the iliac crest at the level of the mid-axillary line. The incision must not be placed too low, as difficulty with proper exposure results.

DETAILS OF PROCEDURE. The dissection is then extended down to the external oblique aponeurosis, and the aponeurosis of the muscle is incised lateral to the border of the rectus muscle. If necessary, the incision is extended laterally to expose more internal oblique. If the tenth and eleventh intercostal nerves are encountered, they are retracted to avoid injury. The internal oblique and transversus muscles are split down to the peritoneum. The ureter is identified and is retracted medially with the peritoneum. The peritoneum is freed posteriorly and medially with blunt dissection to expose the vena cava. Care must be taken not to dissect beneath the psoas muscle, which is in a somewhat anterior position at the depth of the dissection. If difficulty in exposure because of obesity or ascites is anticipated, the muscles should be incised and the incision extended. The right renal vein and two lower right lumbar veins are exposed **(Figure 2)**. Palpation of the aortic bifurcation is a useful point of reference.

Circumferential dissection of the vena cava below the renal vein but above a major lumbar vein allows passage of the ligature and the lower half of the Adams-DeWeese clip around the vessel **(Figure 3)**. The vena cava should be gently palpated to determine if there is proximal extension of the thrombus to this level. If a thrombus is found, the patient is placed in reverse Trendelenburg position. The vena cava is temporarily occluded above the clot, and the vein is opened through a purse-string suture. The thrombus may then be removed before completion of the interruption. After its placement, the clip is closed and its ligature is securely tied **(Figure 4)**. Great care should be exercised to avoid tearing or avulsion of the lumbar veins and to apply the clip above the lower two lumbar veins, which ensure good collaterals should the cava become occluded.

Patients who have had multiple small emboli resulting in pulmonary hypertension may have double ligature of the vena cava with heavy silk sutures instead of partial occlusion with a clip.

CLOSURE. After hemostasis is assured, the patient is returned to an unflexed position, and the incision is closed in layers as usual.

POSTOPERATIVE CARE. In the event of intraoperative arrhythmia or other overt evidence of a new pulmonary embolism, heparin should be administered immediately and continued. Otherwise, heparinization is reinstituted 24 hours after operation. This is indicated to control and limit extension of the distal thrombus as well as to prevent thrombosis at the site of the clip or ligation and to improve collateral flow. Anticoagulation should continue until all pain and tenderness and most of the edema have disappeared in the lower extremities. In general, this means the patient will receive seven to ten days of in-hospital heparinization followed by several months of oral anticoagulant therapy. In the meantime, the legs should be encased in elastic bandages or elastic stockings, which may be necessary for several months.

Any necessary respiratory support and general postoperative care are maintained as after other major operations. Cardiac disease or complications which often accompany thromboembolic phenomena may require special attention and management.

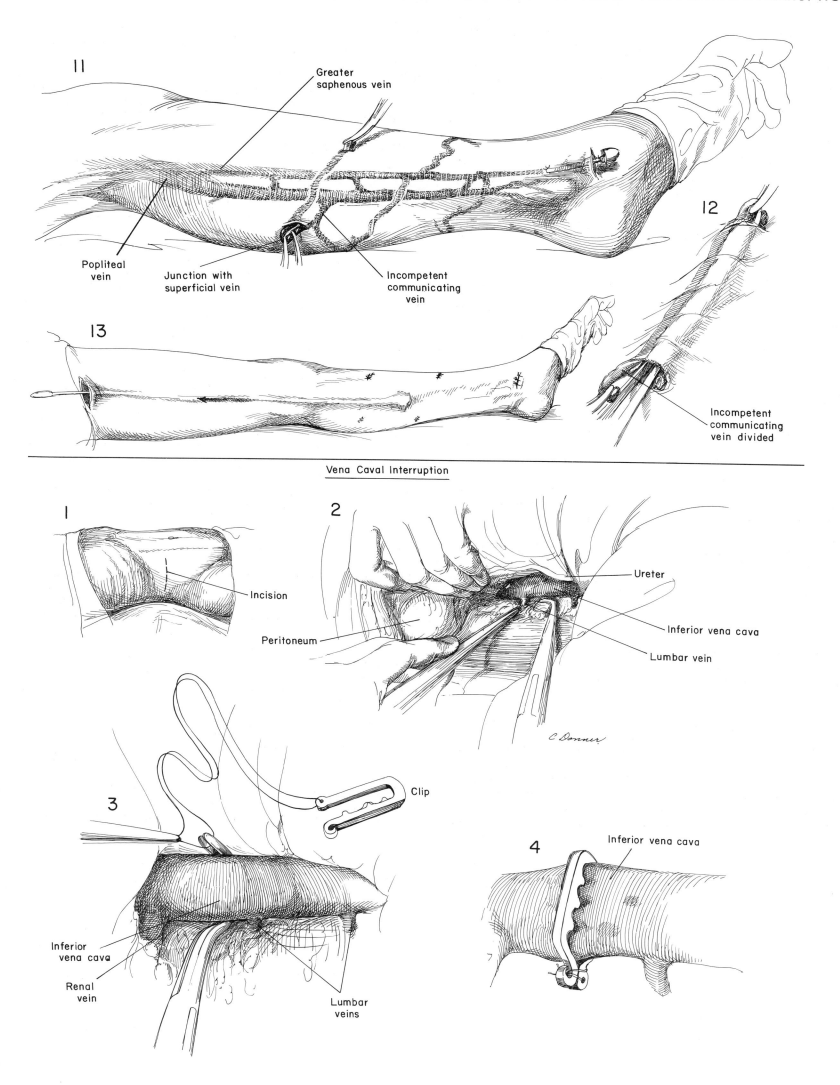

11

Greater
saphenous vein

Popliteal
vein

Junction with
superficial vein

Incompetent
communicating
vein

12

13

Incompetent
communicating
vein divided

Vena Caval Interruption

1

Incision

2

Peritoneum

Ureter

Inferior vena cava

Lumbar vein

3

Clip

Inferior
vena cava

Renal
vein

Lumbar
veins

4

Inferior vena cava

C Donner

PLATE CXIV · LUMBAR SYMPATHECTOMY

INDICATIONS. Lumbar sympathectomy is a well-established procedure, primarily indicated for peripheral vascular insufficiency affecting the skin of the toes, feet, or legs in patients in whom direct arterial surgery is not feasible. The cause of the vascular insufficiency may be atherosclerosis, with or without diabetes mellitus, or disorders such as thromboangiitis obliterans (Buerger's disease), and vasospastic conditions such as Raynaud's disease. The results of sympathectomy for peripheral artery insufficiency are unpredictable preoperatively. In general, the young or diabetic patient with pregangrenous skin changes in toes responds better compared to the patient with intermittent claudication. Patients over 70 respond poorly. Procedures such as measuring temperature rise in the foot after an epidural anesthetic, paravertebral sympathetic block, or indirect heat test are unreliable in predicting the response to a sympathectomy. Lumbar sympathectomy may also be indicated in hyperhidrosis and as ancillary therapy in frostbite and may be done at the time of aortic surgery to decrease spasm of the peripheral vessels to the extremities.

PREOPERATIVE PREPARATION. Before surgery the patient should be informed that the sympathectomy may be effective only for a short period of time and that there is no way to determine this preoperatively. The remainder of the preoperative preparation is the same as for any operative procedure.

ANESTHESIA. Lumbar sympathectomy is a relatively straightforward procedure. Muscle relaxation to ensure easy retraction and good exposure is essential. This is best achieved by an inhalation gas anesthetic with muscle relaxants or a spinal anesthetic. The inhalation anesthetic is preferred, as blood pressure is more easily controlled.

POSITION. The patient is placed in a supine position with a small padded sandbag behind the hip on the side of operation **(Figure 1).** This tilts the patient and the abdominal viscera toward the opposite side, thus facilitating the exposure of the retroperitoneal space. It also extends the back, giving more space between the costal margin and iliac crest.

OPERATIVE PREPARATION. With the patient in satisfactory position the skin is widely prepared. The area is then draped with a plastic skin drape and a sterile sheet. The umbilicus should be left in view, or its position should be marked with a towel clip in the sheet.

INCISION AND EXPOSURE. There are several approaches to the lumbar sympathetic chain. The chain is located retroperitoneally upon the lumbar vertebrae and at the medial edge of the psoas major muscle. It is posterior to the right border of the inferior vena cava and lateral to the aorta on the left **(Figures 2 and 7).** The skin incision extends from the tip of the twelfth rib nearly to the midline **(Figure 1).** The dissection is carried through the superficial fascia to the external oblique muscle and its aponeurosis. The aponeurosis and muscle fibers are then divided transversely **(Figure 3),** or they may be split in the line of their fibers. The anterior rectus sheath may be incised without division of the rectus muscle to facilitate exposure. The internal oblique and transversus muscles along with the transversalis fascia are then split in the direction of their muscle fibers, exposing the peritoneum. Care must be taken to preserve the tenth and eleventh intercostal nerves as they lie between the internal oblique and transversus muscles **(Figure 3).** The peritoneum is then pushed medially by blunt dissection. Care must be taken to stay anterior to the quadratus lumborum and psoas major muscles. The most frequent error is to get behind the psoas major muscle and fail to find the sympathetic chain. The ureter and genital vessels usually remain adherent to the peritoneum and are retracted medially, but they should be identified. The genitofemoral nerve will be seen descending obliquely downward and laterally across the front of the psoas major muscle **(Figure 5).**

DETAILS OF PROCEDURE. Once the retroperitoneal space has been exposed and the vena cava clearly visualized and gently retracted upward and medially, the sympathetic chain is identified by palpating and rolling it between the index finger and body of the third lumbar vertebra. It will feel like a bowstring upon the vertebral body at the medial edge of the psoas major muscle and just behind the vena cava, as described above. Actually, the sympathetic chain is buried in the groove formed by the medial edge of the psoas muscle and is sometimes difficult to identify. It will be found under the edge of the vena cava in the majority of instances. The peritoneum is mobilized medially over to the aorta and is held by a wide Deaver retractor. The vena cava is mobilized by sharp dissection and is tented upward with a small vein retractor. Retraction must be gentle so that a lumbar vein will not be torn off. The upper limit of the chain resection can be exposed by retraction with a narrow Deaver retractor. The sympathetic chain can then be encircled and picked up with a sympathectomy hook **(Figure 4).** The chain is freed carefully to expose the proximal end of the second lumbar ganglion. All branches of the main sympathetic chain are clipped with Weck metal clips, to ensure hemostasis, and divided **(Figure 5).**

The narrow Deaver is then shifted to expose the distal end of the sympathetic chain **(Figure 6).** On the right side the lumbar veins are anterior to the sympathetic chain, while on the left they are posterior **(Figure 7).** Therefore, on the right side, in order to remove the lower lumbar sympathetic chain in continuity, the lumbar vein must be ligated and divided **(Figure 8),** or the chain must be tunneled out from behind the vein. The distal limit of excision of the sympathetic chain is at the distal end of the third lumbar ganglion or pelvic brim. The chain is clipped and excised **(Figure 9).**

Hemostasis is established and the wound irrigated and closed.

CLOSURE. The retroperitoneal space may be drained with a half-inch Penrose drain. The drain is brought out through the lateral aspect of the wound. The fascia, muscles, and skin are then closed in layers with interrupted nonabsorbable sutures of 00 silk. A dry dressing is applied, and the patient is then transported to the recovery room.

POSTOPERATIVE CARE. Immediately postoperatively the patient should be maintained on intravenous therapy until bowel sounds are active and the patient has bowel function. Occasionally, a paralytic ileus will develop, and nasogastric suction will be required. The patient should be ambulated as soon as possible. The drain should be removed on the first postoperative day. The care of the specific disorder of the extremities for which this procedure was performed should be resumed. The wound sutures are removed when the wound is healed, sometime after the seventh postoperative day.

The effect of sympathectomy will be evident immediately. The leg will be warm and dry and the veins distended. The pregangrenous skin changes will disappear over a period of days if the sympathectomy is effective.

PLATE CXIV   LUMBAR SYMPATHECTOMY

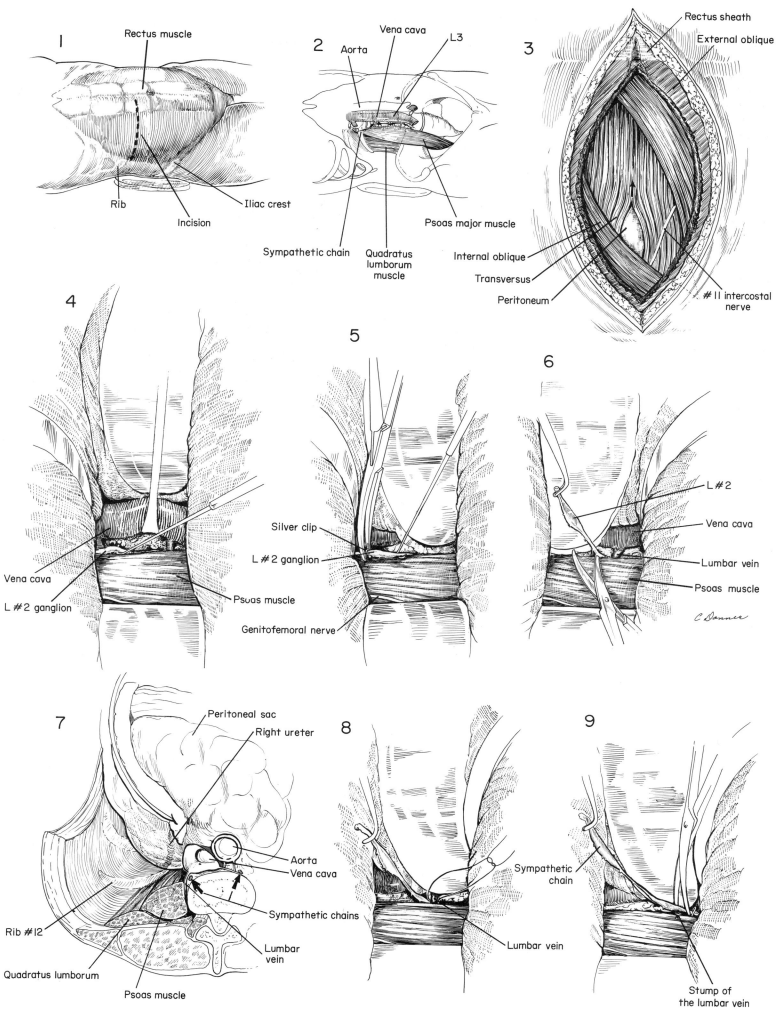

1

Rectus muscle

Rib

Incision

Iliac crest

2

Aorta

Vena cava

L3

Sympathetic chain

Quadratus lumborum muscle

Psoas major muscle

3

Rectus sheath

External oblique

Internal oblique

Transversus

Peritoneum

#11 intercostal nerve

4

Vena cava

L #2 ganglion

Psoas muscle

5

Silver clip

L #2 ganglion

Genitofemoral nerve

Psoas muscle

6

L #2

Vena cava

Lumbar vein

Psoas muscle

C Donner

7

Peritoneal sac

Right ureter

Aorta

Vena cava

Sympathetic chains

Lumbar vein

Rib #12

Quadratus lumborum

Psoas muscle

8

Sympathetic chain

Lumbar vein

9

Sympathetic chain

Stump of the lumbar vein

PLATE CXV · SHUNTING PROCEDURES FOR PORTAL HYPERTENSION

Portal decompression is indicated in patients who have portal hypertension complicated by gastrointestinal hemorrhage from esophageal varices. Some procedures completely interrupt portal venous flow to the liver (end-to-side portacaval shunt), while others selectively decompress the portal system via a collateral shunt (side-to-side portacaval, splenorenal, and mesocaval). The procedure selected will depend upon the patency of the portal and splenic veins, the results of liver function studies, the amount of portal venous blood being shunted, and whether the patient is bleeding acutely.

Selection of patients should be based on their clinical status, results of liver function studies, and interpretation of hepatic hemodynamics as determined by radiologic studies. Patients considered for shunting procedures should generally be under 60 years of age. Ideally, there should be no evidence of encephalopathy, jaundice, ascites, or muscle wasting. Serum albumin should be above 3 Gm. per cent, prothrombin time above 50 per cent, and sodium sulfobromophthalein below 30 per cent at 30 minutes. Deviation from these criteria does not absolutely contraindicate surgery, but the surgical risk is directly proportional to the degree of hepatic decompensation.

Shunting procedures for portal hypertension can be divided into three types: portacaval, splenorenal, and mesocaval. **Figures A** through **F** show diagrammatically the basic surgical choices for diversion of the portal venous flow.

Portacaval Shunt

The primary indication for portacaval shunt is the prevention or control of massive upper gastrointestinal hemorrhage from esophagogastric varices. Portacaval shunts are sometimes preferred when there has been prior splenectomy, splenic vein thrombosis, reversal of flow in the portal vein, thrombosed splenorenal shunt, ascites, and hepatic vein thrombosis. The selection of a direct portacaval shunt, of course, depends upon the demonstration of a patent portal vein preoperatively or at laparotomy.

The side-to-side anastomosis **(Figure A)** has been preferred by some in the presence of portal hypertension with no evidence of a rise in pressure on the hepatic end of the temporarily occluded portal vein. This suggests that the arterial blood supply is going through the liver and that lowering of the portal pressure by the side-to-side anastomosis with the vena cava will not result in diversion of the arterial supply to the liver. Another advantage of this type of shunt is that it decompresses the hepatic sinusoids, and this may be beneficial in the treatment of patients with intractable ascites accompanied by variceal hemorrhage.

The usefulness of the portacaval shunt in the treatment of refractory ascites is not universally accepted, although several studies have suggested that this is an effective mode of therapy. If shunting is indicated to control ascites, the side-to-side shunt or double end-to-side shunt is usually preferred. This is particularly true in unusual cases of hepatic vein thrombosis (Budd-Chiari). No decompressive procedure on the portal system has any beneficial effect on liver function. The end result of any such operation, therefore, will depend largely upon the progress of the basic liver disease.

The end-to-side portacaval shunt **(Figure B)** is the procedure of choice in patients who have had a prior splenectomy, splenic vein thrombosis, or thrombosis of a splenorenal shunt, and in those patients who have reversed flow in the portal vein. In this procedure the portal vein is ligated in the hilus of the liver, and the distal portion of the portal vein is anastomosed to the inferior vena cava. This shunt is particularly indicated when there is no evidence of ascites and when portal blood flow is reversed in the hepatofundal direction, as determined by a rising pressure in the hepatic end of the temporarily occluded portal vein. With the end-to-side anastomosis all of the portal venous blood flow is shunted from the liver, while hepatic artery flow to the liver is preserved.

See Plates CXVI through CXVIII for details of the portacaval shunting procedures.

Splenorenal Shunt

In the presence of extrahepatic block of the portal vein, secondary hypersplenism, prior biliary surgery, and/or cavernomatous changes of the portal vein, a shunt between the splenic vein and left renal vein may be the procedure of choice, provided the splenic vein is patent and of adequate size. If it is necessary or desirable to remove the spleen, a conventional splenorenal anastomosis **(Figure C)** may be performed. The distal splenorenal shunt (Warren shunt, **Figure D)** retains the spleen and, while selectively decompressing the esophageal varices, allows maintenance of portal pressure and perfusion of the liver, thus providing protection against hepatic encephalopathy. This shunt is particularly indicated in the presence of normal liver function, high volume of portal flow to the liver, minimal hepatocellular disease, marked splenomegaly, or idiopathic portal hypertension. The procedure consists of dividing the splenic vein at its junction with the superior mesenteric vein, ligating the proximal portion of the vein, and anastomosing the distal portion to the left renal vein. As an alternative to dividing the splenic vein, as interposition graft may be anastomosed between the splenic vein and the left renal vein, with ligation of the splenic vein proximal to the graft as well as ligation of the coronary and right gastroepiploic veins.

See Plates CXIX through CXXIV for details of the splenorenal shunting procedures.

Mesocaval Shunt

In most instances portal decompression may be accomplished by portacaval or splenorenal shunt procedures. However, the mesocaval shunt **(Figure E)** is necessary in patients who have undergone splenectomy and have either thrombosis or cavernomatous changes of the portal vein. The mesocaval shunt is advisable in patients with excessive bleeding at surgery from periportal or perisplenic vessels. Finally, it should be the procedure of choice in small children in whom the splenic and/or portal veins may be too small for a successful procedure (minimal size approximately 1 cm. in diameter). Elective shunts in children should be postponed, if possible, until the age of four years. The procedure consists of division of the superior vena cava and anastomosis side to end with the superior mesenteric vein.

In cases of emergency a lesser technical procedure without division of the inferior vena cava can be accomplished by the interposition of a large knitted dacron graft between the vena cava and superior mesenteric vein at the level of its first branches **(Figure F)**. This modification of the mesocaval shunt (interposition mesocaval shunt or Drapanas shunt) offers the advantages of a simplified technical approach with minimal blood loss.

See Plates CXXV through CXXVII for details of the mesocaval shunting procedures.

PLATE CXV   SHUNTING PROCEDURES FOR PORTAL HYPERTENSION

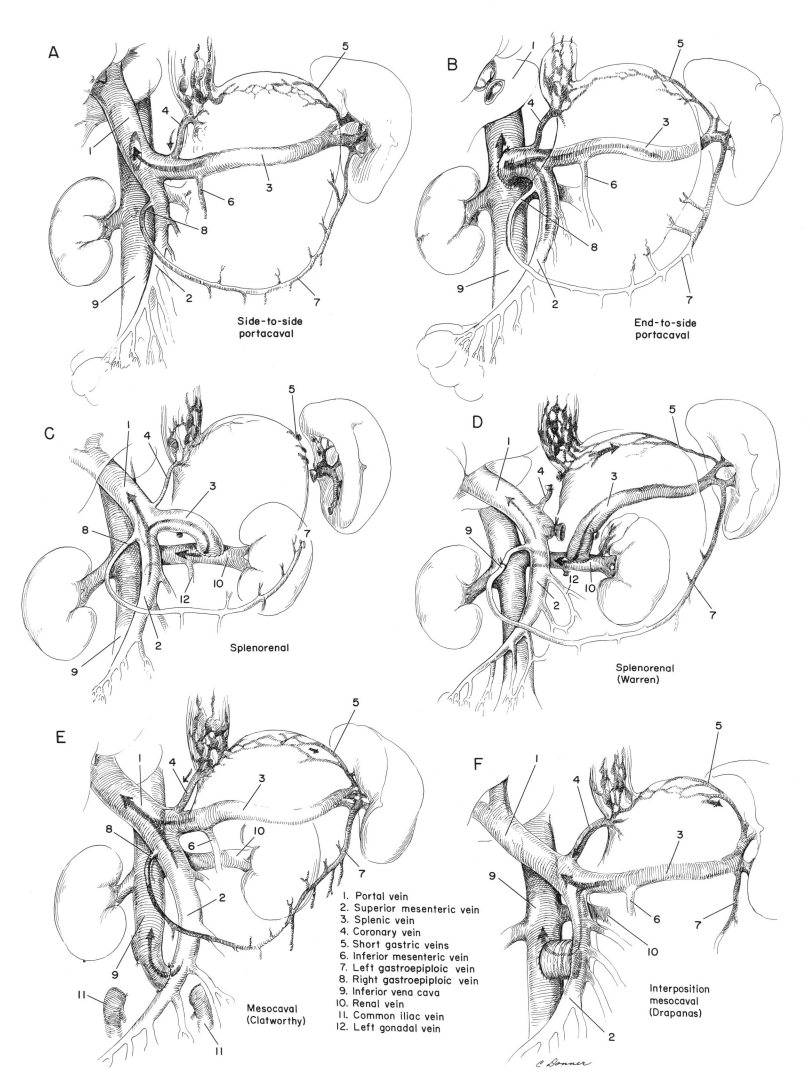

A   Side-to-side
portacaval

B   End-to-side
portacaval

C   Splenorenal

D   Splenorenal
(Warren)

E   Mesocaval
(Clatworthy)

1. Portal vein
2. Superior mesenteric vein
3. Splenic vein
4. Coronary vein
5. Short gastric veins
6. Inferior mesenteric vein
7. Left gastroepiploic vein
8. Right gastroepiploic vein
9. Inferior vena cava
10. Renal vein
11. Common iliac vein
12. Left gonadal vein

F   Interposition
mesocaval
(Drapanas)

C. Donner

PLATE CXVI · PORTACAVAL SHUNT

INDICATIONS. See Plate CXV.

PREOPERATIVE PREPARATION. The patient's ability to tolerate a portacaval shunt procedure depends primarily upon the state of liver function at the time of the procedure. In general, every effort should be made to improve the patient's general nutrition and hepatic state before surgery. Several weeks of careful medical management of diet, diuretics, and activity are often necessary. After a careful history and physical examination, hepatic function studies and hepatosplanchnic hemodynamic determinations are obtained.

If the patient is bleeding, the acute phase of the hemorrhage from the gastrointestinal tract requires prompt control with iced saline lavage and/or with an intraesophageal pressure balloon. Vasopressin may be administered as a continuous intravenous infusion (20 to 40 units/hour) or as a selective intra-arterial infusion (superior mesenteric artery at 0.1 to 0.4 units/minute). In addition to vasopressin's efficiency in reducing portal pressure, it helps evacuate blood and fecal residue from the alimentary tract. If vasopressin is not administered, it is essential to remove old blood by means of colonic irrigation. This simplifies exposure and reduces the risk of ammonia intoxication. Nonabsorbable antibacterial agents are used to control nitrogen-splitting bacteria in the gastrointestinal tract. Blood volume should be restored preoperatively by careful use of whole blood, albumin, and lactated Ringer's solution. Fresh whole blood, platelet transfusion, and vitamin K are sometimes indicated, depending upon the results of coagulation studies.

Liver function must be evaluated using a combination of clinical factors and laboratory studies. A history of jaundice or ascites indicates an increased surgical risk. Serum albumin should be above 3 Gm. per cent and prothrombin time above 50 per cent. The partial thromboplastin time and platelet count should be within normal limits. If there are any deviations from these values, correction should be attempted with vitamin K and parenteral administration of albumin, fresh frozen plasma, or whole blood. Diuretic therapy may be necessary in those patients with ascites. Appropriate steps must be taken to control electrolyte and acid-base balance, especially hypokalemic alkalosis. Coagulation deficits other than those associated with prothrombin may be corrected with fresh frozen plasma and platelet concentrate. At the time of surgery 10 to 12 units of whole blood should be available.

Esophagoscopy and gastroscopy should be obtained routinely along with appropriate barium studies of the esophagus and stomach. Hepatosplanchnic hemodynamics can be determined by estimation of total hepatic blood flow, liver scan, hepatic vein catheterization, splenoportography, indirect portography, and visceral angiography. Total hepatic blood flow can be estimated using radioactive colloidal gold. Via hepatic vein catheterization it is possible to determine the degree of portal hypertension and the amount of hepatopetal portal blood flow. Splenoportography is usually the single best source of estimating portal hemodynamics. Prerequisites for this study are that prothrombin time be above 50 per cent and the operating room available, should trouble from hemorrhage develop. This study will reveal the degree of portal hypertension, and according to the degree of opacification of the portal vein, it can give valuable information concerning the degree of compromise of portal blood flow to the liver. Information obtained from these hemodynamic studies may influence the choice of shunt to be performed.

ANESTHESIA. A general anesthetic is required. The major hazards during anesthesia are anoxia and hypotension. These hazards are more significant than the effect of any particular anesthetic agent commonly employed today. However, there is sufficient reason to suspect the possible danger of using halogenated compounds in patients with impaired liver function, and therefore these agents should not be used during the operation. The other commonly employed general anesthetic agents and the muscle relaxants appear to have no adverse effect on liver function. Provision should be made for the quick administration of blood and fluids in adequate amounts.

POSITION. Elevation of the right side to a 30-degree angle aids in extension of the right subcostal incision into the flank and provides additional exposure for this procedure. If the choice between the portacaval and splenorenal shunt has not been made before operation, the patient should be left in the supine position so that either procedure may be carried out merely by extending the initial central incision in the appropriate direction.

OPERATIVE PREPARATION. The skin is cleansed higher than the nipples and well down to the symphysis. Likewise, the chest, particularly on the left side, should be prepared, since an extension of the incision into the left thorax may be necessary.

INCISION AND EXPOSURE. Along the right subcostal margin an incision is made crossing the left rectus muscle and extending well into the flank (**Figure 1,** A). Satisfactory exposure may also be obtained by a combined thoracoabdominal incision (**Figure 1,** B), but it is less desirable because of the increased morbidity that usually accompanies it.

DETAILS OF PROCEDURE. The routine exploration is carried out after the peritoneal cavity is opened. The diagnosis of portal hypertension is confirmed by catheterization of an omental vein (**Figure 2**), preferably toward the stomach. This is useful even if splenic pulp pressure has been measured preoperatively, since measurement at this time will permit a more valid comparison of pre- and postshunt pressures. The pressure will normally measure 30 cm. of saline or higher above the portal vein level. Considerably lower pressures would not indicate the necessity or desirability of a shunting procedure. If a previous splenoportogram has shown the presence of a satisfactory portal vein, dissection is begun by mobilizing the duodenum. If the presence of a suitable portal vein for shunting is in doubt, this vein should be isolated and surveyed with a portal venogram before exposure of the vena cava. Collateral venous networks are usually considerably enlarged over the posterior peritoneum and subject to increased pressure. Therefore, this normally avascular area may be quite the opposite, and dissection during the Kocher maneuver should progress by clamping and ligating the peritoneal surfaces, rather than by making the usual simple incision lateral to the descending portion of the duodenum (**Figure 3**). This precaution applies to all dissection during this procedure in the retroperitoneal space and in the hepatoduodenal ligament. The inferior vena cava is ordinarily exposed without great difficulty (**Figure 4**). A required additional exposure may be obtained in the presence of an enlarged caudate lobe of the liver by resecting a portion of that lobe. Through-and-through mattress sutures of 00 silk are placed to control the bleeding before the liver is divided. The caudate lobe is freed from the vena cava, and the veins encountered are ligated (**Figures 5** and **6**).

PLATE CXVI   PORTACAVAL SHUNT

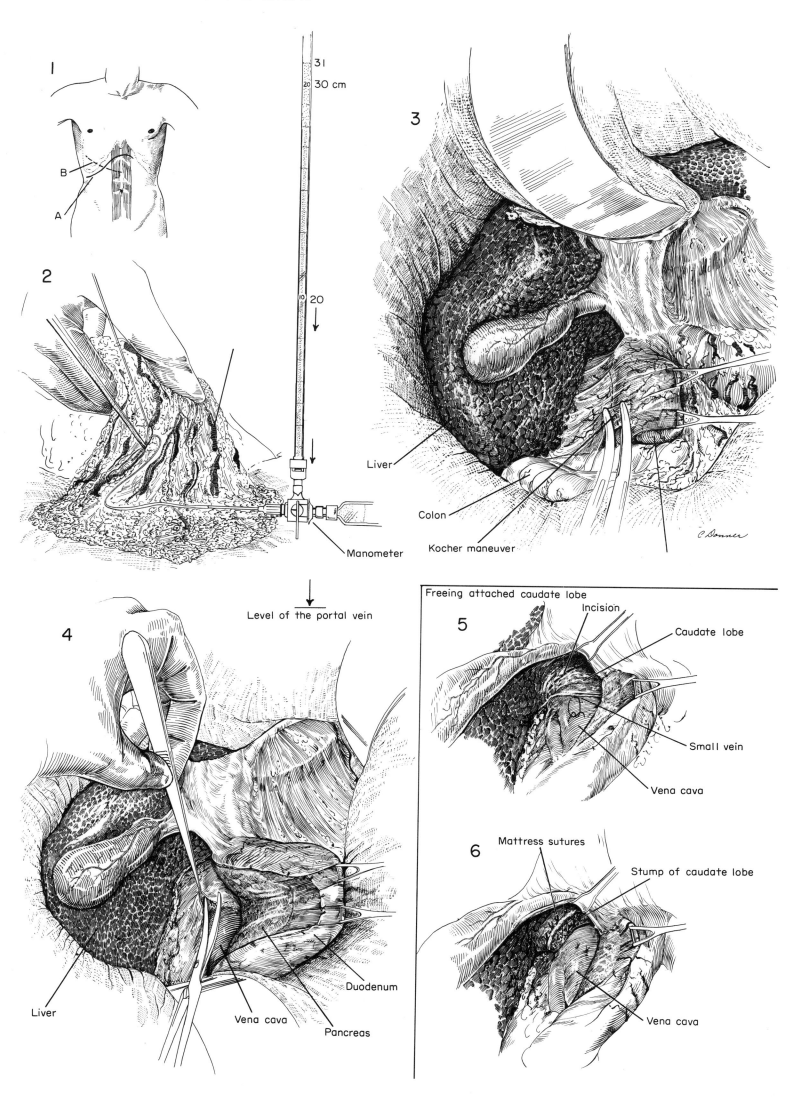

1

2

31

20 30 cm

20

10

Manometer

Level of the portal vein

3

Liver

Colon

Kocher maneuver

C. Donner

4

Liver

Vena cava

Duodenum

Pancreas

5

Freeing attached caudate lobe

Incision

Caudate lobe

Small vein

Vena cava

6

Mattress sutures

Stump of caudate lobe

Vena cava

PLATE CXVII · PORTACAVAL SHUNT

DETAILS OF PROCEDURE (*Continued*). The portal vein is next identified in the hepatoduodenal ligament by the same careful dissection **(Figure 7).** It may be helpful during this dissection to place a tape or rubber tissue drain about the common bile duct in order to facilitate exposure of the portal vein **(Figure 8).** The portal vein should be exposed from the hilum of the liver to the superior surface of the pancreas, where the usual pancreatic tributaries should be located and protected. Once the three structures of the hepatoduodenal ligament have been clearly identified, the remaining adipose tissue containing enlarged venous and lymphatic channels may be divided in order to bring the portal vein in proximity with the vena cava **(Figure 9).** The area at which the portal vein crosses closest to the cava is ordinarily just proximal to the entrance of the renal veins.

At this point, if a side-to-side shunt has been decided upon, two noncrushing clamps are applied to the portal vein so that it may be rotated to expose its inferior surface **(Figure 10).** This is necessary to prevent twisting or angulation of the portal vein as the anastomosis is accomplished. Two points must be borne in mind in preparing the anastomotic sites. The first is that the portal vein and the inferior vena cava are not parallel to each other, and therefore openings in the longitudinal axis of each vein would result in twisting of the anastomotic site when the clamps are released. It is necessary to incise the portal vein obliquely to avoid any twisting **(Figure 11).** Second, a simple longitudinal window, either in the portal vein or in the vena cava, is not adequate for a satisfactory shunt because of the low pressures in the venous system. A simple slit opening will behave more like a valve and tend to close, resulting in a high incidence of shunt failure. The anastomosis should be between windows cut in the veins by excising a definite portion of their walls in an elliptical fashion **(Figure 12).** It is not usually necessary to cross-clamp the vena cava completely. A curved noncrushing clamp, placed to exclude a portion of the lumen, is satisfactory for this purpose **(Figure 13).** The anastomosis should be made so that it is at least as large as the diameter of the portal vein.

PLATE CXVII   PORTACAVAL SHUNT

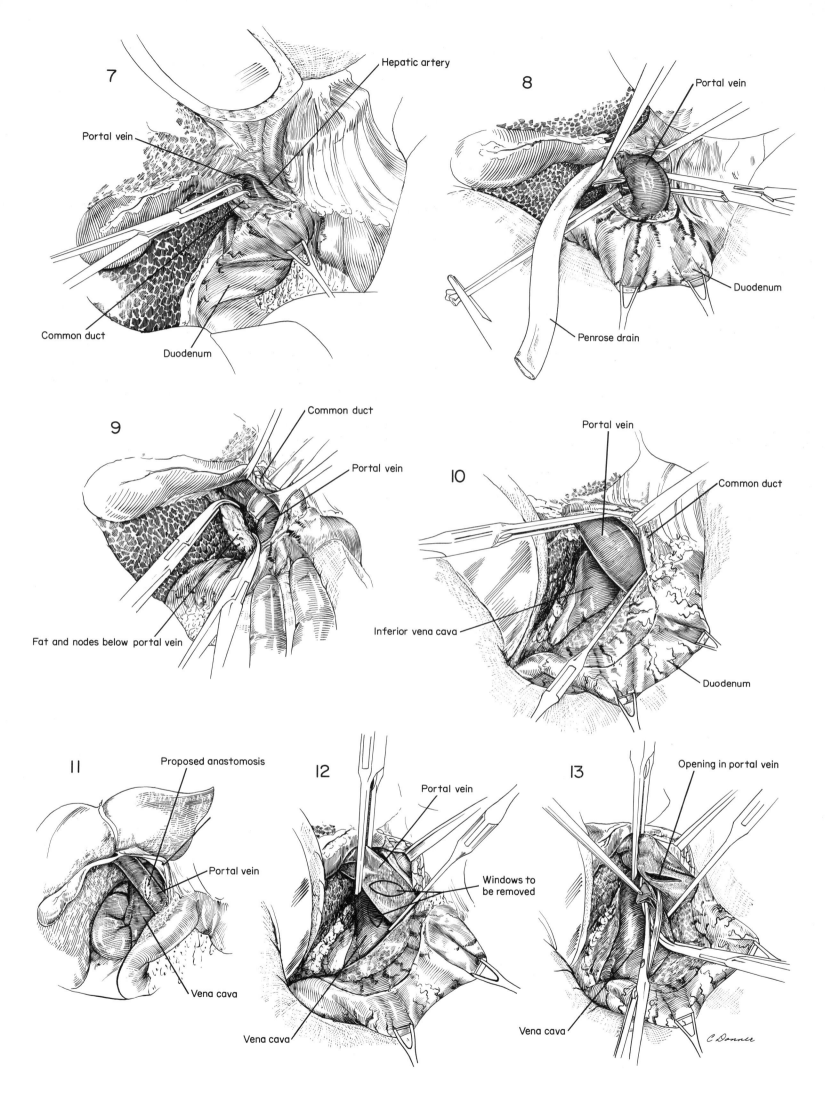

7
Hepatic artery
Portal vein
Common duct
Duodenum

8
Portal vein
Duodenum
Penrose drain

9
Common duct
Portal vein
Fat and nodes below portal vein

10
Portal vein
Common duct
Inferior vena cava
Duodenum

11
Proposed anastomosis
Portal vein
Vena cava

12
Portal vein
Windows to be removed
Vena cava

13
Opening in portal vein
Vena cava

C Donner

PLATE CXVIII · PORTACAVAL SHUNT

DETAILS OF PROCEDURE (*Continued*). The anastomosis itself is usually accomplished by a continuous suture of fine, nonabsorbable suture material on atraumatic needles. Two angle sutures of 00000 arterial silk or synthetic material are placed with knots tied on the outside **(Figure 14)**. Both the portal vein and the inferior vena cava are very fragile. It is therefore necessary to use the utmost caution during the suturing process to avoid trauma to these vein walls. This caution should apply not only to the surgeon doing the actual suturing, but equally, if not more, to his assistant holding the clamps. A very slight shearing force created by shifting the vascular clamps in relation to each other may easily disrupt a partly completed anastomosis. Leaks from the anastomotic site, particularly along the left side of the anastomosis, may be difficult to expose for subsequent resuturing. The anastomosis is completed **(Figures 15 and 16)**, and the occluding clamps are released one at a time to check the adequacy of the suture line. Although the portal vein represents the high pressure system in this anastomosis, it is usually convenient to release one of the portal clamps first, since these are normally easier to reapply if hemostasis is not satisfactory. After all clamps are released, it is frequently possible to detect the functioning of the shunt by visible turbulence in the vena cava. Palpation of the opening between the two veins by invaginating the anterior wall of the portal vein also can be used to verify the patency of the anastomosis. Repeat measurement of pressure in the portal system will normally show that it has been reduced to about half of its preoperative level.

End-to-Side Portacaval Shunt

The completed end-to-side anastomosis is illustrated **(Figure 17)**. This is usually accomplished by dividing the portal vein as close as possible to the liver hilum. It is important not to leave the proximal stump of the portal vein too short, since this is a large vein and under considerable pressure. One should leave room for a double ligature, the second being a transfixion suture ligature with several millimeters of vein cuff to assure adequate control of the hepatic side of the portal vein **(Figure 18)**. A longer stump of portal vein is retained if a double end-to-side shunt is indicated **(Figure 19)**. A noncrushing vascular clamp is placed on the portal vein as close to the pancreas as possible to leave the maximum amount of portal vein free for the anastomosis **(Figure 19)**. Again, the appropriate site on the inferior vena cava is selected, excluded by a partially occluding vascular clamp,

and an ellipse of vein wall is excised. A single-layer continuous anastomosis of arterial silk or synthetic suture is accomplished as described for the side-to-side anastomosis **(Figure 20)**. Although this is an easier anastomosis to accomplish, the same precautions apply here concerning the fragility of the vein walls. After the anastomosis has been completed, the clamps are removed individually. If hemostasis is satisfactory, the procedure is concluded as described above.

CLOSURE. The incision is closed in layers. Drainage of the right upper quadrant is not ordinarily required unless there has been unusual trauma to the liver, pancreas, or biliary system. Retention suturing may be useful.

POSTOPERATIVE CARE. In the immediate postoperative period it is important to prevent hypoxia, and therefore routine administration of oxygen is recommended for the first 24 to 48 hours. Central venous pressure combined with serial hematocrits should be monitored to assure maintenance of an adequate blood volume.

Because this type of shunt has the highest incidence of hepatic coma, postoperative efforts should be continuous to decrease protein catabolism. During the period of no oral intake, the patient should be given a minimum of 200 Gm. of carbohydrate per day to prevent the undue breakdown of protein. When oral intake is resumed, protein should be restricted initially to 30 Gm. per day. If tolerated, gradual increments, usually 10 Gm. every other day, may be instituted until a level of 50 to 75 Gm. of protein is reached. Tolerance of this nitrogen load may be checked with fasting and two-hour postprandial blood ammonia levels. If signs of hepatic insufficiency develop, protein intake should be further restricted and intestinal antibiotics administered.

The prothrombin activity must be monitored and supplemental vitamin K given as indicated. Continued administration of multiple vitamin preparations is also useful.

Ascites may be a distressing, if not a dangerous, problem postoperatively. Careful monitoring of both fluid and sodium intake may prevent or minimize this complication. If ascites develops, it is best managed by severe sodium restriction combined with diuretics.

The increased incidence of peptic ulceration following portacaval shunt should be remembered and appropriate (low Na^+) antacid therapy instituted.

PLATE CXVIII   PORTACAVAL SHUNT

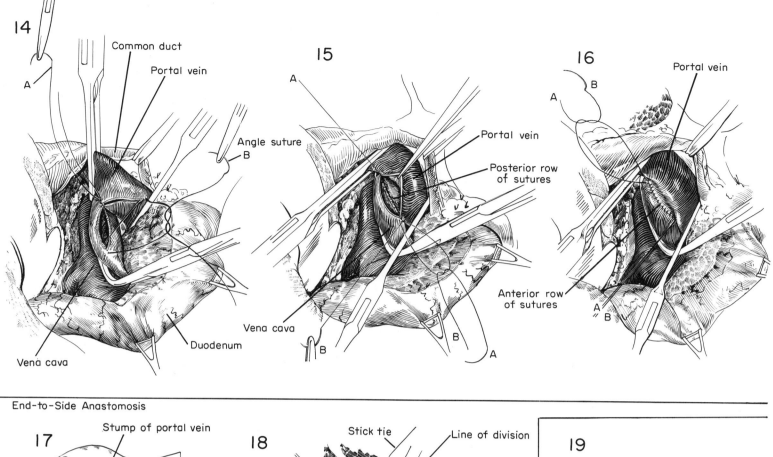

14 Common duct
Portal vein
A
Angle suture
B
Vena cava
Duodenum
Vena cava

15 A
Portal vein
Posterior row
of sutures
Anterior row
of sutures
Vena cava
B
A

16 Portal vein
B
A
A" B

End-to-Side Anastomosis

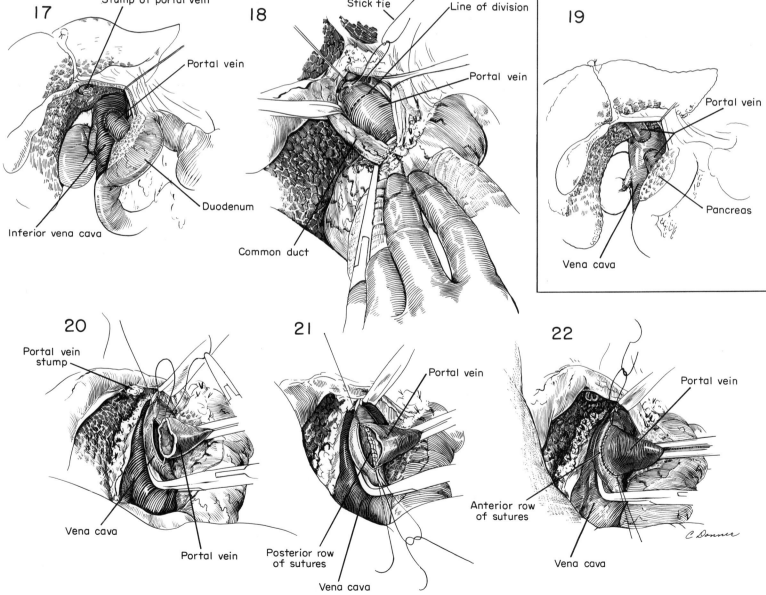

17 Stump of portal vein
Portal vein
Inferior vena cava
Duodenum

18 Stick tie   Line of division
Portal vein
Common duct

19 Portal vein
Pancreas
Vena cava

20 Portal vein
stump
Vena cava
Portal vein

21 Portal vein
Posterior row
of sutures
Vena cava

22 Portal vein
Anterior row
of sutures
Vena cava

C Donner

PLATE CXIX · SPLENORENAL SHUNT

INDICATIONS. See Plate CXV.

PREOPERATIVE PREPARATION. See Plate CXVI. To these preparations evaluation of kidney function and the left renal vein must be added.

ANESTHESIA. See Plate CXVI.

POSITION. The patient is placed in supine position. It may be helpful to place a folded towel under the left flank.

OPERATIVE PREPARATION. The skin is cleansed higher than the nipples and well down to the symphysis. Likewise the chest, particularly on the left side, should be prepared, since an extension of the incision into the left thorax may be necessary.

INCISION AND EXPOSURE. A left paramedian or left subcostal incision is used **(Figure 1).** It may or may not be necessary to excise the xiphoid. When the spleen is quite large, the incision should be extended well below the umbilicus on the left side. All bleeding points should be meticulously clamped and tied. It may be necessary to transfix the enlarged veins about the region of the umbilicus. When the peritoneal cavity is opened, the extent of the attachments of the spleen to the parietes is noted as well as the gross appearance of the liver. If fluid is present in the abdomen, it should be removed by suction and an accurate record made of the amount removed.

On occasion it may be desirable to determine the venous pressure by isolating an available dilated vein in the gastrosplenic ligament or in the omentum for introduction of a catheter and measurement with a water manometer. Usually, this pressure has been taken at the time of splenoportogram. The anticipated pressure is usually about 300 mm. of water.

There is usually less blood loss if a standard technic for the removal of the spleen is followed, as described in Plates CI and CII. Since the tissues tend to be porky and quite vascular, owing to increased venous pressure, it is essential that only small bites be taken during the application of curved clamps in the region of the lowermost portion of the gastrosplenic ligament **(Figure 2).** When the lesser sac has been opened, the incision is carried up along the greater curvature and the contents of the clamps transfixed with 00 silk on both sides. The suture on the gastric side should include a bite of the gastric wall in order to avoid subsequent slipping off of the knot during possible postoperative gastric distention **(Figure 3).**

The incision on the gastrosplenic ligament should be carried up toward the superior pole of the spleen until there is a very liberal exposure of the lesser sac. At that time an S retractor may be placed over the stomach to retract it upward. Downward retraction of the transverse colon or lateral retraction of the huge spleen by a large curved S retractor applied over a Mikulicz pad is necessary to adequately expose the lesser sac before identification and ligation of the splenic artery. An incision is made in the peritoneum over the splenic artery. If the splenic artery cannot be identified, its location should be verified by digital palpation. Since more than the usual amount of bleeding may be incurred if adjacent dilated veins are torn, great care should be taken in isolating the splenic artery before its ligation with 00 silk. Usually, two ligatures are placed on the splenic artery **(Figure 4).**

With the splenic artery tied, the spleen tends to shrink and become firmer, making its retraction and manipulation a little easier. Occasionally, the fundus of the stomach is intimately attached to the uppermost portion of the hilus of the spleen **(Figure 5).** Direct vision of this area is required as the uppermost portion of the gastrohepatic ligament is divided and the contents of these clamps carefully transfixed and ligated with 00 silk. On occasion a very large but short vein may be overlooked at the uppermost portion of the gastrosplenic ligament, with the result that it may be torn with considerable loss of blood and subsequent difficulty in ligating it on the splenic side. The peritoneum up over the superior surface of the spleen is divided if the exposure is adequate.

The surgeon should once again palpate over the surface of the spleen and free any adhesions that are present. If there has been a very firm attachment between the capsule of the spleen and the parietes, it may be advisable to consider incising the peritoneum and leaving it attached to the surface of the spleen. Blood transfusions are given to replace current blood losses, which must be measured accurately.

PLATE CXIX   SPLENORENAL SHUNT

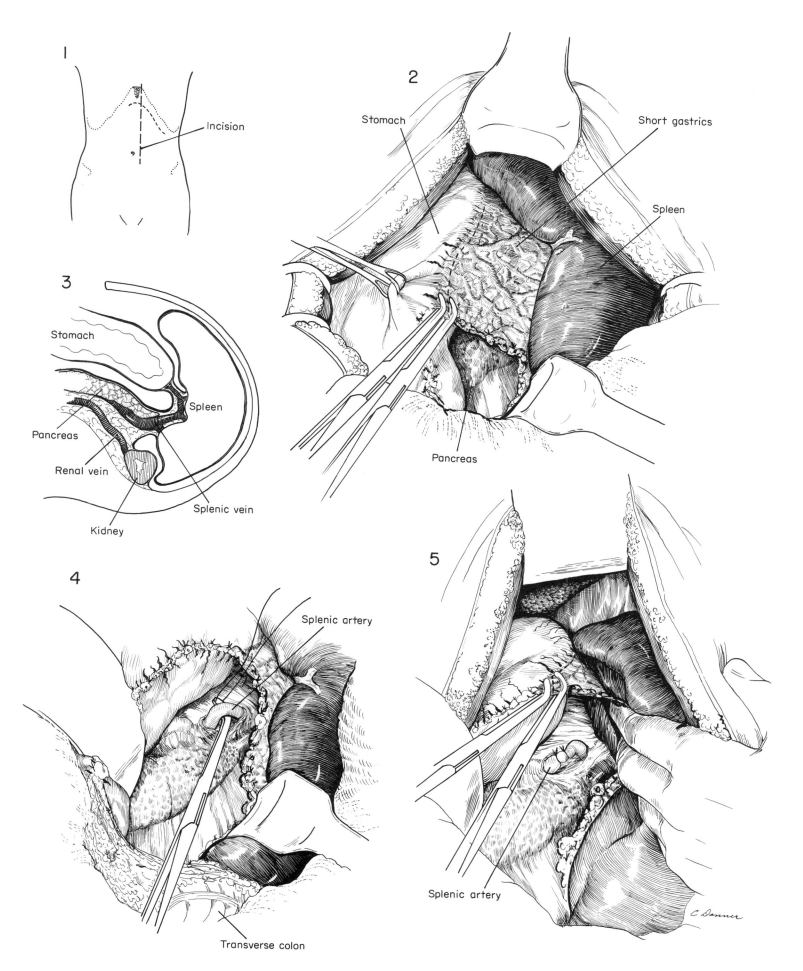

1

Incision

2

Stomach

Short gastrics

Spleen

Pancreas

3

Stomach

Spleen

Pancreas

Renal vein

Splenic vein

Kidney

4

Splenic artery

Transverse colon

5

Splenic artery

C Donner

PLATE CXX · SPLENORENAL SHUNT

DETAILS OF PROCEDURE. After ligation of the splenic artery and the complete division of the gastrosplenic ligament up to and including the region of the fundus, the inferior pole of the spleen is retracted upward in order to define the splenocolic ligament **(Figure 6).** Often there are sizable veins in this area that must be controlled by the careful application of clamps. Any adhesions between the splenic flexure of the colon and the lateral peritoneal wall are separated in order to visualize the splenocolic ligament better. The contents of these clamps are ligated with 00 silk as the incision in the splenocolic ligament is carried around laterally to the region of the splenorenal ligament **(Figure 7).** Because of the increased vascularity and the usual thickening of the splenorenal ligament, it is advisable to apply long right-angle clamps in pairs so that the free peritoneal margins on the lateral side can be ligated. Troublesome bleeding will occur unless all these bleeding points are carefully controlled. The incision in the splenorenal ligament is carried upward to the region of the base of the diaphragm and up around to meet the incision carried from the region of the reflection of the peritoneum off the diaphragm to the fundus of the stomach. This completely frees the spleen, except for the pedicle.

The wound is retracted laterally as the surgeon passes his hand over the enlarged spleen and gently tilts it up into the wound **(Figure 8).** Any restraining peritoneal adhesions between the backside of the hilus of the spleen and the parietes are carefully divided after the application of clamps. The posterior side of the tail of the pancreas, as well as the large splenic vein, gradually comes into view. It may be advisable to use blunt gauze dissection to push away the edematous fatty tissue in order to mobilize the tail and body of the pancreas as far medially as possible. With the spleen retracted medially, the region of the splenic vein and the left kidney is more readily identifiable. The tissues over the renal vein are divided by careful dissection until the region of the left adrenal vein is completely separated from the adjacent tissues. Any bleeding points about the region of the left adrenal should be clamped and ligated. Likewise, the ligatures on the greater curvature of the stomach are inspected from time to time to make sure that there is no slow loss of blood. The same attention should be given to oozing from vessels which have not been ligated in the splenic bed.

PLATE CXX   SPLENORENAL SHUNT

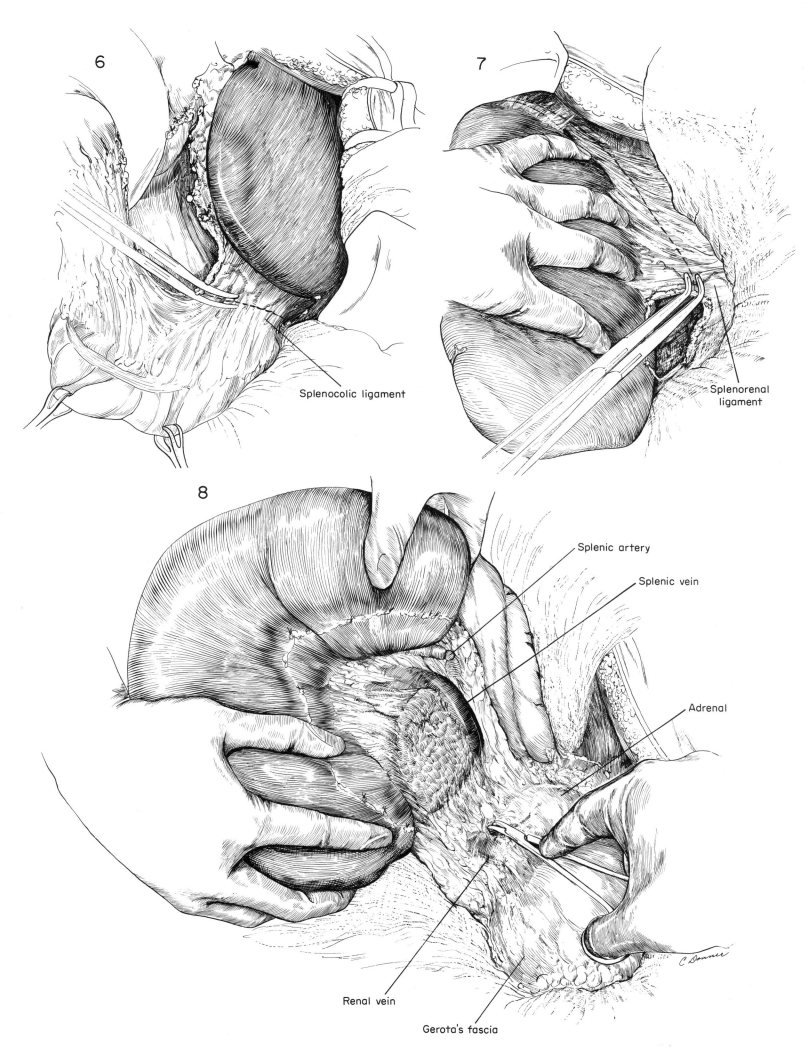

6

Splenocolic ligament

7

Splenorenal
ligament

8

Splenic artery

Splenic vein

Adrenal

Renal vein

Gerota's fascia

PLATE CXXI · SPLENORENAL SHUNT

DETAILS OF PROCEDURE (*Continued*). Unless the capsule of the spleen has been torn and troublesome bleeding occurs, it is helpful to leave the spleen attached to serve as a tractor while the tail of the pancreas and the major vessels in the splenic pedicle **(Figure 9)** are being identified. The tail of the pancreas may be firmly attached deep into the hilus of the spleen, or it may be separated for several centimeters from the hilus. Small curved clamps are used to divide any ligament attachments between the inferior surface of the tail of the pancreas and the splenic pedicle. The contents of these clamps are promptly tied with 00 silk sutures. As a matter of fact, great attention must be paid to these small vessels entering the tail of the pancreas, as troublesome postoperative bleeding may occur if they are not securely controlled. Likewise, the pancreatic tissue itself should not be damaged as the tail of the pancreas is freed to the region of the dilated splenic vein.

The segment of the splenic artery adjacent to the splenic vein is gently dissected free from adjacent tissue and doubly clamped **(Figure 10).** The ligation followed by transfixing suture provides a fourth ligature to control this major vessel. The artery on the splenic side should be ligated to provide ready access to the region of the dilated splenic vein **(Figure 11).** Gentle traction on the spleen tends to define the tissues over the dilated splenic vein better and enhances the surgeon's ability to gently dissect off the overlying tissues **(Figure 11).** On occasion the splenic vein will bifurcate at some distance from the hilus of the spleen, which tends to shorten the length of the splenic vein finally available for the splenorenal anastomosis. As much as possible of the splenic vein up to the point of bifurcation should be gently freed and visualized from the adjacent structures **(Figure 12).** The final adhesions between the hilus of the spleen and the tail of the pancreas are defined and small paired clamps applied. Following the division of these structures, great care must be exercised to avoid tearing the splenic vein as it is maintained on tension to facilitate the removal from the adjacent pancreas **(Figure 13).** Small clamps of the curved mosquito type should be applied to each small vein, regardless of how insignificant it may appear to be. The number of clamps required on both the splenic vein side and the pancreatic side is variable. This is a very critical point in the procedure, and the surgeon must take all the time that is required in carefully freeing the splenic vein from the adjacent pancreas **(Figure 14).** It may be desirable to transfix the small curved clamps on the venous side using French needles and 0000 silk. The region of the tail of the pancreas should be checked from time to time, and any small bleeding points should be meticulously controlled.

PLATE CXXI   SPLENORENAL SHUNT

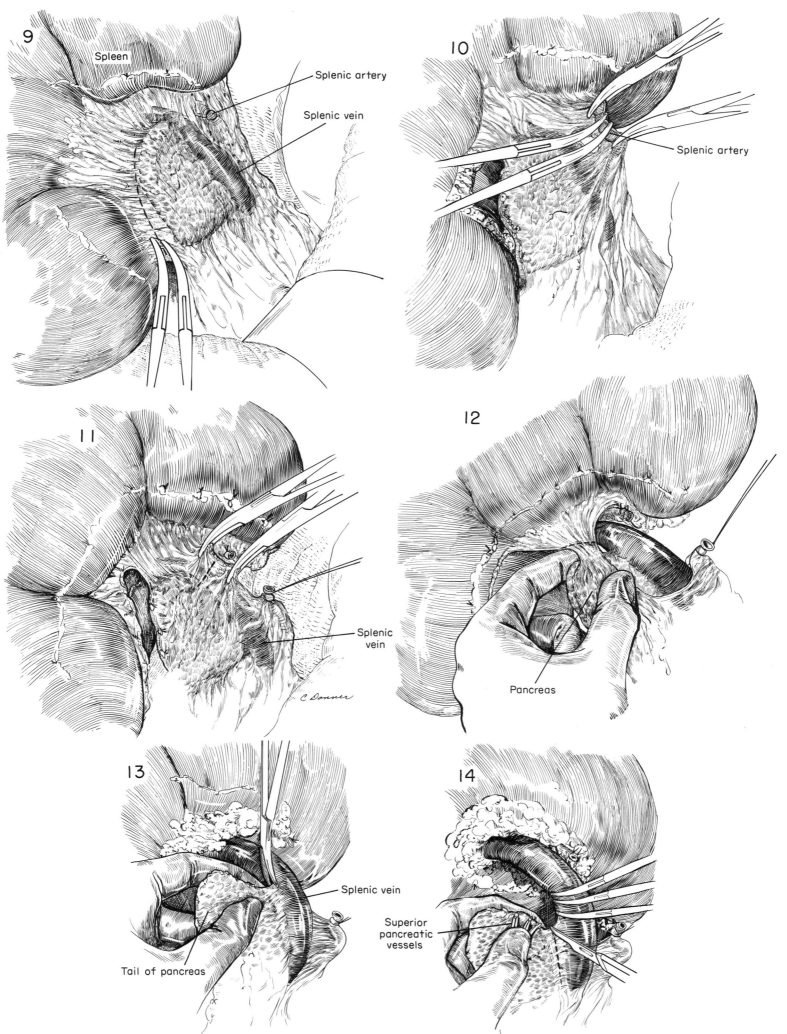

9

Spleen

Splenic artery

Splenic vein

10

Splenic artery

11

Splenic vein

C Donner

12

Pancreas

13

Splenic vein

Tail of pancreas

14

Superior pancreatic vessels

PLATE CXXII · SPLENORENAL SHUNT

DETAILS OF PROCEDURE (*Continued*). Regardless of how much vein seems to be available at first, it is desirable to continue isolating the splenic vein to make absolutely certain it can be subsequently rotated down to the region of the left renal vein without undue tension or angulation **(Figure 15)**. The region of the splenic artery is separated from the vein, and all bleeding points are carefully controlled. Vascular clamps, such as straight Potts clamps, are applied in pairs to the splenic vein at the point of bifurcation. The vein is divided with a knife or sharp scissors. A good segment of freed vein should be apparent. It is estimated that 7 cm. or more should usually be available **(Figure 16)**.

Gerota's fascia, over the anterior surface of the left kidney, is divided with curved scissors, and the kidney is manually delivered up out of its bed. The renal vein is further isolated from the adjacent tissue until there is a long segment well defined. It is usually necessary to divide the sizable left adrenal vein, which empties into the superior surface of the renal vein a short distance from the renal pelvis **(Figure 17)**. In addition, the rather small renal artery is identified in adjacent tissues in order that bulldog forceps can be applied to control the arterial blood supply into the kidney before the renal vein is doubly clamped **(Figure 18, 2 and 3)**. The kidney and the left adrenal vein should be sufficiently mobilized to make certain that an adequate incision can be made in the anterior surface of the renal vein in anticipation of the anastomosis with the splenic vein. The end of the splenic vein **(Figure 18)** should be brought down to the region of the renal vein to make certain that a sufficient amount of splenic vein has already been mobilized. A small, serrated vascular-type bulldog clamp is applied to the very base of the splenic vein. A small window is excised in the anterior wall of the renal vein in anticipation of a direct anastomosis with the splenic vein. Interrupted sutures are taken at either end of the opening in the renal vein with the corresponding side of the splenic vein. When these sutures **(Figure 19)** are tied, the contour of the splenic vein should be surveyed to make sure there is no undue angulation or twisting before the anastomosis progresses. A continuous 0000 silk suture on an atraumatic needle may be used to close the posterior layer **(Figure 20)**. A continuous suture is utilized to close the anterior layer **(Figure 21)**. The bulldog clamp **(Figure 18, 3)** on the renal vein is removed as a check against backbleeding in the region of the anastomosis. Additional interrupted 0000 silk sutures may be required to control any oozing or active bleeding about the anastomosis.

The bulldog clamp on the base of the renal vein is then opened, followed by removal of the bulldog clamp on the renal vein adjacent to the kidney and, finally, the clamp on the splenic vein itself. Interrupted sutures may be required to control leaks about the anastomosis. If difficulties are encountered in the anastomosis with undue prolongation of the operation, it may be advisable to close the opening in the renal vein temporarily with a curved vascular clamp while the remaining bulldog clamps on the renal veins are removed and the arterial supply temporarily reestablished to the left kidney.

At the completion of the procedure it is advisable to insert a needle into the splenic vein and once again determine the portal pressure. It is hoped that the pressure will have fallen to 200 mm. of water or less. The kidney is gently returned to its bed, and a few sutures may be taken to approximate the fascia over the surface of the kidney if desired. If there is any question of angulation of the splenic vein, it may be desirable once again to determine the pressure with the manometer to make certain that the anastomosis is patent and functioning satisfactorily.

The region of the tail of the pancreas is inspected for evidence of bleeding, and all bleeding points, regardless of where encountered, are carefully clamped and ligated. A small biopsy of the margin of the liver is taken for microscopic evaluation of the extent of the liver pathology.

CLOSURE. The wound is closed in layers without drainage.

POSTOPERATIVE CARE. These patients require intensive postoperative care for several days. Hypotension should be avoided with the careful monitoring of hourly urine output and central venous pressure, combined with serial hematocrits. Four units of whole blood should be held in reserve at all times. Careful fluid and salt balance is maintained by the administration of glucose, water, and electrolyte solutions on the basis of daily requirements and accurate intake and output records. If fluid retention has been a postoperative problem, close attention must be paid to serum electrolyte and albumin levels and to urinary salt excretion.

Atelectasis is a common postoperative complication. The patient should be encouraged to cough, deep-breathe, and ambulate early. Tracheal suctioning may be required to clear the respiratory tract. If pleural effusions develop, thoracentesis may be necessary. If this problem recurs, administration of salt-poor albumin of whole blood, salt restriction, diuretics, or digitalis may be indicated.

Oral feedings may be instituted after bowel activity has returned. This is confirmed by an oral dye marker, such as carmine red, and one ounce of mineral oil. Initial feedings should be low in salt and protein, until the patient has proved that further additions can be tolerated, as evidenced by the absence of ascites or edema and stabilization of the blood urea nitrogen. Antibacterial agents or diuretics may be added if signs of mild ammonia intoxication or fluid retention occur. In the absence of postoperative gastrointestinal hemorrhage, severe ammonia intoxication is infrequent. If severe, it is necessary to withdraw all protein feedings, maintain caloric intake with intravenous glucose, and cleanse the bowel by the use of castor oil, antibacterials administered through a nasogastric tube, and enemas. The administration of arginine and glutamic acid has been shown to be of value in reducing blood ammonia levels temporarily. Other recommended measures to combat ammonia intoxication include hemodialysis and the use of ion exchange resins. It should be remembered that because of the shunt and the impaired liver function, the blood urea nitrogen level may not accurately reflect the amount of protein breakdown. Determination of the blood ammonia level is frequently of more value in this regard. After symptoms have cleared and the blood ammonia level has been stabilized, oral feedings are again instituted, with gradual increases of the protein to 50 to 75 Gm. daily. The antibacterial agents are withdrawn slowly. To date, the postoperative complication of hepatic encephalopathy appears minimal following selective distal splenorenal decompression of esophageal varices.

Postoperative hemorrhage may be due to peptic ulceration or bleeding from esophageal or gastric varices. To decrease the possibility of ulceration, prophylactic antacids should be started when oral feedings are instituted. If conservative measures fail to control hemorrhage, it may be necessary to initiate esophageal compression by the insertion of a special tube and balloon. The blood in the gastrointestinal tract should be cleared by cathartics, enemas, and antibacterial drugs. As time elapses after the shunt, the prognosis with a hemorrhage improves as the liver function improves.

Recurrent ascites may indicate thrombosis of the shunt. If persistent, bed rest, salt restriction, and diuretics may be used. Progressive ascites is usually due to advanced and progressive cirrhosis. Administration of salt-poor albumin may be useful, and steroids have been recommended.

PLATE CXXII   SPLENORENAL SHUNT

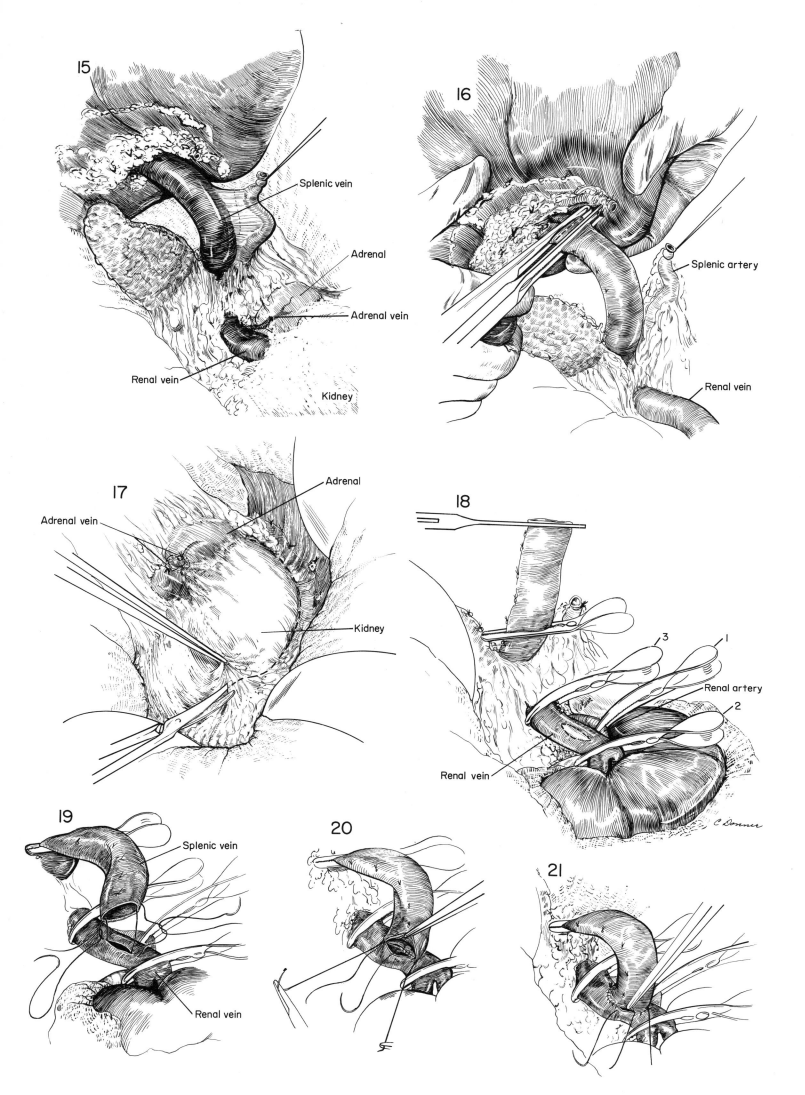

15

Splenic vein

Adrenal

Adrenal vein

Renal vein

Kidney

16

Splenic artery

Renal vein

17

Adrenal

Adrenal vein

Kidney

18

3

1

Renal artery

2

Renal vein

19

Splenic vein

Renal vein

20

21

PLATE CXXIII · SPLENORENAL SHUNT (WARREN)

INDICATIONS. See Plate CXV. The selective distal splenorenal shunt may be indicated in the patient with cirrhosis of the liver without ascites but with evidence of a major hemorrhage from gastro-esophageal varices. The incidence of encephalopathy may be reduced in comparison with other types of portosplenic shunts.

PREOPERATIVE PREPARATION. These patients require detailed evaluation of both hepatic and renal function. Severe ascites contraindicates the procedure. A needle biopsy of the liver evaluates the basic hepatic disease as well as determines the possibility of acute inflammation caused by alcoholic hepatitis or chronic aggressive hepatitis and cirrhosis. The operation is indefinitely delayed if acute alcoholic hepatitis is found. Except in emergency situations, the hepatic disease should be considered stable before the shunting procedure is planned.

Preoperative angiography is essential to establish the presence or absence of portal venous flow to the liver, as well as to obtain a gross estimate of the volume of portal venous perfusion of the liver. The preoperative angiogram also determines the patency and anatomical relationships of the mesenteric, splenic, and portal veins.

In addition, catheterization and visualization of the left renal vein is essential. This permits a preoperative evaluation of the structural relationships and reveals any abnormalities or unusual anatomical variations that would make the proposed shunt impossible.

ANESTHESIA. See Plate CXVI.

POSITION AND OPERATIVE PREPARATION. See Plate CXIX.

INCISION AND EXPOSURE. The surgeon should be familiar with the anatomy of the portal system as well as the veins draining the stomach **(Figure 1).** Maximum exposure is essential. A long midline incision extending from the xiphoid to well below the navel may be used **(Figure 2).** The incision may be made to the right of the navel, and the umbilical vein and round ligament to the liver ligated and divided. A long bilateral curved incision extending from the midrectus on the right to well out into the left flank may be preferred, with the left side of the patient elevated 10 to 15 degrees.

Gentle and limited exploration of the opened abdomen is indicated to avoid possible hemorrhage from delicate torn vascular adhesions. The region of the needle puncture for a splenoportogram is inspected for evidence of continued bleeding. Some type of hemostatic material may be required to control the oozing site. A biopsy of the liver should be taken.

The gastrocolic omentum is detached from the transverse colon, including the flexures, without ligating the gastroepiploic vessels. This ensures good access to the pancreas and, in turn, the splenic and renal veins. Adhesions between the posterior wall of the stomach and the pancreas are divided. The right gastroepiploic vein is divided in the infraduodenal region to interrupt the collateral venous drainage from the pancreas or intestine through the gastroepiploic system **(Figure 3).** The right gastroepiploic artery may also be included in the mass ligature of the veins below the pylorus. Neither the left gastroepiploic nor the short gastrosplenic veins should be interrupted, in order to maintain their pathway for drainage of the varices of the upper end of the stomach and lower esophagus.

The peritoneum along the inferior margin of the body of the pancreas is divided with special attention to possible injury to the underlying inferior mesenteric vein **(Figure 4).** Gentle finger and instrument dissection may be used to mobilize the margin and the posterior surface of the body of the pancreas over a distance of 8 to 10 cm. The vascular retroperitoneal tissue over the superior mesenteric vein is carefully cleared away with good visualization of the several branches, and the middle colic, coronary vein, etc., are visualized. Careful dissection is continued until the junction with the splenic vein has been clearly established. It may be easier to identify the medial portion of the splenic vein first and follow it into the inferior mesenteric vein. The inferior mesenteric vein is not always a reliable landmark, since it may empty into the superior mesenteric vein instead of into the splenic vein.

PLATE CXXIII   SPLENORENAL SHUNT (WARREN)

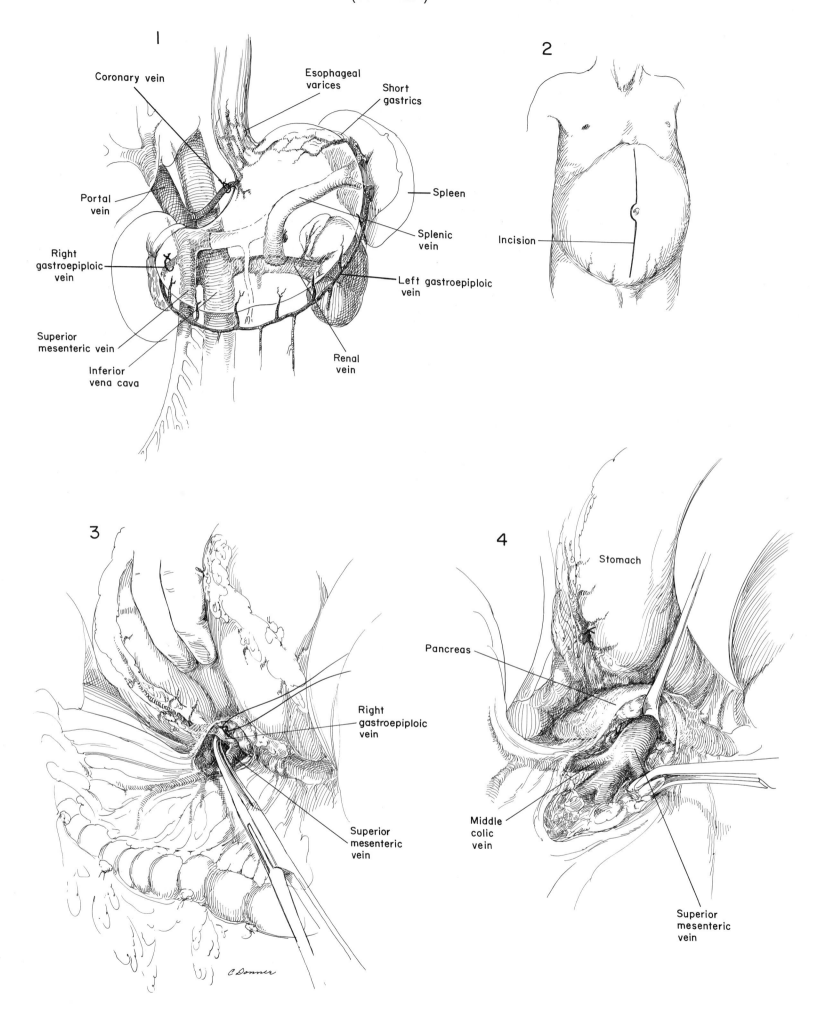

1

Coronary vein

Esophageal varices

Short gastrics

Portal vein

Spleen

Splenic vein

Right gastroepiploic vein

Left gastroepiploic vein

Superior mesenteric vein

Inferior vena cava

Renal vein

2

Incision

3

Right gastroepiploic vein

Superior mesenteric vein

4

Stomach

Pancreas

Middle colic vein

Superior mesenteric vein

C Donner

PLATE CXXIV · SPLENORENAL SHUNT (WARREN)

DETAILS OF PROCEDURE. Freeing up the splenic vein from its pancreatic bed is usually quite difficult because of the many delicate veins draining into it from the pancreas. Less bleeding may occur if the vessels are ligated on both the pancreatic and the splenic vein side before they are divided. Before division of the splenic vein, its relationship to the superior mesenteric vein should be confirmed, and the inferior mesenteric vein should be ligated **(Figure 5).** The mobilization of the splenic vein may be enhanced by dividing it near where it joins the superior mesenteric vein **(Figure 6).** However, before the splenic vein is divided, the renal vein should be completely prepared for the anastomosis, since occlusion of the splenic vein increases the pressure in the retroperitoneal collateral veins in this area. Freeing up the renal vein requires delicate dissection in order to avoid injury to venous collaterals with resultant blood loss. The left adrenal vein and the gonadal vein are usually divided and securely ligated to ensure safe and adequate mobilization of the renal vein. It is not necessary to clamp the renal artery, since there are adequate venous collaterals to decompress the kidney despite complete occlusion of the renal vein.

Following division of the splenic vein, the mesenteric end is carefully closed with a continuous 00000 arterial suture **(Figure 7).** The coronary vein is sometimes readily visualized at this point and may be divided and ligated just above its junction with the portal vein.

One of the major problems in this procedure is the proper placement of the anastomosis between the splenic and left renal veins. The mobility of the splenic vein may need to be increased if it does not easily reach the renal vein at the proposed site of anastomosis. A wide anastomosis is essential, without twisting or angulation of the splenic vein. Following application of an occluding vascular clamp, an oblique window is excised from the wall of the renal vein, unless its size is especially small. The end of the splenic vein is tailored obliquely to fit the opening in the renal vein. It may be wise to split the end of the splenic vein for a centimeter or more to avoid tension on the anastomosis. The splenic vein may be anchored to the renal vein at either angle, and the posterior anastomosis is completed with a continuous 00000 arterial suture **(Figure 8).** Interrupted 00000 arterial sutures are used in the anterior closure to minimize the split-like character of the orifice and allow increased distensibility of the anastomosis **(Figure 9).** The noncrushing vascular clamp on the splenic vein is released just before the final anterior suture is tied to remove air and flush out any blood clots. A suture is taken around the coronary vein above the lesser curvature if it has not been ligated from below. This suture may include the left gastric artery, but it should be far enough away from the stomach to avoid accidental inclusion of the vagus nerves.

Venous pressures are taken in the splenic, renal, and inferior mesenteric veins. Early elevations in pressure are common but do not indicate occlusion of the anastomosis, providing the splenic vein feels soft to compression and palpation reveals a thrill within the renal vein. The field of operation is carefully rechecked for evidence of uncontrolled oozing or active bleeding. The completed venous drainage outlet is illustrated in **Figure 10.**

CLOSURE. Because of the possibility of ascites, a water-tight closure of the peritoneum and general wound closure without drainage are indicated. Retention sutures are frequently employed. These should not penetrate the peritoneal cavity because of the danger of leakage from ascites.

POSTOPERATIVE CARE. Nasogastric suction should be continued after operation. Some gastric bleeding can be anticipated during the early postoperative period. Fluids during operation as well as in the early postoperative period should be restricted, with regulation based on hourly urinary output determinations and central venous pressure measurements. Diuretic therapy may be indicated to ensure a good urinary output. Ascites is a more likely development following this procedure than following other types of portosystemic decompression.

PLATE CXXIV   SPLENORENAL SHUNT (WARREN)

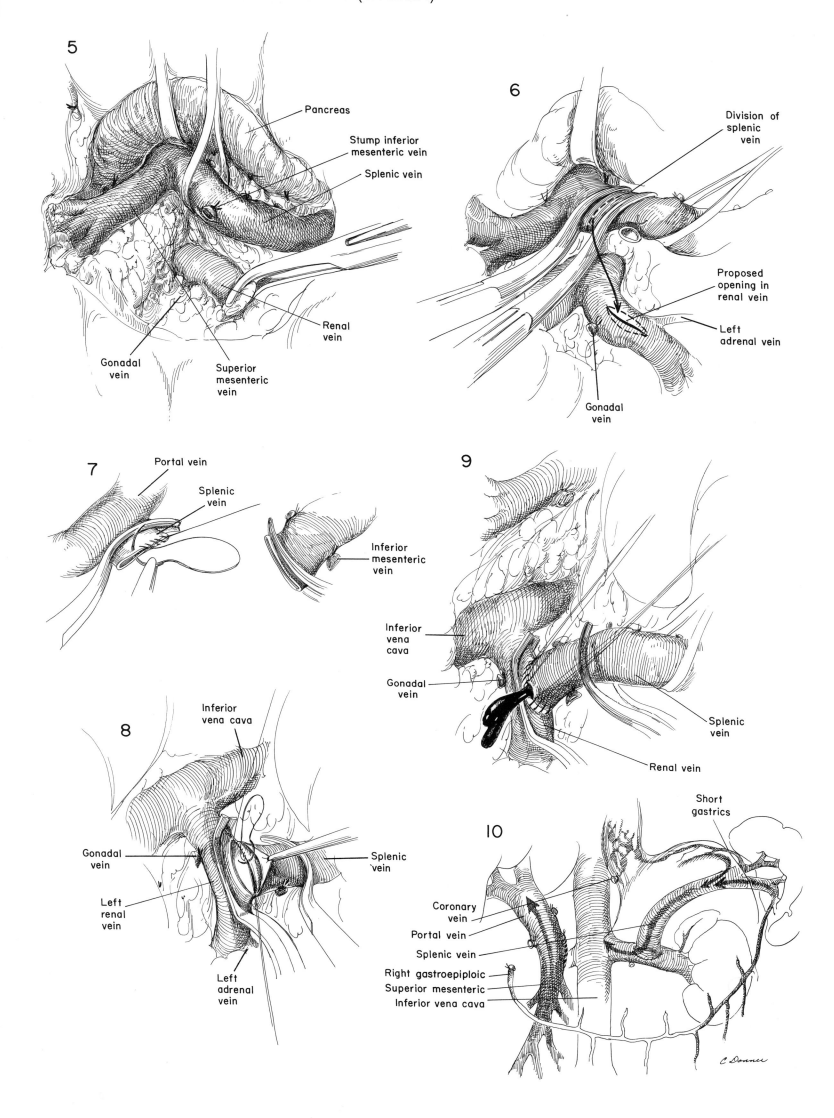

5

Pancreas

Stump inferior
mesenteric vein

Splenic vein

Renal vein

Gonadal
vein

Superior
mesenteric
vein

6

Division of
splenic
vein

Proposed
opening in
renal vein

Left
adrenal vein

Gonadal
vein

7

Portal vein

Splenic
vein

Inferior
mesenteric
vein

9

Inferior
vena
cava

Gonadal
vein

Splenic
vein

Renal vein

8

Inferior
vena cava

Gonadal
vein

Left
renal
vein

Left
adrenal
vein

Splenic
vein

10

Short
gastrics

Coronary
vein

Portal vein

Splenic vein

Right gastroepiploic

Superior mesenteric

Inferior vena cava

C Donner

PLATE CXXV · MESOCAVAL SHUNT (CLATWORTHY)

INDICATIONS. See Plate CXV.

PREOPERATIVE PREPARATION AND ANESTHESIA. See Plate CXVI.

POSITION. The patient is placed supine on the table, and the feet and legs are snugly wrapped or fitted with full-length elastic stockings. A lumbar pad is of value in deep incisions.

OPERATIVE PREPARATION. The skin is prepared and draped in the routine manner after placement of a secure venous catheter for infusion of medications and blood or measurement of central venous pressure.

INCISION AND EXPOSURE. A midline or right paramedian incision, extending from two fingerbreadths below the xiphoid to the lowermost abdominal skin crease, is preferred **(Figure 1).** Troublesome bleeding and interference with collateral return flow through the superficial and deep epigastric plexi are thus avoided. A careful abdominal examination, liver biopsy, and portal venography should precede the performance of the shunt.

DETAILS OF PROCEDURE. The mesocaval shunt requires the presence of either a satisfactory superior mesenteric vein free of venitis and thrombosis or a venous lake in the area of the confluence of the mesenteric and splenic veins. After the abdomen has been opened, the transverse colon is retracted upward as a fan, and one or more large middle colic venous tributaries leading into the depths of the edematous mesentery can be seen. The superior mesenteric vein can be further identified by palpation or, if one wishes, by the passage of a small catheter through a venous tributary into the vein, although in our experience this is rarely necessary.

A T-shaped incision is made at the line where the superior mesenteric vein and the mesentery of the transverse colon meet. The vertical arm of the T is extended downward over the expected site of the superior mesenteric vessels **(Figure 2).** The mesenteric vein is then dissected from its bed for approximately 5 cm. Small tributaries on the right side are individually ligated and divided with 000000 silk. Larger tributaries on the left side are preserved. The difficulty of this dissection varies with the degree of lymphatic engorgement and is most tedious in patients who have extrahepatic portal bed block **(Figure 3).** Small saline-softened umbilical tapes or heavy silk ligatures are then placed around the major unligated tributaries leading into the dissected segment of the superior mesenteric vein **(Figure 4).** These tapes are left loose, and exposure of the vena cava is begun.

Although the vena cava may be approached directly from the anterior position, we have preferred to continue with our initially recommended method of approaching it by mobilizing the right colon mesially. As one dissects the mesocolon from the gutter, multiple collateral vessels are encountered which must be individually clamped and ligated **(Figure 5).**

PLATE CXXV   MESOCAVAL SHUNT (CLATWORTHY)

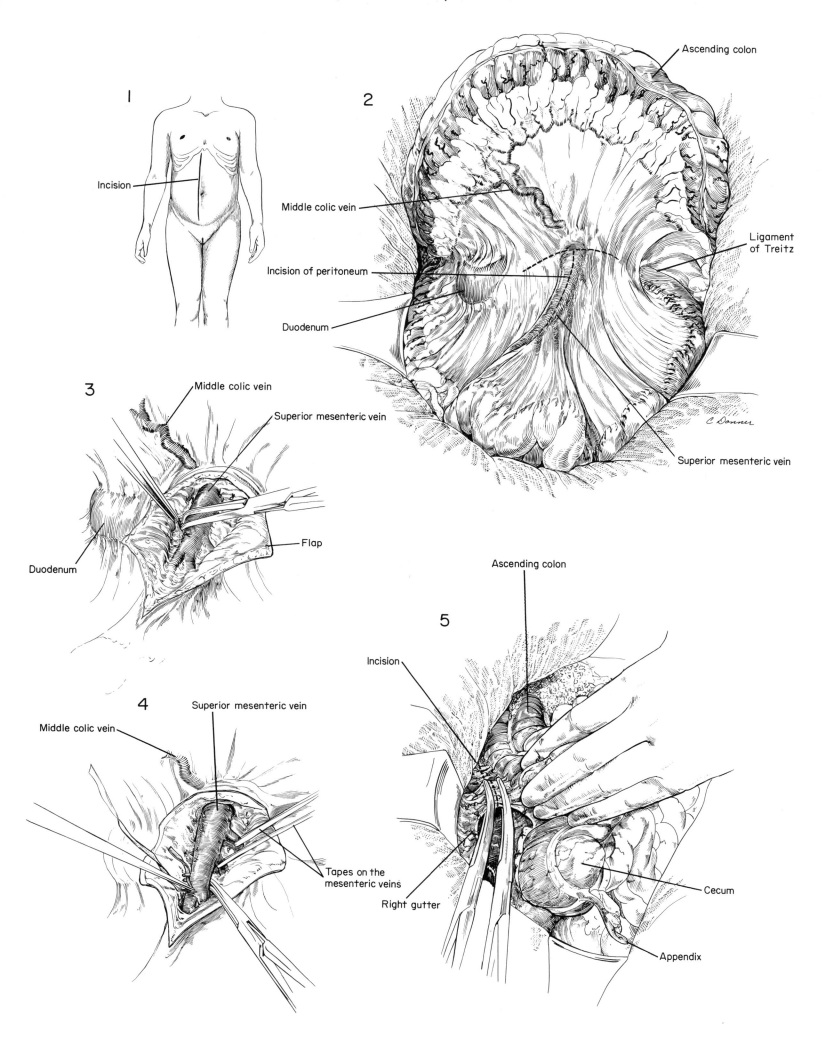

1

Incision

2

Ascending colon

Middle colic vein

Ligament of Treitz

Incision of peritoneum

Duodenum

Superior mesenteric vein

3

Middle colic vein

Superior mesenteric vein

Duodenum

Flap

4

Middle colic vein

Superior mesenteric vein

Tapes on the mesenteric veins

5

Ascending colon

Incision

Right gutter

Cecum

Appendix

PLATE CXXVI · MESOCAVAL SHUNT (CLATWORTHY)

DETAILS OF PROCEDURE (*Continued*). The lower pole of the kidney, the right ureter, and gonadal vessels are exposed and identified **(Figure 6).** As the duodenum has been swept upward by gentle traction, the inferior vena cava and the right side of the aorta come into view. Although in some cases the vena cava below the duodenum is sufficiently long to assure an adequate anastomosis without tension below the duodenum, it is wiser to dissect out the common iliacs on either side as well as the vena cava **(Figure 7).** To accomplish this, tapes are placed around the vena cava and below the right renal vein and the right common iliac at the confluence of the iliacs. The vena cava may then be rolled toward the left, exposing the large lumbar vein (or veins) and the large vertebral veins, all of which may be individually ligated and divided under direct vision. Laceration or bleeding from the vena cava, if such should inadvertently occur, should be dealt with by fine silk suture lest constriction of the vena cava or extensive damage to the shunt segment ensue **(Figure 8).**

It is then necessary to produce a tunnel through the often thick, fibrotic retroperitoneal tissue lying between the superior mesenteric vein and the vena cava. In **Figure 9** one can view the surgeon's left hand placed just beneath and behind the previously dissected superior mesenteric vein and holding the right colon anteriorly. This woody, lymph-filled vascular tissue must be carefully cored out to provide an adequate tunnel for two fingers to slip freely through the new opening **(Figure 9).** A curved bulldog vascular clamp is applied to the vena cava near the newly formed tunnel **(Figure 10).** The tape is removed after the vena cava has been mobilized. The right iliac vein is occluded adjacent to the vena cava by two pairs of straight vascular forceps. They are applied obliquely as shown in **Figure 10.** The vein is divided between the pairs of forceps. The forceps nearest the cut end of the vein are removed, assuring a small cuff of vein, which is closed by an interlocking suture of 00000 or 000000 black silk. The proximal side is similarly closed **(Figures 10 and 11).**

PLATE CXXVI   MESOCAVAL SHUNT (CLATWORTHY)

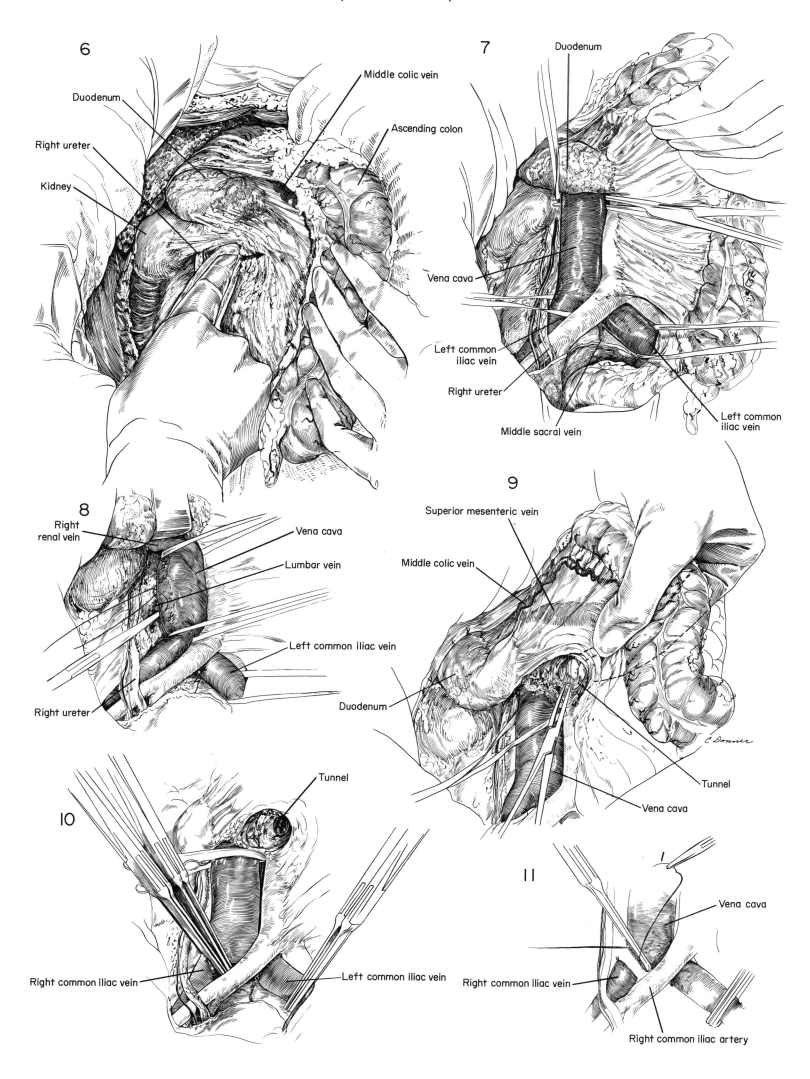

6

Duodenum

Right ureter

Kidney

Middle colic vein

Ascending colon

7

Duodenum

Vena cava

Left common iliac vein

Right ureter

Middle sacral vein

Left common iliac vein

8

Right renal vein

Right ureter

Vena cava

Lumbar vein

Left common iliac vein

9

Superior mesenteric vein

Middle colic vein

Duodenum

Tunnel

Vena cava

10

Tunnel

Right common iliac vein

Left common iliac vein

11

Vena cava

Right common iliac vein

Right common iliac artery

C Donner

PLATE CXXVII · MESOCAVAL SHUNT (CLATWORTHY)

DETAILS OF PROCEDURE (*Continued*). In contrast, the left common iliac is clamped by a pair of vascular forceps as far distally as possible without reaching a major bifurcation. The left iliac vein is divided proximal to the clamps, and the distal end of this is closed **(Figure 12)**. Stay sutures are placed in the divided left common iliac and drawn through the previously prepared tunnel in the mesentery **(Figure 12)**. Diluted heparin is used to wash out and thereafter intermittently bathe the opened venous segments as the vessels are brought into proximity of the superior mesenteric vein without tension, angulation, or torsion. In **Figure 13** a schematic diagram of the proposed anastomosis is shown.

The shunt segment is now tailored by excising any unneeded segment of the left common iliac vein or distal inferior vena cava **(Figure 14)**. Excessive length produces kinking, obstruction, and subsequent thrombosis. Too short a segment will produce compression obstruction as the vessel passes around the duodenum. Occasionally, a tunnel between the pancreas and superior surface of the duodenum has been required to obviate this latter complication when the common iliac has not been available as an extension to the canal segment.

Vascular clamps and snugging-up of the previously placed tapes on the superior mesenteric vein provide a bloodless field through which, on the right posterior lateral surface, an incision may be made and a segment of the superior mesenteric vein may then be excised **(Figure 15)**. After placing stay sutures, A and B, a running 000000 black silk vascular suture row is placed from inside the anastomotic orifice and tied outside the vessel **(Figure 16)**. A third stay suture, C, is placed **(Figure 17)** and, in smaller children, a second anterior over-and-over suture is then completed **(Figure 18)**. The use of the triangulation technic ensures an unconstricted orifice, and breaking the suture line at three points in children encourages anastomotic growth when very fine silk is used. In young children we have preferred 0000000 silk for this anastomosis **(Figure 19)**.

Completion of the anastomosis is followed by removal, first, of the vena caval clamp, then the proximal mesenteric, and finally, the distal mesenteric clamp and tapes **(Figure 20)**. Reperitonealization of the anastomotic area is desirable, and generally the right gutter is also closed with running 000 or 0000 chromic catgut, although this is probably less necessary.

Interposition Mesocaval Shunt (Drapanas)

The interposition mesocaval shunt requires the presence of a satisfactory superior mesenteric vein, which is isolated as previously described. The inferior vena cava is next exposed through the base of the right transverse mesocolon, allowing direct visualization of the anterior inferior vena cava without incurring troublesome bleeding from retroperitoneal venous collaterals. The third and fourth portions of the duodenum, including the ligament of Treitz, are mobilized to prevent possible obstruction by the graft.

The knitted dacron graft used for the shunt should be between 19 and 22 mm. in diameter, with length tailored to avoid undue tension as well as redundancy, usually about 6 or 7 cm.

The caval anastomosis is done first. A partially occluding atraumatic vascular clamp is placed on the inferior vena cava midway between the renals and the iliac bifurcation. A small button of caval wall is removed. With 00000 synthetic vascular suture first the lateral half of the anastomosis is completed and then the medial half. The graft is now trimmed to adequate length and turned clockwise 30 degrees to approximate the normal course of the superior mesenteric vein. The superior mesenteric vein is completely occluded, and anastomosis is performed on the posterior aspect of the vein. The medial side is closed first from within the lumen, and then the lateral side is completed. Completion of the shunt is followed by removal of clamps from the superior mesenteric vein. It has proved both unnecessary and unsafe to tunnel grafts between duodenum and pancreas because of the risk of pancreatitis.

CLOSURE. The abdomen is closed in layers without drainage.

POSTOPERATIVE CARE. Nasogastric or gastrostomy decompression is indicated in these patients to avoid abdominal distention, which may lead to occlusion of the anastomosis in the early postoperative period. Following the cessation of ileus the patient may be started on a diet of increasing caloric value, with protein added sparingly over a period of two weeks in cirrhotic patients. Ambulation with elastic hose or compression bandages is desirable if hypostatic edema of the lower extremities is to be avoided. In the absence of preexisting thrombophlebitis, a leg edema is rare.

PLATE CXXVII   MESOCAVAL SHUNT (CLATWORTHY)

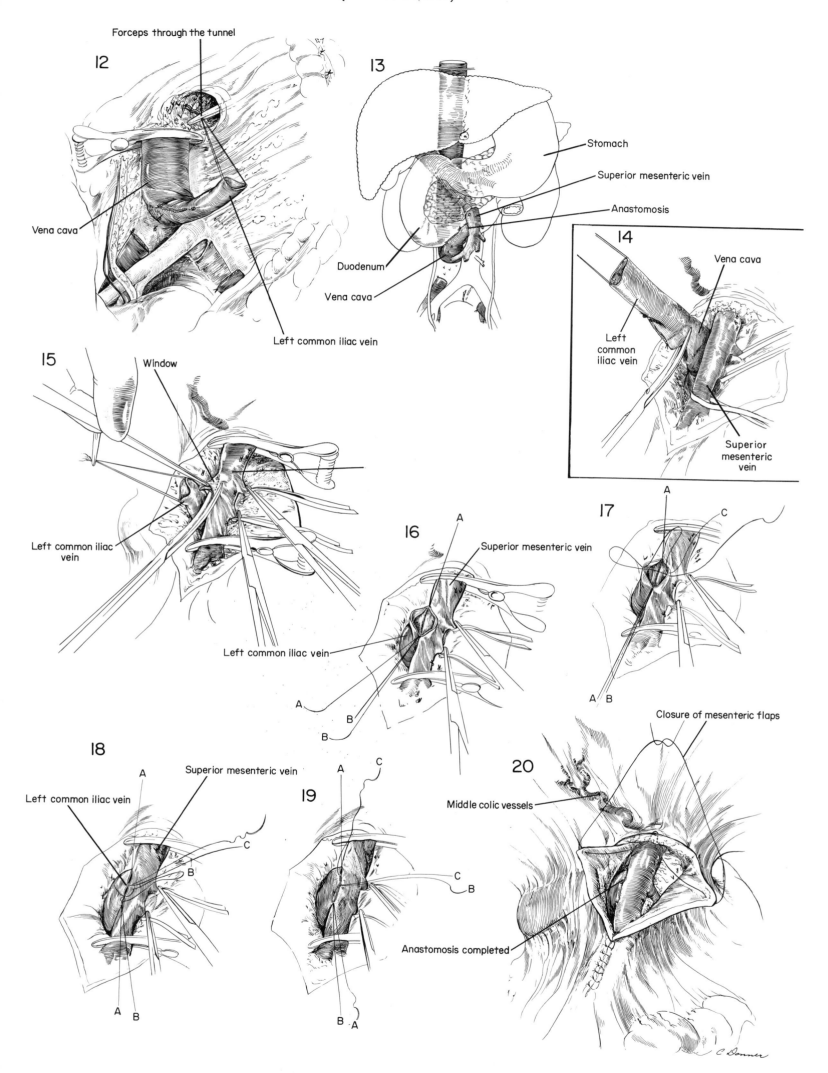

12 Forceps through the tunnel

Vena cava

Left common iliac vein

13 Stomach

Superior mesenteric vein

Anastomosis

Duodenum

Vena cava

14 Vena cava

Left common iliac vein

Superior mesenteric vein

15 Window

Left common iliac vein

16 Superior mesenteric vein

Left common iliac vein

A
B
B

17 A
C

A B

18 Left common iliac vein

A

Superior mesenteric vein

C
B

A B

19 A C

C
B

B A

20 Closure of mesenteric flaps

Middle colic vessels

Anastomosis completed

C. Donner

GYNECOLOGIC PROCEDURES

GYNECOLOGIC SYSTEM–ROUTINE FOR ABDOMINAL PROCEDURES

Gynecologic procedures, in general, carry less risk than other abdominal surgical procedures, because of the minimal amount of manipulative trauma to the alimentary tract and the patient's generally good condition. However, the same general principles apply here as in any major surgical operation, and the patient's condition must be carefully appraised.

PREOPERATIVE PREPARATION. The obese patient should diet sufficiently to obtain a more normal weight before elective procedures are done. Secondary anemia is corrected preoperatively by whole blood transfusions. Urinary complaints are investigated by analysis of the catheterized specimen of urine and endoscopic and roentgenographic studies when indicated. The lower colon is cleansed with saline enemas. Chemotherapy and/or antibiotics are given when sepsis is suspected.

ANESTHESIA. A general anesthetic is satisfactory. Spinal or continuous spinal anesthesia may be used if desired; however, women usually prefer to be rendered unconscious.

The perineal and pubic hair is clipped or shaved.

POSITION. After the induction of the anesthesia, the patient is moved to the lithotomy position for the necessary operative preparation. The table is shifted to a slight reverse Trendelenburg position to facilitate the cleansing of the perineum and vagina with an iodine-containing liquid cleanser, preliminary to catheterization of the bladder. Pelvic examination under anesthesia and often a diagnostic dilatation and curettage as a general principle precede a pelvic laparotomy.

Upon completion of the vaginal procedures, the patient is shifted to the Trendelenburg position. Before this position is continued, the patient's respirations must be entirely satisfactory to the anesthetist.

The maximum illumination of the pelvis must be assured by adjusting both the source of light and the operating table. The surgeon stands on the patient's left side.

INCISION AND EXPOSURE. A lower midline incision is made, and the lower angle of the wound is held open with a superficial retractor to permit a free dissection of the fascia until the location of the midline is absolutely ascertained.

Some operators prefer the transverse incision (Pfannenstiel), which is a convex incision following the lines of skin cleavage just above the symphysis. The upper skin flap may be dissected from the underlying rectus muscles, and the usual midline incision of the muscles and peritoneum is made. When an extensive exposure is required, it is better to cut across the recti muscles as in any classic transverse incision. An increased number of blood vessels require ligation by this approach in comparison to the midline incision.

The fascia is incised, scissors being employed at the lower angle of the wound to open the fascia down to the symphysis. The medial edge of presenting rectus muscles is freed and pushed laterally with the scalpel handle. Although few bleeding points are encountered in the midline, all must be clamped and tied or controlled by electrocoagulation. As the incision progresses, its margins are protected with gauze pads. The peritoneum, before being incised, is picked up to one side of the urachus with toothed forceps alternately by the operator and first assistant as in any abdominal procedure. The urachus, which can be seen through the peritoneum as a thickened cord, should be left intact, since it is not only vascular but also exerts traction on the bladder, inviting its accidental opening.

A self-retaining retractor is substituted for the superficial ones, although deep individual retractors may be used if a shifting of the retraction is desired to procure the maximum exposure as the operation progresses.

Careful inspection is made to ensure that no intestine is caught in the retractor. When a self-retaining retractor is used, the smooth blade is inserted and the whole apparatus is adjusted.

Unless contraindicated by infection in the pelvis, a general abdominal exploration is carried out. The surgeon moistens his hands in saline and systematically explores the abdomen and finally the pelvis. His operative note should contain a description of his findings, especially the presence or absence of gallstones. If a large uterus with extensive involvement by fibromyomata is encountered, it may be advantageous to deliver the uterus through the abdominal opening before the introduction of the self-retaining retractor. Large ovarian cysts, if benign and not grossly adherent, may be reduced in size by aspirating their contents through a trocar, great caution being used to avoid contamination from their contents. A tenaculum is applied to the fundus of the uterus to maintain traction while the intestines are walled off completely with several moist gauze pads. To accomplish this, the intestines are retracted upward by the left hand as the gauze pads are directed inward and upward by long, smooth dressing forceps, the packing being continued until the pelvis is free of small intestine. Douglas' pouch is emptied of intestines, other than the rectosigmoid, and is likewise protected by a gauze pack. To maintain these packs in position, a moderate-sized smooth retractor is sometimes placed in the midline at the umbilical end of the wound.

CLOSURE. Before the abdominal closure is started, the site of operation is finally inspected for evidence of bleeding, and the appendix may be removed. A search is made for needles, instruments and sponges, and a correct count reported before closure is started. The sigmoid and omentum are returned to the pelvis. After the peritoneum has been closed, the patient is gradually returned from the Trendelenburg position to horizontal to release tension on the wound and to permit stabilization of the blood pressure while the patient is under the surgeon's direct supervision. A routine abdominal wall closure is done without suturing the rectus muscles (Plates VI, VII, and VIII). The surgeon inspects, as well as palpates, the fascial suture line to ensure a secure closure. Retention sutures are necessary only in the presence of marked obesity, carcinoma, secondary anemia, chronic cough, or infection. A flat film of the abdomen may be taken to confirm that all foreign bodies have been removed before the patient is transferred to the recovery room.

POSTOPERATIVE CARE. The patient, when conscious, is placed in a comfortable position. The fluid balance is maintained with two liters of glucose and distilled water the day of operation and each day thereafter until fluids and food are tolerated by mouth. Saline and potassium are added after the first day, if constant gastric suction is necessary, to accurately replace the losses by gastric intubation. The measured blood loss during surgery should be replaced if it exceeds 500 ml. and the pulse is elevated. Additional blood or plasma may be required to replace the internal losses from the raw surfaces remaining after extensive procedures. Antibiotics or chemotherapy are not routinely administered.

The patients should be ambulated at the earliest possible time, but no later than the morning after surgery. Ambulation in contrast to dangling is advisable. The inlying Foley catheter is removed in 24 to 72 hours, depending upon the extent of the surgical procedure and the patient's general condition. If repeated catheterizations are necessary, the amount of residual urine should be recorded and the catheterized specimens should be examined for evidence of infection. If infection is found, the appropriate antibiotic or chemotherapy is given. Sterile perineal care is observed. Stockings of cotton webbing are worn, especially if varicose veins are prominent or there has been a past history of phlebitis. Skin sutures are removed on the fifth to seventh day after operation.

PLATE CXXVIII · ABDOMINAL PANHYSTERECTOMY

INDICATIONS. Panhysterectomy is most commonly performed for benign lesions of the uterus, such as fibromyomata, or malignant disease of the body of the uterus. Other indications include adenomyosis, extensive pelvic inflammatory disease, and early malignant lesions of the cervix.

PREOPERATIVE PREPARATION. See Gynecologic System—Routine for Abdominal Procedures.

POSITION. See Gynecologic System—Routine for Abdominal Procedures.

OPERATIVE PREPARATION. Routine vaginal and abdominal preparation is given. The patient is catheterized, and an indwelling Foley catheter, size F 20 to 22, is inserted without inflation of the balloon. The catheter is anchored by adhesive tape to the inner aspect of the thigh. The vagina is cleansed with a soap solution containing hexachlorophene or an iodine-containing liquid cleanser. Usually, a diagnostic dilatation and curettage is performed. A large gaping cervix may be closed with several catgut sutures. No sponge is placed in the vagina.

INCISION AND EXPOSURE. See Gynecologic System—Routine for Abdominal Procedures.

DETAILS OF PROCEDURE. Whenever conditions will permit, the uterus is pulled upward toward the umbilicus, exposing the anterior uterine surface and allowing incision of the peritoneum at the cervicovesical fold **(Figure 1).** This loose layer of peritoneum is picked up with toothed forceps and incised transversely with scissors close to its attachment to the uterus **(Figure 2).** The operator thrusts his index finger through the avascular posterior leaf of the broad ligament and pushes downward and upward until the round ligament and fallopian tube are isolated **(Figure 2).** Should a very large and irregularly shaped uterus be encountered, it may be easier to apply clamps to the adnexa and to start from above downward. It is noteworthy that in many instances the cervicovesical fold of the peritoneum may be incised, and the adnexa may be more easily isolated, even in the presence of an interligamentous fibroid, after the finger has been passed through the avascular space. The top of the broad ligament is grasped in Ochsner clamps along with the tube, the ovarian ligament, and the round ligament adjacent to the uterus, and all are divided between the clamps with a knife. A transfixing suture of 0 chromic catgut on a Ferguson needle is taken to include a bite of the round ligament and a superficial bite of the peritoneum adjacent to the fallopian tube **(Figure 3).** An additional transfixing suture may be added proximal to the first one.

When it is desirable to remove a tube or ovary or both, they are grasped with forceps and reflected medially **(Figure 4).** When the pelvic structures are considerably relaxed, a pair of Ochsner clamps may be applied to include the infundibulopelvic and round ligaments, saving as much of the round ligaments as possible **(Figure 4).** A suture of 00 chromic catgut is taken in the round ligament and the edge of the peritoneum adjacent to the ovarian vessels to prevent retraction of the contents. Usually, curved clamps are applied in pairs beneath the tube and ovary, especially if it appears that there is too much tissue for one clamp **(Figure 4),** and their contents are tied with mattress sutures.

After the vessels have been tied, only the Ochsner clamps on either side of the fundus remain **(Figure 5).** Removal of clamps from the field allows sufficient space for the operator to examine the region of the cervix with two fingers to determine its length and the position of the bladder. The bladder is pushed gently downward with gauze over the right index finger **(Figure 5),** although in some instances it may be advantageous to divide the tissue over the cervix with scalpel or scissors until a definite avascular cleavage plane is established. The blunt dissection should be in the midline directly over the cervix, or troublesome bleeding will be induced from tearing vessels in the broad ligament. This permits the bladder to be directed forward and downward until the operator's thumb and index finger can compress the vaginal wall below the cervix **(Figure 6).**

PLATE CXXVIII   ABDOMINAL PANHYSTERECTOMY

1

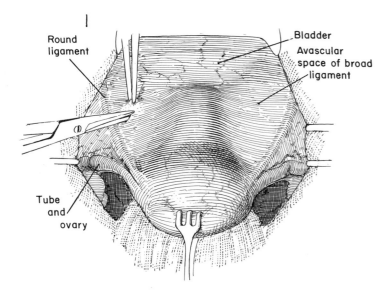

Round
ligament

Bladder

Avascular
space of broad
ligament

Tube
and
ovary

2

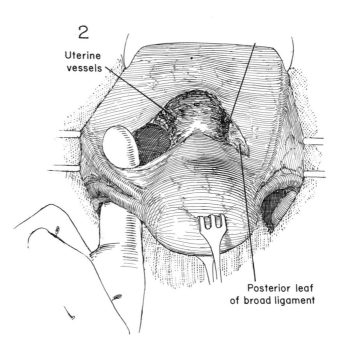

Uterine
vessels

Posterior leaf
of broad ligament

3

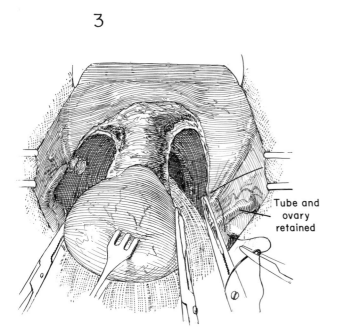

Tube and
ovary
retained

Alternate Method   4

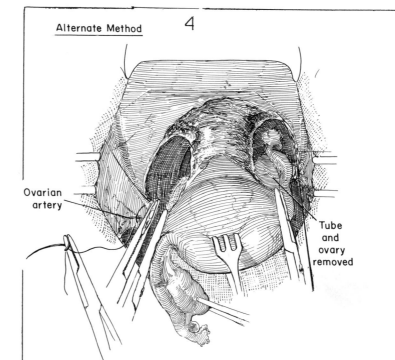

Ovarian
artery

Tube
and
ovary
removed

5

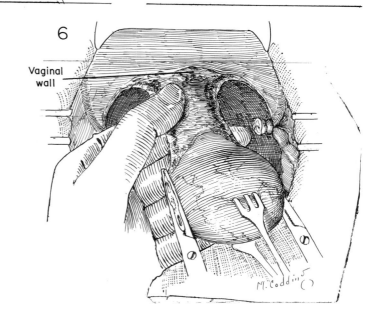

Freeing of
bladder from
cervix

6

Vaginal
wall

M. Coddins

PLATE CXXIX · ABDOMINAL PANHYSTERECTOMY

DETAILS OF PROCEDURE (*Continued*). The surgeon then holds the uterus forward and makes certain that the rectum is not adherent to the upper portion of the vagina. Should the rectum be adherent to the vagina, it is carefully dissected free to avoid possible injury. This is a critical step, if panhysterectomy is to be performed. After the relative position of the ureters has been identified, a moist gauze sponge is loosely introduced into Douglas' pouch to prevent any intestine from coming into the field of operation. The uterus is rotated slightly to the right in preparation for the application of a pair of straight Ochsner clamps **(Figure 7)**. The straight Ochsner clamps are applied from the side at a 45-degree angle to the cervix to include a small bite of cervical tissue. The second clamp is similarly placed 1 to 2 cm. above the first to ensure a good pedicle of tissue for double ligation. The Ochsner clamps should never be directed downward parallel to the cervix because of possible injury to the ureters. Now the uterine vessels are divided with curved scissors **(Figure 7)**. If the uterus is quite large, a half-length clamp may be affixed to the vessels higher up along its wall to prevent troublesome back bleeding as the uterine vessels are divided. The paracervical tissue is divided with scissors to a point just below the level of the lower Ochsner clamp to develop a free pedicle that can be easily tied **(Figure 8)**. Failure to carry the incision beyond the tip of the distal clamp hinders accurate ligation of the uterine vessel pedicle, and troublesome bleeding results. A transfixing suture, a, of 0 chromic catgut is tied as the lower Ochsner clamp is slowly withdrawn, and a second similar suture, b, is taken toward the severed end of the pedicle **(Figure 8)**. The development of an easily tied pedicle that includes the uterine artery is one of the most important steps in abdominal panhysterectomy.

After a similar procedure has been concluded on the opposite side, Teale forceps are applied to the paracervical tissue between the cervix and the uterine vessels **(Figure 9)**. The peritoneum on the posterior cervical wall is incised and pushed gently downward. Frequently, the incision is carried entirely around the anterior wall of the cervix, and the tissues are pushed downward by blunt dissection until the cervix can be palpated easily through the thinned-out vaginal vault. With the uterus held forward, an incision is made into the vagina posteriorly, and the vaginal vault is divided by long, curved scissors as close to the cervix as possible, or desirable, according to the disease present **(Figure 10)**. As the cervix is freed from the vaginal vault, the anterior and posterior vaginal walls are approximated with Teale forceps to include the full thickness of the vaginal wall as well as its posterior peritoneal surface **(Figure 11)**. The lateral angles of the vaginal vault are first closed with figure-of-eight sutures of 00 chromic catgut on cervix cutting needles **(Figure 12)**, following which one or more sutures are placed at the middle portion to ensure complete closure and hemostasis. The most likely place for troublesome bleeding is at the outer angles of the vagina near the ligated uterine vessels. Accurate and firm closure of the angles is imperative **(Figure 12)**. Upward traction on the vaginal vault is released to determine if any bleeding occurs.

PLATE CXXIX   ABDOMINAL PANHYSTERECTOMY

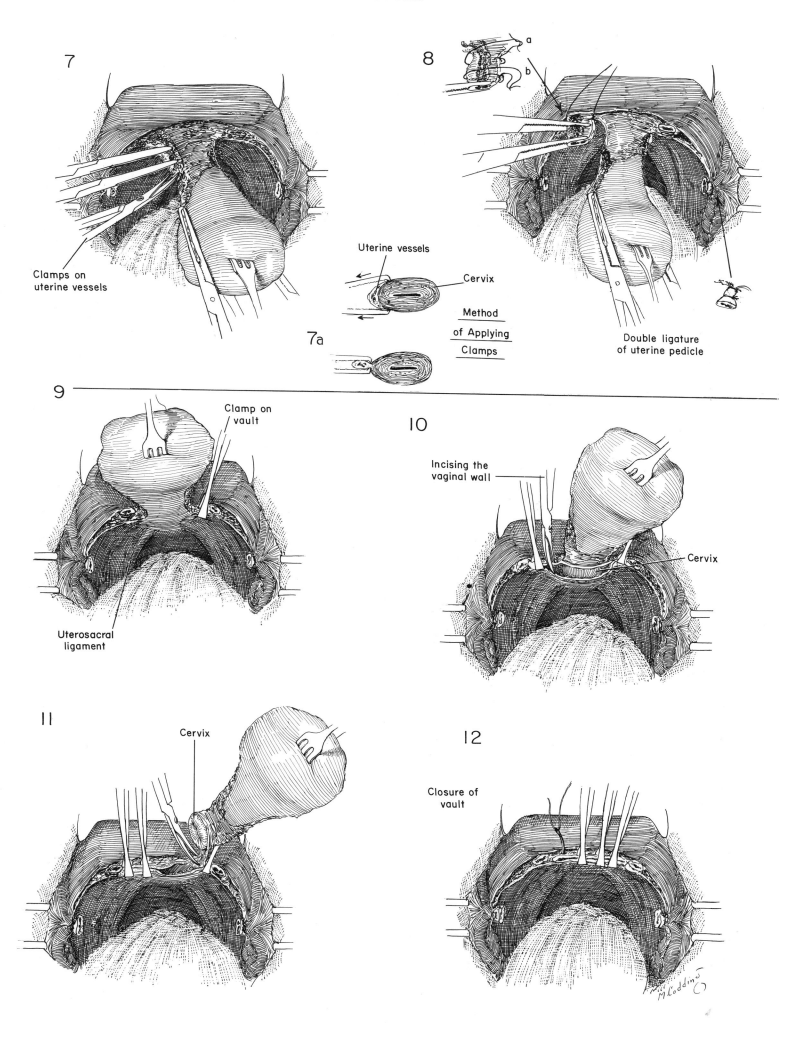

7

Clamps on
uterine vessels

7a

Uterine vessels

Cervix

Method
of Applying
Clamps

8

a

b

Double ligature
of uterine pedicle

9

Clamp on
vault

Uterosacral
ligament

10

Incising the
vaginal wall

Cervix

11

Cervix

12

Closure of
vault

M Codding

PLATE CXXX · ABDOMINAL HYSTERECTOMY

Supravaginal Hysterectomy

DETAILS OF PROCEDURE. For supravaginal hysterectomy the operation proceeds as in panhysterectomy, except that the uterine arteries may be ligated higher on the cervix. The cervix is kept in position by Teale or similar forceps at the lateral margins and is divided at the level of the internal os, or lower **(Figure 13).** In the very unusual instance where the cervix is to remain, the cervical canal must be completely coned out from above for microscopic examination. The procedure also serves as prophylaxis against the eventual development of carcinoma in the retained cervical stump. The cervical stump is then closed transversely by placing with a cervix cutting needle several figure-of-eight sutures of 0 chromic catgut, one in each lateral angle and one or more in the central portion. These sutures must be placed sufficiently deep to secure complete hemostasis **(Figure 14).**

In either panhysterectomy or supravaginal hysterectomy, the sutures, a and b, used to close the cervix or vaginal vault, are left long and retracted upward **(Figure 15).** The ends of the initial suture, c, in the uterosacral ligaments are uncut, since they are used secondarily to anchor the flap of vesical peritoneum backward to the approximated uterosacral ligaments, ensuring a complete covering of all raw surfaces by peritoneum. The sutures, a and b, are released from tension to permit a final inspection for bleeding; and, if necessary to control bleeding, additional sutures are taken. Usually, two or more additional sutures are required. When the field is dry, a long single crown suture of 0 chromic catgut is placed to form the pelvic sling **(Figure 16).** A bite is taken first in the adnexa on the right side adjacent to the point of ligature, then through the right uterine vessel pedicle, the closed vaginal vault or cervix, the left uterine vessel pedicle, and finally in the adnexa on the left side **(Figure 16).** This suture, when tied, pulls the round ligaments together in the midline. In instances where there is too much tension on the supporting structures, the round ligaments are anchored to the lateral margins of the cervix. The long ends of the sutures, a and b, are in turn threaded through a needle, and a small bite of the round ligament is taken on either side to give further support to the vaginal vault **(Figure 17).** The suture, c, is rethreaded and brought forward to include a bite of the bladder flap **(Figure 17),** which is pushed backward as the suture is tied, completely covering all raw surfaces **(Figure 18).** Large raw surfaces left after removal of diseased adnexa are covered by approximating the peritoneum with interrupted chromic catgut sutures. Douglas' pouch is inspected for evidence of bleeding from the vaginal vault. Routine appendectomy is performed unless contraindicated by the patient's poor condition.

CLOSURE. The sigmoid and omentum are returned to Douglas' pouch. After the peritoneum is closed, the patient is returned to the horizontal position while the fascia and skin are being closed. A patient should never be taken from high Trendelenburg position and placed directly in bed. Only in rare instances is drainage instituted either through the vagina or abdominal wall.

POSTOPERATIVE CARE. See Gynecologic System—Routine for Abdominal Procedures.

PLATE CXXX   ABDOMINAL HYSTERECTOMY

13

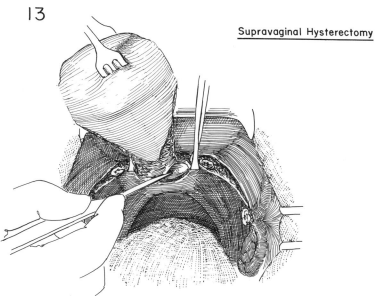

Supravaginal Hysterectomy

Conization of cervix

14

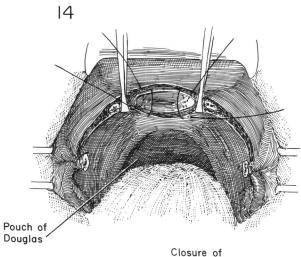

Pouch of
Douglas

Closure of
cervical stump

15

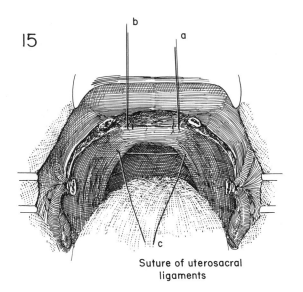

b

a

c

Suture of uterosacral
ligaments

16

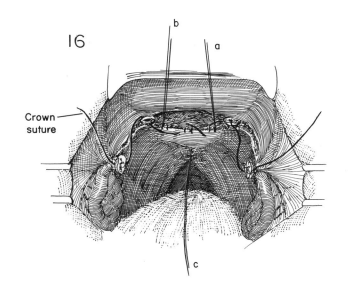

b

a

Crown
suture

c

17

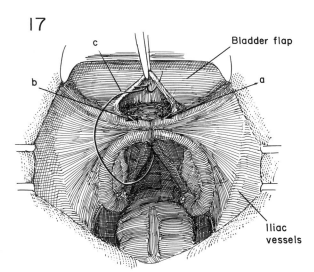

c

b

Bladder flap

a

Iliac
vessels

18

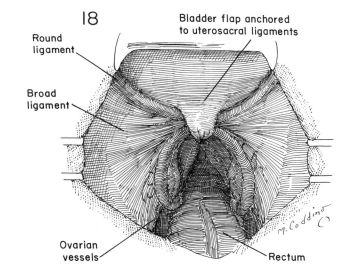

Round
ligament

Broad
ligament

Bladder flap anchored
to uterosacral ligaments

Ovarian
vessels

Rectum

M. Coddino

PLATE CXXXI · SALPINGECTOMY—OOPHORECTOMY

INDICATIONS. Removal of the fallopian tubes or ovaries is indicated for inflammatory involvement of the adnexa which cannot be relieved by the use of conservative measures, including chemotherapy and/or antibiotics, for ovarian cysts, neoplasms, ectopic pregnancies, and so forth. Removal of the ovaries may be indicated in the treatment of carcinoma of the breast occurring in premenopausal patients. Bilateral oophorectomy is advised by some as a desirable procedure in extensive carcinoma of the rectum because of the susceptibility of the ovaries to tumor transplantation from lesions of the gastrointestinal tract. In the absence of malignancies every effort should be made to conserve even remnants of functioning ovarian tissue in the younger age groups.

PREOPERATIVE PREPARATION. See Gynecologic System—Routine for Abdominal Procedures. The skin is covered by a sterile transparent plastic drape.

OPERATIVE PREPARATION. The skin is prepared in the routine manner. The surgeon stands on the patient's left side.

INCISION AND EXPOSURE. See Gynecologic System—Routine for Abdominal Procedures. In the presence of extensive pelvic inflammation, the intestines are often attached to the adnexa by adhesions that must be separated either by blunt or sharp dissection. Haste and roughness must be avoided. By placing the adhesions on tension as they are cut, the cautious surgeon almost always can develop a cleavage plane between the diseased adnexa and the other structures. The intestines are carefully pushed aside and packed away with warm, moist gauze pads, or placed in a plastic bag and moistened with warm saline. The freed adnexa are then held upward with a half-length clamp **(Figure 1)**.

A. Salpingectomy

DETAILS OF PROCEDURE. The uterus is held forward either by a tenaculum applied to the round ligament adjacent to the uterus **(Figure 1)** or by a fine catgut suture through the fundus **(Figure 7)**. The mesosalpinx is clamped with a sufficient number of half-length clamps, usually three pairs, to include its entire length **(Figure 3)**. To avoid possible interference with the blood supply of the ovary, the line of incision is kept near the fallopian tube **(Figure 1)**. As an alternative, the mesosalpinx may be saved by controlling the blood supply with three or four mattress sutures meticulously placed to avoid vessels when the needle is introduced **(Figure 2)**. Regardless of the method used to divide the mesosalpinx, an elliptical incision is made through the thickness of the uterine wall to cone out the interstitial portion of the fallopian tube **(Figure 4)**. Ligatures are applied to the mesosalpinx as the half-length clamps are removed **(Figure 4)**. Brisk bleeding is usually encountered from the cornual artery, which may

be controlled either by placing deep mattress sutures through this area before the interstitial portion of the tube is excised, or by manual compression while mattress sutures are placed **(Figure 5)**. These mattress sutures, which are tied together gently to avoid tearing the friable uterine wall, effect an even approximation and give complete hemostasis.

B. Salpingectomy and Oophorectomy

DETAILS OF PROCEDURE. When both the tube and ovary are to be removed, incision is made as shown in **Figure 6**. The half-length clamps are applied to the infundibulopelvic ligament, which includes the ovarian vessels **(Figure 6)**. The vessels are divided and tied with a transfixing suture of 0 chromic catgut. The leaves of the broad ligament are either doubly clamped with curved, half-length clamps and divided with scissors or scalpel, or ligated with mattress sutures carefully placed so that the needle does not penetrate any of the thin-walled veins between its layers. Now the interstitial portion of the fallopian tube is removed as shown in **Figure 4**. The appearance of the raw surfaces of the broad ligaments after the tubes and one ovary have been resected is shown in **Figure 7**. Where the ovarian ligament is quite long, allowing the ovary to prolapse into the pelvis, it is shortened by means of a mattress suture through the posterior wall of the uterus and the ovarian ligament, thus suspending the ovary adjacent to the posterior wall of the uterus. The raw surfaces remaining after the excision of part or all of the uterine adnexa must be covered with peritoneum. Moreover, some type of suspension is usually advisable after removal of a part or all of the adnexa.

When the suspension of the uterus is to be carried out after removing the tube or tube and ovary, the shortening of the round ligament may be accomplished so as to cover a great part of the raw surface with peritoneum on either side. If the cut surface of the infundibulopelvic ligament is not covered, a suture, s, which includes a bite of the peritoneum on either side of the pedicle, is taken to enfold it with peritoneum **(Figure 8)**. When another type of suspension is used, the raw surfaces remaining after removal of part or all of the adnexa may be buried by approximating the peritoneum over them, using either a continuous suture, a, of 00 chromic catgut, or interrupted mattress sutures, b **(Figure 9)**. Several interrupted sutures are placed to approximate the posterior wall of the fundus of the uterus and the round ligaments **(Figure 8)**. Three or four sutures are usually sufficient to ensure an adequate midline suspension of the uterus and at the same time to cover most of the raw surfaces.

CLOSURE. See Gynecologic Procedures—Routine for Abdominal Procedures.

POSTOPERATIVE CARE. See Gynecologic Procedures—Routine for Abdominal Procedures.

PLATE CXXXI   SALPINGECTOMY—OOPHORECTOMY

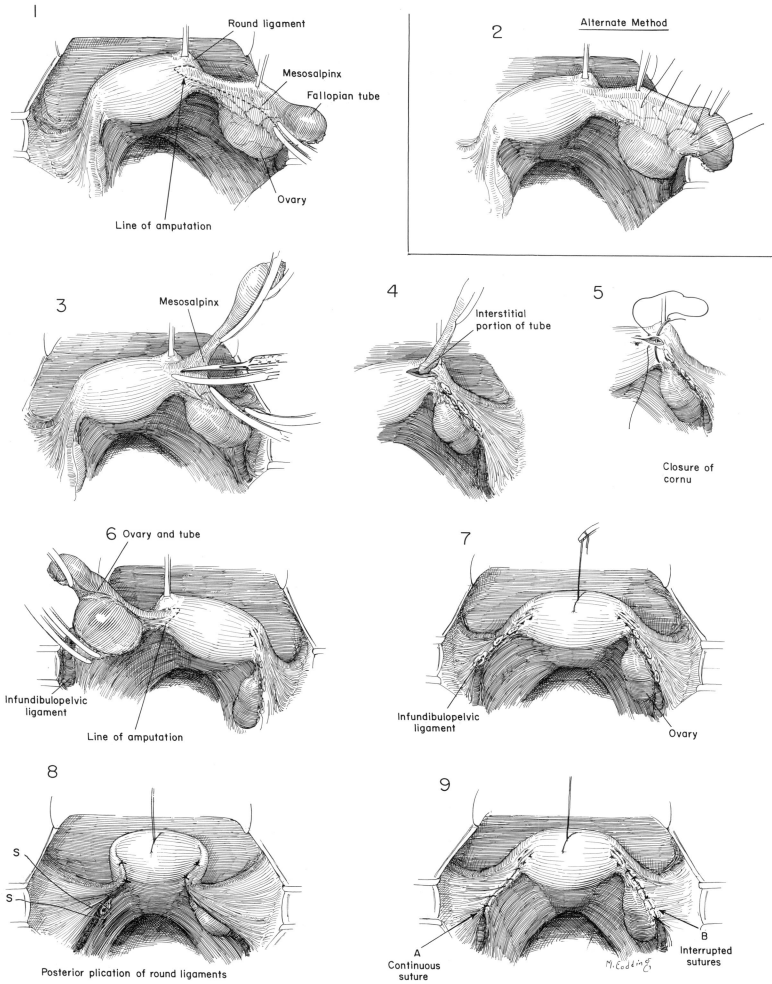

1

Round ligament

Mesosalpinx

Fallopian tube

Ovary

Line of amputation

2   Alternate Method

3   Mesosalpinx

4   Interstitial portion of tube

5   Closure of cornu

6   Ovary and tube

Infundibulopelvic ligament

Line of amputation

7   Infundibulopelvic ligament   Ovary

8   S

S

Posterior plication of round ligaments

9   A   Continuous suture   B   Interrupted sutures

M. Eadding

PLATE CXXXII · MYOMECTOMY—SUSPENSION OF UTERUS

A. Myomectomy

INDICATIONS. Panhysterectomy should not be carried out in young women of childbearing age until it has been definitely ascertained that the fibroid tumors cannot be enucleated and the uterus cannot be satisfactorily reconstructed. A preliminary dilatation and curettage is essential to determine any irregularities of the uterine cavity due to submucous fibroids.

PREOPERATIVE PREPARATION. See Gynecologic System—Routine for Abdominal Procedures.

ANESTHESIA. See Gynecologic System—Routine for Abdominal Procedures.

DETAILS OF PROCEDURE. The pelvis is walled off by gauze, and the uterus is held upward with one suture through the fundus **(Figure 1)** or by half-length clamps applied to the round ligaments. An incision is made through the uterine wall down to the underlying glistening tumor **(Figure 1)**, which is grasped with a forceps and shelled out of its bed with curved scissors or by blunt dissection **(Figure 2)**. In cases of pedunculated fibroids an elliptical incision is made about the base of the pedicle to include as much of the uterine wall as is indicated. Because of the friability of the uterine wall, vessels cannot be clamped and tied but are controlled by deep interrupted sutures of 00 chromic catgut, so placed that they do not enter the uterine cavity **(Figure 3)**. A second layer of interrupted sutures of 00 chromic catgut may be used to approximate the peritoneal surface **(Figure 3)**. Some type of round-ligament suspension is advisable to maintain the uterus in a physiologic position.

CLOSURE. See Gynecologic System—Routine for Abdominal Procedures.

POSTOPERATIVE CARE. See Gynecologic System—Routine for Abdominal Procedures.

B. Suspension of Uterus (Modified Gilliam Suspension)

INDICATIONS. Suspension of the uterus is rarely advised as a primary operation. This procedure is routinely performed after part or all of the adnexa has been removed.

PREOPERATIVE PREPARATION. See Gynecologic System—Routine for Abdominal Procedures.

ANESTHESIA. See Gynecologic System—Routine for Abdominal Procedures.

POSITION. See Gynecologic System—Routine for Abdominal Procedures.

OPERATIVE PREPARATION. See Gynecologic System—Routine for Abdominal Procedures.

INCISION AND EXPOSURE. See Gynecologic System—Routine for Abdominal Procedures. The anterior rectus sheath is carefully cleaned of subcutaneous fat for 3 to 4 cm. on either side of the midline.

DETAILS OF PROCEDURE. About 3 to 4 cm. above the lower angle of the wound, a blunt-nosed half-length or a specially designed clamp is passed under the anterior sheath of the rectus muscle, beyond its outer edge **(Figure 5)**. By rotating the handle of the clamp laterally, its nose is pushed through the aponeurosis of the muscle until the clamp presents beneath the peritoneum. The clamp is advanced slowly underneath the peritoneum as the blades are alternately opened and closed, separating the tissues. With the abdominal wall retracted to permit direct visualization, the nose of the clamp is directed toward the internal ring and is pushed through the peritoneum just anterior to the ring **(Figure 6)**; or, if the surgeon prefers, it may be pushed through the internal ring between the layers of the broad ligament out on the round ligament. The region of the internal ring can be seen better when the round ligament is held under moderate traction. Each round ligament in turn is grasped firmly in the tip of a clamp about 3 to 4 cm. from the fundus and is pulled up through the abdominal wall beneath the anterior sheath of the rectus muscle **(Figure 7)**. The round ligaments are then fastened to the anterior rectus sheaths by interrupted sutures of 0 catgut, which are passed in through the anterior rectus sheath, through each arm of the loop of round ligament, and finally out through the rectus sheath adjacent to the point of entry **(Figure 7)**. These sutures are not tied until both round ligaments have been pulled upward and a symmetric position of the fundus is obtained.

Some prefer to further support the uterus by taking a bite in each uterosacral ligament near the uterus. Three or four such sutures when tied tend to shorten the uterosacral ligaments **(Figure 4)**. Before the abdominal wall is closed, the margins of the wound are retracted sufficiently so that the operator may assure himself that the fallopian tubes were not angulated in shortening the round ligaments. The sigmoid and omentum are returned to Douglas' pouch.

PLATE CXXXII   MYOMECTOMY—SUSPENSION OF UTERUS

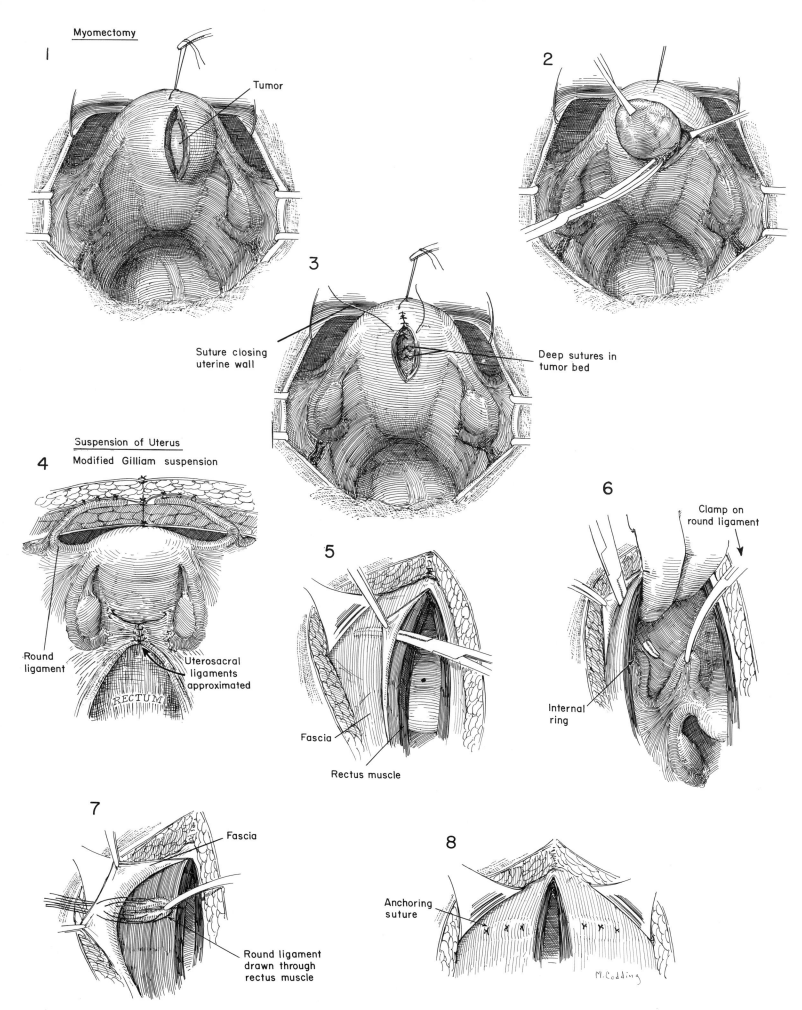

Myomectomy

1

Tumor

2

3

Suture closing
uterine wall

Deep sutures in
tumor bed

Suspension of Uterus

4   Modified Gilliam suspension

Round
ligament

Uterosacral
ligaments
approximated

RECTUM

6

Clamp on
round ligament

5

Fascia

Rectus muscle

Internal
ring

7   Fascia

Round ligament
drawn through
rectus muscle

8

Anchoring
suture

M. Codding

GYNECOLOGIC SYSTEM—ROUTINE FOR VAGINAL PROCEDURES

PREOPERATIVE PREPARATION. In the majority of instances the patient has employed vaginal douches over a prolonged period. The symphysis, perineum, and adjacent surfaces are shaved or clipped carefully the night before operation. That same night a cleansing enema is given and may be followed by an antiseptic vaginal douche. Any secondary anemia which may be present is corrected by blood transfusions. Whole blood should be available at the time of operation.

ANESTHESIA. Light general or intravenous anesthesia may be employed. Saddle block or low spinal anesthesia is very satisfactory.

POSITION. Vaginal procedures are carried out in the lithotomy position (Plate CXXXIII, **Figure 1**). After the induction of the anesthesia, the legs of the patient are raised simultaneously to avoid straining the sacroiliac joints and are fixed in stirrups. Whenever possible, the legs are elevated upward and backward to permit the assistant to be nearer the field of operation. The hips of the patient are lifted well beyond the margin of the table to provide better exposure, to avoid unnecessary wetting of the patient, and to make possible the later introduction of the weighted speculum. The operating table is turned so that the natural light falls upon the field. Additional artificial light, if necessary, is focused on the introitus.

OPERATIVE PREPARATION. The surgeon or first assistant, wearing sterile gloves, places a folded sterile towel over the symphysis of the patient as a guide to the upper margin of the field to be cleaned and a similar towel under the buttocks. The vulvae and adjacent skin areas are scrubbed from above downward with pairs of gauze sponges held in the gloved hands. The gauze sponges are saturated with a solution of water and a detergent with germicidal action, such as iodine-containing scrub. In all, five pairs of sponges are used, each being discarded as it comes in contact with the anus. The vaginal vault is cleansed with six saturated sponges held in long sponge forceps. Four dry sponges are used to remove excess solution from the vaginal vault. The cleansed skin is blotted dry with a sterile towel. The anus is excluded from the operative area by the use of a spray-on adhesive compound and the application of a piece of sterile, transparent plastic film. The footboard of the operating table is raised to a convenient level and serves as an instrument table for the surgeon (Plate CXXXIII, **Figure 1**). A sterile, fenestrated perineal drape is applied, and the bladder is emptied by catheterization.

EXPOSURE. Adequate exposure is obtained by introducing into the vagina either a weighted vaginal speculum or a self-retaining retractor, depending on the type and location of the operation to follow. A thorough pelvic examination is made as a preliminary to the technical procedures.

POSTOPERATIVE CARE. After the completion of the operation, the vagina and perineum are cleaned with sponges moistened with saline or a mild antiseptic solution. A sterile perineal pad is then applied and held in position by a T binder. When constant bladder drainage is desired, a retention catheter is inserted and held by adhesive tape anchored to a labium. The drapes are removed, and the legs are withdrawn slowly and simultaneously from the stirrups to prevent disturbances in blood pressure and straining of the sacroiliac joints.

The immediate postoperative care is similar to that following abdominal procedures with certain added perineal precautions. If there is no indwelling catheter, the patient should be catheterized every four to six hours, depending upon the fluid intake, until she voids voluntarily. Even then, daily catheterization is done until residual urine is less than 50 ml. Patients on constant drainage, although more comfortable, are more subject to cystitis because of the constant trauma to the trigone; therefore, on these patients fluids are forced, bladder irrigations are performed several times daily, and suitable chemotherapy or antibiotics are given. The catheter is removed in three to five days. The daily intake and output are recorded for at least 72 hours.

Blood transfusion may be indicated, depending upon the blood loss at the time of operation. If sepsis is suspected or any cystitis exists, chemotherapy and/or antibiotics are usually indicated.

After every voiding or defecation the perineum is cleaned with cotton pledgets moistened with an antiseptic solution, and a sterile pad is reapplied. The nurse must be careful to do all wiping away from the site of operation. This strict sterile perineal precaution is continued for approximately one week. Warm, moist applications or dry heat to the perineum may be used to relieve pain. Sitz baths promote comfort and stimulate voiding. A stool-softening preparation is given starting either the evening of surgery or the first postoperative morning. After procedures requiring extensive tissue dissection, bowel movements are delayed for three to five days. Douches of saline or a mild antiseptic solution may be started after eight to ten days unless vaginal bleeding is initiated. The principle of early ambulation is followed unless contraindicated by the patient's general condition.

PLATE CXXXIII · ANTERIOR COLPORRHAPHY

INDICATIONS. The decision to perform anterior colporrhaphy depends upon the size of the cystocele, the severity of the symptoms, the associated pathology, and the age of the patient in relation to childbearing. Surgery may be advised if the cystocele is large but asymptomatic, or if it produces symptoms such as a protruding vaginal mass, pelvic pain or pressure, incomplete emptying of the bladder, cystitis, or urinary incontinence. The repair is delayed in women who may have more children, unless the symptoms are marked. Surgery is also delayed until the cystitis is brought under control by medical therapy, which should include the drugs indicated from the bacterial sensitivity studies done on cultures of the urine.

The complaint of urinary incontinence requires additional study, especially if previous correction by surgery has been indicated. Evaluation by cystoscopy and urethrocystograms is indicated. The key features demonstrated by the urethrocystogram include: (1) descent and funneling of the bladder base in the upright position which are aggravated by straining; (2) loss of the posterior urethrovesical angle; and (3) downward as well as backward rotation of the urethra in the more severe cases. Mild degrees of incontinence may respond to pubococcygeal exercises, but those with pronounced difficulty require skillful repair. The routine repair of a cystocele cannot be depended upon to correct urinary incontinence. Basically, there are four different types of operative procedures that may be used to correct this difficulty: (1) plication of the bladder neck muscle and fascia; (2) return of the urethra and bladder neck to a normal position behind the symphysis; (3) lengthening or curving of the urethra; and (4) musculofascial slings placed beneath the urethra.

ANESTHESIA. See Gynecologic System—Routine for Vaginal Procedures.

PREOPERATIVE PREPARATION. See Gynecologic System—Routine for Vaginal Procedures.

POSITION. The lithotomy position is used with the table in slight reverse Trendelenburg **(Figure 1).**

OPERATIVE PREPARATION. See Gynecologic System—Routine for Vaginal Procedures.

EXPOSURE AND INCISION. The assistant stands on the patient's left side to the right of the operator so that his left hand is available for sponging and his right is free to handle instruments. The state of the pelvic organs is determined by careful bimanual examination before the plastic procedures. A self-retaining Friedman's retractor is attached to the labia in a reverse position to give lateral retraction **(Figure 2),** and a weighted vaginal speculum is placed to further the exposure. The cervix is grasped on either side by long bullet or Teale forceps and is brought into view. Only moderate traction is used in order that the supporting structures of the uterus will not be overstretched **(Figure 3).** A routine dilatation and curettage is carried out. With the tissues on traction to facilitate separation of the layers, a small transverse incision, which is made at the junction of the vaginal mucosa and the cervix, is carried down to the cervical tissue dividing the vesicovaginal fascia **(Figure 4).**

DETAILS OF PROCEDURE. The surgeon elevates the upper part of the vaginal mucous membrane with mouse-toothed forceps in the left hand and inserts straight Mayo dissecting scissors immediately beneath to prevent injury to the bladder **(Figure 5).** The blades are alternately opened and closed to develop a cleavage plane and are progressively advanced upward. The anterior vaginal wall is maintained under moderate tension between the Teale forceps on the cervix and the one applied at the midline about 1 to 2 cm. below the urethra **(Figure 5).** With each angle of the vaginal flap held with hemostats or Allis forceps, the mucous membrane is divided in the midline with straight scissors to a point 1 to 2 cm. below the urethral meatus **(Figure 6).** In the presence of a large cystocele, the lower portion of the mucous membrane is more easily divided before the cleavage plane has been entirely freed up to the Teale forceps beneath the urethra. While the clamps on the mucous membrane are held taut, the bladder is freed laterally from the vaginal flaps by the use of gauze over the surgeon's index finger; however, it should not be separated so far laterally that troublesome bleeding results. The bladder wall is grasped with thumb forceps to place the surrounding tissues under tension, and the uterovesical ligament is divided with scissors, the points of which are directed toward the cervix to avoid puncturing the bladder **(Figure 7).** The bladder itself is pushed up off the cervix by blunt gauze dissection, usually with very little bleeding if the proper cleavage plane has been developed and the dissection maintained on the midline over the cervix **(Figure 8).** Occasionally, it may be necessary to incise the bladder pillars to permit this upward displacement. The index finger of the left hand is placed behind the vaginal flap to aid in developing the proper cleavage plane, and the vesicovaginal fascia is now dissected from the mucous membrane first with a knife **(Figure 9)** or scissors.

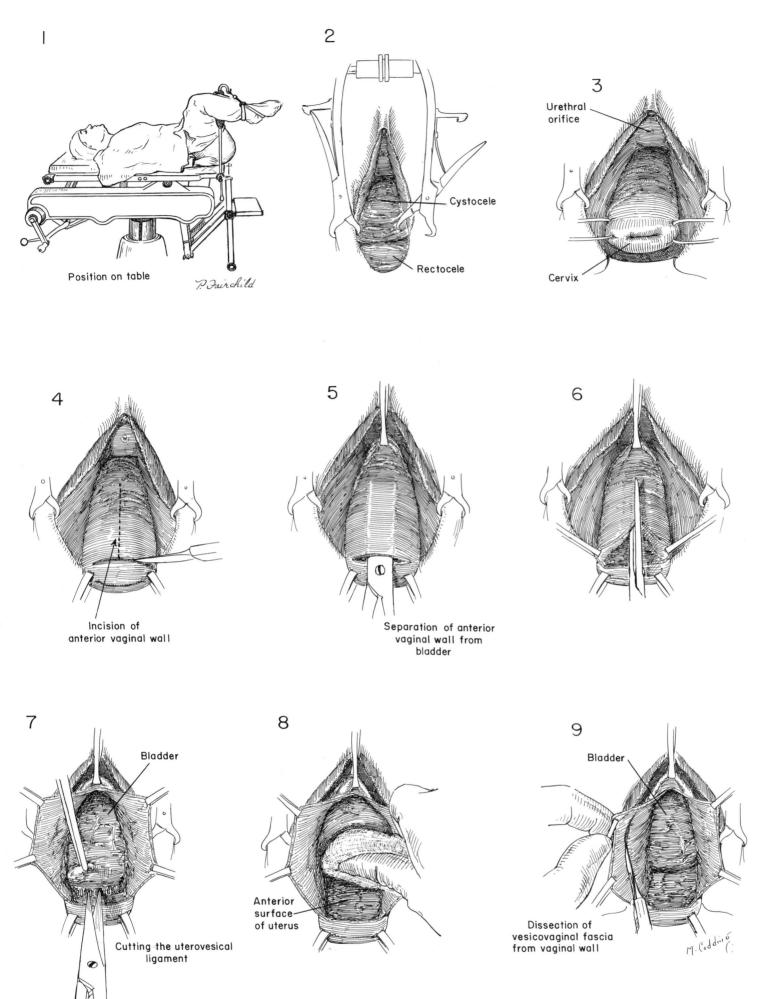

1

Position on table

P. Fairchild

2

Cystocele

Rectocele

3

Urethral orifice

Cervix

4

Incision of anterior vaginal wall

5

Separation of anterior vaginal wall from bladder

6

7

Bladder

Cutting the uterovesical ligament

8

Anterior surface of uterus

9

Bladder

Dissection of vesicovaginal fascia from vaginal wall

M. Codding

PLATE CXXXIV · ANTERIOR COLPORRHAPHY

DETAILS OF PROCEDURE (*Continued*). Frequently, a definite layer of vesicovaginal fascia can be developed by sharp and blunt dissection **(Figure 10).** In patients with incontinence this dissection should be carried well up to free the urethra on either side. A Foley catheter, No. 20 or 22, is inserted into the bladder and kept under moderate traction, pulling the traumatized sphincter muscle upward. Sutures of 00 chromic catgut are placed with small, curved Mayo needles to include a bite of tissue on either side of the urethra **(Figure 11).** Further sutures may be added in the opposite direction to pull the tissues defined by the Foley catheter upward in the direction of the urinary meatus. Several additional interrupted sutures may be taken to plicate the bladder neck in this location **(Figure 12).**

The bladder is separated upward from the anterior surface of the cervix to the vesicouterine pouch of peritoneum and may be held by several sutures in this location **(Figure 13).** However, it should not be anchored too high on the uterine wall, since this may produce too great a shortening of the anterior vaginal wall.

CLOSURE. Interrupted 00 chromic catgut sutures on No. 8 Ferguson needles are placed to approximate the vesicovaginal fascia **(Figure 14).** If this tissue layer has not been well defined, the fascia over the bladder wall is plicated. Sutures, a and b, are taken routinely in the vesicovaginal fascia to include a bite of the anterior wall of the cervix about the level of the internal os **(Figure 14).** When the cystocele is associated with descensus of the uterus, additional sutures, c and d, are taken in the tissues lateral to the cervix to incorporate the cardinal ligaments and a bite of the cervix **(Figure 15).** The placement of these sutures is facilitated by pulling the cervix to the side opposite that to which the suture is to be taken, while the operator's left index finger is held behind the flap of mucous membrane to guide the needle through the perimetric tissue yet not entirely through the mucous membrane. The degree of prolapse of the uterus determines the necessary amount of plication of the cardinal ligaments. These sutures, c and d, are allowed to remain long and are not tied until all others in the vesicovaginal fascia have been tied **(Figure 15).** As the sutures in the cardinal ligaments are tied, the cervix is drawn upward and backward toward the hollow of the sacrum **(Figure 16).** All bleeding points are controlled by transfixing sutures of fine chromic catgut. After the amount of vaginal mucosa necessary to permit easy approximation has been gauged by first overlapping the flaps, the redundant tissue is excised **(Figure 17).** The vaginal mucous membrane is closed by interrupted 00 chromic catgut sutures on No. 8 Ferguson needles, which include a bite of the underlying fascial layer, thus closing all dead space **(Figure 18).** These sutures are tied gently to avoid blanching the mucous membrane, for if they are tied tightly, the blood supply is cut off, producing sloughing along the suture line. The incision is often closed in a straight line instead of by the inverted T closure to increase the length of the anterior vaginal wall.

POSTOPERATIVE CARE. See Gynecologic System—Routine for Vaginal Procedures.

PLATE CXXXIV   ANTERIOR COLPORRHAPHY

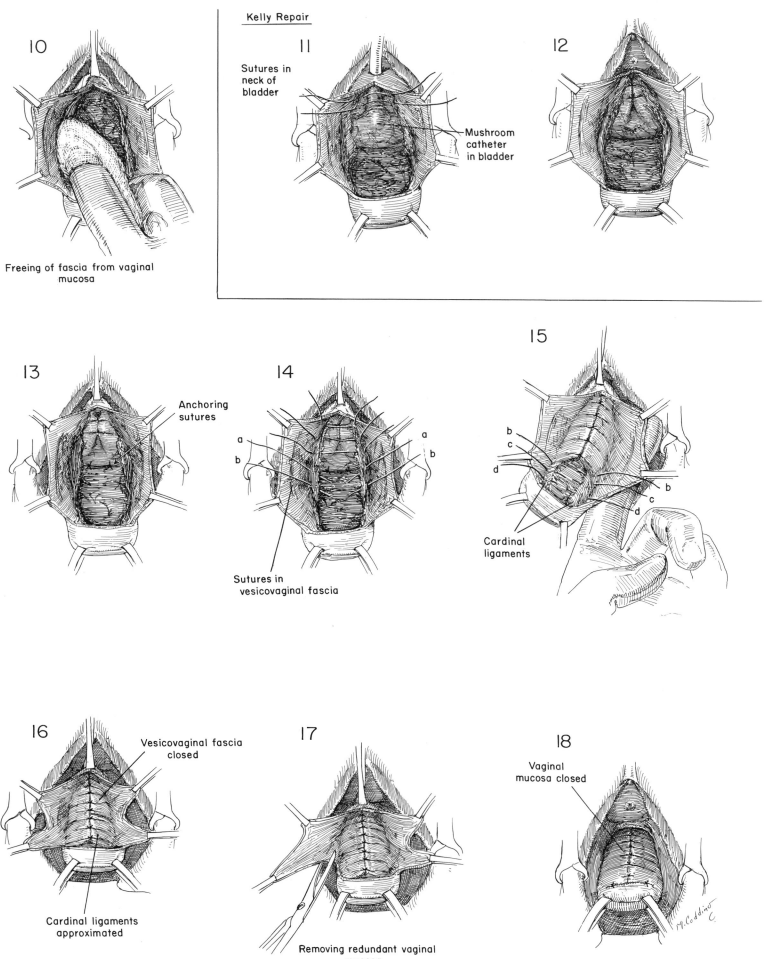

10

Freeing of fascia from vaginal mucosa

Kelly Repair

11

Sutures in neck of bladder

Mushroom catheter in bladder

12

13

Anchoring sutures

14

a
b

a
b

Sutures in vesicovaginal fascia

15

b
c

d

b
c
d

Cardinal ligaments

16

Vesicovaginal fascia closed

Cardinal ligaments approximated

17

Removing redundant vaginal mucosa

18

Vaginal mucosa closed

M.Coddino C.

PLATE CXXXV · AMPUTATION OF CERVIX AND COLPORRHAPHY (MANCHESTER)

INDICATIONS. The Manchester operation may be used in patients with prolapse requiring repair or with a diseased or elongated cervix requiring amputation. This procedure can be carried out judiciously in women of childbearing age by leaving intact a sufficient amount of the cervix to ensure against a precipitate birth in the event of pregnancy. It also has the advantage of limiting the entire operation to the vagina as well as removing the most likely site of cancer in the female.

PREOPERATIVE PREPARATION. See Gynecologic System—Routine for Vaginal Procedures.

ANESTHESIA. See Gynecologic System—Routine for Vaginal Procedures.

POSITION. See Gynecologic System—Routine for Vaginal Procedures.

OPERATIVE PREPARATION. See Gynecologic System—Routine for Vaginal Procedures.

EXPOSURE AND INCISION. The anterior vaginal wall, the bladder, and the vesicovaginal fascia are defined and exposed as described for anterior colporrhaphy (Plates CXXXIII and CXXXIV).

DETAILS OF PROCEDURE. The level of amputation of the cervix is indicated in **Figure 1.** The site for amputation, however, may be at a much higher level, depending upon the measured length of the cervical canal and the degree of prolapse. The cervix must be well dilated to aid in the placement of sutures following the amputation. The posterior incision in the mucous membrane may be outlined, if preferred, when the T incision is made (Plate CXXXIII, **Figure 4).** After the dissection of the anterior vaginal wall has been completed, the posterior vaginal wall is freed as the cervix is held upward **(Figure 2).** The mucous membrane is pushed downward by blunt dissection with gauze over the right index finger until the posterior cervical wall is exposed slightly beyond the proposed level of amputation.

CLOSURE. Sutures, a to e, of 0 chromic catgut are placed with No. 8 Ferguson needles in the vesicovaginal fascia **(Figure 3),** as in anterior colporrhaphy (Plate CXXXIV), two or more of which should include a bite of the anterior surface of the upper cervix as well as the vesticovaginal fascia **(Figure 4).** With the index finger held at the side of the cervix, behind the flap of the vaginal mucosa to guard against its inclusion, deep sutures are taken to incorporate the cardinal ligaments and blood vessels in the paracervical tissue slightly above the proposed level of amputation. Now the paracervical tissue, which includes the bases of the broad ligaments, is doubly clamped or ligated close to the cervix, divided, and subsequently tied anterior to the cervix **(Figure 3).** These sutures, f and g, are left untied until just before the final closure of the mucous membrane, because when the sutures are tied, the cardinal ligaments are shortened and the uterus is pulled upward, decreasing the exposure for the subsequent technical procedures on the cervix.

The cervix is amputated at the desired level **(Figure 4),** and the upper cervical segment is held by Teale or bullet forceps on either side **(Figure 5).** It has been found beneficial in covering the raw surface of the upper cervical segment to make the coning out obliquely forward; in other words, the margin of the cervical canal forms the apex. A Sturmdorf stitch is placed with a cervix needle to draw the apex of the posterior flap of vaginal mucous membrane into the cervical canal **(Figure 5).** The placement of this intricate and effective suture is enhanced if a Hegar dilator is maintained in the cervical canal. The dilator tends to direct the needle out through the cervical canal and ensures a patent and adequate cervical canal. The needle passes from without in through the cervical canal, out through the apex of the mucous membrane on the vaginal side adjacent to the forceps, then back into the cervical canal, and out again through the mucous membrane adjacent to its point of entry. When the suture is pulled taut and tied, the mucous membrane is drawn well into the cervical canal **(Figure 6).** The sutures through the cardinal ligaments, f and g, are now tied, and the excess vaginal mucous membrane is excised **(Figure 7).** A crown suture of the Sturmdorf type, c, is placed at the lower angle of each anterior flap of vaginal mucous membrane to pull the flaps into the cervical canal, covering the raw surfaces **(Figure 8).** While a right-angle hook keeps the mucous membrane under tension laterally, a sufficient number of interrupted sutures, which include a bite of cervix, are placed to approximate the vaginal flaps lateral to the os **(Figure 9).** These sutures are permitted to remain long and untied until lateral tension is released and satisfactory coaptation of the wound edges is attained. The vaginal mucous membrane is closed routinely with interrupted 00 chromic catgut sutures on No. 8 Ferguson needles, which should include a bite of the underlying vesicovaginal fascia. The patency of the cervical canal is finally proved by reinsertion of a Hegar dilator. Frequently, a posterior colporrhaphy will follow.

POSTOPERATIVE CARE. See Gynecologic System—Routine for Vaginal Procedures.

PLATE CXXXV   AMPUTATION OF CERVIX AND COLPORRHAPHY (MANCHESTER)

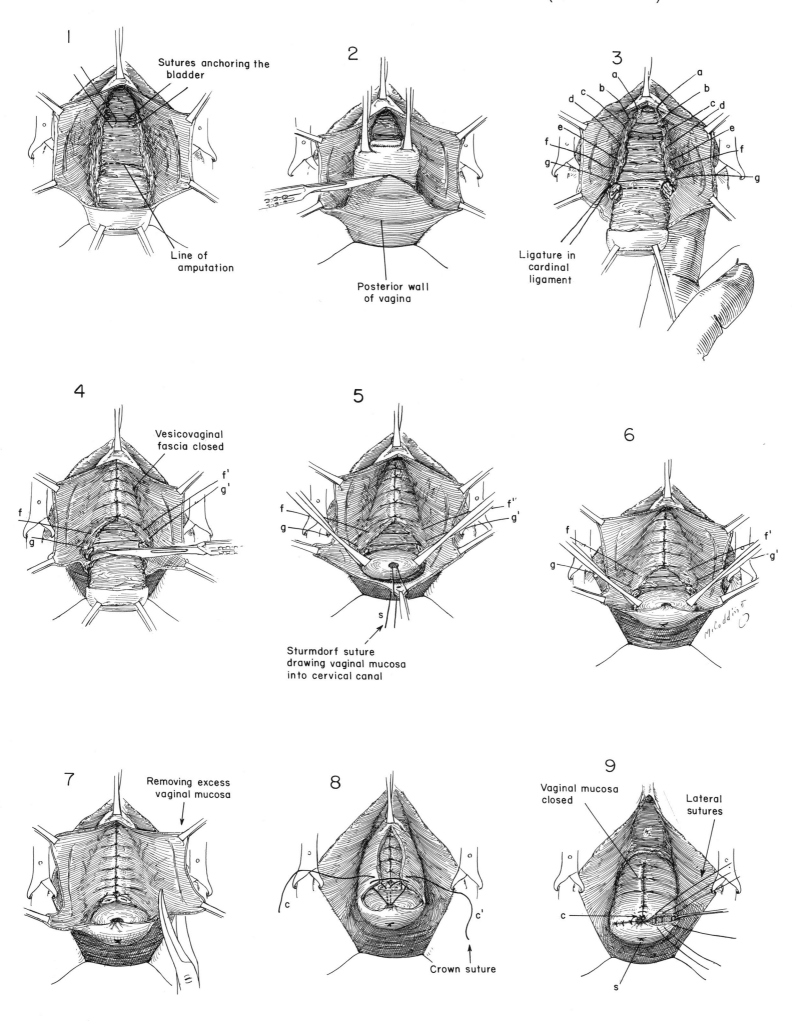

1. Sutures anchoring the bladder / Line of amputation

2. Posterior wall of vagina

3. Ligature in cardinal ligament

4. Vesicovaginal fascia closed

5. Sturmdorf suture drawing vaginal mucosa into cervical canal

6.

7. Removing excess vaginal mucosa

8. Crown suture

9. Vaginal mucosa closed / Lateral sutures

PLATE CXXXVI · POSTERIOR COLPORRHAPHY

INDICATIONS. Posterior colporrhaphy is advised to correct the classic symptoms of relaxed pelvic floor in women beyond childbearing age or with the desired number of children. If the symptoms are pronounced or the sphincter ani muscles are sufficiently lacerated to give anal incontinence, earlier repair is advised.

PREOPERATIVE PREPARATION. See Gynecologic System—Routine for Vaginal Procedures. When there is an extensive laceration necessitating repair of the sphincter ani muscles or anterior anal wall, the patient is placed on a low-residue diet for several days, and the intestines are cleansed with saline purges and enemas.

ANESTHESIA. See Gynecologic System—Routine for Vaginal Procedures.

POSITION. See Gynecologic System—Routine for Vaginal Procedures.

OPERATIVE PREPARATION. See Gynecologic System—Routine for Vaginal Procedures.

EXPOSURE AND INCISION. A self-retaining retractor is attached at the base of the labia minora on either side or at the level of the openings of Bartholin's ducts and is regulated until the mucocutaneous border is under sufficient tension to form a ridge **(Figures 1 and 2)**. As an alternative method of retraction, interrupted sutures may be taken to include a bite of the labia minora and the skin of the buttock, which, when tied, give retraction of the labia. However, this technic is not so satisfactory as the use of the self-retaining retractor, since the latter permits a gradual decrease in retraction as the operation progresses. A pad of gauze moistened in saline is anchored just below the mucocutaneous border with several Teale or Allis forceps to aid in walling off the anus **(Figure 2)**.

DETAILS OF PROCEDURE. The posterior vaginal wall is grasped with forceps in the midline at the planned apex of the denudation of the mucous membrane. When traction is applied at this point, the mucous membrane will lift upward to the region of the urethra **(Figure 2)**. A narrow strip of the mucocutaneous ridge, formed by the self-retaining retractor, is excised with curved scissors **(Figure 2)**. The incised margin of the vaginal mucosa is grasped in toothed thumb forceps in the operator's left hand, while a pair of straight Mayo dissecting scissors, with the blades directed away from the rectum, is inserted beneath the mucous membrane. By alternately opening and closing the blades as the scissors are advanced, the surgeon is able to develop a cleavage plane between the rectum and the posterior vaginal wall **(Figure 3)**. The flap of the posterior vaginal wall is grasped transversely with a blunt-nosed, curved, half-length forceps. With several fingers of the operator's left hand inserted into the vagina for counterpressure, the rectum is pushed gently away by blunt gauze dissection **(Figure 4)**, but frequently it is necessary to use sharp dissection to separate the lateral borders of the mucous membrane from the underlying muscle. If the proper cleavage plane has been entered, the rectum is easily freed from the posterior vaginal wall as high as desired with only a limited amount of bleeding. Vessels actively bleeding are clamped and tied with 000 chromic catgut. A narrow, triangular-shaped fragment of posterior vaginal wall is excised up to the midline clamp with right- and left-curved scissors **(Figure 5)**. To avoid unnecessary tension at closure, it is preferable to remove too little rather than too much mucous membrane, since the mucosa adds nothing to the support of the repair.

CLOSURE. A continuous 00 chromic catgut suture on a large Mayo needle is used to approximate the apex of the denuded area in the posterior vaginal wall. The suture, a, is tied gently, lest it interfere with the blood supply of the mucous membrane along the suture line, and its long free end, a', weighted with a hemostat, is allowed to dangle over the perineum **(Figure 6)**. Suture a' will be buried beneath the levator ani muscles and, at the completion of the operation, will be tied to the suture a, compressing the newly made perineal body gently and anchoring the mucous membrane at the apex of the suture line. Suture a is continued as a lock suture to include small bites of mucous membrane for a short distance, after which the suture, with needle attached, is placed over the patient's symphysis. In placing sutures, the operator must be constantly alert to the possibility of injury to the rectum. This may be averted if the operator's index finger, while depressing the rectum, is so held that the needle point presents itself anterior to the finger. With the operator's index finger in position, interrupted 0 chromic catgut sutures are taken laterally to include liberal bites of the levator ani muscles **(Figure 7)**. These sutures, placed obliquely so that the perineum is elevated from within outward, are not tied but are retracted firmly upward by the assistant to aid in defining the muscles and in placing subsequent sutures and to decrease the chance of possible injury to the rectal wall **(Figure 7)**.

The uppermost suture in the levator ani muscles is now tied gently. When the levator ani muscles have been approximated high enough, the upper vagina will admit three fingers. If the topmost suture is determined by digital examination to be placed satisfactorily, the remainder of the sutures in the levator ani muscles are tied. The lock suture, a, is now continued in the mucous membrane to include an occasional superficial bite of the underlying levator ani muscles **(Figure 8)**. Note that suture a' is buried at the bottom of the wound **(Figure 8)**. The surgeon tests the vaginal canal from time to time to make sure that, as the levator ani muscles are approximated, the vagina will not be constricted beyond the easy width of two fingers. Additional interrupted 0 chromic catgut sutures may be taken in the levator ani muscle and urogenital trigone, if necessary, to decrease the lumen of the vagina **(Figure 9)**. Traction by the self-retaining retractor is gradually decreased as these sutures are tied **(Figure 9)**. All Teale forceps are removed, but one is reapplied in the midline of the mucocutaneous border of the perineal wound. The skin of the perineum adjacent to the mucocutaneous border is undercut to permit suture a, which has been a continuous lock suture in the mucous membrane, to be continued over the perineum as a subcuticular suture **(Figure 10)**. In placing this suture, it is essential that the sensitive tissue at the mucocutaneous junction should not be drawn into a constricting band. The skin margins are accurately approximated, and gentle traction is placed on suture a' to compress the perineal body, obliterate dead space, and express any blood that may have collected **(Figure 11)**. The continuous suture a is then tied gently to its original partner, a', and the ends are cut on the knot, burying it beneath the margins of the incision.

In the presence of an enterocele the posterior vaginal wall is divided until the peritoneal cavity is opened. The deep Douglas' pouch is dissected free and closed as a hernial sac.

POSTOPERATIVE CARE. See Gynecologic System—Routine for Vaginal Procedures. When extensive plastic procedures have been carried out on the sphincter muscles and anterior rectal wall, daily heat lamp therapy and sitz baths usually are effective in alleviating the discomfort of the first few postoperative days. Stool softeners are given routinely, and instillation of warm oil several hours before the first bowel movement is also comforting. Troublesome hemorrhoids often appear following extensive posterior colporrhaphy and are managed by aggressive local therapy of heat, astringents, and anesthetic ointments.

PLATE CXXXVI   POSTERIOR COLPORRHAPHY

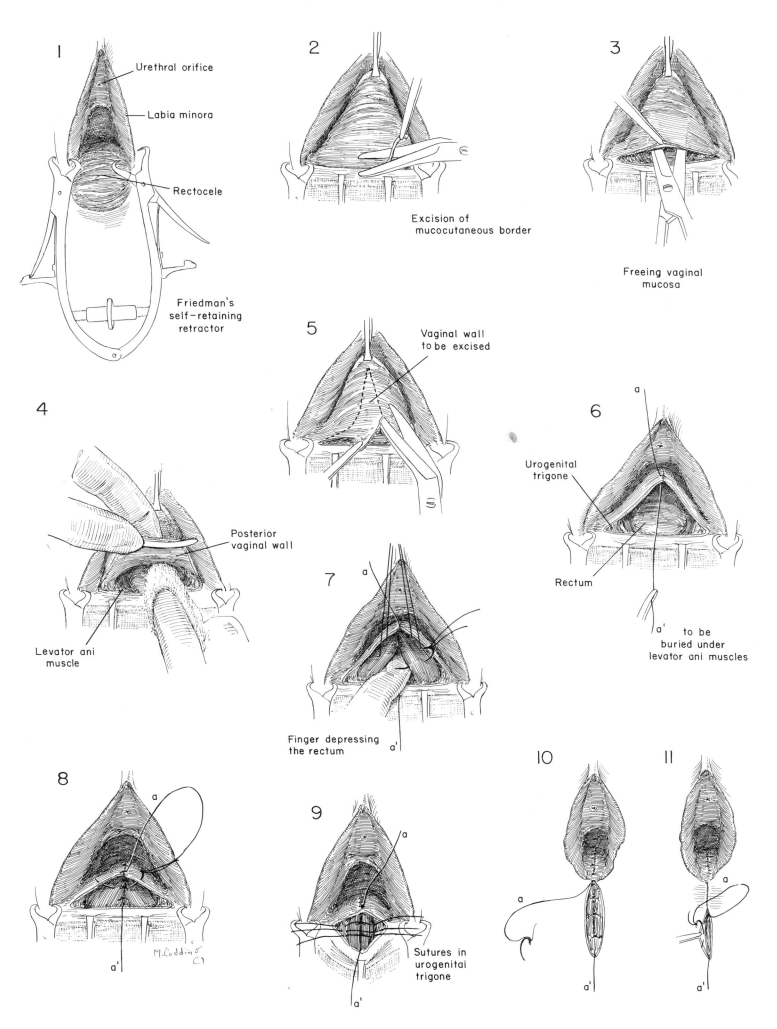

1
Urethral orifice
Labia minora
Rectocele
Friedman's self-retaining retractor

2
Excision of mucocutaneous border

3
Freeing vaginal mucosa

4
Posterior vaginal wall
Levator ani muscle

5
Vaginal wall to be excised

6
a
Urogenital trigone
Rectum
a' to be buried under levator ani muscles

7
a
Finger depressing the rectum   a'

8
a
a'
M.Coddino C)

9
a
Sutures in urogenital trigone
a'

10
a
a'

11
a
a'

INDICATIONS. Cold knife conization is indicated for suspicious lesions of the uterine cervix to confirm or exclude the diagnosis of cervical cancer. Certain out-patient procedures usually precede conization and are useful in the investigation of cervical lesions. The Papanicolaou smear taken with an Ayerst applicator is an efficient method of establishing the diagnosis of gross or microscopic lesions of the uterine cervix. In the event of a suspicious Papanicolaou smear or an obvious lesion of the cervix, the cervix is sprayed with Graham's 7 per cent iodine solution. A punch biopsy is taken in the area which does not stain in an otherwise deep-mahogany stained cervix **(Figure 1)**. After exposure of the cervix the punch biopsy forceps is introduced, and a piece of unstained cervical tissue is removed with inclusion of a small bite of surrounding healthy tissue.

A suspicious or positive Papanicolaou smear and/or positive punch biopsy necessitates hospitalization for cold knife conization, the definitive diagnostic procedure for malignant lesions of the cervix.

PREOPERATIVE PREPARATION. See Gynecologic System—Routine for Vaginal Procedures. Douches are omitted.

ANESTHESIA. Either general or spinal anesthesia is given.

POSITION. The patient is placed in a dorsal lithotomy position.

OPERATIVE PROCEDURE. The usual preparation of the perineum is carried out, but preparation of the vagina and cervix is avoided, lest loosely attached epithelium essential for diagnosis be destroyed. Even during the pelvic examination under anesthesia, the examiner's gloved fingers avoid the surface of the cervix. Following the pelvic examination a speculum is inserted into the vagina, and the anterior lip of the cervix is grasped with a single-toothed tenaculum. Dilatation and curettage is not performed before conization because it interferes with the lining of the endocervical canal and the squamocolumnar junction, making a pathologic diagnosis more difficult.

DETAILS OF PROCEDURE. The cervix may be sprayed with a 7 per cent iodine solution for evidence of possible carcinoma. A Garret retractor can be placed in the cervix for traction purposes. The surgeon maintains traction on the tenaculum as an incision is made with a No. 11 triangular-shaped blade at a 45-degree angle toward the endocervical canal. The involved portion of the cervix is excised **(Figure 2)**. The proximal 1.5 cm. of the endocervix is also removed **(Figure 3)**. The removed tissue, which appears as a cone, is immediately placed in a fixative to avoid loss of diagnostic epithelium through contact with gauze, etc. It is important to remove the endocervical canal, since carcinoma of the cervix is frequently of multicentric origin and over 50 per cent of invasive lesions occur in the endocervical canal. It is advisable not to do too deep a conization which would involve the internal os, as stenosis could result **(Figure 3A)**.

After the cone is removed, some prefer to smooth surgical margins by using the cutting current with the triangular wire loop completely encircling the coned area. This often is satisfactory in establishing hemostasis. The wire triangle is kept quite superficial. No effort is made to cut deeply into the body of the cervix. Individual points of hemorrhage are coagulated if

necessary. The complete cone can be excised with the triangular wire loop **(Figures 4** and **4A)**. Persistent bleeding is controlled by interrupted figure-of-eight fine sutures.

In the presence of extensive chronic cystic cervicitis, especially when the cervix is hypertrophied, a more extensive conization or amputation of the cervix should be considered. A rim of mucosa at least 1 cm. wide should be mobilized from the entire margins of the amputated cervix. The mobilized mucosa will be necessary to reconstruct the new cervix. This can be accomplished by the placement of anterior and posterior Sturmdorf sutures **(Figures 5** and **6)**.

The proper placement of the rather complicated Sturmdorf stitch can be enhanced if a moderate-sized Hank's dilator is inserted into the cervical canal. A cervical cutting needle is introduced approximately 2 cm. from the cervical margin in the midline anteriorly and directed out over the Hank's dilator **(Figure 5)**. The mobilized mucosa in the midline anteriorly is grasped with forceps and a transverse bite taken with the same needle **(Figure 5)**. The Hank's dilator is reinserted in order to assist mechanically in the proper placement of the needle within the cervical canal and back out in the midline anteriorly.

The efficiency of this suture in everting the anterior wall is tested by traction on the suture. Accuracy is essential, and the surgeon should not hesitate to replace the suture **(Figure 7)**.

The patency of the reconstructed cervical canal is tested by the insertion of a Hank's dilator **(Figure 7A)**. A similar Sturmdorf suture is placed in the midline posteriorly. Again, with the Hank's dilator in the cervical canal to ensure its patency, the lateral margins of raw surface are closed with interrupted catgut sutures. These lateral sutures should include the margins of the mucosa and a bite in the underlying cervix. One or two sutures on either side are usually sufficient **(Figure 8)**. It is preferred to leave no pack in the vagina, as good hemostasis should be obtained at the completion of the procedure.

The patency and direction of the cervical canal are determined by the passage of a uterine sound. The cervix is dilated gently with a series of lubricated, graduated Hegar dilators, and a systematic curettage is carried out **(Figures 9** and **10)**. For diagnostic curettage dilatation up to a No. 8 or No. 10 Hegar is adequate. The largest sharp curette that can pass through the dilated cervix is gently inserted and passed to the fundus. The anterior wall is scraped until all endometrium is removed from the posterior wall. Curettage is then repeated on the right and left walls, the fundus, and finally the uterine cornua. Following curettage of the uterus, persistent bleeding from the cold knife conization is controlled with figure-of-eight sutures. Diagnostic conizations are of such limited scope that plastic reconstruction of the cervix is not required.

POSTOPERATIVE CARE. Postoperative care in a cervical conization is most important. Wide and deep conizations of the internal os may be the source of cervical stenosis. Postconization stenosis may be associated with the development of dysmenorrhea as well as sterility. Postconization patients should be seen in the office in six weeks for dilatation of the cervix. Under no circumstances should a stem pessary be left in the cervix at the time of conization, since infection may supervene in the presence of a foreign body. On occasion patients develop a perimetritis. They usually respond very well to a bactericidal antibiotic agent.

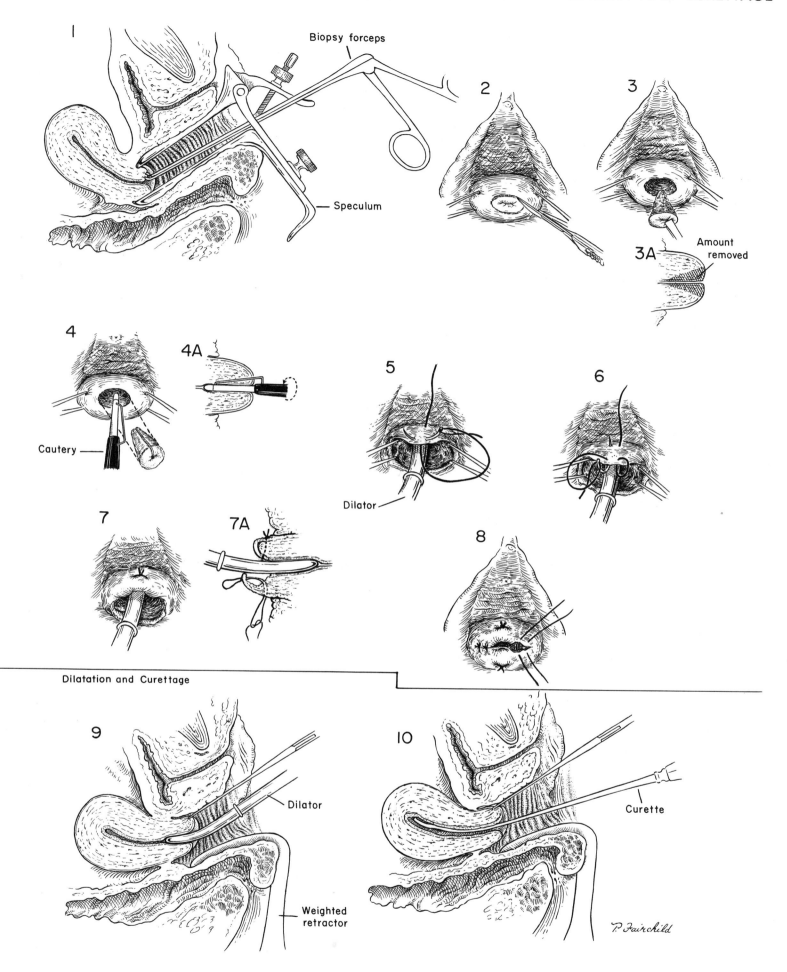

1   Biopsy forceps

Speculum

2

3

3A   Amount removed

4   4A

Cautery

5   Dilator

6

7   7A

8

Dilatation and Curettage

9   Dilator

Weighted retractor

10   Curette

P. Fairchild

PLATE CXXXVIII · VAGINAL HYSTERECTOMY

INDICATIONS. Vaginal hysterectomy is frequently recommended in elderly women with procidentia and may also be used in prolapse of a moderate degree where there is a pathologic process requiring removal of the uterus. Although the mortality from this procedure is extremely low, the reconstructed vagina may be shortened and its function altered.

PREOPERATIVE PREPARATION. See Gynecologic System—Routine for Vaginal Procedures. In addition, it is often advisable for the patient to remain in bed a few days with the prolapse reduced until the general condition of the vagina has improved and the congestion of the tissues is relieved. Since the operation is usually carried out in elderly women, special attention should be given to the state of the circulatory and respiratory systems.

ANESTHESIA. See Gynecologic System—Routine for Vaginal Procedures.

POSITION. See Gynecologic System—Routine for Vaginal Procedures.

OPERATIVE PREPARATION. See Gynecologic System—Routine for Vaginal Procedures.

EXPOSURE AND INCISION. When vaginal hysterectomy has been decided upon, the lips of the cervix are sewed together to prevent contamination from the cervical secretions in the later stages of the operation **(Figure 1).** These sutures closing the cervix may be tied to form a hammock for the weighted retractor, which pulls the cervix downward over the perineum and maintains firm, even traction during the early stages of the operation. The anterior vaginal wall is dissected as in anterior colporrhaphy (Plate CXXXIII).

DETAILS OF PROCEDURE. The bladder is freed from the anterior surface of the cervix until the vesicouterine peritoneum is well exposed. It is then pushed upward behind the symphysis by the insertion of a moist gauze sponge and is maintained there by a small, smooth retractor held by an assistant **(Figure 1).** After the vesicouterine peritoneum has been incised carefully to avoid injuring any intra-abdominal structures **(Figure 1),** the index and middle fingers of the operator's left hand are introduced into the peritoneal cavity to serve as internal retractors while the peritoneal opening is extended laterally as far as the broad ligaments. The body of the uterus and the adnexa are then palpated by several fingers of the left hand through this opening, and the fundus is delivered **(Figure 2).** Delivery of an enlarged fundus may necessitate the application of bullet forceps or specially designed hooks. If so, this procedure may be facilitated if traction on the cervix is discontinued and if the cervix is reintroduced into the vagina before delivery is attempted. The posterior vaginal wall may be incised either in the initial stages of the operation or after the fundus has been delivered. The vaginal mucous membrane is pushed away from the cervix by blunt gauze dissection until the uterosacral ligaments are visualized, as well as the peritoneum of Douglas' pouch **(Figure 3).** The fingers of the operator's left hand then may be inserted down into Douglas' pouch behind the uterus to place the peritoneum under tension and to eliminate possible accidental trauma to the intestines when the peritoneum is incised **(Figure 3).** Now the peritoneum is opened laterally as far as the uterosacral ligaments on either side, and a weighted speculum is introduced into

Douglas' pouch **(Figure 4).** The contents of the abdominal cavity may be prevented from entering the field either by shifting the patient to a moderate Trendelenburg position or by introducing a moist sterile pack behind the fundus of the uterus and by bringing it out through the opening in Douglas' pouch. When the uterosacral ligaments are well defined, a curved half-length forceps is applied to either side, and the ligaments are divided **(Figure 4).** Straight Ochsner clamps are placed at the top of the left broad ligament, usually in pairs, because occasionally troublesome back bleeding may occur from the uterus **(Figure 5).** A similar pair of clamps grasps the base of the broad ligament, often including the uterosacral ligaments as well as the cardinal ligaments and the uterine vessels. With several fingers of the surgeon's left hand serving as an intra-abdominal retractor, the broad ligaments are then divided between the clamps **(Figure 5).** The broad ligaments on the opposite side may be similarly clamped and divided, but in order to avoid too many clamps in the wound, it may be safer to reflect the uterus to the opposite side and ligate the broad ligament, which has just been divided, before proceeding with division of the opposite ligaments **(Figure 6).** Should there be considerable tension on the broad ligaments, only small bites of tissue are included in the clamps, and they are reapplied as necessary. Traction on these clamps is carefully avoided because of the possibility of retraction of their contents, with resultant troublesome hidden bleeding. The region of the uterine vessels is usually doubly tied with transfixing 0 chromic catgut sutures on No. 8 Ferguson needles. If two ties have been placed, one end of the outer suture is allowed to remain long so that it may be tied to the corresponding suture of the opposite side at closure. A small bite in the round ligament is included when the uppermost part of the broad ligament is ligated **(Figure 6).** After the opposite side has been similarly divided, a careful check is made to ensure that the uterine vessels are adequately secured and that there is no bleeding into the broad ligaments. If pathology exists in the tube and ovary, each is removed.

At times, when the fundus cannot be freely delivered, the uterus may be removed from the cervix upward. Douglas' pouch is opened, and the operator's left finger is thrust through the avascular space and pulled downward, isolating the base of the broad ligament including uterine vessels **(Figure 7).** This procedure is repeated on the opposite side, following which the uterine vessels are doubly tied. In the presence of a large mass of tissue or considerable tension, it is wiser to divide this step by repeatedly applying clamps and ligating their contents before proceeding further. The top of the broad ligament, including the round ligament and tube, is divided in the final step **(Figure 8).**

CLOSURE. The broad ligaments are approximated by one of several methods. The ends of the sutures that have been allowed to remain long are tied together, approximating the corresponding portions of the broad ligaments **(Figure 9),** or, if preferred, additional interrupted sutures may be used for this purpose. A second method is to approximate the clamps, the contents of which have not been previously tied, and to place a continuous through-and-through suture of 0 chromic catgut starting at the top of the broad ligament. After this suture is tied, it is continued downward, and the clamps are removed as their contents are secured by the continuous suture. This suture is finally tied at the lower end of the broad ligaments. If hemostasis is not complete, additional interrupted sutures may be taken. The uterovesical flap of peritoneum is then anchored to the top of the round ligaments by an interrupted suture **(Figure 9).**

PLATE CXXXVIII   VAGINAL HYSTERECTOMY

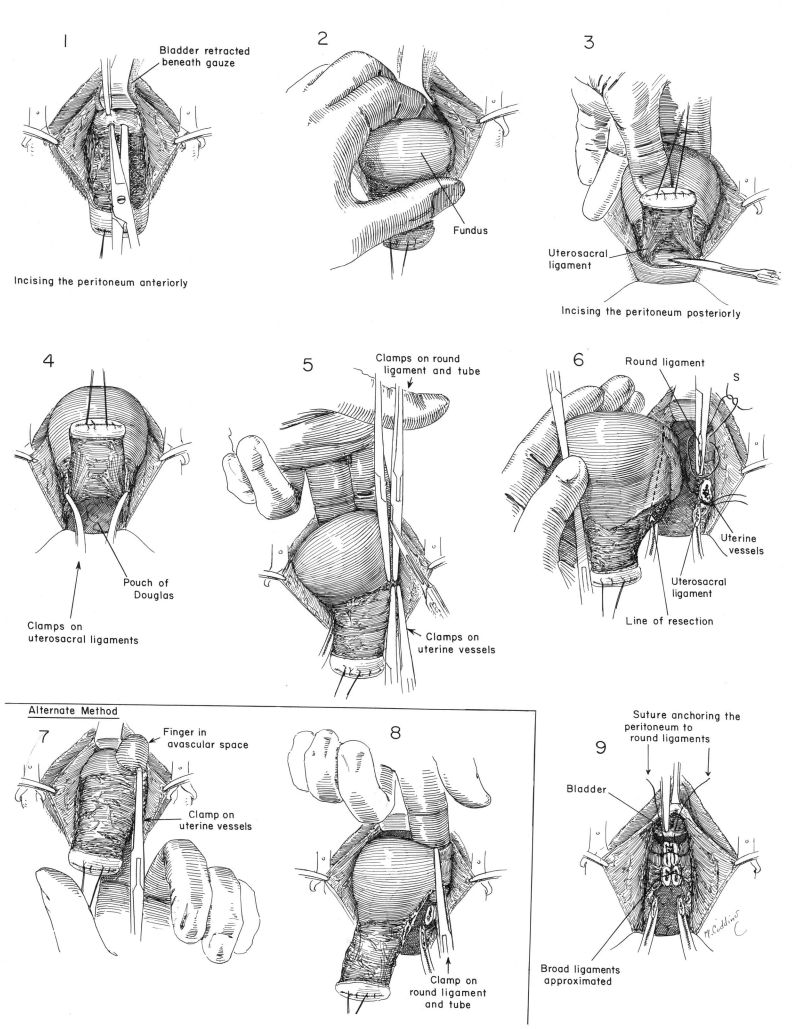

1

Bladder retracted beneath gauze

Incising the peritoneum anteriorly

2

Fundus

3

Uterosacral ligament

Incising the peritoneum posteriorly

4

Pouch of Douglas

Clamps on uterosacral ligaments

5

Clamps on round ligament and tube

Clamps on uterine vessels

6

Round ligament

S

Uterine vessels

Uterosacral ligament

Line of resection

Alternate Method

7

Finger in avascular space

Clamp on uterine vessels

8

Clamp on round ligament and tube

9

Suture anchoring the peritoneum to round ligaments

Bladder

Broad ligaments approximated

PLATE CXXXIX · VAGINAL HYSTERECTOMY

CLOSURE. (*Continued*). In cases of urinary incontinence, one or more Kelly-type stitches are placed as in anterior colporrhaphy (Plate CXXXIV, **Figures 11** and **12**). The round ligaments are approximated to the pubic arch on either side of the urethra with interrupted sutures, a-a', b-b' **(Figure 10)**. The uterosacral ligaments are approximated to the base of the broad ligaments, and the excessive vaginal mucous membrane is excised **(Figure 11)**. If the vesicovaginal fascia is well defined, it is closed as a separate layer, such as sutures x-x', including a bite of the underlying approximated broad ligaments **(Figure 11)**. Otherwise the mucous membrane is held upward by a Teale forceps applied to the midline, and interrupted 00 chromic catgut sutures on No. 8 Ferguson needles, which incorporate the vaginal mucous membrane, the vesicovaginal fascia, and a small bite of the approximated broad ligaments, are placed to close the anterior wall **(Figure 12)**. This not only anchors the vaginal mucous membrane to underlying supporting structures but also aids in approximating the vesicovaginal fascia and obliterating dead space.

The depth of Douglas' pouch is gauged by the index and middle fingers of the surgeon's left hand **(Figure 13)**. Where there is a deep Douglas' pouch or enterocele, it is advisable to divide the mucous membrane of the posterior vaginal wall out to the mucocutaneous border, because it will be necessary to effect a high approximation of the levator ani muscles in the posterior colporrhaphy. The mucocutaneous border is excised with scissors, and the cleavage plane is established between the rectum and posterior vaginal wall by blunt dissection **(Figure 14)**. While the peritoneum is fixed by several fingers of the surgeon's left hand, Douglas' pouch is dissected free, using blunt dissection, and is treated as a hernial sac **(Figure 15)**. The peritoneum is dissected up as high as possible. Now a purse-string suture is taken to close the neck of the hernial sac and fasten it forward to the base of the broad ligaments **(Figure 16)**. Occasionally, additional sutures are taken in the uterosacral ligaments to permit further approximation and to aid in obliterating Douglas' pouch. The excess peritoneum is excised subsequently. The rectum may be pulled upward toward the point of closure of Douglas' pouch by placing a suture to include the fascia on either side of it and a small bite of fascia over the anterior rectal wall about 2 to 3 cm. lower **(Figure 17)**. When these sutures are tied, the anterior rectal wall is fixed. The excess vaginal mucosa is excised from either side **(Figure 17)**. An extensive, high posterior colporrhaphy (Plate CXXXVI) is then performed **(Figure 18)**. Upon its completion, a number of catgut sutures are placed using a large Mayo needle inserted obliquely to build up the perineal body gradually from above outward. The surgeon by repeated digital examination makes certain that the vaginal vault is not shortened and that the vaginal orifice is not constricted more than two fingers in diameter.

POSTOPERATIVE CARE. See Gynecologic System—Routine for Vaginal Procedures.

PLATE CXXXIX   VAGINAL HYSTERECTOMY

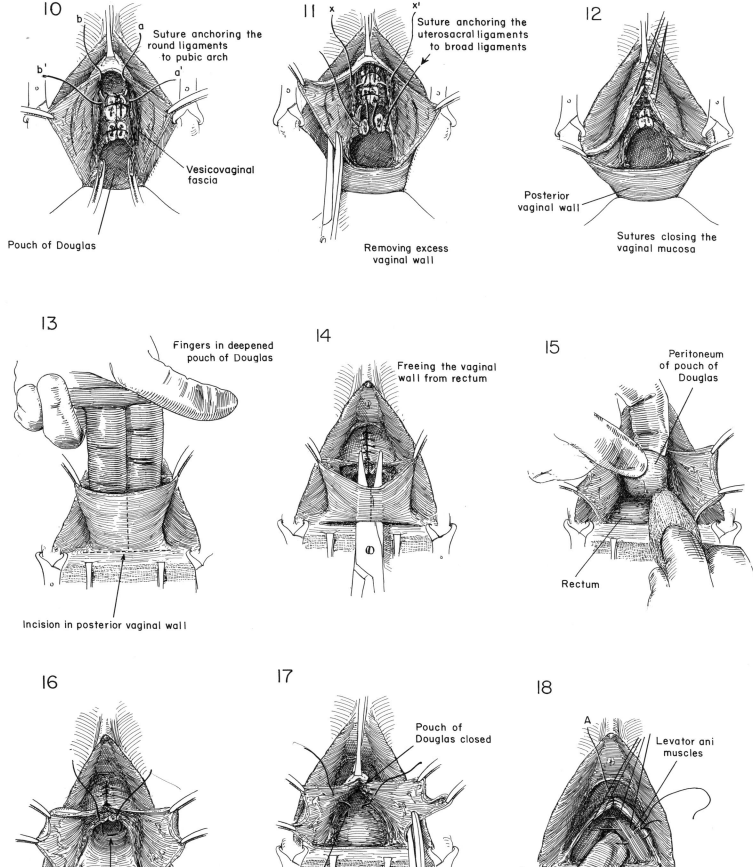

10

b a

b' a'

Suture anchoring the
round ligaments
to pubic arch

Vesicovaginal
fascia

Pouch of Douglas

11 x   x'

Suture anchoring the
uterosacral ligaments
to broad ligaments

Removing excess
vaginal wall

12

Posterior
vaginal wall

Sutures closing the
vaginal mucosa

13

Fingers in deepened
pouch of Douglas

Incision in posterior vaginal wall

14

Freeing the vaginal
wall from rectum

15

Peritoneum
of pouch of
Douglas

Rectum

16

Purse-string suture
closing the pouch of Douglas

17

Pouch of
Douglas closed

Rectopexy
suture

Removing the
excess vaginal wall

18

A

Levator ani
muscles

A'

M. Coddino

PLATE CXL · PARTIAL CLOSURE OF VAGINA (LE FORT)

INDICATIONS. Partial closure of the vagina may be indicated in elderly, poor-risk patients with marked prolapse. If it is desirable to retain the function of the vagina, only the upper third, or shaded area, X, is obliterated **(Figure 9).**

PREOPERATIVE PREPARATION. In addition to the usual preparation for vaginal procedures, special attention is given to the chief cause for the patient's being a poor surgical risk.

ANESTHESIA. See Gynecologic System—Routine for Vaginal Procedures.

POSITION. See Gynecologic System—Routine for Vaginal Procedures.

OPERATIVE PREPARATION. See Gynecologic System—Routine for Vaginal Procedures.

EXPOSURE AND INCISION. Teale forceps are attached to the cervix to secure adequate tension while a rectangular area on the anterior vaginal wall is outlined with a scalpel **(Figure 1).** The enclosed vaginal mucous membrane is removed with knife or scissors **(Figures 2 and 3).** The denudation should be as superficial as possible. The cervix is then held upward, and a similarly shaped portion of the posterior vaginal mucosa is removed **(Figure 4).** Instead of the rectangular area as shown, a much smaller triangular area may be removed near the cervix so that a septum is formed in only the uppermost part of the vagina.

CLOSURE. After the cervix has been partially replaced, interrupted sutures of 0 chromic catgut are taken on No. 8 Ferguson needles to approximate the posterior margins of the denuded area **(Figure 5).** To make certain that a canal is maintained permitting drainage of cervical secretions, these sutures are laid over a small rubber drain **(Figure 5).** Mattress sutures are placed to approximate the lateral margins of the denuded areas **(Figure 6)** and subsequently the anterior margins **(Figure 7),** until all dead space between the two surfaces has been entirely obliterated **(Figure 8).** This may be carried through the entire length of the vagina **(Figure 9)** or may include only the vaginal wall for a short distance adjacent to the cervix. The rubber drain may be removed immediately or after several days. It is frequently advisable to supplement this procedure with an approximation of the levator ani muscles as in a routine posterior colporrhaphy (Plate CXXXVI).

POSTOPERATIVE CARE. See Gynecologic System—Routine for Vaginal Procedures. It must be remembered that douches cannot be given unless the newly made septum is limited to the upper portion of the vagina.

PLATE CXL   PARTIAL CLOSURE OF VAGINA (LE FORT)

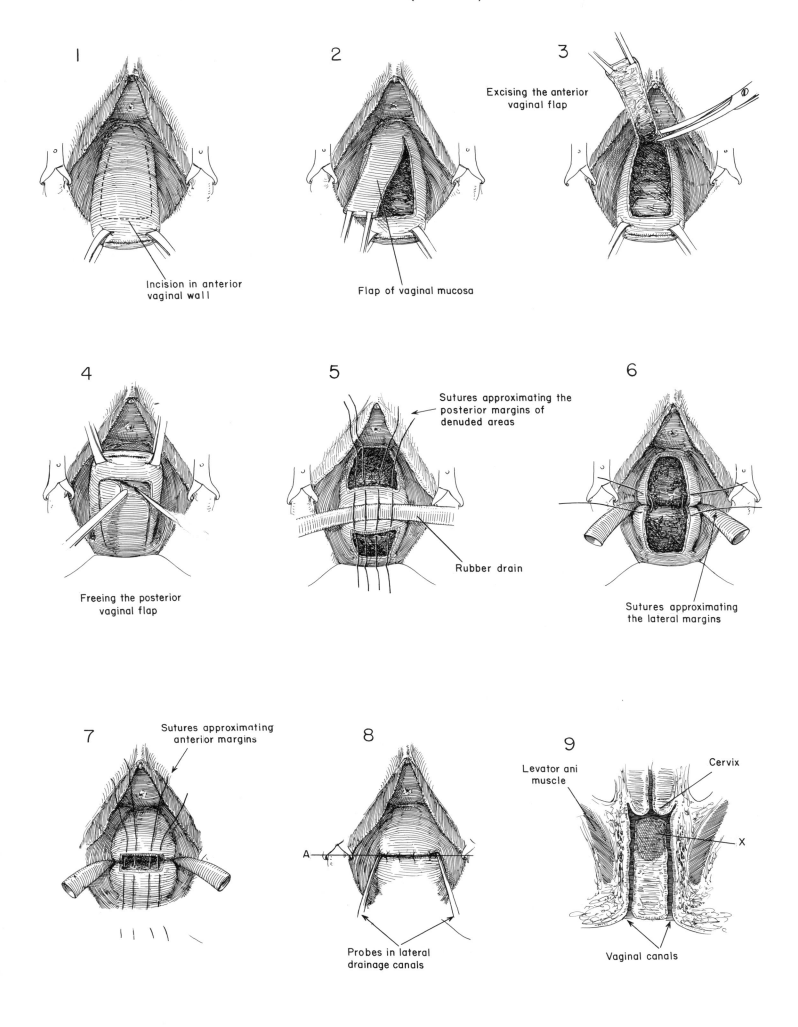

1

Incision in anterior
vaginal wall

2

Excising the anterior
vaginal flap

Flap of vaginal mucosa

3

4

Freeing the posterior
vaginal flap

5

Sutures approximating the
posterior margins of
denuded areas

Rubber drain

6

Sutures approximating
the lateral margins

7

Sutures approximating
anterior margins

8

A

Probes in lateral
drainage canals

9

Levator ani
muscle

Cervix

X

Vaginal canals

MISCELLANEOUS PROCEDURES

PLATE CXLI · THYROIDECTOMY, SUBTOTAL

INDICATIONS. The indications for subtotal thyroidectomy are decreasing because of the smaller incidence of endemic goiters, both colloid and nodular, and the increasing effectiveness of medical therapy in patients who present with thyrotoxicosis, whether this is due to Graves' disease or to nodular toxic goiter.

A definite indication for subtotal thyroidectomy is the removal of a solitary nodule in a young person, especially female, when the mass does not take up radioiodide on thyroid scan and hence is suspect of being malignant. Some surgeons may simply excise the nodule with a surrounding cuff of normal thyroid tissue if they feel on direct inspection that the mass is either a colloid cyst or benign adenoma. However, the subtotal thyroidectomy or lobectomy ensures a better margin and allows pathologic examination of the excised thyroid lobe for multicentric foci should a malignant tumor be found.

The controversy as to whether surgical or medical treatment for thyrotoxicosis is desirable in patients under 35 to 40 years of age and in pregnant patients has yet to be resolved, but it is generally agreed that the use of radioactive iodine is contraindicated. Surgical removal should be considered if antithyroid drugs are poorly tolerated or required in large prolonged doses and if thyrotoxicosis recurs after an apparently successful medication regimen. In the poor-risk patient or one who has had a recurrence of toxicity following previous thyroid surgery, medical therapy is usually the treatment of choice. Also, some pregnant patients may be best treated with antithyroid drugs in order to defer surgery until after the patient has delivered. However, thyroid replacement is given daily once the patient is euthyroid to prevent the development of a goiter in the fetus.

Subtotal thyroidectomy is also performed for an enlarged thyroid gland that produces pressure symptoms or an undesirable cosmetic effect (endemic goiter), for toxic goiters, and occasionally for inflammatory conditions such as Riedel's struma and Hashimoto's disease.

PREOPERATIVE PREPARATION. The only indication for emergency thyroidectomy is in that exceedingly rare situation where pressure symptoms develop rapidly due to intrathyroidal hemorrhage. In all other situations thyroidectomy should be considered an elective procedure performed when the patient is in optimal physical health. This is particularly true in thyrotoxicosis.

Patients with thyrotoxicosis should be treated with antithyroid drugs until an euthyroid state is reached. Because the (thiourea) compounds block the synthesis of thyroxine but do not inhibit the release of the hormone from existing colloid stores, the time required for symptomatic improvement may vary widely from two weeks to as long as three months. The variability is in part related to the size of the gland, as large goiters usually contain more colloid. When the patient has become euthyroid, iodine given as Lugol's solution, potassium iodide solution, or tablets or syrup of hydriodic acid is administered for ten days before surgery. If this procedure is followed, almost any thyroidectomy can be performed under optimal conditions. If significant tachycardia due to an increased intraoperative or postoperative release of thyroid hormone is encountered, propranolol should be used to control it.

ANESTHESIA. Endotracheal intubation is preferred, particularly if there has been long-standing pressure against the trachea, substernal extension, or severe thyrotoxicosis. For the severely toxic or for the apprehensive patient, rectal thiopental sodium, tribromethanol, or a short-acting intravenous barbiturate may be given in the patient's room to avoid undue excitement. General anesthetic agents used are intravenous thiopental sodium combined with nitrous oxide and oxygen or halothane.

POSITION. The patient is placed in a semierect position with a folded sheet underneath the shoulders so that the head is sharply angulated backward **(Figure 1).** The headrest of the table can be lowered to hyperextend the neck further. The anesthetist should make certain that the head is absolutely straight with the body before the line of incision is marked. Any deviation to the side may cause the surgeon to make an inaccurately placed incision.

OPERATIVE PREPARATION. The patient's hair has been previously covered completely by a snug gauze or mesh cap to avoid contamination of the field. The skin is prepared routinely. Before the incision is scratched, it may be accurately outlined by compressing a heavy silk thread against the skin. The incision should be made about two fingers above the sternal notch and should be almost exactly transverse, extending well onto the borders of the sternocleidomastoid muscles **(Figure 2).** In the presence of large goiters it should be made a little higher in order that the final scar will not lie in the suprasternal notch. A short midline crosshatch may be made across the outlined incision to provide a guide to accurate approximation of the skin at closure **(Figure 2).** The site for the incision is then draped with sterile towels secured with towel clips at the four corners, similar to a routine abdominal draping. Silk transfixing sutures may then be placed through the towel into the skin in the middle of the incision on either side. This secures the towel at the center of the incision and avoids contamination when the flaps are reflected upward and downward. Skin towels sutured or clipped to the field may be eliminated by the use of a sterile transparent plastic drape that is made adherent to the skin with an adhesive spray. After the skin is prepared, the incision may be scratched and crosshatched before applying the adhesive spray. A large sterile sheet with an oval opening completes the draping.

INCISION AND EXPOSURE. The surgeon stands at the patient's right side, since it is customary to commence the procedure at the right upper pole. He should be thoroughly familiar with the anatomy of the neck, especially with the blood supply and anatomic relationships of the thyroid gland **(Figures 3, 4, and 5).** A thorough understanding of the anatomy of this region should lessen the complications of hemorrhage, injury to the recurrent laryngeal nerve, which may course through the bifurcation of the inferior thyroid artery, and injury to the parathyroids. A dry field is maintained if the various fascial planes are carefully considered during the procedure **(Figure 3).** The locations of the major blood vessels, the parathyroid, and recurrent laryngeal nerve are shown in **Figures 3 and 5.**

The surgeon applies firm pressure over gauze sponges to one margin of the wound, while the first assistant applies similar pressure to the opposite margin. In this manner the active bleeding from subcutaneous tissue is controlled, and the margins of the wound are evenly separated. The skin incision is made with a deliberate sweep of the scalpel, dividing the skin and subcutaneous tissue simultaneously if the panniculus is not too thick. The belly of the scalpel should be swept across the tissues but not pressed into them. Bleeding vessels in the subcutaneous tissues are seized with hemostats; the large vessels are ligated, while small vessels are merely clamped and released. Hemostats with finely tapered jaws that can be applied to the vessel alone are the best type to use, because they permit ligation without strangulation of a tab of surrounding fat. One or two mass ligatures may do no harm, but many strangulated bits of tissue cause induration and inflammation during healing since the avascular tabs must be absorbed.

The incision is deepened to the areolar tissue plane just below the platysma muscle where an avascular space is reached. All active bleeding points are grasped with curved, pointed hemostats that are reflected upward or downward depending upon to which side of the incision they have been applied **(Figure 6).** Active bleeding and danger of air embolus may occur from accidental openings made into the anterior jugular vein if too deep an incision is made. Sharp dissection may be used alternately with blunt gauze dissection to facilitate the freeing of the upper flap **(Figures 7 and 8).** Usually, a small blood vessel will be encountered, high up beneath the flap on either side, which will produce troublesome bleeding unless it is doubly ligated **(Figures 8 and 9).** The dissection goes up to the thyroid notch, exposing all of the thyroid cartilage, as well as down to the suprasternal notch. Outward and downward traction is then applied to the lower skin flap as it is freed from the adjacent tissue down to the suprasternal notch **(Figure 9).** At the very lowest part of the wound, care should be taken to avoid damage to the communicating arch connecting the two anterior jugular veins. The ascending branches of these veins should be ligated below the communicating arch with a transfixing suture to prevent the complication of air embolism **(Figure 9).**

PLATE CXLI   THYROIDECTOMY, SUBTOTAL

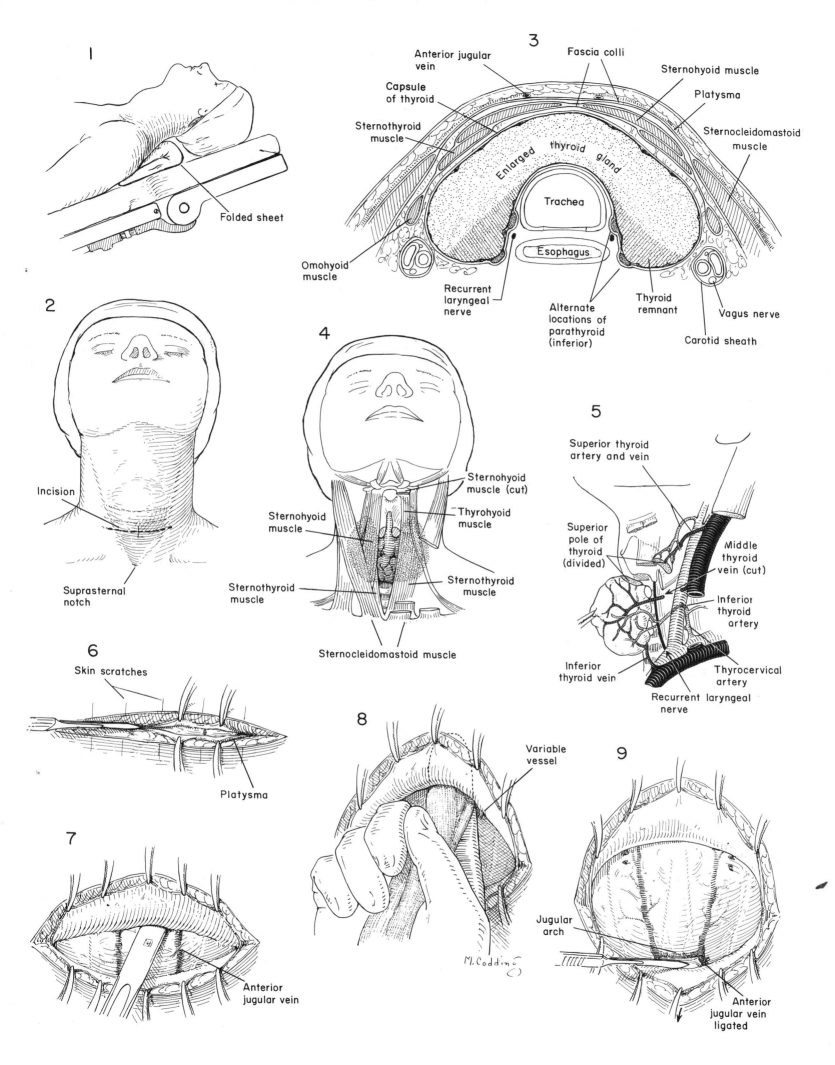

1

Folded sheet

3

Anterior jugular vein
Capsule of thyroid
Sternothyroid muscle
Fascia colli
Sternohyoid muscle
Platysma
Sternocleidomastoid muscle
Enlarged thyroid gland
Trachea
Esophagus
Omohyoid muscle
Recurrent laryngeal nerve
Alternate locations of parathyroid (inferior)
Thyroid remnant
Vagus nerve
Carotid sheath

2

Incision
Suprasternal notch

4

Sternohyoid muscle (cut)
Thyrohyoid muscle
Sternohyoid muscle
Sternothyroid muscle
Sternothyroid muscle
Sternocleidomastoid muscle

5

Superior thyroid artery and vein
Superior pole of thyroid (divided)
Middle thyroid vein (cut)
Inferior thyroid artery
Inferior thyroid vein
Thyrocervical artery
Recurrent laryngeal nerve

6

Skin scratches
Platysma

8

Variable vessel

9

7

Anterior jugular vein

Jugular arch
Anterior jugular vein ligated

M. Codding

PLATE CXLII · THYROIDECTOMY, SUBTOTAL

DETAILS OF PROCEDURE. Some type of self-retaining retractor is inserted to hold apart the skin flaps. In the presence of a large thyroid gland that necessitates division of sternohyoid and sternothyroid muscles, it is advisable to free the anterior margins of the sternocleidomastoid muscles. The margins of these muscles run diagonally across the outer limits of the wound and can be easily identified. The incision is made into the fascia along the margins of the sternocleidomastoid muscle **(Figure 10).** The handle of the scalpel is used as a dissecting tool to develop the correct plane of cleavage between the sternocleidomastoid muscle and the outer boundaries of the sternothyroid muscle **(Figures 11 and 12).**

To avoid bleeding, a vertical incision is placed exactly in the midline of the neck between the sternohyoid muscles, extending from the thyroid notch to the level of the sternal notch. All bleeding points are controlled by the application of hemostats. The tissues on either side of the incision are lifted up so that the incision is not carried directly through into the thyroid gland **(Figure 13).** The blunt handle of the knife is inserted beneath the exposed sternohyoid muscles **(Figures 14 and 15).** At this point the loose fascia over the thyroid gland should be picked up with forceps and incised with the scalpel in order to develop a cleavage plane between the thyroid gland and the sternothyroid muscle **(Figures 16, 17, and 18).** This is one of the most important steps in a thyroidectomy. Many difficulties may be encountered unless the proper cleavage plan is entered at this time. When the fascia of the sternothyroid muscle has been completely incised and reflected, the blood vessels in the capsule of the thyroid gland are clearly visible **(Figure 18).** After the proper cleavage plane is developed, the sternohyoid and sternothyroid muscles are pulled outward from the thyroid gland by means of a retractor, so that any unusual blood vessel communication between the sternothyroid muscle and the thyroid gland can be clamped and ligated **(Figure 18).** Once the surgeon is working in the proper cleavage plane, the delivery of the gland may be facilitated by inserting the two forefingers side by side to the outer edge of the thyroid gland and separating them, thus freeing the gland without injuring blood vessels **(Figures 19 and 20).** If an effort is made to free the entire lateral surface of the gland by finger dissection, it must be remembered that in some instances the middle thyroid vein is quite large and may be accidentally torn by this maneuver, resulting in troublesome bleeding.

If the thyroid is only moderately enlarged, retraction of the prethyroid muscles forward and laterally by narrow retractors will give adequate exposure for the subsequent procedure; however, if the mass of thyroid tissue is large, it may be wiser to divide the prethyroid muscles between muscle clamps. There is no difficulty with healing or function after transverse incision of the prethyroid muscles if this is done in the upper third to avoid injury to the motor nerve supply. The freed margin of the sternocleidomastoid muscle on either side is retracted laterally to avoid its inclusion in the muscle clamp **(Figures 20 and 21).** The muscle clamps are applied over the surgeon's finger as a guide to avoid including any part of the contents of the carotid bundle. The muscle is divided between the clamps, and an incision is made upward and downward from the end of either clamp to facilitate the retraction of the divided muscles **(Figure 21).** If large anterior jugular veins are present, it is advisable first to ligate them with transfixing sutures of fine silk adjacent to the upper and lower clamps. The muscle clamps can then be lifted out of the wound and will not hinder the subsequent procedure. The muscles on the left side are similarly divided.

PLATE CXLII   THYROIDECTOMY, SUBTOTAL

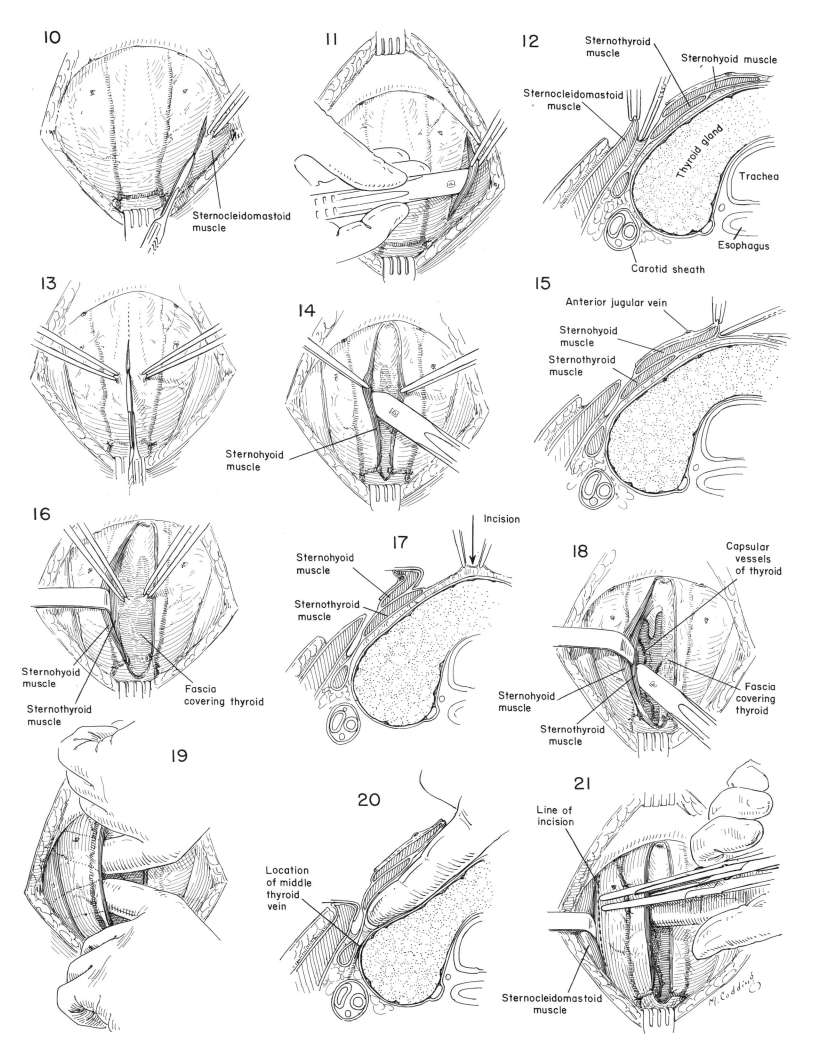

10

Sternocleidomastoid muscle

11

12
Sternothyroid muscle
Sternohyoid muscle
Sternocleidomastoid muscle
Thyroid gland
Trachea
Esophagus
Carotid sheath

13

14
Sternohyoid muscle

15
Anterior jugular vein
Sternohyoid muscle
Sternothyroid muscle

16
Sternohyoid muscle
Sternothyroid muscle
Fascia covering thyroid

17
Incision
Sternohyoid muscle
Sternothyroid muscle

18
Capsular vessels of thyroid
Sternohyoid muscle
Sternothyroid muscle
Fascia covering thyroid

19

20
Location of middle thyroid vein

21
Line of incision
Sternocleidomastoid muscle

M. Codding

PLATE CXLIII · THYROIDECTOMY, SUBTOTAL

DETAILS OF PROCEDURE (*Continued*). Occasionally, as the upper muscle clamp is retracted upward and outward, a branch of the superior thyroid artery may be encountered, extending from the muscle to the surface of the thyroid gland in the region of the upper pole. This vessel should be carefully clamped and tied **(Figure 22)**.

It is customary to begin a subtotal thyroidectomy at the right upper pole or on the larger side. A narrow retractor is placed in the wound at the superior pole. Blunt dissection, which allows the thyroid capsule to be pushed away from the larynx, is best accomplished by opening a small, curved hemostat in the membranous tissue at this point **(Figure 23)**. At the uppermost portion of the gland there is a thin fascia that almost encircles the trachea. This area must be carefully clamped, since it contains a small blood vessel which, if allowed to retract, is very dangerous to secure because of its proximity to the superior laryngeal nerve. Traction should be maintained on the thyroid gland by means of a curved hemostat or a specially devised tenaculum applied to the gland in the region of the upper pole. There is less chance of tearing a friable gland if curved hemostats rather than a toothed tenaculum are used for traction. By sharp and blunt dissection the superior thyroid vessels are exposed well above their point of entry into the gland **(Figure 23)**. The surgeon now decides whether to leave any thyroid tissue at the upper pole region and places his next clamp either at the upper limits of the gland or in the substance of the gland, perhaps 1 cm. below the top of the pole. Hemostasis is more easily effected if the superior thyroid arteries are ligated extracapsularly. Moreover, if much glandular tissue is to be retained, it should be on the posterior surface at the level of the inferior thyroid arteries, as there is more likely to be a recurrence at the superior pole. Three small, straight or curved hemostats are applied to the superior thyroid vessels. The vessels are divided, leaving one clamp on the thyroid side and two clamps on the vessels **(Figure 24)**. The application of two clamps to the upper pole vessels permits a double ligation and lessens the possibility of active troublesome bleeding. If possible, the second ligature should be a transfixing suture of fine silk **(Figure 25)**.

If the middle thyroid vein has not already been identified and ligated, an effort should be made to locate this vessel. Often it is stretched to a thin strand as a result of traction applied to the gland in order to displace it **(Figure 26)**. After the superior vessels and middle thyroid vein have been ligated, the narrow retractor is moved to the right lower pole, where the lower pole vessels enter the gland. These vessels are carefully freed from the adjacent structures either with a small, curved clamp or by finger dissection **(Figure 27)**. Care must be taken not to injure the trachea at the

time these vessels are divided and doubly tied **(Figure 28)**. Occasionally, a venous plexus (or thyroidea ima) is found over the trachea entering the inferior surface of the gland in the region of the isthmus. This is carefully separated from the trachea with a blunt-nosed hemostat and ligated in the usual fashion.

As an alternate method the surgeon may decide to start at the lower pole and luxate the gland before the upper pole is ligated. The thyroid tissue over the trachea is divided, and the right lobe is reflected outward **(Figure 29)**. The lower pole vessels are then clamped and ligated. The middle thyroid vein is brought into view by medial retraction and can easily be tied. The upper pole is now freed by pushing the index finger behind the superior thyroid vessels. As the superior pole is pushed forward with the finger, a curved clamp may be inserted between the trachea and the medial surface of the superior pole, and the vessels can be doubly clamped **(Figure 30)**.

After the middle and inferior veins have been ligated and the superior pole freed by either method, the next step is exposing the inferior thyroid artery. Traction is maintained anteriorly and medially as the artery is exposed on the lateral inferior surface of the gland **(Figure 31)**. A narrow retractor is inserted laterally, and by gauze dissection the lateral aspect of the gland in the region of the inferior thyroid artery is clearly visualized. It should be remembered, especially in the presence of a large gland which has been displaced outward, that the recurrent laryngeal nerve may be much higher in the wound than is ordinarily anticipated. If a very extensive removal of thyroid tissue is indicated, it is necessary by careful dissection to identify this nerve, which may run between the bifurcation of the inferior thyroid artery as it enters the gland. The fossa posterior to the gland should also be inspected to determine, if possible, the location of the parathyroid glands, which are usually a pinkish chocolate color. Before commencing this dissection, it is wise to place hemostats on the vessels at the margins of the gland where the major branches of the inferior thyroid artery lie. The application of paired clamps to the major blood vessels at a safe distance from the region of the recurrent laryngeal nerve **(Figure 32)** defines the amount of thyroid tissue that will remain and lessens the chance of accidental injury to the nerve. With the trachea in view and the gland lifted into the wound, another row of small, curved hemostats is placed well into the parenchyma so that the desired amount of thyroid tissue is retained along with the posterior capsule **(Figure 33)**. The amount of thyroid tissue allowed to remain in relation to recurrent laryngeal nerve is illustrated in Plate CXLI, **Figure 3**.

PLATE CXLIII   THYROIDECTOMY, SUBTOTAL

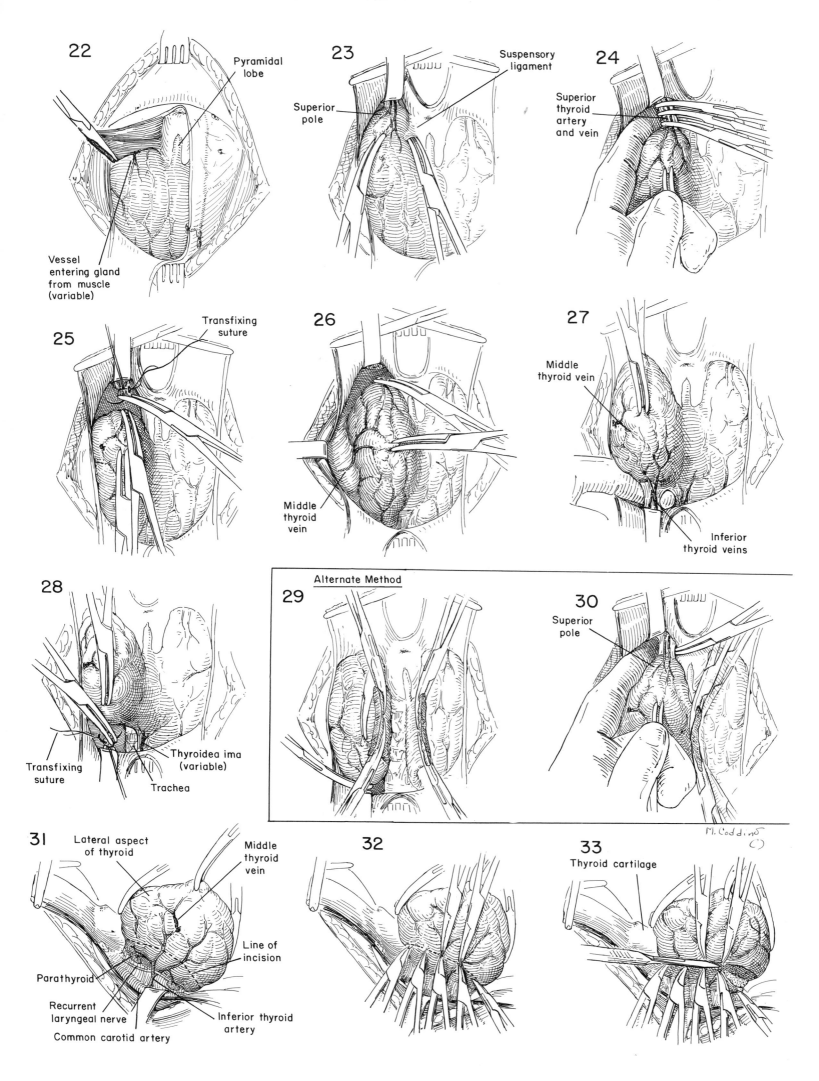

PLATE CXLIV · THYROIDECTOMY, SUBTOTAL

DETAILS OF PROCEDURE (*Continued*). With the lateral hemostats in place, the right lobe is pushed laterally, and the isthmus is exposed. The isthmus is divided, if this has not already been done. The inferior border immediately over the trachea is grasped with mouse-toothed forceps and pulled upward as a curved clamp is inserted between the trachea and the posterior portion of the gland **(Figure 34)**. A similar clamp is inserted from the upper side. After the cleavage plane between the thyroid gland and the anterior surface of the trachea has been developed, the entire isthmus is divided between curved clamps. If the clamps enter the tracheal fascia, there will be added discomfort in the postoperative period. The isthmus is divided close to the right side of the clamps **(Figure 35)**. The clamps remain on the left portion of the thyroid as the right lobe margin is retracted laterally **(Figure 36)**. Curved clamps are inserted across the trachea into the parenchyma of the gland and pointed toward the lateral row of clamps (Plate CXLIII, **Figure 32**). If the clamps are placed horizontally across the trachea, the points will not injure the recurrent laryngeal nerve **(Figure 37)**. The portion to be removed is now lifted and dissected free **(Figure 38)**. The bleeding points in the center of the remnant are clamped. Only small amounts of tissue are included. Actively bleeding points that retract, especially along the tracheal margin of the remnant, are controlled by lateral compression with the index finger. Blind clamping of thyroid tissue, particularly at the superior edge, may result in injury to the recurrent laryngeal nerve **(Figure 39**, point x). All bleeding points are carefully ligated. Blind, deep placement of transfixing sutures is avoided because of the likelihood of danger to the underlying structures. The surgeon must tie beneath these clamps with great care, preferably using a surgeon's knot on the first throw of the tie, so that the subsequent knots can be tied without keeping the ligature under tension. As a rule, the tissues have been clamped under tension, and the vessels tend to retract unless securely held by the first throw of the tie. If transfixion is required, it should be done with a small, curved needle, and great care should be exercised to prevent penetration of the posterior capsule and possible injury to the recurrent laryngeal nerve.

When no bleeding points remain, the cavity may be irrigated with saline. The pyramidal lobe, which may be variable in size, is entirely removed. There is usually a bleeding point at the top of this lobe, and hemostats are applied and the vessel is ligated **(Figure 40)**. When freeing the isthmus, great care is taken to avoid injury to the thin tracheal fascia. If this fascia is torn, postoperative tracheitis and undue soreness may be encountered.

The left side is freed similarly. The additional space left by the removal of a large right lobe somewhat simplifies the removal of the left lobe. The surgeon moves to the left side and takes every precaution to protect the recurrent laryngeal nerve and to effect complete hemostasis. The field is inspected for evidence of bleeding **(Figure 41)**.

CLOSURE. The folded sheet is removed from beneath the neck, and the tension on the chin is relaxed. The wound is repeatedly irrigated with large amounts of saline, and the field is again inspected for any bleeding.

The wound is carefully protected while the anesthetist introduces the laryngoscope to inspect the position of the vocal cords. If the position of the vocal cords suggests injury to either nerve, the surgeon should visualize the nerve on the involved side throughout its course and release any sutures that may have included or damaged the nerve. While the anesthetist is inspecting the vocal cords, the surgeon should inspect the specimen very carefully for adherent parathyroid glands. Questionable tissue must be closely inspected; any parathyroid substance found should be transplanted, preferably into the sternocleidomastoid muscle.

The operator must familiarize himself with the appearance of the parathyroid gland, which is a pinkish-brown, flattened node about 3 to 4 mm. in diameter. The superior glands are usually found on the posterior surface of the thyroid about the level of the lower portion of the thyroid cartilage. The inferior glands are seen at the lower portion of the thyroid, usually underneath the inferior pole or lying in the fat a little below and deeper than the thyroid substance. Usually, the inferior parathyroids are seen and

can be left behind when the small inferior thyroid veins and the thyroidea ima vessels are first divided. Regardless of the fact that the surgeon may be certain that the parathyroid glands remain in the wound, any suspected tissue attached to the specimen is transplanted into the wound.

The prethyroid muscles are then approximated. If the anterior jugular veins have not previously been ligated, they should be tied with a transfixing suture adjacent to the muscle clamps. The anterior margins of the sternocleidomastoid muscles are retracted laterally as the sutures are placed beneath the muscle clamps **(Figure 42)**. After closure of the transverse incision, the prethyroid muscles are approximated in the midline with interrupted sutures **(Figure 43)**. Drainage is unnecessary in a dry field; however, if a large cavity has resulted following the removal of a large nodular gland, a small rubber tissue drain may be brought out through the center of the incision or through a small stab wound beneath the incision.

The hemostats are removed from the subcutaneous tissue, and all active bleeding points are ligated with fine 0000 silk ligatures. The skin flaps are approximated, and the platysma and the subcutaneous tissue are repaired in separate layers in order to mound up the tissues and obviate the necessity for tension on the skin sutures **(Figure 44)**. The very fine skin sutures are introduced close to the margin of the incision and are tied loosely so that circulation is not jeopardized. A light sterile dressing consisting of a flat piece of gauze is sufficient and is held in position by a long piece of adhesive tape which encircles the neck and is crossed over the dressing with the ends anchored to the chest wall on either side.

POSTOPERATIVE CARE. The patient is immediately placed in a semi-sitting position. Adequate precautions should be taken to prevent hyperextension of the neck. Oxygen therapy is administered, 4 to 5 liters per minute, until the patient has reacted. A sterile tracheotomy set should always be available in the event of acute collapse of the trachea. Parenteral fluids are given until the patient can take adequate fluids by mouth. The addition of sodium iodide and calcium gluconate depends upon the patient's general condition. Liquids by mouth are permitted as tolerated. Opiates or sedatives are used as necessary. Blood loss is replaced by blood transfusions.

Early complications include hemorrhage into the wound, hoarseness and temporary aphonia, vocal cord paralysis, and postoperative thyroid "storm."

The most important postoperative complication is hemorrhage in the wound. If wound hemorrhage is suspected, the dressing is removed, several skin sutures are taken out, the blood is evacuated under aseptic conditions, and major bleeding points are ligated.

Bilateral injury of the recurrent laryngeal nerve may result in paralysis of both vocal cords and may require tracheotomy.

The salient symptoms of postoperative crisis are high fever, severe tachycardia, extreme restlessness, excessive sweating, sleeplessness, vomiting, diarrhea, and delirium. Ice caps or cooling blankets, sedation, and parenteral high-calorie fluids, to which 1 Gm. of sodium iodide and 100 mg. of corticoids have been added, are indicated. The continued administration of approximately 15 mg. of a satisfactory corticoid preparation per hour in an intravenous drip is recommended. Oxygen, antipyretics, and multivitamin preparations are also administered.

Postoperative hypoparathyroidism requires calcium chloride 5 per cent or calcium gluconate 10 per cent intravenously. Vitamin D_2 is administered at a dosage sufficient to maintain a normal serum calcium level. No added oral calcium other than a glass of milk with each meal is required. Two or three grains of desiccated thyroid are given daily to prevent the recurrence of nontoxic nodular goiter.

Any drains are removed on the first postoperative day, and the skin sutures are removed, half on the second day, the remainder on the fourth day. The patient is permitted out of bed on the first postoperative day and sent home on the fifth day unless some complication occurs.

PLATE CXLIV   THYROIDECTOMY, SUBTOTAL

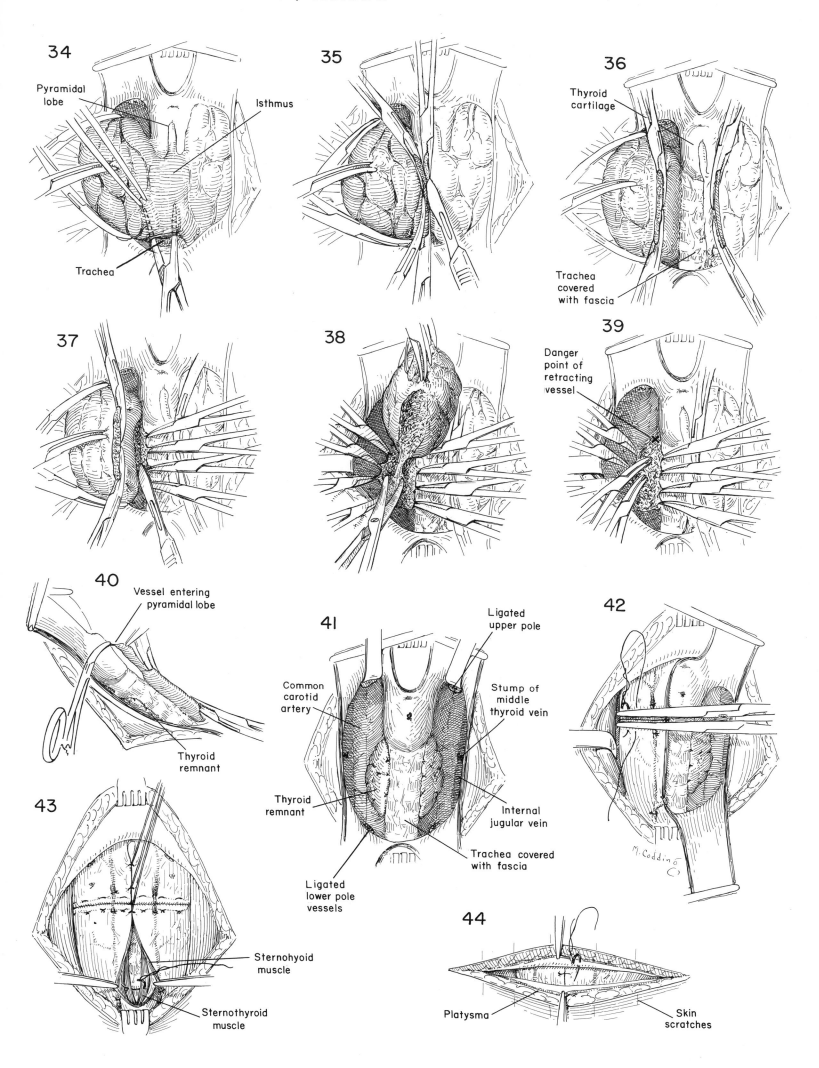

34
Pyramidal lobe
Isthmus
Trachea

35

36
Thyroid cartilage
Trachea covered with fascia

37

38

39
Danger point of retracting vessel

40
Vessel entering pyramidal lobe
Thyroid remnant

41
Ligated upper pole
Common carotid artery
Stump of middle thyroid vein
Thyroid remnant
Internal jugular vein
Trachea covered with fascia
Ligated lower pole vessels

42
M. Coddino

43
Sternohyoid muscle
Sternothyroid muscle

44
Platysma
Skin scratches

PLATE CXLV · TRACHEOTOMY

INDICATIONS. Tracheotomy is performed for two groups of patients. In the first group are those with an obstruction of the airway at or above the level of the larynx. Such obstruction may result acutely from laryngeal tumors, edema, fracture, foreign bodies, burns about the oropharynx, or severe throat and neck infections.

In the second group are patients with chronic or long-term respiratory problems. Inability to cough out tracheobronchial secretions in paralyzed or weakened patients may be an indication for tracheotomy, which allows frequent and easy endotracheal suctioning. This group of patients includes those with prolonged unconsciousness after drug intoxication, head injury, or brain surgery, and those with bulbar or thoracic paralysis as in poliomyelitis. To this group are added patients with general debility, especially in the presence of pulmonary infection or abdominal distention, where a temporary course of respiratory support with an endotracheal tube and mechanical ventilator for three to six days must be converted into a longer course of pulmonary assistance. In these patients inability to maintain an adequate gas exchange or oxygen or carbon dioxide may dictate conversion of the endotracheal tube to a tracheotomy one. Frequently, checks of arterial blood gases will reveal hypoxemia or hypercarbia, while simple measurements of vital capacity and negative inspiratory force will detect insufficient respiratory muscular effort. These tests are important in the decision to continue tracheal intubation with ventilator assistance. Other candidates for tracheotomy may include patients undergoing major operative or radical resections of the mouth, jaw, or larynx, where this procedure is often done as a precautionary measure.

PREOPERATIVE PREPARATION. Because the patient is usually in respiratory difficulty, preoperative preparation is generally not possible.

ANESTHESIA. In cooperative patients, in both elective and emergency situations, local infiltration anesthesia is preferred. In patients who are comatose or are choking, no anesthesia may be necessary or possible. Because it helps to ensure a good airway during tracheotomy, endotracheal intubation is especially useful in patients whose laryngeal airway is very poor and who may obstruct at any moment. It is also an aid in palpating the small, soft trachea of infants.

POSITION. A sandbag or folded sheet under the shoulders helps extend the neck **(Figure 1),** as does lowering the headrest of the operating table. The chin is positioned carefully in the midline.

OPERATIVE PREPARATION. In emergency tracheotomy sterile preparation is either greatly abbreviated or omitted entirely. In routine tracheotomy a sterile field is prepared in the usual manner.

A. Emergency Tracheotomy

INCISION AND EXPOSURE. Emergency tracheotomy is done when there is not time to prepare for a routine tracheotomy. There may be no sterile surgical instruments available and no assistants.

An emergency airway is made by a transverse cut or stab through the circothyroid membrane. Here the airway is immediately subcutaneous, yet the level is still under the vocal cords **(Figure 2).** The wound is held open by twisting the handle of the knife blade in the wound. Later, with the airway assured, the patient is removed to the operating room, and a routine tracheotomy is done.

B. Elective Tracheotomy

INCISION AND EXPOSURE. A vertical incision is made in the midline of the neck from the middle of the thyroid cartilage to just above the suprasternal notch **(Figure 3).** The skin, subcutaneous tissues, and strap muscles are retracted laterally to expose the thyroid isthmus **(Figures 4 and 5).** The isthmus may be either divided and ligated or retracted upward after the pretracheal fascia is cut. Usually, upward retraction is the better method.

After the cricoid cartilage is identified **(Figure 6),** the trachea is opened vertically through its third and fourth rings **(Figures 7** and **8).** In order to facilitate insertion of the tracheotomy tube, either a cruciate incision is made, or a very narrow segment of one ring may be removed **(Figure 9).** The transverse incision, preferred by some surgeons for cosmetic reasons, is more time consuming. The difference in the final cosmetic result is negligible since it is the tube and not the incision that causes scarring.

DETAILS OF PROCEDURE. A tracheal hook is used to pull up the trachea and steady it for incision **(Figure 9).** Great care must be taken not to cut through the trachea too deeply since the posterior wall of the trachea is also the anterior wall of the esophagus.

After the trachea has been incised, a previously selected tracheotomy tube is inserted. A No. 6 tube is ordinarily suitable for an adult male and a No. 5 or 6 tube for an adult female. Correspondingly smaller tubes are used in children and infants. The trachea of a newborn will accept only a No. 00 or 0 tube. The assistant must be careful to keep the tube in the trachea by holding one finger on the flange; otherwise, the patient may cough it out. Plastic endotracheal tubes with an inflatable cuff usually of the size similar to oral intubation are used.

CLOSURE. Closure should be loose to prevent subcutaneous emphysema. Only skin sutures are used. Ties hold the tube in place **(Figure 10).** A dressing is made by cutting a surgical gauze and pulling the gauze under the flange of the tube.

POSTOPERATIVE CARE. Special and frequent attention is very desirable in the first few postoperative days. The inner tube must be cleaned every hour or two; otherwise, it may block off with accumulated secretions. After a tract has formed, usually in two or three days, the outer tube may be removed, cleaned, and replaced. Even then, however, the tube should be replaced rapidly since the stoma constricts sufficiently in only 15 or 20 minutes to make replacement difficult. An obturator is provided with each tracheotomy tube to make insertion of the outer tube easier. There must always be a duplicate trachea tube at the patient's bedside.

Suctioning of the trachea is done as needed. In the alert patient who can cough, suctioning may not be needed at all, but in the comatose patient suctioning may be required every 15 minutes. It is essential that moisture be added to the air, since the nasal chambers are bypassed and the usual means by which the body moistens the air are lost. This can be accomplished by the use of aerosol bubblers or ultrasonic nebulizers.

Blood gases and blood pH should be monitored frequently until stable and satisfactory levels have been attained.

PLATE CXLV   TRACHEOTOMY

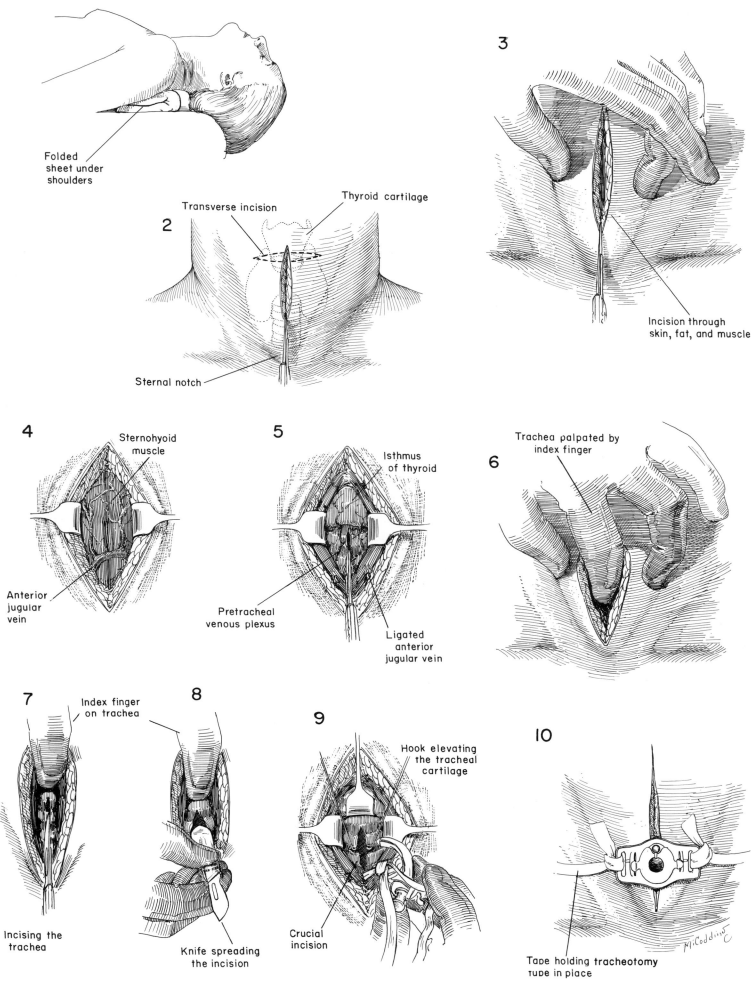

Folded sheet under shoulders

2

Transverse incision

Thyroid cartilage

Sternal notch

3

Incision through skin, fat, and muscle

4

Sternohyoid muscle

Anterior jugular vein

5

Isthmus of thyroid

Pretracheal venous plexus

Ligated anterior jugular vein

6

Trachea palpated by index finger

7

Index finger on trachea

Incising the trachea

8

Knife spreading the incision

9

Hook elevating the tracheal cartilage

Crucial incision

10

Tape holding tracheotomy tube in place

PLATE CXLVI · RADICAL NECK DISSECTION

INDICATIONS. There are two major indications for radical neck dissection. The first is for the removal of palpable metastatic cervical lymph nodes, and the second is for the removal of presumed occult metastatic disease in the neck. The latter indication has been termed "prophylactic neck dissection." "Elective neck dissection" better describes this operation, since it is not intended to prevent metastasis but to remove occult metastatic lymph nodes.

Before radical neck dissection is performed, the surgeon must have assurance that the primary lesion can be controlled either by simultaneous *en bloc* removal with the radical neck dissection or by radiation therapy. However, curative radiation for cervical metastases must be confined to a single node or small group of nodes, because patients cannot tolerate cancericidal radiation to the entire neck. Node fixation, invasion of adjacent tissues, bilateral or contralateral, and distant metastases are relative contraindications to this procedure. In general, radical dissection of the cervical lymph nodes in a patient who is a reasonable surgical risk remains the preferred treatment for metastatic disease of the neck.

The usual patient with metastatic cancer in the neck from an unknown primary source should be treated as if the primary tumor were controlled. If surgical treatment of the cervical metastasis is deferred until the primary neoplasm becomes obvious, the opportunity to control the neck disease is lost.

PREOPERATIVE PREPARATION. The patient's general medical status should be assessed and corrective measures instituted for any treatable abnormalities. Intraoral ulcerations represent a potential source of pathogenic material. The liberal preoperative use of nonirritating solutions (e.g., diluted hydrogen peroxide) can significantly reduce the danger of postoperative infection.

Only rarely will primary cancers of the hypopharynx, cervical esophagus, larynx, etc., produce respiratory obstruction or interference with alimentation significant enough to require preoperative tracheostomy or insertion of a feeding tube.

On the morning of surgery the face, neck, and upper chest are cleanly shaved.

ANESTHESIA. The major consideration is a free airway. The equipment should allow free movement of the head and easy access to the endotracheal tube.

The choice of anesthetic agents varies. Consideration must be given to the individual needs of the patient and to the need for cautery. General endotracheal anesthesia is preferred.

Complications at surgery are the carotid sinus syndrome, pneumothorax, and air embolus. The carotid sinus syndrome, consisting of hypotension, bradycardia, and cardiac irregularity, usually can be corrected by infiltrating the carotid sinus with a local anesthetic agent. Intravenous atropine sulfate usually will control the syndrome if the local anesthetic fails. Pneumothorax may result from injury of the apical pleura. It is treated with a closed-tube thoracostomy through the second intercostal space anteriorly.

POSITION. The patient is placed in a dorsal recumbent position. The head of the table is somewhat elevated to lessen the blood pressure, particularly the venous pressure, in the head and neck and thus reduce blood loss. The bend of the neck should be placed on the hinge of the headpiece so that the head may be either flexed or extended as needed. A small sandbag should be placed under the shoulders so that the head and neck are extended while the chin remains on a plane horizontal with the shoulders.

OPERATIVE PREPARATION. The patient's hair should be completely covered by a snug gauze cap to avoid contamination of the operative field. Once the patient has been correctly positioned on the table, the skin is prepared routinely. The preparation should include a large portion of the face on the side of the dissection, the neck from the midline posteriorly to the sternocleidomastoid muscle of the opposite side of the neck, and the anterior chest wall down to the nipple. The entire field of dissection is outlined with sterile towels secured by either towel clips or sutures. A large sheet about the head and neck area completes the draping.

INCISION AND EXPOSURE. The surgeon stands on the side of the proposed dissection. Many types of incision have been used. The most useful incision is a modification of the double trifurcate incision **(Figure 1),** in which the angles of the skin flaps are obtuse and connected by a short vertical incision. The upper arm of the double Y extends from the mastoid process to just below the midline of the mandible. The lower arm extends from the trapezius in a gentle curve to the midline of the neck. This incision allows the greatest exposure of the neck area while producing a good cosmetic result. Creation of the skin flaps includes the platysma muscle **(Figure 2).** In most instances if the skin flaps are developed without inclusion of the platysma muscle, poor wound healing and uncomfortable scarring with fixation of the skin to the deep neck structures will result. The two lateral skin flaps are turned back, the posterior flap extended as far as the anterior edge of the trapezius muscle, and the anterolateral flap extended to expose the strap muscles covering the thyroid gland. In developing the superior skin flap, care must be taken to preserve the mandibular marginal branch of the facial nerve **(Figure 2).** This branch of the facial nerve innervates the lower lip. In the majority of cases the nerve can be identified as it crosses over the external maxillary artery and the anterior facial vein beneath the platysma muscle. Usually, it lies parallel to the lower border of the mandible. Occasionally, the nerve will lie much higher, and it may not be visualized during the neck dissection. As suggested by others, a useful maneuver to preserve this nerve is to identify the external maxillary artery and the anterior facial vein at least a centimeter below the lower border of the mandible **(Figure 2).** After identification the nerve is retracted and covered by securing the upper end of the vascular stump to the platysma muscle. If obvious or strongly suspected tumor is present in this area, the branches of this nerve are voluntarily sacrificed. The inferior skin flap should be reflected down to expose the superior aspect of the clavicle.

DETAILS OF PROCEDURE. Once the four skin flaps have been created, the inferior limits are outlined. The sternocleidomastoid muscle is severed just above its insertion into the clavicle and the sternum **(Figure 3).** The dissection is then shifted to the posterior cervical triangle. Using both sharp and blunt dissection, the surgeon exposes the anterior border of the trapezius muscle **(Figure 4).**

PLATE CXLVI   RADICAL NECK DISSECTION

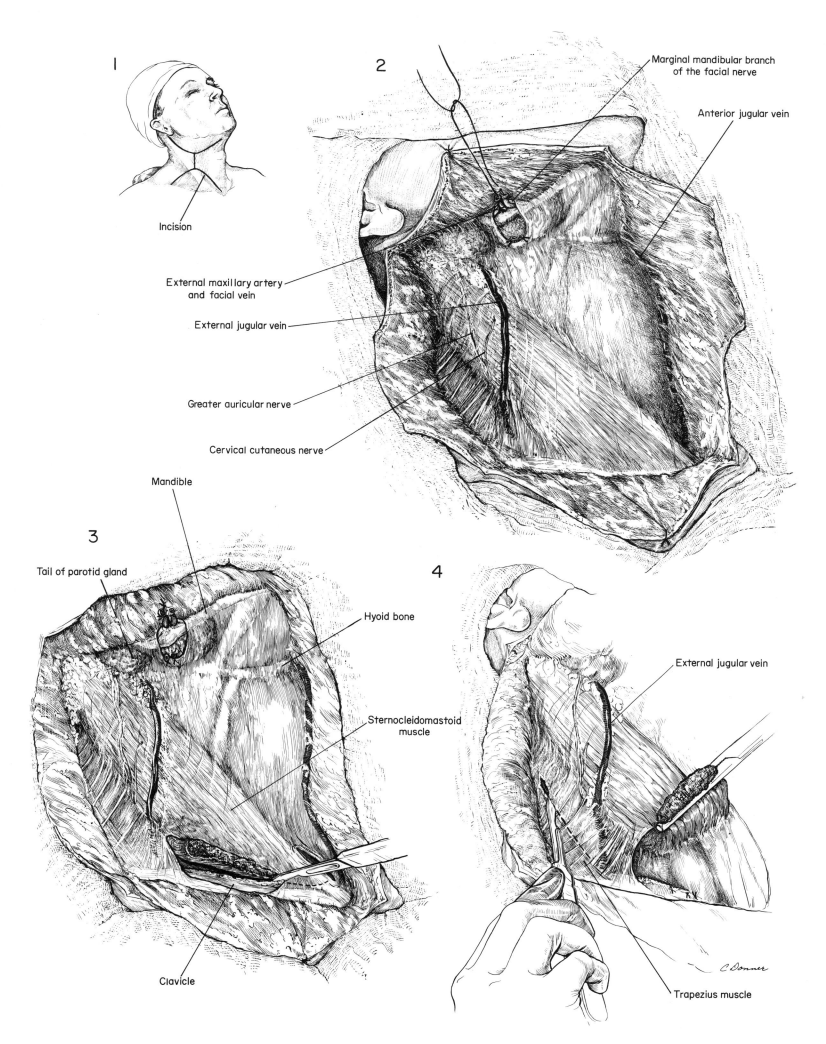

1

Incision

2

Marginal mandibular branch of the facial nerve

Anterior jugular vein

External maxillary artery and facial vein

External jugular vein

Greater auricular nerve

Cervical cutaneous nerve

Mandible

3

Tail of parotid gland

Hyoid bone

Sternocleidomastoid muscle

Clavicle

4

External jugular vein

Trapezius muscle

PLATE CXLVII · RADICAL NECK DISSECTION

DETAILS OF PROCEDURE (*Continued*). As one approaches the most posteroinferior angle of the neck dissection, the first important structure to be seen is the external jugular vein. It is ligated and divided at the posteroinferior corner **(Figure 5).** Then the posterior cervical triangle can be completely cleaned of its areolar and lymphatic tissues. The spinal accessory nerve must be divided **(Figure 6),** or clean dissection of this area is impossible. Dissection is carried forward along the superior aspects of the clavicle. The posterior belly of the omohyoid muscle and the transverse cervical artery and vein are visualized **(Figure 6).** The posterior belly of the omohyoid muscle is severed **(Figure 7)** to allow greater exposure of the deep muscles and the brachial plexus. The phrenic nerve is found lying upon the anterior scalene muscle between the brachial plexus and the internal jugular vein **(Figure 8A).** To avoid paralysis of the corresponding leaf of the diaphragm, this nerve should be preserved unless invaded by the cancer. The phrenic nerve lies upon the scalenus anticus muscle. Its exposure has been facilitated by the previous transection of the lower end of the sternocleidomastoid muscle. Just medial to the phrenic nerve the internal jugular vein is seen **(Figure 8A).** This vessel, which lies within the carotid sheath **(Figure 8B),** is dissected free **(Figure 9),** doubly ligated by a stick tie on the inferior ligation, and then divided **(Figure 10).** By division of the internal jugular vein, avoiding the thoracic duct on the left side, the dissection has been carried down to the prevertebral fascia overlying the deep muscle structures of the neck. The inferior compartment of the neck is then outlined medially by division of the pretracheal fascia just lateral to the strap muscles of the thyroid **(Figure 11).** This facilitates exposure of the common carotid artery, which permits the dissection to be carried superiorly. With the lateral limits of the dissection defined and the common carotid artery exposed, dissection is started inferiorly and extended superiorly following the floor of the neck or the prevertebral fascia.

PLATE CXLVII   RADICAL NECK DISSECTION

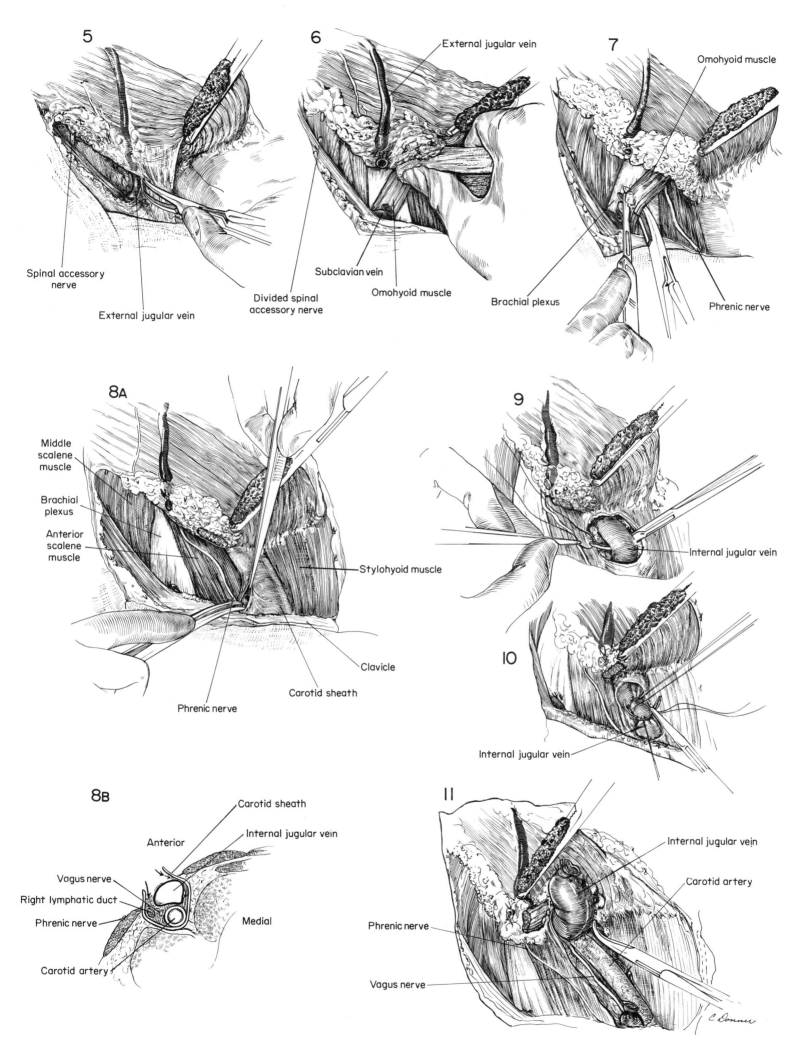

5
Spinal accessory nerve
External jugular vein

6
External jugular vein
Subclavian vein
Omohyoid muscle
Divided spinal accessory nerve
Brachial plexus

7
Omohyoid muscle
Phrenic nerve

8A
Middle scalene muscle
Brachial plexus
Anterior scalene muscle
Stylohyoid muscle
Clavicle
Carotid sheath
Phrenic nerve

9
Internal jugular vein

10
Internal jugular vein

8B
Carotid sheath
Internal jugular vein
Anterior
Vagus nerve
Right lymphatic duct
Phrenic nerve
Medial
Carotid artery

11
Internal jugular vein
Carotid artery
Phrenic nerve
Vagus nerve

PLATE CXLVIII · RADICAL NECK DISSECTION

DETAILS OF PROCEDURE (*Continued*). This dissection consists of turning up the areolar and lymphoid tissues of the neck lying along the course of the internal jugular vein, which is reflected upward with these structures **(Figure 12).** All loose areolar tissue about the carotid artery is completely removed. This dissection may be carried out without danger to any of the vital structures, since both the vagus nerve and the common carotid artery are in full view and the other important nerve structures—namely, the phrenic nerve and the brachial plexus—are covered by the prevertebral fascia **(Figure 12).** As the dissection proceeds superiorly, branches of the cervical plexus are seen penetrating the fascia; they should be divided as they emerge through the fascia.

In the anterior part of this phase of the dissection, tributaries of the superior thyroid, superior laryngeal, and pharyngeal veins are seen as they cross the operative field to enter the jugular vein. These may be ligated as the dissection proceeds. The carotid bifurcation usually can be identified by the appearance of the superior thyroid artery **(Figure 12).** With reasonable care this vessel can be preserved. After exposure of the bifurcation dissection proceeds superiorly with some caution to expose the hypoglossal nerve as it crosses both the internal and external carotid arteries a centimeter or so above the carotid bifurcation **(Figure 12).** The surgeon should watch for this nerve as it emerges deep to the posterior belly of the digastric muscle. The hypoglossal nerve continues forward into the sub-maxillary triangle, where it lies inferior to the main submaxillary salivary duct.

After identification of the hypoglossal nerve, attention should be directed to the submental area of the neck. The fascia from the midline of the neck is divided **(Figure 13).** This facilitates exposure of the anterior belly of the digastric muscle and the underlying mylohyoid muscle. Complete exposure of the digastric muscle in the submental compartment is necessary to remove the paired submental nodes **(Figure 13 or 14).** By following the anterior digastric muscle from anterior to posterior, the submaxillary gland is exposed. The submaxillary gland is dissected from its bed by approaching the gland anteriorly **(Figure 15).** By mobilizing the gland from its bed from anterior to posterior, the lingual nerve, which lies in the most superior aspect of the submaxillary space; the submaxillary duct, which lies in the midportion of the compartment; and the hypoglossal nerve, which lies in the most inferior aspect of the area, are identified **(Figure 16).** This exposure may be eased by traction on the submaxillary gland with a tenaculum. This allows the surgeon to visualize the posterior edge of the mylohyoid muscle and to retract this muscle anteriorly **(Figure 16),** thereby exposing the three important structures: the lingual nerve, the salivary duct, and the hypoglossal nerve. To facilitate removal of the submaxillary gland, the major salivary duct is divided and ligated.

PLATE CXLVIII   RADICAL NECK DISSECTION

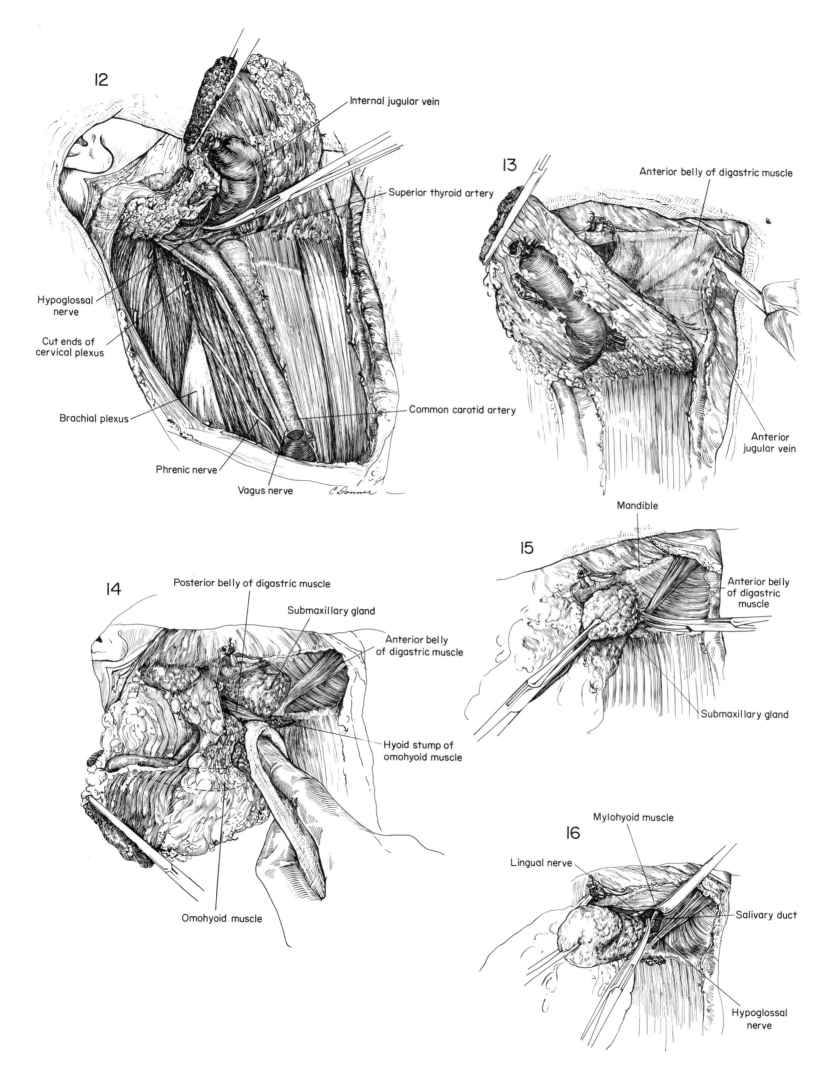

12

Internal jugular vein

Superior thyroid artery

Hypoglossal nerve

Cut ends of cervical plexus

Brachial plexus

Phrenic nerve

Vagus nerve

Common carotid artery

13

Anterior belly of digastric muscle

Anterior jugular vein

14

Posterior belly of digastric muscle

Submaxillary gland

Anterior belly of digastric muscle

Hyoid stump of omohyoid muscle

Omohyoid muscle

Mandible

15

Anterior belly of digastric muscle

Submaxillary gland

Mylohyoid muscle

16

Lingual nerve

Salivary duct

Hypoglossal nerve

PLATE CXLIX · RADICAL NECK DISSECTION

DETAILS OF PROCEDURE (*Continued*). The anterior belly of the omohyoid muscle is divided from the sling of the digastric muscles, and the dissection then can be completed after the posterior belly of the digastric muscle is exposed **(Figure 17).** Retraction of the posterior belly of the digastric superiorly exposes the internal jugular vein for clamping and division **(Figure 18).** Retraction of the posterior belly of the digastric muscle also allows complete exposure of the hypoglossal nerve **(Figure 18).** The internal jugular vein must be clamped high, since the upper limit of the internal jugular chain of lymphatics is one of the most frequent areas for metastatic cancer in the neck. To ensure that it has been divided high, the tail of the parotid **(Figure 19)** is sacrificed as the complete surgical specimen is excised. If extensive node involvement is present in the upper jugular chain of lymphatics, additional exposure can be obtained by total division of the posterior belly and its subsequent total removal. The dissection is completed with the division of the sternocleidomastoid muscle at the mastoid process.

CLOSURE. Hemostasis is secured in all areas of the neck. The platysma is closed using interrupted 0000 silk sutures. The skin is approximated with interrupted 0000 silk sutures. Before closure of the platysma and the skin, catheters are placed beneath both the anterior and posterior skin flaps and connected to suction **(Figure 20).** The placement of the catheters is important to ensure complete removal of fluid from beneath the flaps and to eliminate dead space in the area of dissection. A vacuum-type suction source can be attached to the patient, thus permitting early ambulation. Such catheters have eliminated bulky and uncomfortable pressure dressings.

POSTOPERATIVE CARE. The patient is immediately placed in a semi-sitting position to reduce venous pressure within the neck. Oxygen therapy is administered at 4 to 5 liters per minute until the patient has reacted. The most immediate danger is airway obstruction, especially when the neck dissection has been combined with an intraoral resection. Elective tracheostomy is done when either radical neck dissection is combined with removal of a portion of the mandible or the patient has had significant intraoral excision. If tracheostomy has not been performed, it is advisable to have a sterile tracheostomy set at the bedside.

Another early complication is hemorrhage. The wound should be inspected frequently for such a difficulty. Only moderate analgesia is necessary to control the patient's pain, since the operative site has been almost completely denervated by division of the cervical cutaneous nerves. Excessive sedation is unwise owing to the dangers of asphyxia by airway obstruction.

The suction catheters usually can be removed by the fourth or fifth postoperative day, and the skin sutures can be removed on the seventh postoperative day.

Tube feedings are necessary only in those patients who have had a combined neck dissection with intraoral dissection.

PLATE CXLIX   RADICAL NECK DISSECTION

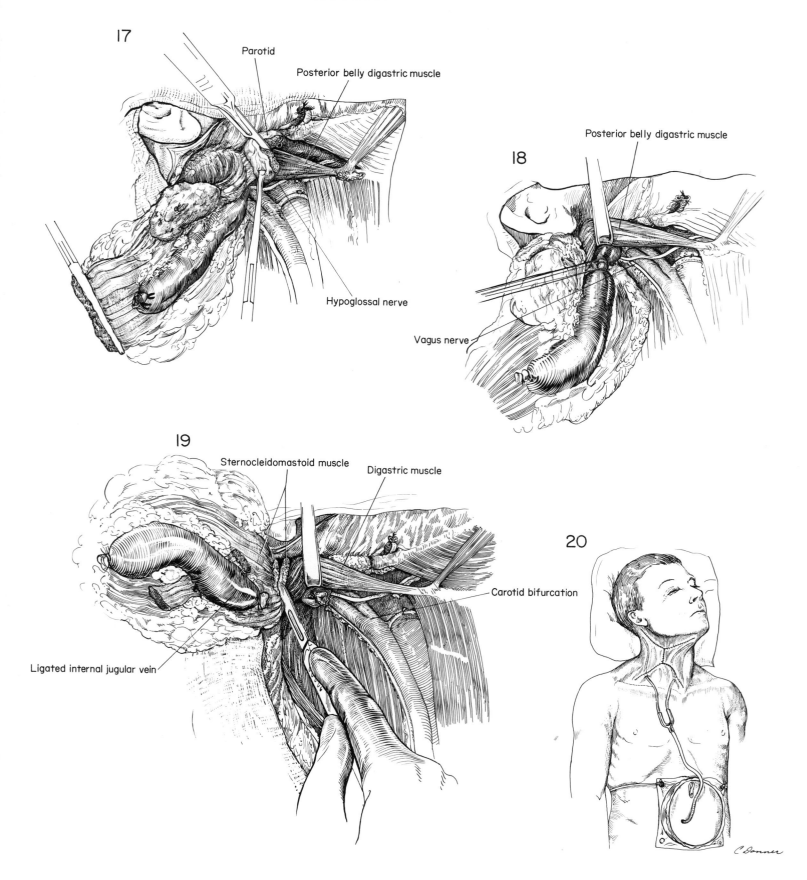

17   Parotid   Posterior belly digastric muscle

Hypoglossal nerve

18   Posterior belly digastric muscle

Vagus nerve

19   Sternocleidomastoid muscle   Digastric muscle

Carotid bifurcation

Ligated internal jugular vein

20

C Donner

PLATE CL · ZENKER'S DIVERTICULECTOMY

INDICATIONS. The indications for repairing a Zenker's diverticulum are partial obstruction, dysphagia, a choking sensation, pain on swallowing, or coughing spells associated with aspirations of fluid from the diverticulum. The diagnosis is confirmed by a barium swallow. The pouch appears suspended by a narrow neck from the esophagus. Zenker's diverticulum is a hernia of mucosa through a weak point located in the midline of the posterior wall of the esophagus where the inferior constrictors of the pharynx meet the cricopharyngeal muscle **(Figure 1).** The neck of the diverticulum arises just above the cricopharyngeal muscle, lies behind the esophagus, and usually projects left of midline. The barium collects and remains in the herniated mucosa of the esophagus.

PREOPERATIVE PREPARATION. The patient should be on a clear liquid diet for several days before operation. He should gargle with an antiseptic mouthwash. Antibiotic therapy may be initiated.

ANESTHESIA. Endotracheal anesthesia is preferred through a cuffed endotracheal tube which is inflated to prevent any aspiration of material from the diverticulum. If general anesthesia is contraindicated, the operation can be performed under local or regional infiltration with 1 per cent procaine.

POSITION. The patient is placed in a semierect position with a folded sheet under his shoulders. The head is angulated backward **(Figure 2).** The chin may be turned toward the right side if the surgeon wishes.

OPERATIVE PREPARATION. The patient's hair is covered with a snug gauze or mesh cap to avoid contamination of the field. The skin is prepared routinely, and the line of incision is marked along the anterior border of the sternocleidomastoid muscle, centered at the level of the thyroid cartilage **(Figure 2).** Skin towels may be eliminated by using a sterile adherent transparent plastic drape. A large sterile sheet with an oval opening completes the draping.

INCISION AND EXPOSURE. The surgeon stands on the patient's left side. He should be thoroughly familiar with the anatomy of the neck and aware that a sensory branch of the cervical plexus, the cervical cutaneous nerve, crosses the incision 2 or 3 cm. below the angle of the jaw **(Figure 3).** The surgeon applies firm pressure over the sternocleidomastoid muscle with a gauze sponge. The first assistant applies similar pressure opposite him. The incision is made through the skin and platysma muscle along the anterior border of the sternocleidomastoid muscle. Bleeding in the subcutaneous tissues is controlled by hemostats and ligation with fine 0000 silk sutures.

DETAILS OF PROCEDURE. As the surgeon approaches the upper extent of the wound, he must avoid dividing the cervical cutaneous nerve, which lies in the superficial investing fascia **(Figure 3).** The sternocleidomastoid muscle is then retracted laterally, and its fascial attachments along the anterior border are divided. The omohyoid muscle crosses the lower portion of the incision and is divided between clamps **(Figure 4).** Hemostasis is obtained by a 00 silk ligature. The inferior end of the omohyoid muscle is retracted posteriorly, while the superior end is retracted medially **(Figure 5).** As the middle cervical fascia investing the omohyoid and strap

muscles is divided in the upper portion of the wound, the superior thyroid artery is exposed, divided between clamps, and ligated **(Figures 4 and 5).** The cervical visceral fascia containing the thyroid gland, trachea, and esophagus is entered medial to the carotid sheath. The posterior surfaces of the pharynx and esophagus are exposed by blunt dissection. The diverticulum is then usually easy to recognize, unless inflammation is present which causes adhesions to the surrounding structures **(Figures 6 and 7).** If difficulty is encountered in outlining the diverticulum, the anesthesiologist can pass a rubber or plastic catheter down into it. Air is injected into this catheter to distend the diverticulum. The lower end of the diverticulum is freed from its surrounding structures by blunt and sharp dissection, its neck is identified, and its origin from the esophagus located **(Figures 6, 7, and 8).** Special attention is given to the removal of all connective tissue surrounding the diverticulum at its origin. This area must be cleaned until there remains only the mucosal herniation through the defect in the muscular wall between the inferior constrictors of the pharynx and the cricopharyngeal muscle below. Care must be taken not to divide the two recurrent laryngeal nerves which may lie on either side of the neck of the diverticulum or in the tracheoesophageal groove, more anteriorly **(Figure 8).** Two stay sutures are then placed at the superior and inferior sides of the neck of the diverticulum **(Figure 9).** These are tied, and straight hemostats are applied to the ends of the sutures for retraction and orientation. The diverticulum is opened at this level **(Figure 10),** care being taken not to leave any excess mucosa and, on the other hand, not to remove too much mucosa to prevent narrowing of the esophageal lumen. At this time the anesthesiologist passes a nasogastric tube through the esophagus into the stomach. It can be seen within the esophagus as the diverticulum is divided **(Figure 10).** A two-layer closure of the diverticulum is begun. The first row of interrupted 0000 silk is placed longitudinally to invert the mucosa with the knot tied on the inside of the esophagus, gentle traction being used on the diverticulum to enhance the exposure. The diverticulum is gradually excised as the closure progresses **(Figure 11).** Then a second row of horizontal sutures closes the muscular defect between the inferior constrictors of the pharynx and the cricopharyngeal muscle below. These muscles are brought together by interrupted 0000 silk sutures.

CLOSURE. After thorough irrigation careful hemostasis is obtained. A small Penrose or rubber slip drain may be placed, and the omohyoid is rejoined with several interrupted sutures. Interrupted 0000 silk sutures are used to reapproximate individually the platysma and skin. Finally, a lightweight sterile gauze dressing is applied, but it must not be circumferential about the neck.

POSTOPERATIVE CARE. The patient is kept in a semisitting position and is not allowed to swallow anything by mouth. Water and tube feedings are provided through the nasogastric tube to maintain fluid and electrolyte balance for the first three days. The drain is removed on the second postoperative day unless contraindicated by excessive serosanguineous drainage or by saliva draining from the wound. The nasogastric tube is removed on the fourth postoperative day, and the patient is started on clear fluids. The diet is advanced as tolerated. One-half of the skin sutures are removed on the second day and the remainder on the fourth day. The patient is permitted out of bed on the first postoperative day and may ambulate with his nasogastric tube in place but clamped off. Antibiotic coverage is optional, depending upon the amount of contamination.

PLATE CL   ZENKER'S DIVERTICULECTOMY

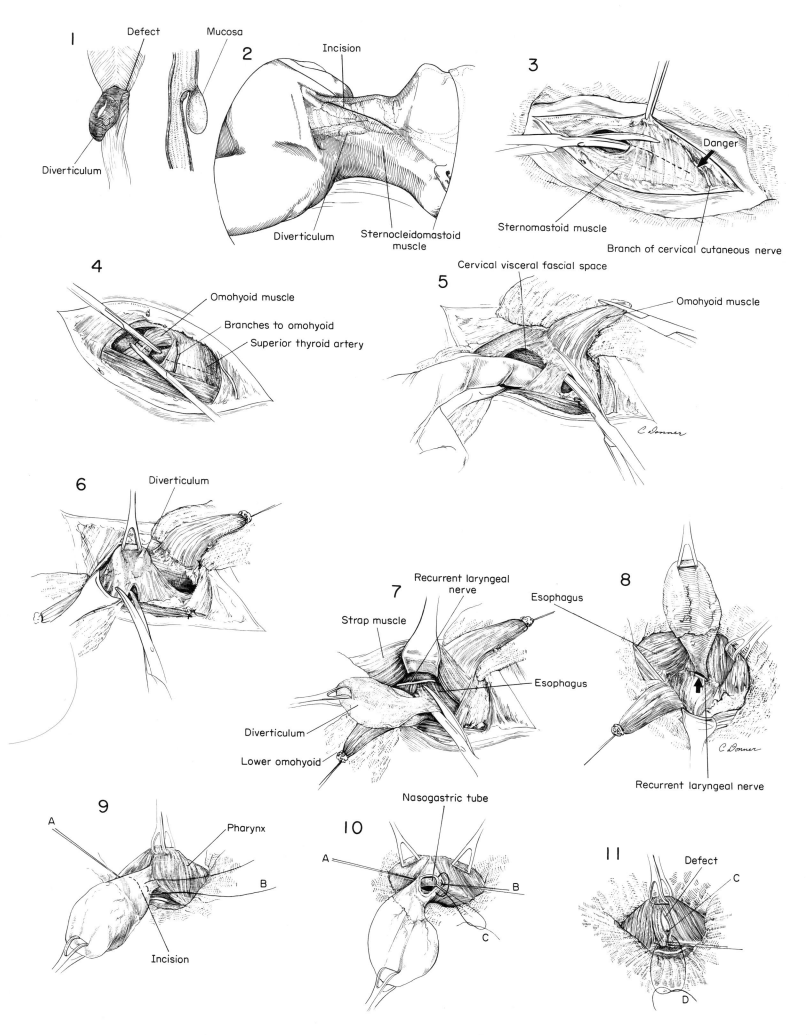

1 Defect   Mucosa
Diverticulum

2 Incision
Diverticulum   Sternocleidomastoid muscle

3 Danger
Sternomastoid muscle
Branch of cervical cutaneous nerve

4 Omohyoid muscle
Branches to omohyoid
Superior thyroid artery

5 Cervical visceral fascial space   Omohyoid muscle

6 Diverticulum

7 Recurrent laryngeal nerve   Esophagus
Strap muscle
Esophagus
Diverticulum
Lower omohyoid

8 Recurrent laryngeal nerve

9 A   Pharynx
B
Incision

10 Nasogastric tube
A   B
C

11 Defect
C
D

PLATE CLI · PAROTIDECTOMY, LATERAL LOBECTOMY

INDICATIONS. Tumors are the most frequent indication for surgical exploration of the parotid gland. Most are benign mixed tumors that arise in the lateral lobe and are treated with wide excision of the tumor, including a margin of normal tissue to prevent local recurrence. Exploration of the parotid area must include careful identification of the facial nerve and its branches, thus avoiding the major complication, facial nerve palsy. Malignant tumors are also seen and require a wide excision, which may include all or a portion of the facial nerve if it is involved. Lesions of the medial lobe may necessitate a total parotidectomy; a superficial parotidectomy is carried out first to identify and preserve the facial nerve before the medial lobe is explored.

PREOPERATIVE PREPARATION. It is essential that all patients undergoing parotid surgery be made aware of the possible loss of facial nerve function with its resultant functional and cosmetic disability. Men should shave themselves early on the morning of surgery, and the hair about the ear may be cleared by the surgeon before draping.

ANESTHESIA. Oral endotracheal anesthesia with a flexible coupling is utilized so that the anesthesiologist may be located at the patient's side, thus giving the surgeon adequate room. Long-acting muscle relaxants, which will be active while the facial nerve is being dissected, should be avoided. Abnormal responses to direct nerve stimulation may result from the use of these drugs, causing difficulty in identifying the nerve.

POSITION. The patient is positioned on his back, and the face is turned to the side opposite the lesion. The head and neck are placed in slight extension, and the head of the table is elevated to reduce venous pressure in the head and neck.

OPERATIVE PREPARATION. After appropriate skin preparation with detergents and antiseptic solutions, sterile towel drapes are positioned to allow visualization of the entire ipsilateral side of the face.

INCISION AND EXPOSURE. The incision is carried in the crease immediately in front of the ear, around the lobule and up in the postauricular fold (**Figure 1**). It then curves posteriorly over the mastoid process and swings smoothly down into the superior cervical crease. The superior cervical crease is located approximately 2 cm. below the angle of the mandible. It should be remembered that with the patient's neck extended and head turned to the side, the facial skin is pulled down onto the neck, and the incision should be made low enough that when the patient's head is returned to normal position, the incision does not lie along the body of the mandible. No incisions are made on the cheek itself. The cervical-facial skin flap is then elevated with sharp dissection to adequately expose the area of the tumor. This elevation takes place to the anterior border of the masseter muscle. A traction suture may be placed through the earlobe to hold this out of the operator's visual field (**Figure 2**). The masseteric parotid fascia has then been exposed, and the parotid gland can be seen within its capsule, bounded superiorly by the cartilages of the ear, posteriorly by the sternocleidomastoid muscle, and medially by the digastric and stylohyoid muscles.

DETAILS OF PROCEDURE. The surgeon must clearly understand the surgical anatomy of the facial nerve. The main trunk of the facial nerve emerges from the stylomastoid foramen. It courses anteriorly and slightly inferiorly between the mastoid process and the membranous portion of the external auditory canal. The main trunk of the nerve usually bifurcates into the temporofacial and cervicofacial divisions after it enters the gland, but occasionally this occurs before entrance. The parotid gland is commonly described as being divided into superficial and deep lobes, the nerve passing between the two. These lobes are not anatomically distinct, as the separation is defined by the location of the nerve, which actually passes directly through the glandular parenchyma. The cervicofacial division bifurcates into the small platysmal or cervical branch and the marginal mandibular branch at the inferior margin of the gland. The latter courses within the platysma muscle just inferior to the horizontal ramus of the mandible, where it innervates the lower lip. Whereas most other branches of the facial nerve have numerous cross-anastomoses, the marginal mandibular branch has none, and therefore division of this branch will always result in paralysis of half of the lower lip. Identification of the marginal mandibular branch before the main nerve trunk is defined is facilitated by the fact that 97 per cent of the time it lies superficial to the posterior facial vein.

The buccal zygomatic division emerges from the anterior margin of the gland with numerous filamentous branches that innervate the muscles of facial expression, including the periorbital muscles and circumoral muscles of the upper lip. The temporal branch runs superiorly and innervates the frontal muscles. This branch has poor regenerative potential and no cross-anastomosis; injury to it will lead to permanent paralysis of the frontalis muscle.

The safest way of identifying the facial nerve is to locate and expose the main trunk. The anterior border of the sternocleidomastoid muscle is identified, as are the posterior facial vein and the greater auricular nerve, in the inferior portion of the incision (**Figures 2** and **3**). The capsule of the parotid gland is then mobilized from the anterior border of the sternocleidomastoid muscle, and dissection is carried down in an area inferior and posterior to the cartilaginous external auditory canal.

Several landmarks are utilized here in the search for the main trunk of the facial nerve. The sternocleidomastoid muscle is retracted posteriorly and the parotid gland anteriorly. The posterior belly of the digastric can be visualized as it pushes up into its groove (**Figure 4**), and the nerve lies anterior to this. The membranous portion of the canal is the superior landmark, and the nerve lies approximately 5 mm. from the tip of this cartilage. By using these landmarks, as well as a Faradic stimulator or gentle mechanical stimulation with forceps, the surgeon can safely locate the main trunk of the nerve (**Figure 5**). If mechanical stimulation is used, the instruments must not be clamped firmly on the tissue as a form of testing, but rather the tissue should be gently pinched as the muscles of the face are observed for motion. If an electrical nerve stimulator is used, it must be tested regularly to be certain that it is functioning in each test situation. A final landmark is a branch of the postauricular artery just lateral to the main trunk of the facial nerve. If the position or bulk of the tumor makes exposure of the main trunk of the facial nerve difficult, it may be identified distally. As indicated previously, the marginal mandibular branch lies superficial to the posterior facial vein in most circumstances. The buccal branch lies immediately superior to Stensen's duct, and identification of this duct will lead the operator to the buccal branch of the nerve. Dissection from distal to proximal must be carried out carefully, as the junction of other branches of the nerve may not be as easily seen as divisions of the nerve when the dissection is carried out in the opposite direction.

Numerous methods have been described for freeing the gland from the nerve. The safest dissection technic is the hemostat-scissors dissection. By dissecting bluntly with a fine hemostat and then cutting only the tissue exposed in the open jaws, the surgeon can protect the nerve (**Figure 6**). The gland may be elevated by clamping the tissue or by the use of holding sutures, and the two major divisions of the facial nerve are identified. Dissection may proceed anteriorly along any or all of the major divisions, depending upon the tumor's position. Since the majority of tumors occur in the lower portion of the lateral lobe, the upper segment of the gland is usually mobilized first (**Figure 7**). A moderate amount of bleeding may be expected, but this will be controllable with finger pressure, electrocoagulation, or fine ligatures. Once the tumor has been freed from the facial nerve, Stensen's duct will appear in the midanterior portion of the gland (**Figure 8**). The lateral lobe tributary only is ligated, as medial lobe atrophy will occur if the main duct is tied. After removal of the lateral lobe, the isthmus and the medial lobe remain deep to the facial nerve; they will appear as small islands of parotid tissue and should represent only 20 per cent of the total parotid gland. The lobe may be transected when the tumor and a surrounding portion of normal tissue have been completely separated from the facial nerve.

CLOSURE. The wound is thoroughly irrigated and meticulous hemostasis obtained. A small Penrose drain may be placed in the wound and brought out through the most inferior margin, or a perforated plastic catheter may be brought out through a stab wound and attached to a suction apparatus. The subcutaneous tissue is approximated with fine absorbable suture material, and fine nonabsorbable suture material is used for the skin.

POSTOPERATIVE CARE. Alternate sutures may be removed on the second day and the remainder of the sutures removed on the fourth day along with the drain. Temporary paresis from traction may occur and usually clears in a few days to a week. If the greater auricular nerve has been divided in the course of the procedure, anesthesia in its distribution will be permanent.

PLATE CLI   PAROTIDECTOMY, LATERAL LOBECTOMY

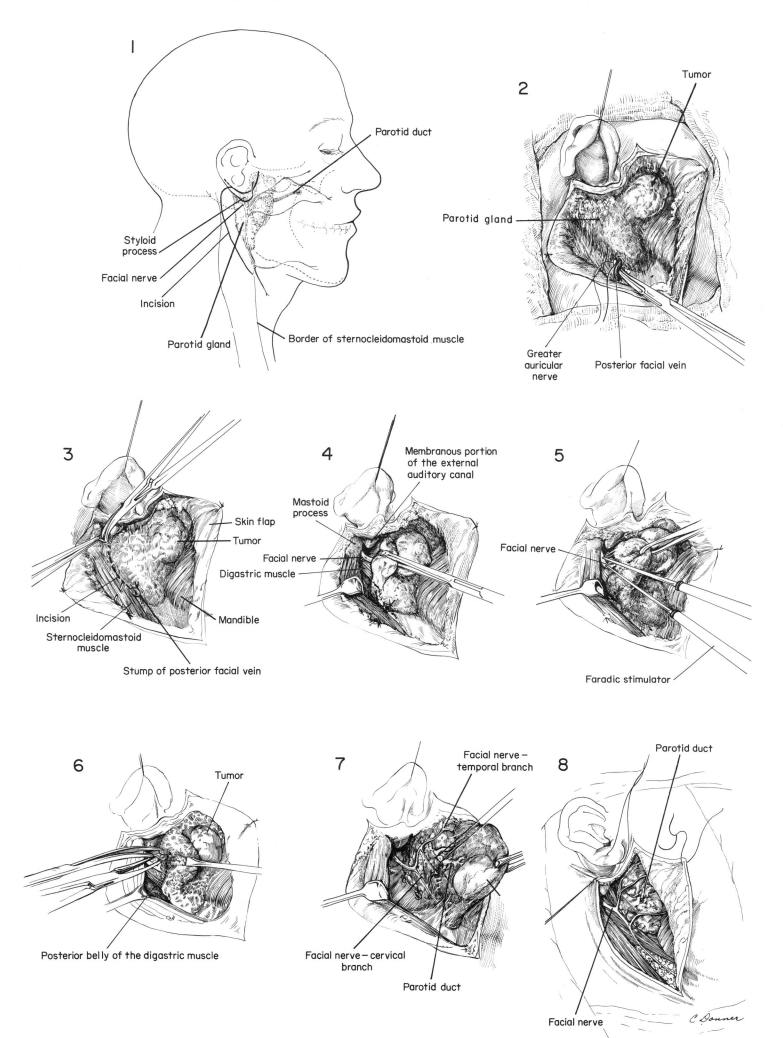

1

Parotid duct

Styloid process

Facial nerve

Incision

Parotid gland

Border of sternocleidomastoid muscle

2

Tumor

Parotid gland

Greater auricular nerve

Posterior facial vein

3

Skin flap

Tumor

Incision

Sternocleidomastoid muscle

Stump of posterior facial vein

Mandible

4

Membranous portion of the external auditory canal

Mastoid process

Facial nerve

Digastric muscle

5

Facial nerve

Faradic stimulator

6

Tumor

Posterior belly of the digastric muscle

7

Facial nerve – temporal branch

Facial nerve – cervical branch

Parotid duct

8

Parotid duct

Facial nerve

C Donner

PLATE CLII · THORACOSTOMY, RESECTION OF RIB

INDICATIONS. Thoracostomy with resection of a rib is performed for the evacuation of loculated purulent material in a walled-off pleural area. In critically ill patients and in the aged the intercostal catheter method may be used as a preliminary procedure. Despite systemic chemotherapy as well as repeated aspirations of the abscess cavity with introduction of a chemotherapeutic agent and/or antibiotic drugs, it is frequently necessary to provide free drainage by rib resection. After several weeks of conservative therapy the intercostal spaces become too small to allow a catheter of sufficient size to be introduced. Thoracostomy with rib resection is also indicated in patients with bronchopleural fistula after fixation of the mediastinum has occurred, and prompt evacuation of the empyema cavity is essential to prevent flooding of the contralateral lung.

PREOPERATIVE PREPARATION. The exact location of the empyema cavity is verified by physical and roentgenologic examinations, the offending organism identified, and the character of the pus determined by aspiration. After aspiration the extent of the cavity, particularly its lower limit, should be determined by the injection of air and a radiopaque medium. Fluoroscopy is carried out, and posteroanterior and lateral films of the chest are taken. Parenteral chemotherapy is maintained, and secondary anemia is corrected by whole blood transfusion.

ANESTHESIA. General anesthesia is preferred, although local infiltration anesthesia is suitable. Following infiltration of the tissues of the skin and tissues of the thoracic wall, an effort should be made to introduce an anesthetic agent into the area of the intercostal nerve, which is located along the inferior margin of the rib **(Figure 1)**. Intercostal or paravertebral blocks of the nerves adjacent to the area of operation may provide a more satisfactory anesthesia. For children and uncooperative patients general anesthesia with endotracheal intubation is preferred.

POSITION. It is usually most convenient to place the patient in a semirecumbent position on the operating table with the arm on the affected side raised over the head **(Figure 2)**. If general anesthesia is used, the patient is placed in Fowler's position with the arm on the affected side across the face.

OPERATIVE PREPARATION. The skin is prepared in the routine manner.

INCISION AND EXPOSURE. To assure the success of this operation, drainage must be accomplished at the most dependent portion of the empyema cavity. Although this is usually at the bottom of the pleural space, the pocket may be walled off anteriorly and high; or in long-standing infection, particularly if the diaphragm is pulled up and adherent, it may be interlobar.

Irrespective of previous aspirations, the presence of pus must be verified at the point where drainage is to be instituted. Cultures are taken routinely. It may be necessary to attempt aspiration in several interspaces to determine the most dependent portion of the abscess cavity **(Figure 2)**. A different sterile needle must be used for each aspiration to avoid introducing sepsis into uninfected regions. The aspirating needle should be introduced over the top surface of the rib to avoid injury to the intercostal nerve and blood vessels **(Figure 1)**. **Figure 2** illustrates a vertical incision over the rib to be removed. A parallel incision over the rib is equally satisfactory. If the removed rib is later found not to be at the bottom of the cavity, the next lower rib can be removed by additional traction. The rib is reached by blunt separation of the muscles in the direction of their fibers, and the margins of the wound are retracted **(Figure 3)**.

DETAILS OF PROCEDURE. It is wise to infiltrate the periosteum, the area of the intercostal nerve, and the pleura with anesthetic agent as each is reached in the dissection. It is particularly difficult to anesthetize the periosteum adequately. An H-shaped incision is made into the periosteum

(Figure 3). An Alexander periosteal elevator is advantageously employed to free the periosteum from the rib. On the superior rib margin the elevator should be swept from the spine anteriorly; on the inferior rib margin, in the opposite direction. In this way the periosteal attachments of the intercostal muscles are divided with the least effort **(Figures 4** and **5)**. Using a relatively sharp periosteal elevator, the surgeon carefully pushes the periosteum away from the superior as well as the inferior margins of the rib to avoid further bleeding and particularly to prevent any injury to the intercostal vessels and nerves.

The elevator is cautiously introduced behind the rib **(Figure 6)**. A Doyen periosteal elevator is then inserted beneath the rib, and with a gentle back and forth motion the rib is further freed from its bed **(Figure 7)**. With the periosteum completely free, both superficially and next to the pleura, about 2 to 4 cm. of rib are removed by a bone-cutting instrument **(Figure 8)**. Any roughness or irregularities of the cut margin of the rib are evened by a blunt rongeur, and any bleeding from the cut end of the rib is controlled by the application of bone wax **(Figure 9)**. The periosteum and the underlying pleura are now between the operator and the exudate. Before proceeding further, it is wise to aspirate again with a needle to ascertain that exudate is present in the anticipated incision area **(Figure 10)**. This needle is left in place, and an incision is made adjacent to it, ensuring an opening directly into the cavity **(Figure 10)**. The pleural opening is enlarged, and the exudate is removed by suction or drainage **(Figure 11)**. The cavity is then carefully explored with the finger, making certain that the drainage point is at the bottom of the infected area **(Figure 12)**. If it is not, the incision is extended downward, and the adjacent rib is resected until the bottom of the infected cavity is reached **(Figures 12** and **13)**. The full reach of the finger is used to break up any loculations. A malleable spoon may be employed to remove debris from the parietal pleura. If no bronchopleural fistula is suspected, the cavity may be washed out cautiously with sterile saline. One or more soft rubber tubes about 2 cm. in diameter are inserted into the cavity and held in position either with sutures through the skin **(Figure 14)** or by safety pins so large that the tubing cannot be sucked into the chest, or a multiple-lumen plastic sump drainage tube may be used. The loss of drainage tubes in empyema cavities is a well-recognized cause of chronic pleurocutaneous sinus.

CLOSURE. Sutures should be unnecessary, but if the wound seems unduly large, several subcutaneous sutures may be used. Several silk sutures on large needles close the skin loosely.

POSTOPERATIVE CARE. Petrolatum gauze is frequently used to make the incision airtight, so that if suction should be desirable, it may be placed directly on the tubes. The patient may blow water from one bottle into another or blow into balloons in order to increase the intrathoracic pressure and assist in evacuating the exudate. Chest wall exercises speed up the re-expansion of the lung. The patient must also be taught to sit and walk with the spine straight to avoid scoliosis, which may follow a long-standing empyema. By the third or fourth day the cavity may be irrigated with saline solution. If a bronchopleural fistula is present, the patient will cough up the saline. If large pieces of fibrin block the opening and no bronchopleural fistula is present, irrigation with saline or debriding enzymes may hasten the breaking down and discharge of such masses. A record of the capacity of the cavity as well as of the daily vital capacity serves to check on the progress of obliterating the empyema cavity. The tubes should never be removed until the instillation of radiopaque substances has ascertained that the cavity no longer exists and the only fistula present is due to the retained tube. The large tubes may then be removed and small rubber tubes substituted to facilitate healing of the tract. The parenteral administration of chemotherapeutic or antibiotic agents or the application of such agents locally into the abscess should be governed by the identity of the offending organism. Nutrition is sustained by high-protein, high-carbohydrate, and high-vitamin diet. The patient should be weighed frequently. In the presence of prolonged sepsis repeated blood and plasma transfusions are generally indicated to control secondary anemia.

PLATE CLII   THORACOSTOMY, RESECTION OF RIB

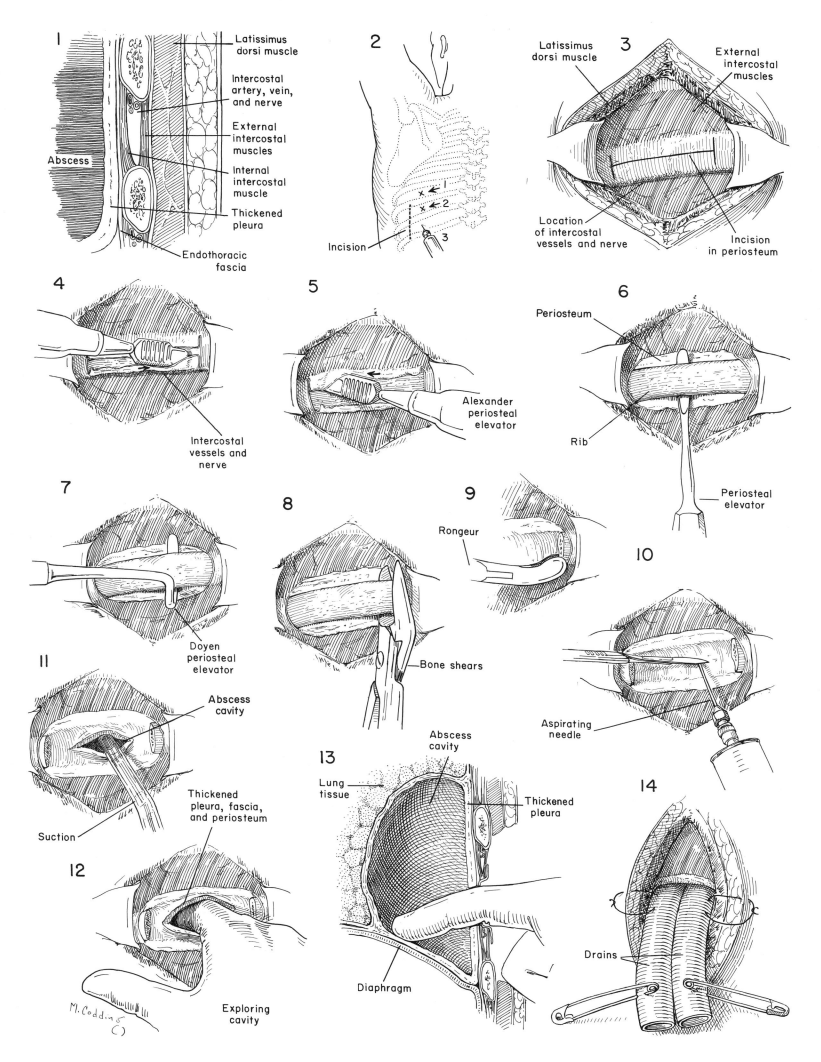

1   Latissimus dorsi muscle
Intercostal artery, vein, and nerve
External intercostal muscles
Internal intercostal muscle
Thickened pleura
Abscess
Endothoracic fascia

2   Incision

3   Latissimus dorsi muscle
External intercostal muscles
Location of intercostal vessels and nerve
Incision in periosteum

4   Intercostal vessels and nerve

5   Alexander periosteal elevator

6   Periosteum
Rib
Periosteal elevator

7   Doyen periosteal elevator

8   Bone shears

9   Rongeur

10   Aspirating needle

11   Abscess cavity
Suction

12   Thickened pleura, fascia, and periosteum
Exploring cavity

13   Abscess cavity
Lung tissue
Thickened pleura
Diaphragm

14   Drains

M. Codding

PLATE CLIII · POSTEROLATERAL THORACOTOMY INCISION

INDICATIONS. This incision is ideal for a wide variety of elective as well as emergency procedures. Through the left side, the heart, descending aorta, lower esophagus, vagus nerves, and diaphragmatic hiatus are well exposed; whereas both vena cavas, the superior exposure of the hepatic veins, and the upper esophagus are approached through the right chest.

The height of the incision on the chest wall varies with the nature of the procedure to obtain optimum exposure of either the apex, the middle, or the basal portions of the chest cavity. One or more ribs may be divided posteriorly and occasionally removed, depending on the mobility of the chest wall and the exposure required. (Resection of a rib provides no better exposure than transection and makes the closure more difficult.)

For optimum exposure of the upper portion of the chest cavity, such as in closure of a patent ductus or resection of a coarctation, the chest is entered at the level of the fifth rib. This may be divided posteriorly, along with the fourth rib, if necessary. For procedures on the diaphragm and lower esophagus, the thoracic cavity should be entered at the level of the sixth or seventh rib. If still wider exposure is desired, one or two ribs above and below may be transected at the neck.

PREOPERATIVE PREPARATION. Except in acute emergencies, the patient must be prepared for optimal pulmonary function by cleansing the tracheobronchial tree with postural drainage, expectorants, and antibiotics, which may be given both systemically and by inhalation. Patients should be advised not to smoke for several weeks before an elective operation. Pulmonary function studies should be performed on all patients being considered for thoracotomy. A further evaluation can be obtained by noting the patient's tolerance to climbing stairs. For practical purposes, any patient able to walk up three flights of stairs will tolerate a thoracotomy. When a patient has borderline pulmonary function, bronchospirometry may be indicated. Because technical difficulties may arise necessitating more extensive resection than planned, the surgeon must be thoroughly familiar with the patient's respiratory reserve.

The evening before surgery the patient's chest should be shaved, including the axilla, and his chest scrubbed. It is helpful to instruct the patient in individual breathing exercises of each hemithorax separately, so that postoperatively he can increase the excursion of the ribs.

ANESTHESIA. All thoracotomies require endotracheal anesthesia. In cases of marked suppuration of one lung, the normal lung can be isolated by selective intubation with a Carlen endobronchial tube.

POSITION. The patient is placed in a lateral decubitus position with the hips secured to the table by wide adhesive tape **(Figure 1).** The lower leg is flexed at the knee, and a pillow is placed between it and the upper leg, which is extended. A rolled sheet or blanket is placed under the axilla to support the shoulder and upper thorax. The arm on the side of the thoracotomy is extended forward and upward and placed in a grooved arm holder in line with the head, permitting access to the veins. The lower arm is extended forward and rested on an arm board perpendicular to the operating table.

OPERATIVE PREPARATION. The skin is cleansed with antiseptic, and the area of incision is either draped with towels or covered with an adhesive plastic drape, followed by the large sterile thoracotomy sheet.

INCISION AND EXPOSURE. The surgeon makes the incision while standing posterior to the patient, with the second assistant on his right. (The surgeon makes the incision while standing on the right; for procedures in the left hemithorax, the surgeon changes sides after entering the pleural space.) The incision begins midway between the medial border of the scapula and the spine, proceeding downward parallel to these two structures for the first few inches and then curving in a gentle S two fingerbreadths below the tip of the scapula, and finally extending down into or just below the submammary crease. In exposures of the fourth or fifth interspace the medial end of the incision is extended transversely toward the sternum. For lower openings of the seventh or eighth interspace, or ones involving transection of the costal cartilages for maximum exposure, the medial end of this incision curves gently toward or into the epigastrium. The surgeon then carries the incision directly down through the latissimus dorsi and the serratus anterior muscles **(Figure 2).** During this process each of the muscles may be individually elevated by the surgeon's index and middle fingers. This is accomplished by entering the auscultatory triangle formed by the superior border of the latissimus dorsi, the inferior border of the trapezius, and the medial border of the scapula.

The incision is extended anteriorly and posteriorly through the borders of the trapezius and rhomboid muscles. Care must be taken to make this posterior incision parallel to the spinal column and thus lessen the chance of dividing the spinal accessory nerve, which innervates the trapezius. Bleeders are clamped as they appear. They may be secured by electrocautery or 00 silk ligatures. Wound drapes of triangularly folded Mikulicz pads are then placed, and the scapula is retracted superiorly. By palpating the widened interspace between the first and second ribs and the insertion of the posterior scalene muscle on the first rib, the surgeon may count down to the appropriate rib level **(Figure 3).** It is preferable to enter the pleural space through the bed of a rib, because there is less bleeding and the subsequent closure is more stable. The periosteum is incised directly over the midportion of the rib. The sacrospinalis muscle and fascia are elevated by a periosteal elevator, and a Richardson retractor is inserted in this space. A Coryllos periosteal elevator is swept anteriorly along the upper half of the rib **(Figure 5).** The Hedblom periosteal elevator is then inserted under the bared portion of the rib and slipped upward along the rib, stripping the remaining periosteum from the upper half of the rib in a posterior to anterior direction **(Figure 6).** A small incision is made through the periosteal bed into the pleura **(Figure 7).** The lung drops away, thus allowing the incision to be extended for the desired length.

PLATE CLIII   POSTEROLATERAL THORACOTOMY INCISION

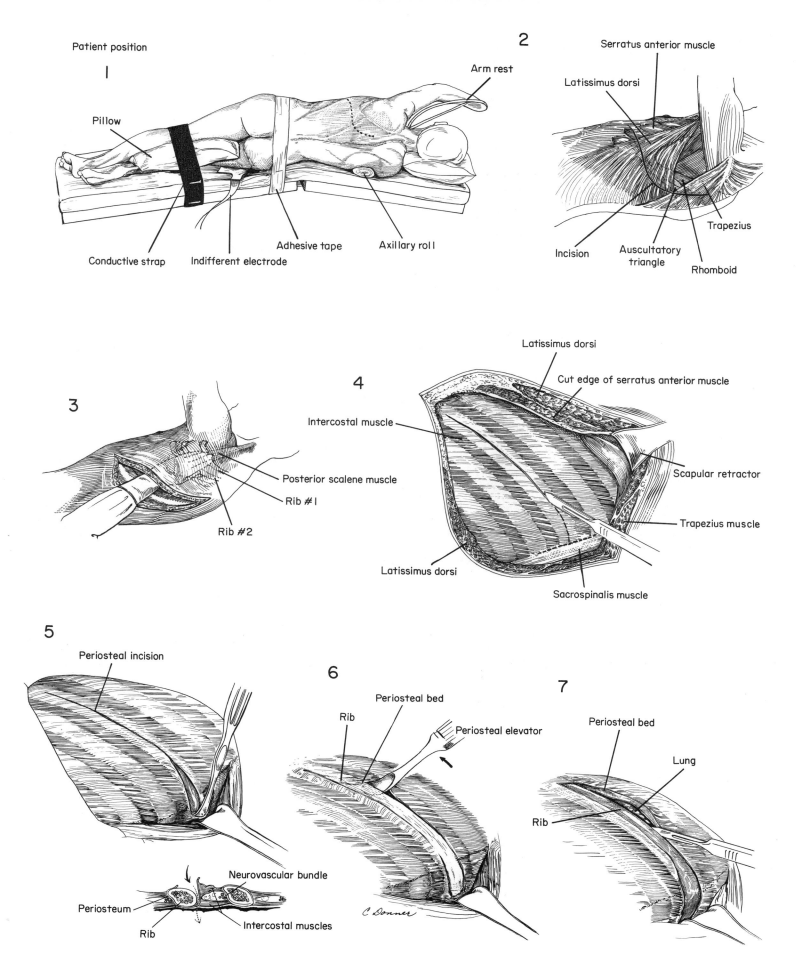

1

Patient position

Pillow

Arm rest

Conductive strap

Indifferent electrode

Adhesive tape

Axillary roll

2

Serratus anterior muscle

Latissimus dorsi

Incision

Auscultatory triangle

Trapezius

Rhomboid

3

Posterior scalene muscle

Rib #1

Rib #2

4

Latissimus dorsi

Cut edge of serratus anterior muscle

Intercostal muscle

Scapular retractor

Trapezius muscle

Latissimus dorsi

Sacrospinalis muscle

5

Periosteal incision

Neurovascular bundle

Periosteum

Rib

Intercostal muscles

6

Rib

Periosteal bed

Periosteal elevator

C Donner

7

Periosteal bed

Lung

Rib

PLATE CLIV · POSTEROLATERAL THORACOTOMY INCISION

INCISION AND EXPOSURE (*Continued*). An alternate method is direct incision into the intercostal space. The incision is made through the intercostal muscles along the superior border of the rib to avoid injuring the neurovascular bundle, which runs along the inferior margin of the rib above. At a point about one-third of the way from the posterior end of the incision, the main bundle sends several small twigs across the interspace to the rib below. Simple ligation of these is sufficient. Dissection is carried directly down and into the pleura. The incision in the pleura is extended anteriorly and posteriorly with scissors. The internal mammary vessels, which join the intercostals at the sternum, lie medial and deep to the costal cartilages and should not be injured during this incision **(Figure 8).** If additional exposure is required, a rib may be divided or resected. The periosteum along the lower border of the rib is stripped to isolate the neurovascular bundle, which is grasped between right-angle forceps, ligated, and divided. The rib is then transected at the costal cartilage of the neck with rib shears **(Figure 9).** A self-retaining retractor is inserted **(Figure 10)** and opened gradually.

CLOSURE. The closure of the thoracotomy incision requires stabilization of the thorax for the entire length of the incision. Encircling No. 1 chromic catgut sutures (A) are placed; these are then tied while the ribs are held in position by a rib approximator **(Figure 11A).** If any ribs were transected or fractured during spreading, sutures (B) must encircle both ribs and immobilize all rib fragments **(Figure 11A).** Chromic catgut is preferred for this purpose, as it produces less postoperative intercostal pain than silk. Further stabilization may be acquired by using a rib peg between the ends of the transected ribs. This is accomplished by excising a 2-cm. fragment from the superior margin of the transected rib with rib shears; after a right-angle clamp has been introduced into the ends of the transected rib, the peg is inserted and wedged tightly into place **(Figure 11B).** Further hemostasis and stabilization of the transected rib are accomplished by placing a suture (C) through the sacrospinalis muscle, fixing it to the neck of the transected rib and the rib above **(Figure 11A).** The chest muscles are approximated by running 0 chromic catgut sutures or interrupted sutures of 00 silk **(Figure 12).** Care must be taken to approximate each of the layers separately—i.e., rhomboids and the serratus anterior above the trapezius and latissimus dorsi. Subcutaneous sutures of 000 silk will prevent disruption of the incision when the skin sutures are removed in seven or eight days.

All patients undergoing thoracotomy should have postoperative drainage of the pleural space. The catheters used must be of adequate size, and anything less than a 26 French catheter will obstruct with blood clots. It is often advantageous to have two catheters in the postoperative chest—one lying in the posterior gutter along the spine and the other directed anteriorly. The posterolateral catheter is brought out through stab wounds in the skin as low as possible in a posterolateral position **(Figure 12).** The position of the greater trochanter of the elevated hip often serves as a landmark through the heavy drapes. A line between it and the shoulder indicates the midaxillary line. Single untied skin silks may be placed through the stab wound before the tube is inserted to aid in closing when the chest tubes are withdrawn. In placing the chest tube, the surgeon first grasps the lower cut edges of the latissimus dorsi and the serratus anterior, and the assistant retracts them superiorly. The surgeon forms a tunnel through the chest wall with Kelly forceps, grasps the chest tube, and draws it out through the wall. The catheter serves two main purposes: to remove air escaping from multiple bronchial fistulas usually present after lung resection, and to remove the blood that accumulates after all thoracotomies. Should excessive air leakage be present, another chest tube is placed in the second or third interspace anteriorly at the level of the midclavicular line **(Figure 13).** A smaller catheter of soft rubber will suffice and will be the last chest tube to be removed. The catheters allow expansion of the lung with approximation of pleural surfaces and thus prevent postoperative atelectasis and fluid accumulation with infection. The catheters are usually attached to an underwater-seal bottle with or without negative suction through a water-trap bottle for as long as there is marked bleeding within the pleural space or persistence of air leakage **(Figure 14).**

POSTOPERATIVE CARE. Analgesics should be held to a minimum; when maximum relief of postoperative pain is desired, the intercostal nerve may be anesthetized for several interspaces above and below the incision. This is easily accomplished by administering a long-acting local anesthetic before the chest is closed. When these nerves are exposed, the surgeon may inject them through the parietal pleura quite near their origin.

The patient should be encouraged to cough vigorously. Expectorants should be used in the form of iodides and steam generated by an ultrasonic nebulizer. The patient should be helped in coughing by the attendant, who supports the operated side of the chest wall. The patient should be encouraged to change positions frequently. Ambulation should be early, and active exercise should be encouraged.

Antibiotics are used in all cases of suppurative disease and esophageal resection. Intermittent positive pressure oxygen inhalation, with or without bronchodilators, can be used in most patients having thoracotomies. The thoracotomy tubes are usually removed when they have served their purpose, as evidenced by normal breathing sounds on the operative side and X-ray films showing complete expansion of the lung and the absence of air spillage and fluid accumulation. This is usually on the second or third postoperative day. Persistent air leakage may indicate improper position of the catheter, leakage around the entrance of the thoracotomy tube, or large bronchial air leaks. Patients with emphysema and resection of a portion of lung should receive postoperative suction in varying degrees for as long as ten days. Occasionally, rotation of the catheter or partial withdrawal will bring about closure of peripheral bronchial fistulas.

To prevent splinting of the thorax, the dressing applied should be minimal. Four layers of gauze over the line of incision held with perforated elastic adhesive tape will be adequate.

PLATE CLIV   POSTEROLATERAL THORACOTOMY INCISION

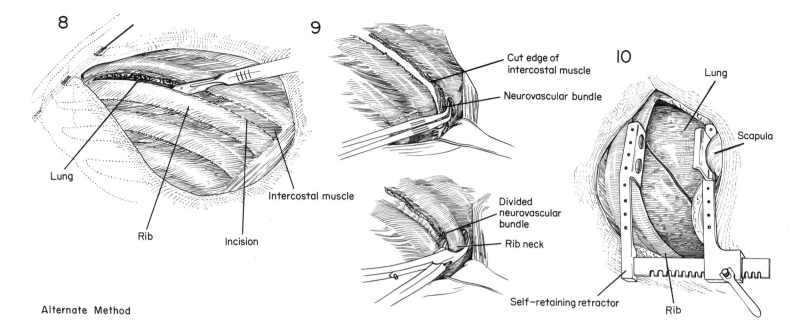

8

Lung

Rib

Incision

Intercostal muscle

Alternate Method

9

Cut edge of intercostal muscle

Neurovascular bundle

Divided neurovascular bundle

Rib neck

Self-retaining retractor

10

Lung

Scapula

Rib

THORACOTOMY CLOSURE

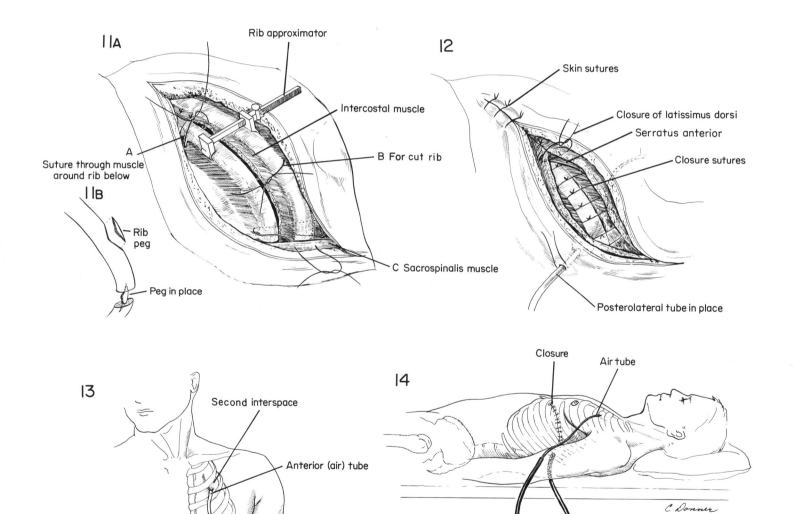

11A

Rib approximator

Intercostal muscle

B For cut rib

A

Suture through muscle around rib below

11B

Rib peg

Peg in place

C Sacrospinalis muscle

12

Skin sutures

Closure of latissimus dorsi

Serratus anterior

Closure sutures

Posterolateral tube in place

13

Second interspace

Anterior (air) tube

To waterseal

14

Closure

Air tube

Posterolateral tube

To suction

Waterseal

1 cm

15 cm

C Donner

PLATE CLV · MINOR PROCEDURES UPON THE BREAST

A. Simple Mastectomy

INDICATIONS. Simple mastectomy may be considered in the presence of extensive malignant disease in a large breast preliminary to heavy irradiation or in elderly, poor-risk patients with a localized lesion, as well as in the patient who resists a radical amputation of the breast. See Plate CLVI.

PREOPERATIVE PREPARATION. The chest, breast, and axilla on the side of the operation are shaved. The patient should be in good general condition before operation.

ANESTHESIA. Any general anesthetic technic not contraindicated by preoperative study of the patient may be used.

POSITION. The patient is placed in a comfortable supine position with the arm on the involved side abducted **(Figure 1)**.

OPERATIVE PREPARATION. After a gentle skin preparation, sterile towels are anchored about the breast, and sterile drapes are applied. Transparent plastic surgical drapes may be used.

INCISION AND EXPOSURE. Usually, an elliptical incision is made about the nipple **(Figure 1)**; however, if the nipple is to be saved for cosmetic reasons, a thoracomammary incision is made in the inframammary fold **(Figure 2)**. The glandular tissue is removed by a subcutaneous mastectomy. The skin and subcutaneous tissue are undermined to the outer margins of the breast tissue **(Figure 1)**.

DETAILS OF PROCEDURE. The breast tissue is grasped with an Allis forceps or a tenaculum, freed from the underlying pectoral fascia at any desired point, and removed, keeping within this well-defined cleavage plane throughout. The axillary contents, insofar as possible, should be included with the breast tissue if malignancy is present. All bleeding points are controlled. The major blood supply will be encountered coming down from the axilla or in the upper inner quadrant from the intercostal vessels. The wound is irrigated with warm saline solution before final inspection for bleeding points.

CLOSURE. The overlying skin is anchored to the pectoral fascia, and all redundant portions are removed, so that the margins of the incision give a good approximation. Occasionally, it is wise to insert a rubber tissue drain through a small stab wound made in a dependent area to ensure good drainage. This should be sutured to the skin.

POSTOPERATIVE CARE. Several thicknesses of sterile gauze are placed over the site of operation and held in position by a binder or elastic adhesive tape to give good compression. Sutures are removed in seven days. Unlimited arm motion may be resumed at this time.

B. Excision of Benign Tumor

INDICATIONS. Any tumor of the breast should be removed for pathologic examination. Although some prefer to aspirate obvious cysts, unless the mass completely disappears, local excision and biopsy are advised. The benign type of tumor usually encountered may be a fibroadenoma, an isolated cyst, an intracanalicular fibroma, or a ductal papilloma.

INCISION AND EXPOSURE. A curved incision in the line of skin cleavage ensures a satisfactory cosmetic result **(Figure 2)**. If the tumor is in the upper or medial quadrant of the breast, the cosmetic result insignificant, and the possibility of a radical amputation likely, a similar radial incision may be made directly over it. Otherwise, a thoracomammary incision in the inframammary fold will adequately expose almost any benign tumor of the breast **(Figure 2)**. The breast is retracted upward and medially by the surgeon's left hand, while the incision is made in the inframammary crease, which usually shows up as a definitely pigmented line **(Figure 3)**. The incision is carried down to the underlying muscle, and all bleeding points are controlled.

DETAILS OF PROCEDURE. The margins of the incision are retracted, and the posterior surface of the breast is isolated from the underlying fascia in a definite cleavage plane over the pectoralis major muscle **(Figure 4)**. The incision is lengthened, and the posterior surface of the breast is exposed to enable the surgeon to evert the undersurface of the breast with the fingers of his left hand through the incision. The incision is then made through the posterior capsule of the breast until the tumor is exposed **(Figure 4)**. The encapsulated, glistening tumor is grasped with forceps and dissected from its bed by a scalpel or curved scissors **(Figure 5)**. The tumor is sectioned, and a frozen section is made. If malignancy is found, preparation for a radical mastectomy is begun immediately.

CLOSURE. The defect in the breast tissue itself is closed with interrupted sutures **(Figure 6)**. Several silk sutures are taken to anchor the posterior surface of the breast to the underlying fascia of the pectoral muscle. Interrupted silk sutures are taken in the subcutaneous tissue and skin. A drain is not inserted. Subcuticular closure of the skin with fine white silk ensures a good cosmetic result for those incisions in an exposed area.

POSTOPERATIVE CARE. Several thicknesses of sterile gauze are applied over the wound. The breast is immobilized with strips of adhesive tape to the adjacent chest wall and is supported either with a binder or an elastic bandage as long as there is tenderness or discomfort. In five to seven days the sutures are removed. Free arm motion may then be resumed.

C. Incision and Drainage for Abscess of Breast

INDICATIONS. Abscesses about the nipple or in the breast tissue require exceptionally free drainage. If they are associated with a retracted nipple, the latter condition will also require correction.

PREOPERATIVE PREPARATION. Chemotherapy and/or antibiotics are administered. Hot applications are used until the abscess is well localized. The breast is immobilized by a proper support.

ANESTHESIA. Any general anesthetic technic is used that is compatible with the patient's preoperative condition.

INCISION AND EXPOSURE. In the majority of instances radial incisions extending outward from the nipple are made to avoid sectioning the mammary ducts **(Figure 2)**. These incisions may be long or short. Localized abscesses about the nipple or in the breast tissue may be drained more readily through a circumareolar incision. If an inverted nipple is associated with the abscess near the areola, the tissue beneath the nipple should be divided and the nipple everted. Deep breast abscesses, especially in the lower or outer quadrants, may be incised and drained through a short thoracomammary incision in the inframammary fold **(Figure 2)**. This assures adequate dependent drainage with minimum scar formation.

DETAILS OF PROCEDURE. Once the skin incision is made, the wound is deepened until pus is encountered. A curved hemostat is inserted to determine the extent of the abscess cavity. The opening is enlarged sufficiently to ensure adequate drainage. A culture should be taken as well as a biopsy of the abscess wall.

CLOSURE. Sutures are not used in the tissue. Rubber tissue drains should be inserted into the abscess cavity and secured there with a skin suture.

POSTOPERATIVE CARE. Sterile dressings are applied, and the breast is supported by a binder. Chemotherapy and/or antibiotics are continued until the patient becomes afebrile. Hot applications may be resumed if indicated. Starting the second day, the drains are shortened a little on each successive day. Arm motion may be resumed at this time. The patient is made ambulatory as soon as her general condition permits.

PLATE CLV   MINOR PROCEDURES UPON THE BREAST

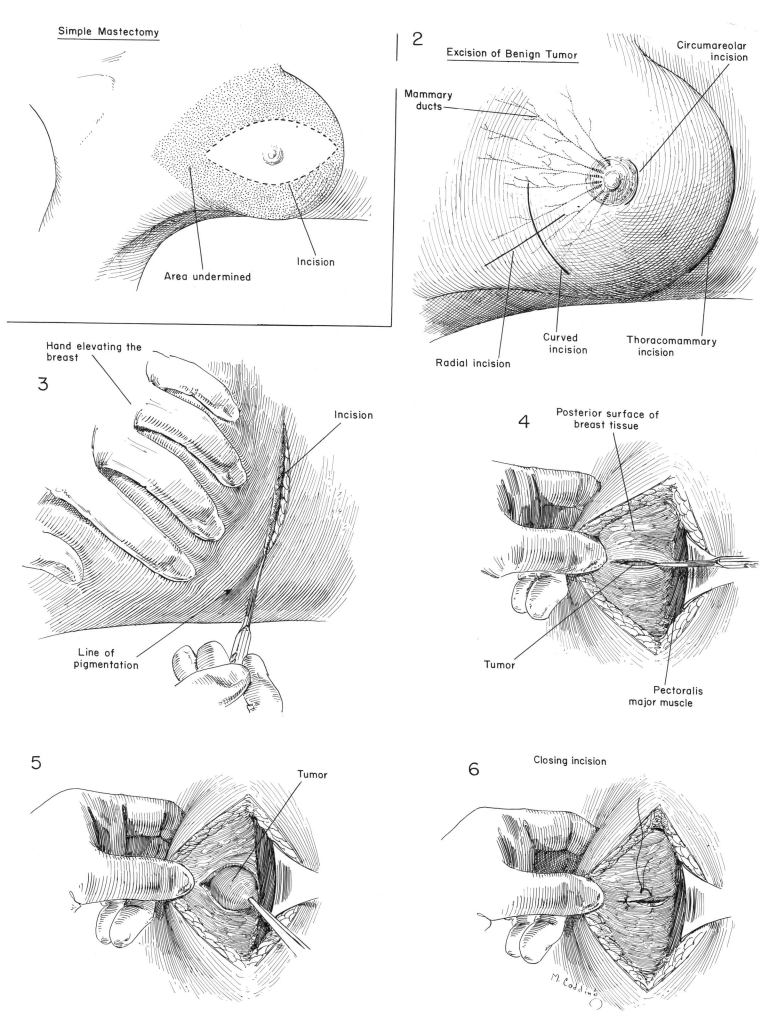

Simple Mastectomy

Area undermined

Incision

2

Excision of Benign Tumor

Circumareolar incision

Mammary ducts

Radial incision

Curved incision

Thoracomammary incision

3

Hand elevating the breast

Incision

Line of pigmentation

4

Posterior surface of breast tissue

Tumor

Pectoralis major muscle

5

Tumor

6

Closing incision

M. Codding

PLATE CLVI · RADICAL MASTECTOMY

INDICATIONS. Carcinoma of the breast is the common indication for removal of the breast, both pectoral muscles, and the axillary fat and lymph nodes by the classical radical mastectomy. All or part of the pectoral muscles may be retained when a modified radical mastectomy is performed. Local excision of a large tumor may be justified as a palliative procedure, despite the presence of extensive metastases, to avoid a foul-smelling ulceration; but before such a decision is made, it is first determined whether the patient is more likely to benefit by radical mastectomy; by hormone therapy, chemotherapy, or X-ray therapy; or by some combination of these treatments. Evidence of metastases to the lungs, skeletal system, and liver should be determined by roentgenograms and appropriate radioisotope scans, and by liver function studies.

PREOPERATIVE PREPARATION. The chest wall, the upper third of the arm, the axilla, and the upper abdomen on the involved side are shaved before operation. The skin is prepared in the usual manner. Whole blood should be available for transfusion.

ANESTHESIA. Same as for simple mastectomy. However, for prolonged operative procedures, endotracheal intubation is indicated.

POSITION. The patient is placed in a comfortable supine position near the margin of the operating table, with the arm on the involved side abducted on an arm board and the table tilted so that the feet are slightly lower than the head. The operating table is moved so that the maximum amount of natural as well as artificial light will fall on the region of the axilla.

OPERATIVE PREPARATION. The skin over the sternum, involved breast, chest wall, upper abdomen, supraclavicular region, shoulder, axilla, and lateral chest wall is gently cleansed with appropriate antiseptic solutions. In order to minimize the dissemination of free tumor cells by manipulation, the usual vigorous scrub of the skin is avoided. After the skin has been prepared, the arm is elevated by an assistant, permitting a sterile half sheet to be placed under the axilla and lateral wall of the chest. The arm is then anchored in abduction to a support, and sterile drapes are applied. A slight Fowler's position and tilt of the table away from the operator ensure the best approach for the surgeon and his assistants.

INCISION AND EXPOSURE. Regardless of how typical of malignancy the lesion appears to be, a diagnostic biopsy is taken in all cases. If the tumor mass is small (that is, 2 cm. or less), total excision, including the overlying skin and adjacent tissue, is carried out for examination by frozen section. If the lesion is appreciably larger, a simple wedge of tumor may be removed from the surface for frozen section examination. Hemostasis is secured, and the wound is tightly approximated and further sealed by a plastic spray or drape. All instruments, drapes, gloves, and gowns are discarded. If the lesion is proved to be cancerous, the skin is again carefully prepared with the appropriate antiseptic solution and the biopsy incision sealed by a plastic surgical drape. The proposed incision for radical mastectomy is outlined, and sterile drapes are reapplied. This procedure must be carried out religiously to avoid any chance of seeding of the tumor as a result of taking a biopsy.

Some prefer to prove the presence of neoplasm by needle aspiration rather than excisional biopsy. Following the usual preparation of the skin, the mass is entered with an 18-gauge needle attached to a 20-ml. syringe.

The syringe is rotated as the needle enters the tumor to ensure obtaining a core of tissue that can be aspirated as the plunger of the syringe is withdrawn. If the frozen section is positive, the radical removal of the breast and axillary contents is carried out.

While radical mastectomy may be performed through many types of incision, as shown in **Figure 2,** A and B, removal of a wide margin of skin at the level of the tumor, regardless of where that may be and without respect to the location of the nipple, is the chief consideration. Further, the incision must permit exposure of the axillary and supraclavicular regions and must extend down below the costal margin to permit exposure of the upper part of the anterior sheath of the rectus muscle. The shaded areas in **Figure 2** indicate the extent to which the skin and subcutaneous tissues are dissected free from the underlying structures.

An improved cosmetic result may be attained with a less restrictive scar by a more transverse incision **(Figure 2,** B). The incision may be started at the base of the axillary hair region and extended well around the lesion, ending up medially in the epigastrium.

Modified Radical Mastectomy

This alternate procedure involves simple mastectomy including the adjacent axillary contents up to the lower border of the axillary vein. A transverse incision **(Figure 2,** B) can be used, extending from the midsternal region around the nipple to the hairline of the axilla. As much skin over the tumor as permits closure of the wound without excess tension is included with the specimen. The exposure of the axilla is enhanced by upward and medial retraction of the margin of the pectoralis major. Some prefer to divide the pectoralis minor near its attachment to the coracoid process to improve the exposure of the axillary contents. The extent of the dissection about the axillary vessels and the inclusion of varying portions of the pectoral muscles immediately beneath the neoplasm vary with the judgment of the individual surgeon. Drainage by rubber tissue drain or suction catheter is usually advisable.

DETAILS OF PROCEDURE. The vascular and lymphatic supply of the breast is illustrated in **Figure 1.** The incision A is usually started at the upper angle. Medial and lateral skin flaps are developed in a plane superficial to the superficial fascia, that is, to the midsternum medially, to the clavicle superiorly, to the latissimus dorsi muscle laterally, and below the costal margin inferiorly. Care should be taken that the skin flaps remain thin; this is especially important as the axilla is approached, since the breast tissue very often lies immediately beneath the superficial fascia and may be inadvertently incised. The completed skin flaps should be 1 to 2 mm. thick at the skin edge and no more than 6 mm. thick at the base. Bleeding may be controlled with electrocautery or fine silk. The margins of the skin flaps are covered with gauze sponges soaked in saline solution. Now the lateral margin of the pectoralis major muscle is freed by sharp dissection. Following this the operator's index finger is passed upward beneath the narrow, tendinous portion of the muscle, and the muscle is divided as near the humerus as possible **(Figure 3).** Any bleeding points are clamped and tied. The cephalic vein is identified and dissected free, so that it is not injured during the further excision of the pectoralis major muscle **(Figure 3).** The cut end of the pectoralis major muscle is grasped with curved half-length clamps or tenacula to aid in retracting it downward, while its clavicular attachment is separated as close to the clavicle as possible **(Figure 4).** The thoracoacromial artery and vein will probably require ligation during the dissection **(Figure 4).**

PLATE CLVI   RADICAL MASTECTOMY

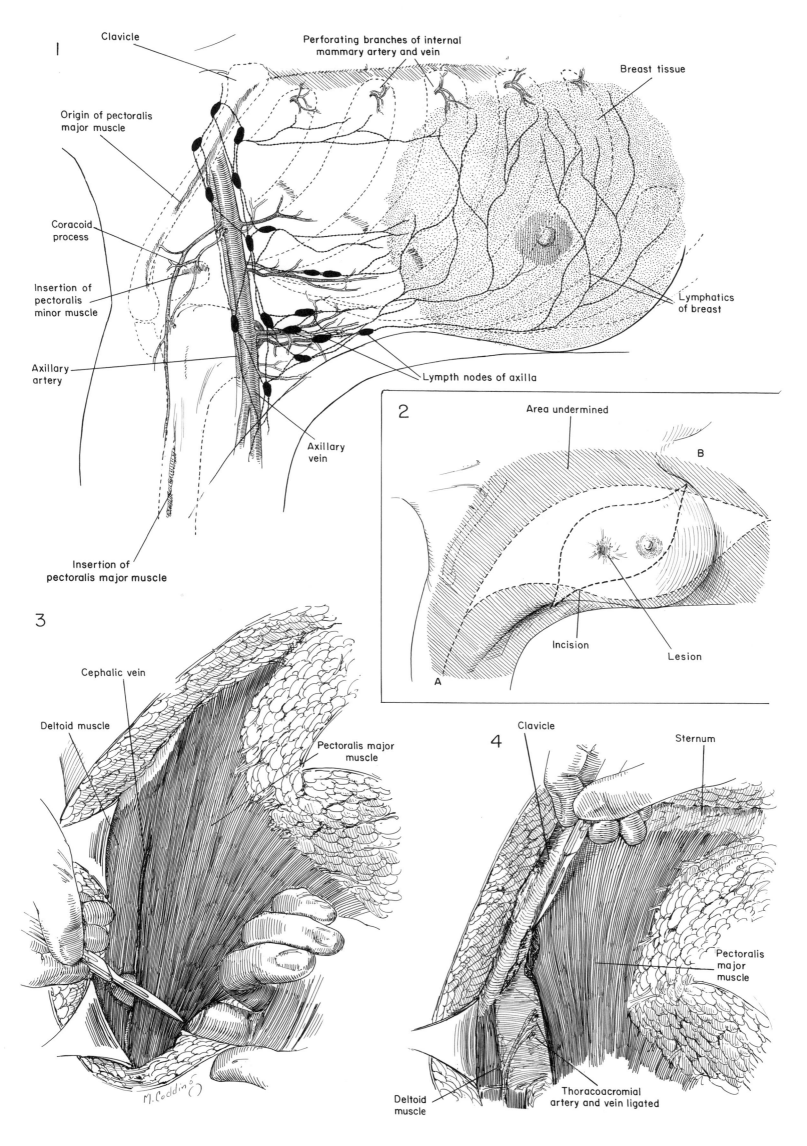

1

Clavicle

Perforating branches of internal
mammary artery and vein

Breast tissue

Origin of pectoralis
major muscle

Coracoid
process

Insertion of
pectoralis
minor muscle

Axillary
artery

Lymphatics
of breast

Lympth nodes of axilla

Axillary
vein

Insertion of
pectoralis major muscle

2

Area undermined

B

Incision

Lesion

A

3

Cephalic vein

Deltoid muscle

Pectoralis major
muscle

M. Codding

4

Clavicle

Sternum

Pectoralis
major
muscle

Deltoid
muscle

Thoracoacromial
artery and vein ligated

PLATE CLVII · RADICAL MASTECTOMY

DETAILS OF PROCEDURE (*Continued*). After the pectoralis major muscle has been freed from its attachments to the humerus and the clavicle, it is pulled downward, exposing the pectoralis minor muscle. The thin fascia over the pectoralis minor muscle is incised, and the index finger is passed beneath its attachments to the coracoid process to permit its division as near this as possible **(Figure 5).** Several bleeding points usually require ligation in the remaining tendinous attachment of the pectoralis minor muscle. With both muscles retracted downward, the axilla is exposed and prepared for dissection of its contents. The axillary vessels lie beneath a thin layer of fascia **(Figure 6).**

PLATE CLVII RADICAL MASTECTOMY

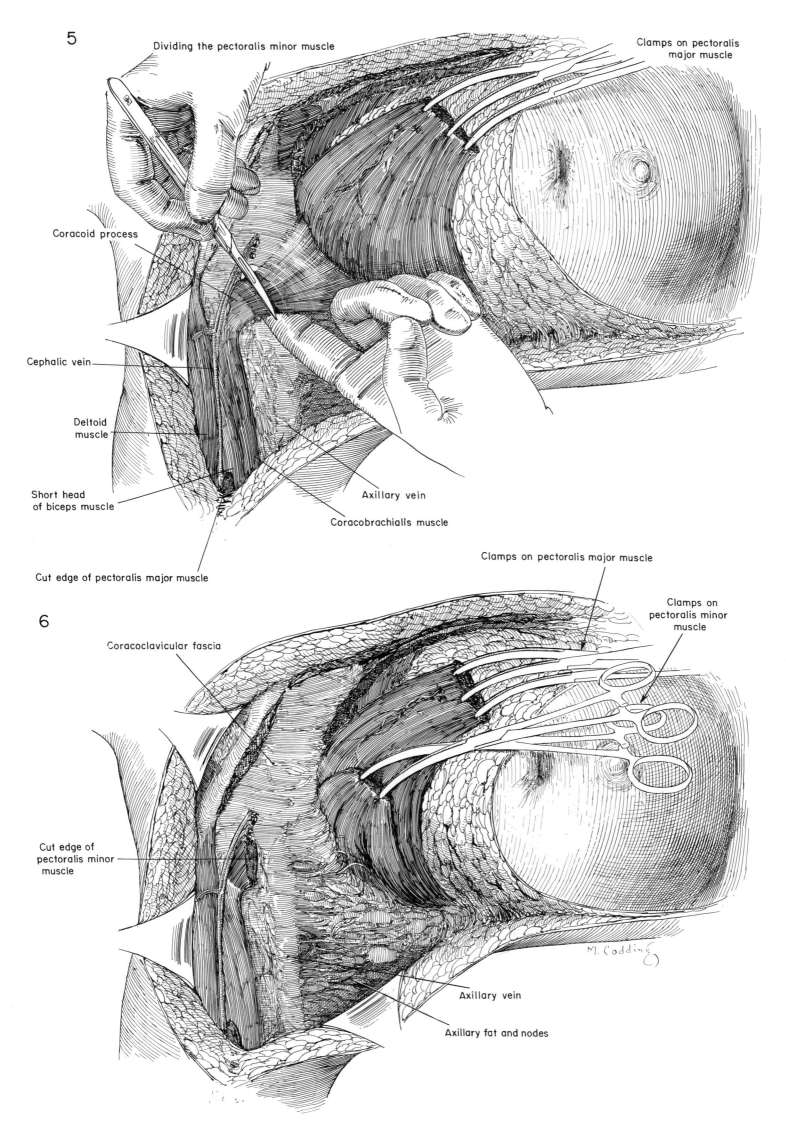

5

Dividing the pectoralis minor muscle

Clamps on pectoralis major muscle

Coracoid process

Cephalic vein

Deltoid muscle

Short head of biceps muscle

Axillary vein

Coracobrachialis muscle

Cut edge of pectoralis major muscle

Clamps on pectoralis major muscle

Clamps on pectoralis minor muscle

6

Coracoclavicular fascia

Cut edge of pectoralis minor muscle

M. Codding

Axillary vein

Axillary fat and nodes

PLATE CLVIII · RADICAL MASTECTOMY

DETAILS OF PROCEDURE. (*Continued*). The costocoracoid membrane, identified beneath the clavicle as a distinct layer, is removed, and the fascia over the axillary vein is incised carefully, using a scalpel or small curved scissors **(Figure 7).** In the course of this maneuver the vascular and nerve supply to the pectoral muscles is divided. The tissues above and below the vein are carefully separated by sharp dissection, and the various vascular branches are individually cut and tied very close to the major vessel **(Figure 8),** but the vein itself should not be traumatized by hemostats or forceps. Portions of the brachial plexus and the underlying artery are exposed above the vein, and as much as possible of the fatty and glandular contents of the axilla is removed from around and beneath the axillary vessels and nerves. The axillary contents, including the lymph nodes, may be dissected from beneath the axillary vessels downward **(Figure 9).** The long thoracic nerve, found about 2 cm. posterior and almost parallel to the pulsating lateral thoracic artery, and the thoracodorsal nerve are identified and protected from injury unless enlarged lymph nodes along their course make their sacrifice imperative **(Figure 9).** Sacrifice of the long thoracic nerve produces a "winging" of the scapula due to the loss of the serratus anterior muscle. The anterior border of the latissimus dorsi is freed for the length of the wound by sharp dissection. After the axilla has been thoroughly cleaned of fat and nodes, it is packed with a gauze pad moistened in warm saline solution; this remains while the dissection of the pectoral muscles is continued. The origins of the pectoralis major and minor muscles are cut with sharp dissection as the breast is retracted downward and outward **(Figure 10).** Perforating vessels, found in the intercostal space about 5 mm. lateral to the sternum, must be clamped and tied with transfixing sutures of fine 0000 silk on small French needles. Blunt-nosed clamps, however, are always applied parallel to the chest wall in an effort to grasp a perforating vessel, since the application of a hemostat, which has a sharp point, at right angles to the chest wall may perforate the pleura and result in the postoperative complication of pneumothorax.

PLATE CLVIII   RADICAL MASTECTOMY

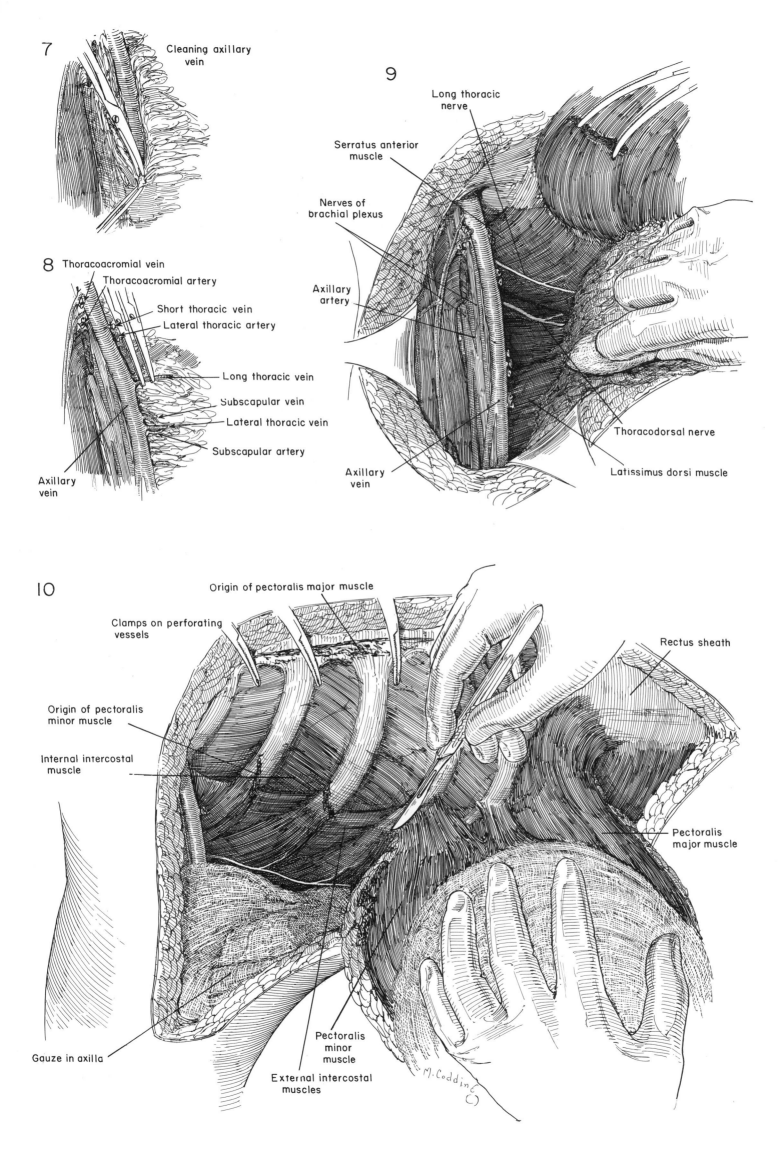

7 Cleaning axillary vein

8 Thoracoacromial vein
Thoracoacromial artery
Short thoracic vein
Lateral thoracic artery
Long thoracic vein
Subscapular vein
Lateral thoracic vein
Subscapular artery
Axillary vein

9 Long thoracic nerve
Serratus anterior muscle
Nerves of brachial plexus
Axillary artery
Axillary vein
Thoracodorsal nerve
Latissimus dorsi muscle

10 Origin of pectoralis major muscle
Clamps on perforating vessels
Origin of pectoralis minor muscle
Internal intercostal muscle
Rectus sheath
Pectoralis major muscle
Gauze in axilla
Pectoralis minor muscle
External intercostal muscles

M. Codding

PLATE CLIX · RADICAL MASTECTOMY

DETAILS OF PROCEDURE (*Continued*). As the pectoralis major and minor muscles are removed, the dissection should not include any fibers of the serratus anterior muscle **(Figure 11)**. The fascia over the anterior sheath of the rectus abdominis muscle on the affected side is dissected off for a distance of about 6 cm. The axilla and as much of the wound as possible are covered with warm, moist pads as the dissection progresses **(Figure 11)**. The field is carefully inspected for evidence of bleeding points. All gauze packs are removed, and the axilla is irrigated repeatedly with warm saline solution.

CLOSURE. Small curved forceps may be applied to the subcutaneous tissue, and the mobility of the skin flaps tested by manually attempting to approximate the skin margins **(Figure 12)**. If the margins do not approximate, the medial flap may be undercut well beyond the midline, and the lateral flap may be undercut to the posterior limits of the axilla. If drainage is desired, a stab wound is made through the lateral flap about 7 to 8 cm. below the axilla, and a rubber tissue drain, which is anchored to the skin with a transfixing suture of fine silk, is inserted upward **(Figure 12)**. A small mushroom catheter may be used instead of a drain, and constant suction attached to the catheter. Many interrupted sutures should be placed, especially in the axilla, to anchor the skin flaps to the underlying chest wall in order to obliterate all dead space and prevent the accumulation of serum. An additional Penrose drain may be placed in the most inferior portion of the medial skin flap along the sternal border. The subcutaneous tissue is approximated with interrupted sutures. It should be recognized that sutures placed at some distance from the cut edge prevent the elasticity of the intervening skin from helping in covering the defect. The whole axilla is carefully compressed to make certain that all the enclosed air is expressed from beneath the flaps and all dead space is obliterated. The skin margins are accurately approximated with interrupted silk sutures **(Figure 13)**. It may be necessary to adduct the arm to permit better approximation of the flaps.

In the case of an extensive lesion a sufficient amount of skin may have been excised so that, even after undercutting, the skin flaps cannot be approximated. Then it is necessary to graft the exposed, raw surface. Appropriate nonadherent dressings are placed on the grafts. Fluffed gauze is carefully inserted into the axilla and beneath the clavicle to make certain that there is an even distribution of pressure on the skin flaps. A considerable amount of gauze is placed about the drain, and combination pads complete the dressing, held in place by elastic adhesive tape. An elastic stocking fitted over the arm may help to reduce the amount of postoperative lymphedema. The arm itself is then immobilized with a sling.

POSTOPERATIVE CARE. Normal blood volume is restored by transfusion. Fluid balance is maintained by the intravenous route. Unless there is an unusual amount of drainage, the dressing remains unchanged for three to five days to permit fixation of the skin flaps to the chest wall and to prevent the formation of serum pockets. The patient is gotten out of bed on the first day if her postoperative condition permits. The patient's comfort is enhanced during the early postoperative days if an overhanging trapeze is provided which the patient can use to shift position. Later the trapeze is useful in mobilizing the arm on the side of the operation. Sutures are removed in seven to ten days. If fluid accumulates under the flaps, it is removed by aspiration under strict conditions of asepsis, and the cavity is compressed by a dressing to prevent a reaccumulation of fluid. Gradual activity of the arm is permitted. The patient is encouraged to practice reaching behind her head for the opposite ear at the end of five to seven days. Frequent short-term follow-ups are essential to evaluate the range of motion of the shoulder and to institute early measures against swelling of the arm should lymphedema develop. A survey of the patient for possible recurrence is performed at the same time.

When positive lymph nodes have been found, subsequent long-term therapy may involve systemic chemotherapy, regional X-ray therapy, or endocrine alteration therapy.

PLATE CLIX   RADICAL MASTECTOMY

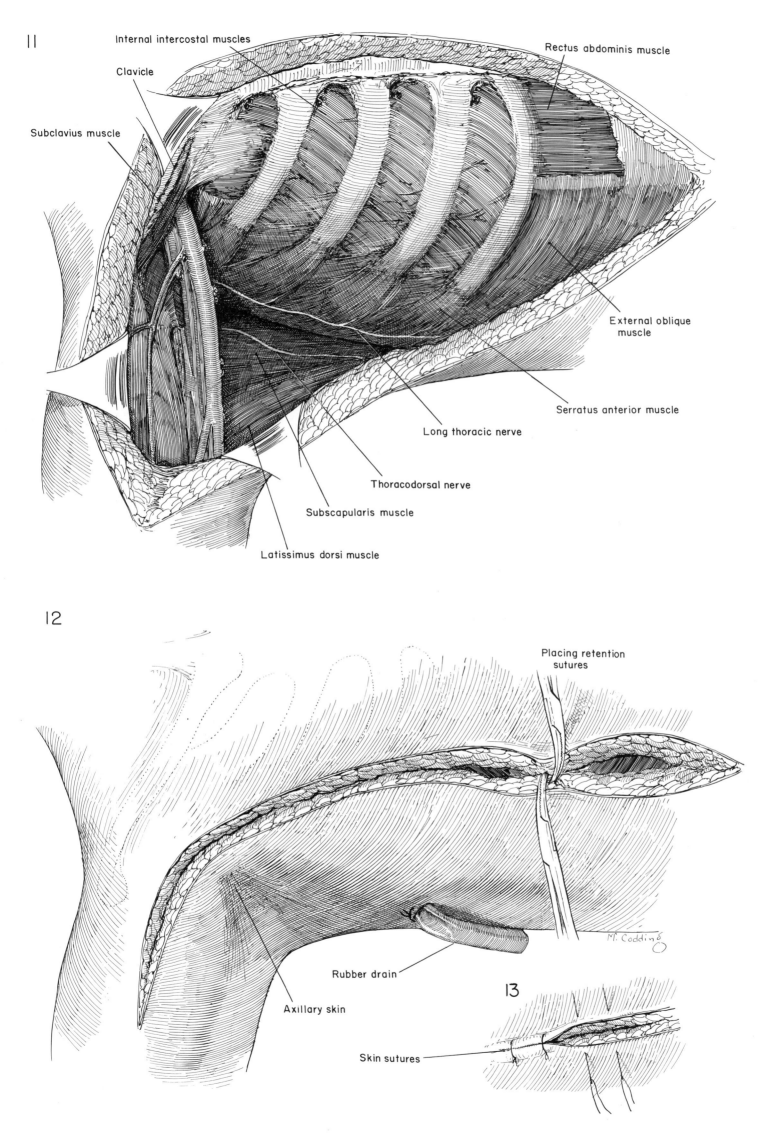

11

Internal intercostal muscles

Rectus abdominis muscle

Clavicle

Subclavius muscle

External oblique muscle

Serratus anterior muscle

Long thoracic nerve

Thoracodorsal nerve

Subscapularis muscle

Latissimus dorsi muscle

12

Placing retention sutures

Rubber drain

Axillary skin

M. Codding

13

Skin sutures

PLATE CLX · REPAIR OF POSTOPERATIVE HERNIA

INDICATIONS. Ventral hernia occurs most frequently at the site of previous surgical wounds where obesity, malnutrition, or sepsis has complicated healing; however, postoperative pulmonary complications, abdominal distention, etc., may be etiologic factors. The hernia should be repaired if the patient's general condition is satisfactory. As an example, we have chosen to depict an upper paramedian incision.

PREOPERATIVE PREPARATION. The major factors in the occurrence of each hernia should be assayed and remedied before repair is undertaken. When the hernia is very large, and a portion of the intestinal tract has been resident in the sac outside the true peritoneal cavity for years, attempts at repair are likely to fail unless, through restricted diet with considerable loss of weight, omental fat is reduced and space is made available within the peritoneal cavity for the contents of the hernial sac.

Patients with large hernias are hospitalized several days before operation in order that respiratory infections, chronic cough, urinary obstruction, and other factors that contraindicate repair may be discovered. Smoking is forbidden to those with a chronic productive cough. In addition, intravenous pyelograms and radiographs of the chest are taken, and barium studies are done of the entire gastrointestinal tract as well as sigmoidoscopic examination. The patient is given a low-residue diet and mild catharsis to reduce abdominal distention. During this time the patient should become accustomed to the use of a bedpan and urinal.

ANESTHESIA. For large hernias spinal anesthesia is often preferable because of the excellent muscle relaxation it provides. General anesthesia is used, however, unless contraindicated. Muscle relaxants secure the same degree of relaxation possible with spinal anesthesia. Some prefer to avoid excessive muscle relaxation in order to approximate the tissues at a more normal tension.

POSITION. The patient is placed in a supine position with the hips moderately flexed to aid in relaxing the abdominal wall. The patient's head is lowered to help in reducing the contents of the sac in repair of hernias occurring in the middle and lower abdomen.

OPERATIVE PREPARATION. Routine preparation of the skin is carried out, with special attention to the folds about the limits of the hernia.

INCISION AND EXPOSURE. Through an elliptical incision encircling all of the old scar **(Figure 1)**, the subcutaneous tissue is divided, and the scarred skin flap is turned back and excised **(Figure 2)**. Following this the underlying sac and the surrounding fascia are cleaned of fat **(Figure 3)**. If there is a thin layer of fascia over the sac, it is dissected back to the point where tissue with good blood supply and sufficient substance to hold suture material is found **(Figure 4)**.

DETAILS OF PROCEDURE. After the scarred fascia is removed, the subcutaneous fat is dissected from the anterior surface of the strong fascia for 5 to 10 cm. preparatory to reuniting it **(Figure 5)**. The lateral flaps are defined and dissected away from the rectus muscle and peritoneum **(Figure 6)**. The peritoneum is now opened, and the adherent intra-abdominal contents are carefully separated from the area before a general abdominal exploration. The hernial sac is then excised, leaving sufficient peritoneum for easy approximation. In the presence of a very large hernia it is advisable to extend the dissection a considerable distance. When the defect is quite large, wide dissection of the subcutaneous fat is indicated. Multiple relaxing incisions 2 to 4 cm. long are made in the fascia at some distance on both sides until the margins of the defect can be approximated without tension.

CLOSURE. The peritoneum is closed with interrupted mattress 00 silk sutures placed to approximate its inner surfaces **(Figure 7),** which should completely obliterate the sac. Care is exercised that tension is not great enough to cut the tissues. To remove undue tension at any particular point, it may be necessary to add further interrupted sutures. The surgeon should remember that multiple silk sutures give a stronger closure than a few heavy sutures on which there is great tension and which will eventually cut through the sustaining tissue in which they are placed. When the peritoneum is closed, the excess beyond the suture line is removed **(Figure 8)**. The decision is made whether the fascia is to be approximated by a figure-of-eight suture, as in an ordinary closure (Plates VI, VII, and VIII), or whether it is to be overlapped as in the procedure for umbilical hernia (Plate CLXI, **Figure 10**). All bleeding points must be carefully tied and the wound irrigated repeatedly with saline to minimize the collection of blood in the dead space beneath the subcutaneous tissue. The insertion of a rubber tissue drain through a separate stab wound should be considered if the hernia was quite large and the patient obese.

POSTOPERATIVE CARE. Constant gastric suction is maintained for several days to prevent abdominal distention. A temporary gastrostomy may be worth while. The patient may be gotten out of bed on the first postoperative day. The wound should be adequately supported; however, the dressing should not interfere with respiration, and great care is taken to guard against tight pressure dressing in the groins as prophylaxis against the occurrence of deep venous thrombosis. All drains are removed within 72 hours. The patient is warned against heavy lifting for six to eight weeks.

PLATE CLX   REPAIR OF POSTOPERATIVE HERNIA

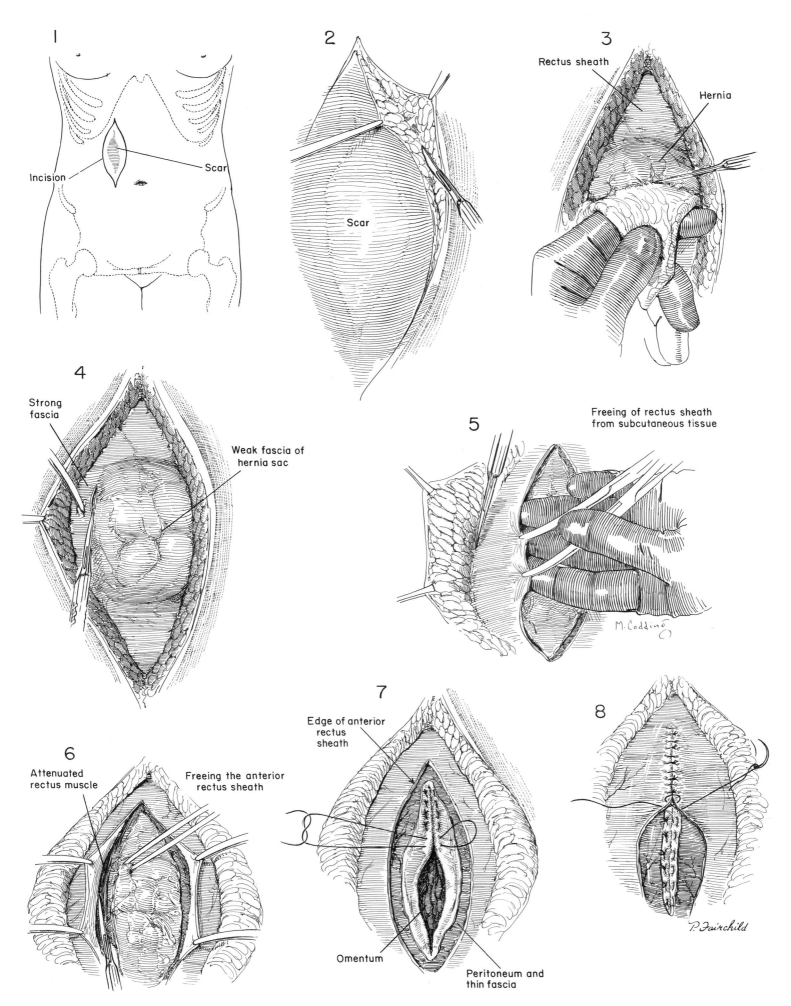

1

Incision
Scar

2

Scar

3

Rectus sheath
Hernia

4

Strong fascia
Weak fascia of hernia sac

5

Freeing of rectus sheath from subcutaneous tissue

M. Codding

6

Attenuated rectus muscle
Freeing the anterior rectus sheath

7

Edge of anterior rectus sheath
Omentum
Peritoneum and thin fascia

8

P. Fairchild

PLATE CLXI · REPAIR OF UMBILICAL HERNIA

INDICATIONS. An umbilical hernia is usually a congenital defect, although it may follow surgery in this region. The increased susceptibility to strangulation of an umbilical hernia in an adult necessitates repair if the patient's condition permits.

There is rarely any indication for repair of an umbilical hernia in the very young child, since 80 per cent of these fascial defects will close by the age of two years. In addition, the incidence of incarceration and strangulation in umbilical hernias in this age group is extremely low. However, if supportive measures such as the "keystone" type of strapping during infancy have failed and the fascial ring is sufficiently large to admit the index finger, then the hernia should be repaired before school age.

PREOPERATIVE PREPARATION. Since this defect is usually seen either in children or obese adults, the preoperative preparation depends entirely on the patient's general condition and age. Obese persons are placed on a reducing diet before such a procedure. A general medical survey, which should include X-rays of the chest and barium studies of the gastrointestinal tract, is indicated. In all cases the patient is placed on a low-residue diet for a few days, and the bowels are emptied by a mild saline purgative. During this period the patient should learn to use a bedpan and urinal. Repair is delayed in the presence of acute respiratory infections, chronic coughs, or infection about the navel. Special attention is given to cleansing of the navel.

ANESTHESIA. In large hernias spinal anesthesia may be preferred because of the excellent relaxation it provides; however, inhalation anesthesia can be used unless it is contraindicated. Muscle relaxants have the advantage of securing muscular relaxation without deep anesthesia.

For children inhalation anesthesia is the method of choice.

POSITION. The patient is placed in a comfortable supine position.

OPERATIVE PREPARATION. The skin is prepared in the usual manner after the umbilicus has been carefully cleansed. The latter may require cotton applicators saturated with the germicide solution used in preparing the skin in order to reach the deep crevices that may be present.

INCISION AND EXPOSURE. An elliptical transverse incision is made that includes the umbilicus at its central point. In stout persons it should be continued laterally as far as the outer borders of the rectus sheaths **(Figure 1)**. In those who wish to retain the umbilicus, either a curved subumbilical or a vertical incision may be utilized, and the umbilicus may be retained in the skin flap **(Figure 2)**. The incision is carried down to the rectus sheaths, which should be carefully defined. The subcutaneous fat in obese patients is fully protected and kept moist with gauze pads. The neck of the hernial sac is then dissected free from all adjacent tissues by a combination of blunt and sharp dissection.

In the child a curved incision is made around the superior half of the umbilical depression.

Adults

DETAILS OF PROCEDURE. A horizontal incision should be made in the rectus sheaths, releasing the neck of the sac and permitting the return of its contents to the abdominal cavity. Frequently, the omentum or intestine is densely adherent to the sac. Sharp dissection is required to detach these structures from the sac as well as from the peritoneum around its base. When there is strong suspicion of gangrenous intestine within the sac, the peritoneal cavity should be entered directly through the incision made in the rectus sheaths. If bowel is seen entering the sac, crushing clamps can be applied and the peritoneal cavity walled off to avoid possible gross contamination. The major portion of the sac, including the overlying skin, is subsequently removed **(Figure 3)**. The opening in the remaining sac is increased as the sac is held taut with clamps **(Figure 4)**. If there is a great deal of omentum in a huge sac that has been long resident outside the peritoneal cavity, it is wise to resect it, since unnecessary and undesirable abdominal tension can be created by replacing it. When the contents of the sac have been reduced and the neck has been well defined, the peritoneum is closed with catgut sutures or interrupted 00 silk sutures **(Figure 5)**. It is

very important to ensure a firm, complete closure of the sac to avoid recurrence of the hernia. Consequently, if a continuous catgut suture is used, it may be judicious to reinforce this single suture with a few interrupted ones, which, when possible, should include transversalis fascia. With the neck of the sac thus closed, any excess peritoneum is trimmed away. The anterior sheaths of the rectus muscles on either side of the linea alba are further defined and cleaned of fat, both above and below, by sharp dissection **(Figure 6)**. The rectus sheaths are freed from underlying muscle for a sufficient distance to permit overlapping of the flaps **(Figure 7)**. If there is an associated large diastasis of the rectus muscles, the muscles may be brought together in the middle with a few interrupted sutures, unless the approximation results in their fraying **(Figure 8)**. When the muscles have been joined, it may be wise to flex the body of the patient further to remove tension from the anterior abdominal wall. The upper rectus sheath is imbricated over the lower rectus sheath by a single row of interrupted mattress 00 silk sutures **(Figure 9)**, following which the margin of the sheath that is now overlapping is anchored with interrupted mattress sutures of 00 silk **(Figure 10)**.

CLOSURE. The subcutaneous sutures are carefully placed to obliterate all dead space. The skin sutures are taken as usual. When the hernia is quite large and the patient obese, rubber tissue drainage through an adjacent dependent stab wound tends to prevent postoperative fluid collection in the subcutaneous space.

POSTOPERATIVE CARE. Special attention is given to the avoidance of abdominal distention. Constant gastric suction is necessary. In the very obese, elderly, or those prone to pulmonary difficulties, a temporary gastrostomy should be considered. The patient is maintained in fluid balance with 5 per cent glucose in distilled water or saline until this is no longer necessary. The patient may be out of bed the first day postoperatively if the abdominal wound is properly supported. Adhesive tape or an abdominal binder may be used and continued for an indefinite period, depending upon the preoperative size of the hernia and on the obesity and general condition of the patient. The patient is warned to avoid heavy lifting and straining for six to eight weeks.

Children

DETAILS OF PROCEDURE. Following the curved incision around the superior half of the umbilical depression, the hernial sac is freed down to the anterior rectus fascia superiorly, and this dissection is then carried laterally on either rectus side, staying close to the hernial sac. It is then possible to pass a blunt instrument around the inferior margin of this sac. The umbilical skin is then held downward, and by countertraction on the hernial sac the attachment of the sac to the umbilical skin is freed by sharp dissection. It is important during this part of the procedure to avoid buttonholing the umbilical skin. Following this the anterior rectus fascia is cleared on all sides of the hernial ring for a short distance. The hernial sac may then be opened and any omentum reduced. The neck of the sac is closed with a few interrupted sutures of fine silk. The edges of the anterior rectus fascia making up the borders of the fascial defect are then closed with interrupted sutures of fine silk. This may be done either vertically or horizontally, depending upon the shape of the fascial defect.

CLOSURE. The skin margins are then approximated with interrupted subcuticular 000000 black silk sutures or a continuous absorbable suture. A short length of umbilical tape is folded into the umbilical depression in order to approximate the umbilical skin to the underlying fascia and thus have a normal-appearing umbilicus. A dry sterile dressing is then applied.

POSTOPERATIVE CARE. No special postoperative care is ordinarily required in these patients. They are usually able to tolerate fluids within four to six hours after the operation and are discharged home on a normal diet the following day. The type of incision and closure described leaves a fine scar in the umbilical depression which blends into the normal skin folds in this region in such a fashion as to make the operative incision virtually invisible after a few weeks.

PLATE CLXI   REPAIR OF UMBILICAL HERNIA

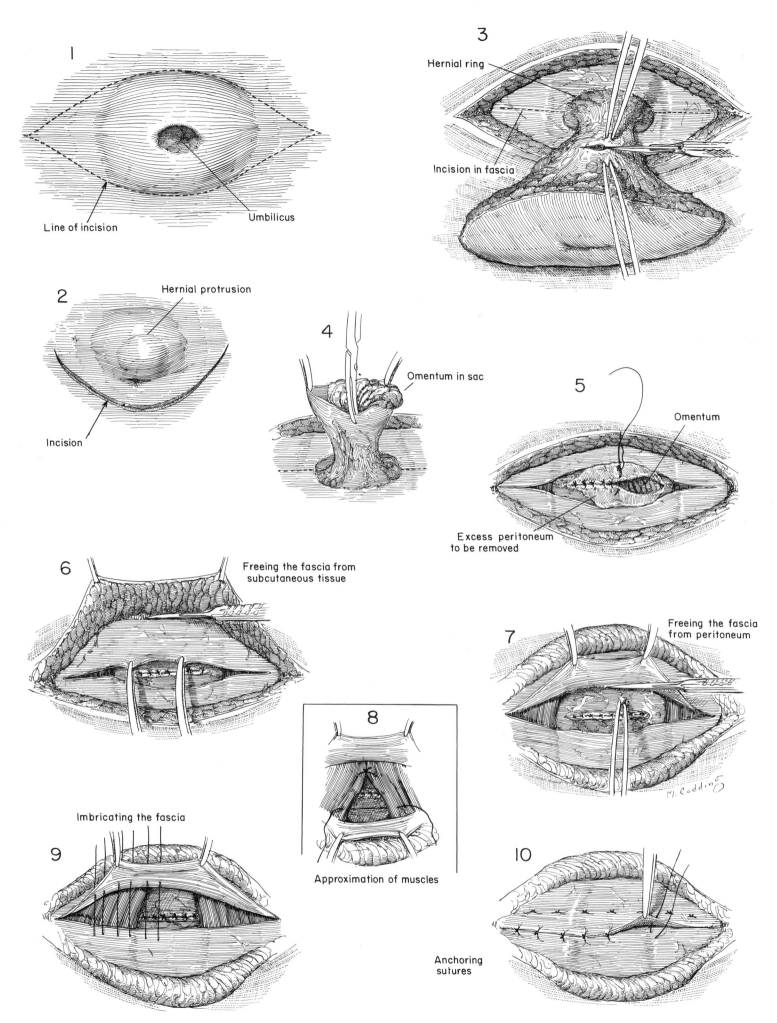

1

Line of incision   Umbilicus

2

Hernial protrusion

Incision

3

Hernial ring

Incision in fascia

4

Omentum in sac

5

Omentum

Excess peritoneum
to be removed

6

Freeing the fascia from
subcutaneous tissue

7

Freeing the fascia
from peritoneum

M. Codding

8

Approximation of muscles

9

Imbricating the fascia

10

Anchoring
sutures

PLATE CLXII · REPAIR OF INDIRECT INGUINAL HERNIA

INDICATIONS. Any indirect inguinal hernia should be repaired unless contraindicated by the tremendous size of the hernia or by the age or poor physical condition of the patient. The appearance of indirect inguinal hernia in middle-aged or elderly patients requires thorough medical investigation, including a roentgenologic examination of the gastrointestinal tract and chest, as well as urologic investigation, before repair is advised. It is wise to rule out any other source of pathology as a cause for the patient's complaint rather than to ascribe it to the presence of an indirect inguinal hernia.

Repair of an inguinal hernia in an infant or child is indicated as soon as practical after the diagnosis is made. In the presence of an undescended testicle, the repair, which includes an orchidopexy, should be delayed until three to five years of age to permit maximum spontaneous descent. The orchidopexy is indicated at any age if there is strong indication for repairing the hernia due to incarceration, etc.

PREOPERATIVE PREPARATION. Obese persons should be refused repair until their weight has been substantially reduced to a point within the range of their calculated ideal weight, in order to assure a low recurrence rate. Repair should be delayed also in patients with acute upper respiratory infections or a chronic cough until these conditions have been remedied. Smoking is curtailed or stopped, and frequent intermittent positive pressure breathing, with appropriate drugs added, should be instituted several days before surgery. During the period of preoperative study the patient should be trained to use the urinal and bedpan and practice a simplified method of getting in and out of bed.

In the presence of strangulation, the operation is delayed only long enough for fluid and electrolyte balance to be established by the intravenous administration of 5 per cent dextrose in a balanced electrolyte solution. Systemic antibiotic therapy is instituted. Whole blood and plasma transfusions may be advisable, especially if gangrenous bowel is suspected. A small stomach tube is passed intranasally, and constant gastric suction is maintained before, during, and for several days after operation. Sufficient time must be taken to ensure a satisfactory urine output of at least 30 to 50 ml. per hour, a pulse under 100 per minute, and an appropriate blood pressure with a normal central venous pressure. Repeated electrolyte values should be approaching normal. Adequate preparation may require from several hours to a much longer period for the administration of several liters of fluids and electrolytes, especially potassium and blood, in the patient who has had intestinal obstruction for several days. Operative intervention before stabilization may have disastrous results.

A child two years of age or older should be prepared psychologically in advance for his hospital experience. Booklets that describe in simple narrative style the various details of hospitalization and operation can be read to the child before operation. Such preparation undoubtedly serves to diminish the incidence of emotional trauma as a complication of elective surgery.

ANESTHESIA. General anesthesia is used unless contraindicated by the patient's physical condition. Local infiltration anesthesia should be considered more frequently, since it allows approximation of the tissues at a more normal tension and also makes it possible for the patient to increase the intra-abdominal pressure by coughing, which will aid in identifying the sac and in testing the adequacy of the repair. Note the position of the nerves for local anesthesia **(Figure 1)**. If obstruction is present, general anesthesia with an endotracheal tube and cuff is recommended to avoid the ever-present threat of tracheal aspiration.

Inhalation anesthesia is the method of choice in children. Open drop vinethene for induction followed by ether and oxygen is satisfactory.

POSITION. The patient is placed in a supine position with a pillow beneath the knees so that slight relaxation at the groin is achieved. The table is tilted with the head down slightly to aid in reducing the contents of the hernial sac and in retracting a thick abdominal wall by gravity.

OPERATIVE PREPARATION. The skin preparation is routine.

INCISION AND EXPOSURE. A skin incision, extending from just below and medial to the anterior superior iliac spine to the pubic spine, is made 2 to 3 cm. above and parallel to Poupart's ligament **(Figure 1, A)**. A more comfortable and cosmetic incision results if the major crease in the lines of skin cleavage is followed **(Figure 1, B)**. This may be defined by gentle downward traction on the abdominal wall, which demarcates the natural crease in the skin beneath the plastic drape. Either incision is carried down to the external oblique fascia. Several blood vessels, especially the superficial epigastric vein and the external pudendal vein, are usually encountered in the subcutaneous tissue in the lower portion of the incision. These must be clamped and tied **(Figure 2)**.

DETAILS OF PROCEDURE. The external oblique is carefully cleaned of all fat by sharp dissection throughout the length of the wound, and the external ring is visualized **(Figure 2)**. After the margins of the wound have been covered with gauze moistened in isotonic saline, a small incision is made in the direction of the fibers of the external oblique which extend into the medial side of the external inguinal ring **(Figure 2)**. The edges of the external oblique are held away from the internal oblique muscle to avoid injury to the underlying nerves as the incision is continued through the medial side of the external ring **(Figure 3)**. The nerves are most commonly injured at the external ring. The lower side of the external oblique is freed by blunt dissection down to include Poupart's ligament. The upper margin is similarly freed for some distance. As the ilioinguinal nerve is dissected free from the adjacent structures, a bleeding point is commonly encountered as it passes over the internal oblique **(Figure 4)**. This bleeding vessel, if encountered, must be carefully tied; otherwise, a hematoma may develop in the wound. When the ilioinguinal nerve has been carefully dissected free, it is pulled to one side over a hemostat placed at the edge of the incision **(Figure 5)**. The cremasteric fibers are grasped with toothed forceps and divided in order to approach the sac **(Figure 6)**. The sac itself is seen as a definite white membrane that lies in front and toward the inner side of the cord; it is usually differentiated easily from surrounding tissues. If the hernia is small, the sac lies high in the canal. The vas deferens can be recognized by palpation because it is firmer than the other structures of the cord. The wall of the sac is lifted up gently and opened with care to avoid possible injury to its contents **(Figure 7)**. While the margins of the opened sac are grasped with hemostats, the contents are replaced within the peritoneal cavity. With the index finger of his left hand introduced into the sac to give counterresistance, the surgeon frees the sac with the right hand by either blunt or sharp dissection **(Figure 8)**. If the dissection is kept close to the sac, an avascular cleavage plane will be found. Sharp dissection is advisable to separate the vas deferens and adjacent vessels from the sac **(Figure 9)**. If this is carefully done, fewer bleeding points will be encountered than if an effort is made to sweep these structures away from the sac by means of blunt dissection with gauze. The dissection is then continued until the properitoneal fat is displaced and the peritoneum beyond the narrow neck of the sac is visualized.

PLATE CLXII   REPAIR OF INDIRECT INGUINAL HERNIA

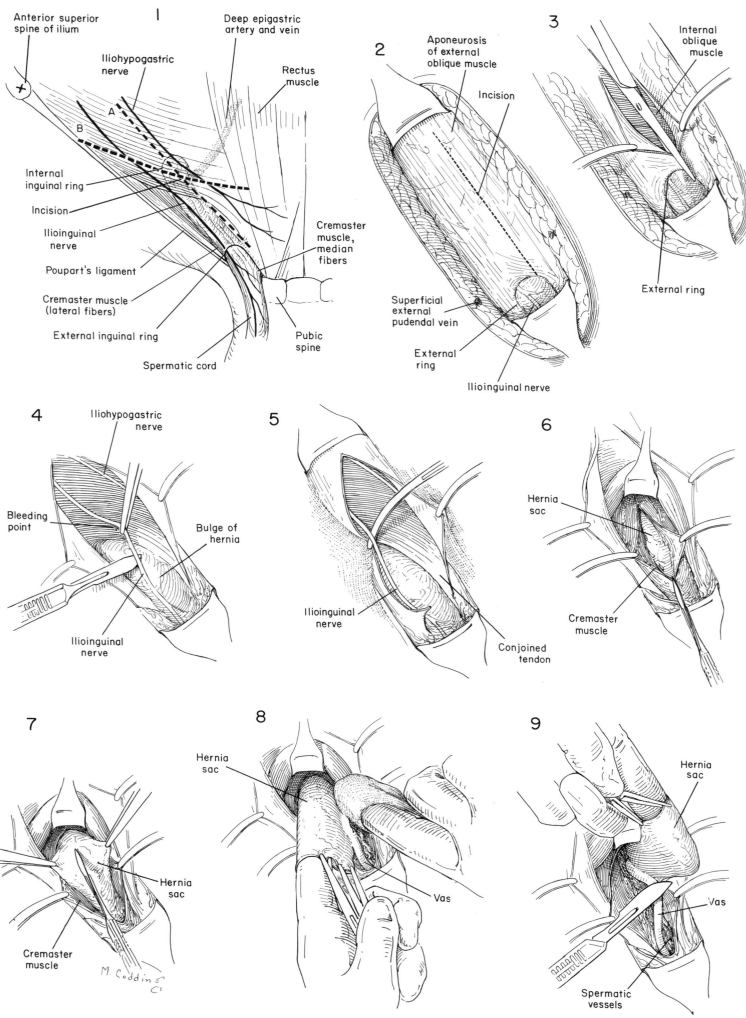

1

Anterior superior spine of ilium

Iliohypogastric nerve

Internal inguinal ring

Incision

Ilioinguinal nerve

Poupart's ligament

Cremaster muscle (lateral fibers)

External inguinal ring

Spermatic cord

Deep epigastric artery and vein

Rectus muscle

Cremaster muscle, median fibers

Pubic spine

A

B

2

Aponeurosis of external oblique muscle

Incision

Superficial external pudendal vein

External ring

Ilioinguinal nerve

3

Internal oblique muscle

External ring

4

Iliohypogastric nerve

Bleeding point

Bulge of hernia

Ilioinguinal nerve

5

Ilioinguinal nerve

Conjoined tendon

6

Hernia sac

Cremaster muscle

7

Hernia sac

Cremaster muscle

M. Codding

8

Hernia sac

Vas

9

Hernia sac

Vas

Spermatic vessels

PLATE CLXIII · REPAIR OF INDIRECT INGUINAL HERNIA

DETAILS OF PROCEDURE (*Continued*). The sac is opened within 2 to 3 cm. of its neck, and exploration is carried out with the index finger to rule out the presence of a "pantaloon" or secondary direct or femoral hernia **(Figure 10)**. To ensure obliteration of the sac, a purse-string suture is placed at the inner side of the neck **(Figure 11)**, or several transfixing sutures may be used if preferred. The lumen of the neck of the sac must be visualized as sutures are placed or tied to avoid possible injury to omentum or intestine. This suture should include the transversalis fascia with the peritoneum. The neck of the sac can sometimes be identified as a slightly thickened white ring. The sac should be ligated proximal to this ring. After the purse-string suture is tied, the excess sac is amputated with scissors **(Figure 12)**.

If desired, the ligated sac may be anchored to the overlying muscle. In this instance the long ends of the suture used to close the neck of the sac are rethreaded. The needle is inserted beneath the transversalis fascia and brought up in the edge of the internal oblique muscle, the two ends being brought through separately and tied **(Figure 13)**. Care should be taken to avoid injuring the inferior deep epigastric vessels.

CLOSURE. There are various methods of repair after the sac has been removed. Large or recurrent hernias in older persons or hernias in patients doing very heavy work may be corrected by a method that either partially or completely transplants the cord and narrows the internal ring. On occasion permission is obtained to remove the cord and testicle, especially in the case of recurrent hernias, where the musculature is poor and the testicle already atrophied.

Nontransplantation of Cord (Ferguson Repair)

The cremasteric fibers, which may or may not be well developed, are approximated with interrupted 00 silk sutures **(Figure 14)**. This covers the raw surface remaining after removal of the sac and restores the structures to a normal appearance. The cremaster muscle may at times be united and pulled beneath the conjoined tendon to assist in pulling Poupart's ligament mesially to relieve strain on the next layer of sutures, and to increase the efficiency of the repair **(Figure 15)**. Sutures are then placed to approximate the conjoined tendon and the internal oblique muscle to Poupart's ligament, the sutures being tied anterior to the cord **(Figure 16)**. The sutures in Poupart's ligament are placed from below upward, unequal portions of the ligament being taken to avoid fraying. All sutures are placed and then tied from below upward. The first suture should be tied loosely enough so that the cord is not constricted and so that there is sufficient space about the cord to permit an instrument as large as a lead pencil to pass; moreover, care should be taken to avoid injury to or inclusion of the ilioinguinal nerve by the sutures. The external oblique fascia is approximated with interrupted sutures **(Figure 17)**. Here again, the external ring should not constrict the cord. If it does, the adjacent fascia may be incised to give additional room, or the lowest suture may be replaced **(Figure 18)**. The subcutaneous tissue is carefully approximated with interrupted 0000 silk sutures; likewise, interrupted 0000 silk sutures are utilized to close the skin **(Figure 19)**. The wound is covered with a layer of gauze and a transparent adhesive spray.

Repair in Children

A short (3 cm.) skin incision is made in the suprapubic crease above the inguinal ligament and centered over the internal inguinal ring.

After the incision has been made through the skin, a small curved mosquito hemostat is placed in the subcutaneous tissue on either side of the midportion of the incision for traction. Scarpa's fascia is exposed and divided. The underlying aponeurosis of the external oblique is cleared down to the external inguinal ring and the inguinal ligament by sharp dissection. The aponeurosis of the external oblique is then opened upward from the external inguinal ring. If there is no associated scrotal hydrocele, the incision through the external oblique aponeurosis may be placed just above rather than through the external ring. Superior and inferior flaps of the aponeurosis of the external oblique are developed with the scalpel handle, and a small right-angle retractor is placed under the superior flap to expose the inguinal canal. The cremasteric muscle fibers are separated by blunt dissection. The hernial sac is identified on the anteromedial aspect of the cord structures, lifted up, and gently separated in the midportion of the inguinal canal from the vas and the vessels. The cord structures themselves should not be mobilized from the inguinal canal. The sac is divided between two straight mosquito hemostats in the midportion of the inguinal

canal, and the proximal portion is freed well above the level of the internal ring. The neck of the sac is then closed with a suture ligature of fine silk and the sac amputated. Ordinarily, it is not necessary to open the sac during this process. However, if omentum or a loop of intestine is within the sac, the sac is opened, and these structures are returned to the peritoneal cavity before the neck of the hernial sac is closed. The distal portion of the sac is freed below the level of the external ring and excised.

If a hydrocele of the tunica vaginalis is present, it can be delivered in most instances by traction on the distal segment of the processus vaginalis. It may be necessary to aspirate fluid from the hydrocele sac and/or to apply upward pressure from the scrotum. It is neither necessary nor desirable to remove such a hydrocele entirely. All that is necessary is to clear the areolar tissue over the bulk of the hydrocele sac and to excise this, leaving the portion that is intimately attached to the testis. All bleeding points must be ligated lest a hematoma develop within the scrotum.

The testis and cord structures are repositioned into their normal anatomic bed if they have been disturbed, and an anatomic closure is performed. The aponeurosis of the external oblique and Scarpa's fascia are closed with interrupted sutures of fine silk. A subcuticular closure with fine silk is used in children. Because of the high incidence of a patent processus vaginalis on the opposite side in instances of a clinical inguinal hernia on one side, it is common practice to perform an inguinal exploration on the opposite side.

It is advisable to resect an intra-abdominal testicle that cannot be brought into the scrotum, providing there is a normal testicle on the opposite side. After the sac, testicle, and cord structures have been separately identified and freed from the canal, an effort is made to determine how far the testicle will extend downward into the bed prepared for it in the scrotum. Added distance can be gained by dividing and ligating the deep epigastric vessels as well as the transversalis fascia over to the pubic bone. The spermatic vessels must also be freed by blunt dissection from the surrounding retroperitoneal tissues. Numerous fibrous bands are divided until the vessels are well mobilized up toward the region of the kidney. One method of preventing the immediate return of the testicle from the scrotum is to pass a 00 silk suture through the capsule of the lower pole of the testicle and out through the bottom of the scrotum. Traction is maintained on the testicle for seven to ten days by tying this suture to a rubber band fastened to the inner aspect of the thigh with adhesive tape.

Repair in Females

The round ligament is usually closely attached to the sac, making sharp dissection necessary for separation. After the neck of the sac is freed and ligated, the repair proceeds as in the operation on the male, except that the round ligament may be included in the sutures that bring the conjoined tendon to Poupart's ligament. If the round ligament is divided, it must be ligated, since it contains a small artery; and the proximal end must be anchored in order to give support to the uterus.

In female children the incision and initial stages of the procedure are as described above. However, in a high proportion of cases a congenital indirect hernia in a female is a sliding type of hernia, with the fallopian tube and its mesenteric attachments making up a portion of the hernial sac. In such instances the hernial sac and round ligament are closed with a suture ligature of fine silk distal to the attachment of the mesosalpinx. The remainder of the procedure is identical with that done in the male.

POSTOPERATIVE CARE. Postoperative care is as follows:

Adult. The patient is placed flat in bed with the thighs somewhat flexed either by a pillow beneath the knees or, if in an adjustable bed, with the lower part of the bed somewhat elevated, in order to prevent undue tension upon the sutures in the wound. However, undue constriction of the groins from tight dressings or position in bed, which might predispose to venous thrombosis, is avoided. Support to the scrotum should be furnished by an adhesive-plaster sling or suspensory. An ice pack may be applied to the scrotum. Coughing must be controlled by sedation. Laxatives are given in sufficient dosage to avoid undue straining at stool. Patients should be permitted out of bed at any time after operation in order to void, rather than be subjected to catheterization. Physical activity should be drastically curtailed for at least three weeks after operation. A period of six weeks should elapse before the patient is permitted to perform heavy physical work; in certain situations a convalescent period of eight weeks should be allowed. Special abdominal supports are usually not necessary.

Child. The infant or child is fed four to six hours after operation and by the evening of operation should be taking a normal diet. These patients may be discharged home the evening of the day of operation.

PLATE CLXIII   REPAIR OF INDIRECT INGUINAL HERNIA

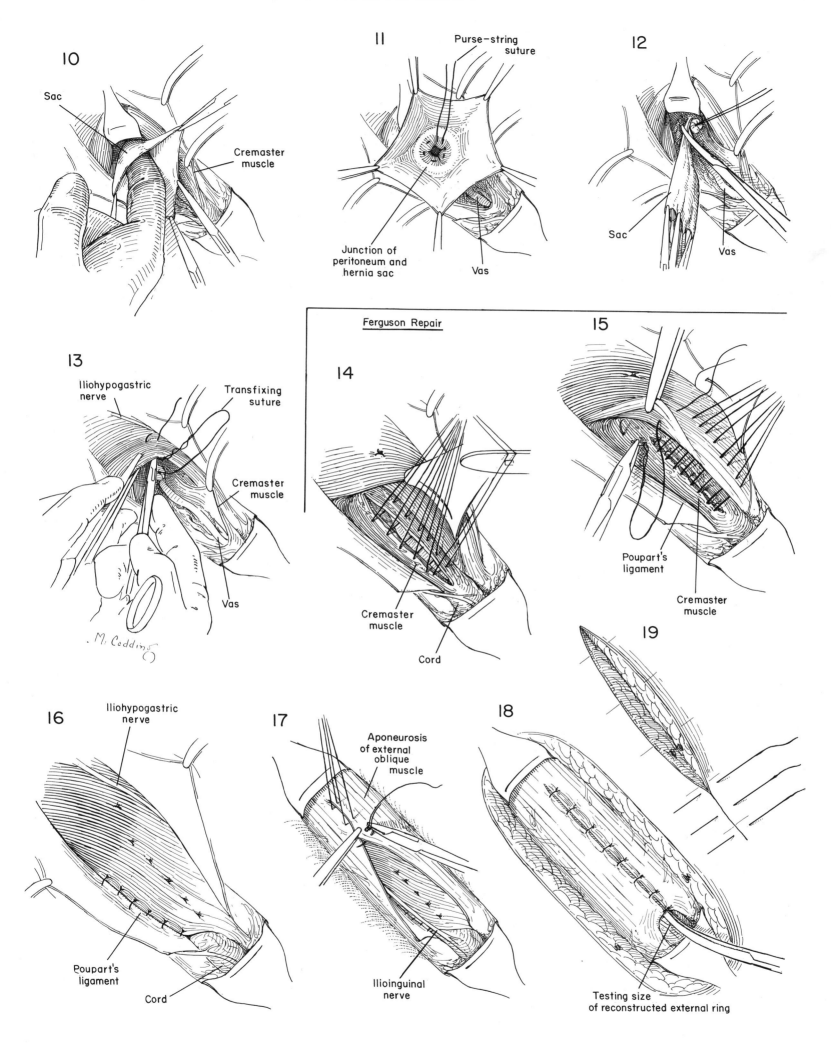

10

Sac

Cremaster muscle

11

Purse-string suture

Junction of peritoneum and hernia sac

Vas

12

Sac

Vas

13

Iliohypogastric nerve

Transfixing suture

Cremaster muscle

Vas

M. Coddins

Ferguson Repair

14

Cremaster muscle

Cord

15

Poupart's ligament

Cremaster muscle

19

16

Iliohypogastric nerve

Poupart's ligament

Cord

17

Aponeurosis of external oblique muscle

Ilioinguinal nerve

18

Testing size of reconstructed external ring

PLATE CLXIV · REPAIR OF INDIRECT INGUINAL HERNIA

Bassini Repair

DETAILS OF PROCEDURE. The cord is visualized by the approach described in Plate CLXII. Since the structures of the cord are to be transplanted, it may be easier to separate the cord from the surrounding structures before the hernial sac is identified and opened. The index finger may be inserted beneath the cord from the medial side just above the pubic tubercle in order to assist in the blunt dissection and freeing of the cord from the underlying Poupart's ligament **(Figure 20).** A curved half-length clamp directed over Poupart's ligament and toward the pubic spine is then passed beneath the cord and guided by the index finger **(Figure 21).** A tube of soft rubber (Penrose drain) is drawn through beneath the cord for traction **(Figure 22).** Many times blood vessels that course downward beneath the cord must be clamped and tied to ensure a dry field. The cremaster muscle is divided, and the hernial sac is grasped with toothed forceps preliminary to opening it **(Figure 23).** Some prefer to completely divide the cremaster muscle near the internal oblique muscle, leaving the vas and its accompanying vessels exposed. The sacrifice of the cremaster muscle at this level permits a more accurate closure of the internal ring. The hernial sac is opened, and traction is maintained by curved or straight hemostats applied to its margin. With the surgeon's index finger in the hernial sac, the vas deferens and accompanying vessels are dissected free by sharp and blunt dissection **(Figure 24).** With the surgeon's finger in the neck of the hernial sac to ensure that all abdominal contents are completely reduced, a purse-string suture is placed at the inner side proximal to the neck of the sac, or several transfixing mattress sutures of 00 silk are used, as preferred **(Figure 25).** Care must be taken that the adjacent epigastric vessels are not injured. If there is a large mass of spermatic veins, especially on the left side, it may be wiser to divide and ligate most of these, leaving a few of the veins to be preserved with the vas to ensure an adequate vascular supply.

CLOSURE (Transplantation of Cord, Bassini). The first step in the closure is to provide adequate retraction of the cord as well as the internal oblique muscle, so that the deep-lying aponeurosis of the transversus abdominis and the transversalis fascia can be identified **(Figure 26).** It is important to reinforce the weakened area over the ligated hernial sac by approximating the thickened fascia just below the free edge of Poupart's ligament, the so-called iliopubic tract, and the edge of the aponeurosis of the transverse abdominal muscle **(Figure 26, suture x).** The remaining opening in the cremaster muscle is closed with interrupted sutures unless it has been completely divided adjacent to the internal oblique muscle. The transversalis fascia may appear to be very thinned out adjacent to Poupart's ligament, but an aponeurosis, the strong white membrane forming the inferior margin of the transversus abdominis, is exposed **(Figure 26)** by retracting the internal oblique sharply upward. The hernia repair is strengthened if an effort is made to approximate the latter structure to the iliopubic tract beyond the margins of Poupart's ligament. The conjoined tendon is retracted upward so that each bite of the needle includes a good portion of the aponeurosis of the transversus muscle **(Figure 27)** and the thickened fascia adjacent to the margin of Poupart's ligament. Several sutures between the iliopubic tract and the aponeurosis of the transversus muscle are taken lateral to the cord to close the redundancy of the internal ring **(Figure 28).**

PLATE CLXIV   REPAIR OF INDIRECT INGUINAL HERNIA

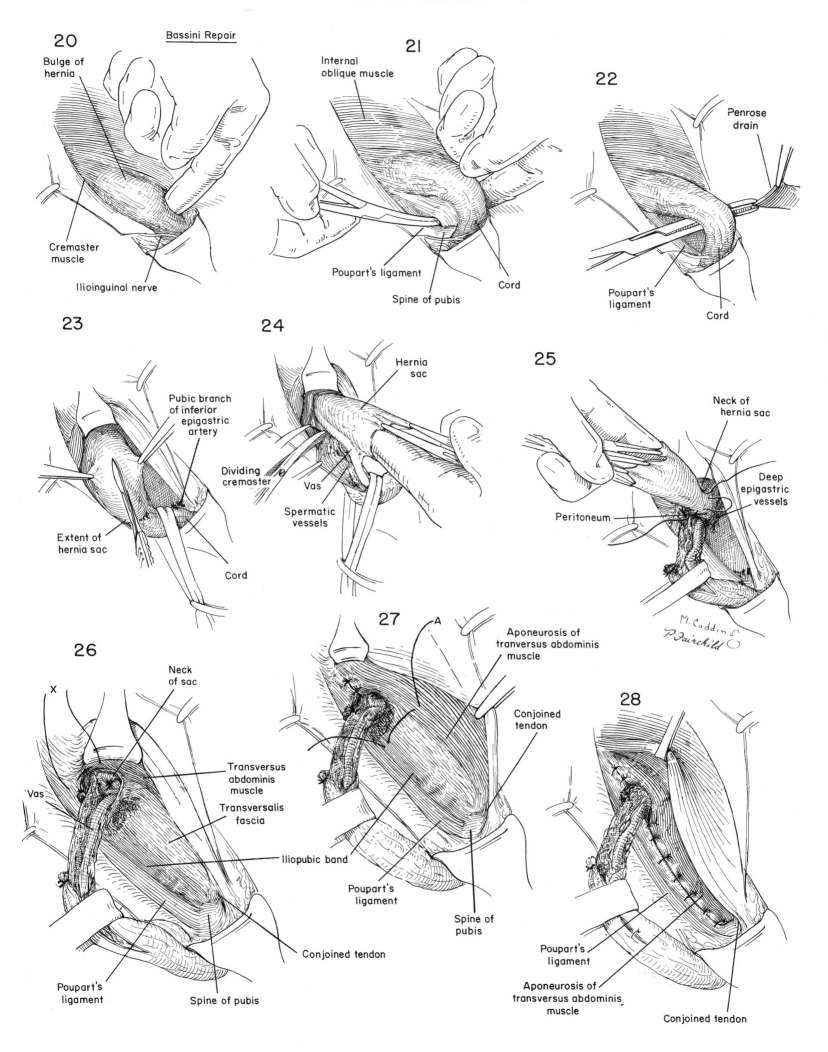

20 Bassini Repair

Bulge of hernia

Cremaster muscle

Ilioinguinal nerve

21

Internal oblique muscle

Poupart's ligament

Spine of pubis

Cord

22

Penrose drain

Poupart's ligament

Cord

23

Pubic branch of inferior epigastric artery

Extent of hernia sac

Cord

24

Hernia sac

Dividing cremaster

Vas

Spermatic vessels

25

Neck of hernia sac

Deep epigastric vessels

Peritoneum

M. Coddin E
P. Fairchild

26

X

Neck of sac

Vas

Transversus abdominis muscle

Transversalis fascia

Iliopubic band

Conjoined tendon

Poupart's ligament

Spine of pubis

27 A

Aponeurosis of tranversus abdominis muscle

Conjoined tendon

Poupart's ligament

Spine of pubis

28

Poupart's ligament

Aponeurosis of transversus abdominis muscle

Conjoined tendon

PLATE CLXV · REPAIR OF INDIRECT INGUINAL HERNIA

CLOSURE (*Continued*). A second layer of 00 silk sutures includes unequal portions of the shelving edge of Poupart's ligament and a bite of the conjoined tendon. This suture line extends from the pubic tubercle outward over the deep epigastric vessels until the cord appears to be angulated laterally. Before these sutures are placed, the mobility and composition of the tendon should be determined. In many instances the conjoined tendon cannot be brought down to Poupart's ligament except under a great deal of tension. A preliminary trial should be carried out by attempting to approximate the conjoined tendon to Poupart's ligament at the proposed suture line to determine the amount of tension that will be present **(Figure 29)**. The medial leaf of the external oblique fascia is retracted medially, and by blunt dissection the underlying sheath of the rectus is exposed **(Figure 30)**. If the tension appears to be excessive, relaxation of the fascia with retained support of the underlying rectus muscle is achieved by multiple incisions in the rectus sheath **(Figure 31)**. The incisions can be made about 1 cm. apart and 1 cm. in length. Eight or ten or even more may be required to produce the desired relaxation **(Figures 31 and 32)**. The number required can be judged by the spread of the tissues as the incisions are made and as traction on the fascia is maintained. The conjoined tendon is sutured to the lower edge of Poupart's ligament adjacent to the suture line that has approximated the aponeurosis of the transverse abdominal muscle to the iliopubic tract. The initial suture should include the periosteum of the pubic spine and the medial portion of the conjoined tendon. Several sutures are taken to approximate the muscles to Poupart's ligament above the point of exit of the cord, but these must not constrict

the cord, especially if its size has been markedly decreased by the excision of some of the dilated veins and the cremaster muscle **(Figure 33)**. The ilioinguinal nerve is replaced, and the external oblique aponeurosis is closed over the cord, either by imbricating the mesial flap of the external oblique muscle over the lower flap by two rows of mattress sutures **(Figures 34 and 35)** or by a simple approximation of the edges of the external oblique by interrupted 00 silk sutures. The newly constructed external ring should be tested to make certain that the cord is not unduly constricted.

Transplantation of Cord (Halsted)

Some surgeons prefer the method of transplanting the cord to the subcutaneous fatty layer **(Figure 36)**. Here the cord is brought out through the upper third of the incision in the external oblique fascia **(Figure 36)**, and the fascia is closed beneath the cord, leaving it entirely in the superficial fatty tissue **(Figure 37)**. The size of the cord is usually decreased by the excision of many of the spermatic veins as well as the cremaster muscle; however, sufficient blood supply to the testicle must be retained. The cord must not be constricted, or atrophy of the testicle will occur. The size of the external ring is tested with a curved clamp, and, if necessary, a small incision is made just through the margin to release the constriction about the cord **(Figure 36)**.

POSTOPERATIVE CARE. Care is routine. See Plate CLXIII.

PLATE CLXV   REPAIR OF INDIRECT INGUINAL HERNIA

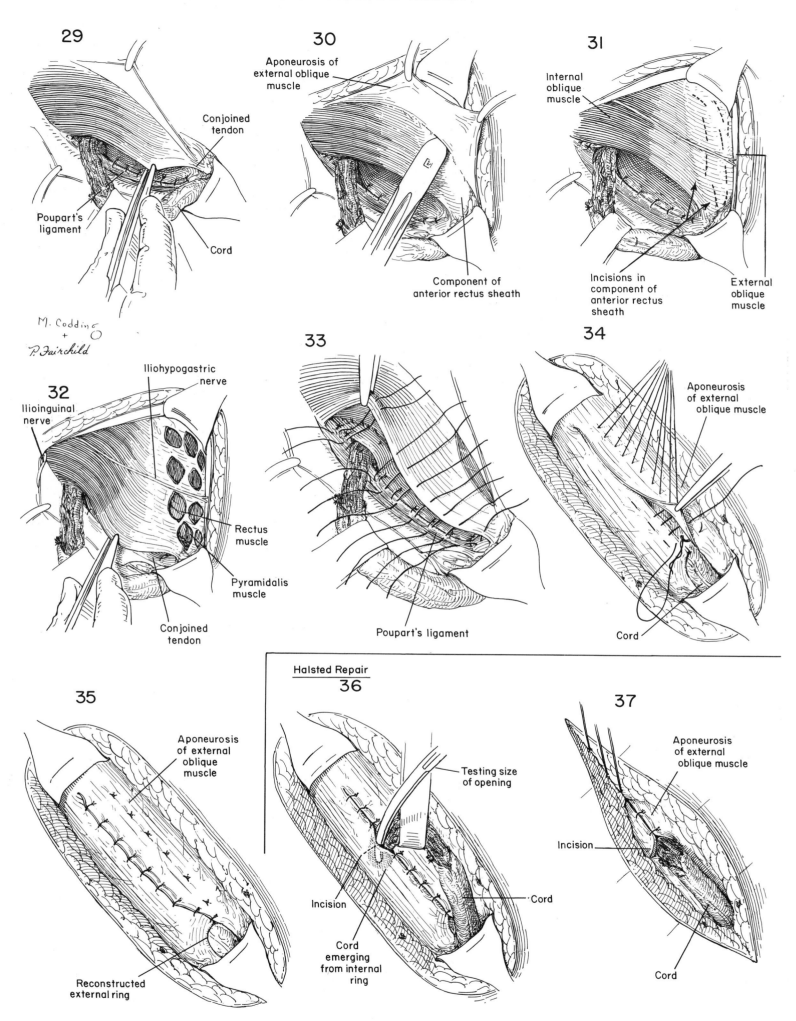

29

Conjoined tendon

Poupart's ligament

Cord

M. Codding
+
P. Fairchild

30

Aponeurosis of external oblique muscle

Component of anterior rectus sheath

31

Internal oblique muscle

Incisions in component of anterior rectus sheath

External oblique muscle

32

Ilioinguinal nerve

Iliohypogastric nerve

Rectus muscle

Pyramidalis muscle

Conjoined tendon

33

Poupart's ligament

34

Aponeurosis of external oblique muscle

Cord

35

Aponeurosis of external oblique muscle

Reconstructed external ring

Halsted Repair
36

Testing size of opening

Incision

Cord

Cord emerging from internal ring

37

Aponeurosis of external oblique muscle

Incision

Cord

PLATE CLXVI · REPAIR OF DIRECT INGUINAL HERNIA

INDICATIONS. The surgeon should remember that this defect is more common in older persons, who will invariably require a general evaluation before operation. Regardless of the care exercised, the incidence of recurrence tends to be higher following a direct inguinal hernia repair than following repair of an indirect inguinal hernia. In such a patient pathologic conditions, including hypertrophy of the prostate, emphysema, chronic cough, and so forth, may be present, the importance of which may greatly outweigh that of the hernia; therefore, not all direct hernias are repaired. A complete gastrointestinal examination should be made before the hernia is repaired regardless of whether the patient complains of any symptoms referable to this system. New gastrointestinal symptoms in patients with long-standing hernias are particularly unlikely to be a result of a reducible hernia. Every effort must be made to explain the symptomatology and to rule out any disease that may be, indirectly, the etiologic factor in the production of the hernia. X-rays of the chest are routine and clearance of the lower genitourinary tract mandatory before repair to ensure the best results.

PREOPERATIVE PREPARATION. See Plate CLXII.

ANESTHESIA. See Plate CLXII.

POSITION. The patient is placed in a comfortable supine position, with thighs slightly flexed. The table is tilted in a mild Trendelenburg position to reduce the contents of the sac and provide gravity retraction of the abdominal wall away from the incision.

OPERATIVE PREPARATION. The skin is prepared in the routine manner.

INCISION AND EXPOSURE. The usual incision for inguinal hernia is made just above and parallel to Poupart's ligament or in the line of skin cleavage (Plate CLXII).

DETAILS OF PROCEDURE. The conjoined tendon is pulled upward with a small retractor, bringing into view the bulging peritoneum through the weakened transversalis fascia mesial to the cord and the deep epigastric vessels **(Figure 1).** The cord is isolated from the surrounding tissues and retracted downward with the rubber tissue drain. By sharp and blunt dissection the hernial sac is freed from the adjacent structures **(Figure 2).** Where there is no definite sac but a diffuse bulge, it may be sufficient to plicate the transversalis fascia, after the cord has been retracted to one side, without making any attempt to excise the pseudosac. The bulge is everted with forceps while the defect in the transversalis fascia is repaired by interrupted 00 sutures **(Figure 3).** Care must be taken while plicating the sac that the point of the needle does not injure the bladder, intestines, or deep epigastric vessels **(Figure 4).** After the defect in the transversalis fascia has been completely repaired, there should be no evidence of a bulge or weakness in this area.

A common finding is a definite sac with a wide base **(Figure 5).** In this instance the sac is explored as in the operation for simple indirect inguinal hernia **(Figure 6).** It is not uncommon to find that the wall of the bladder forms part of the medial side of the direct hernial sac. This can be identified as a thickened, somewhat vascular structure **(Figure 7).** The neck of the sac is amputated, and the margins of the peritoneum are grasped with small forceps **(Figure 8).** This is done only after it has been carefully ascertained that the thickened vascular bladder wall does not form a part of the neck of the sac. Following exploration with the index finger in the peritoneal cavity for either an indirect or a femoral sac, the neck of the sac is closed with interrupted 00 silk mattress sutures, which include transversalis fascia, in order to strengthen the tissues against recurrence of the hernia **(Figure 9).**

When dissected free of surrounding tissues, the sac of a direct hernia may have the gross appearance of a diverticulum with a narrow, well-defined neck **(Figure 10).** Great care should be exercised in making certain that the bladder is carefully dissected away from the neck of the sac; otherwise, it may be accidentally opened. After the bladder has been dissected away from the sac and reduced, the neck of the sac is ligated, and the defect in the transversalis fascia is repaired with interrupted sutures. Sometimes there is a protrusion both above and below the inferior deep epigastric artery **(Figure 11).** The condition should always be verified by opening the indirect sac as well and by exploring with the finger for "pantaloon" or accessory sacs. It is best to join the two sacs into a single one by pulling the lower one above the deep epigastric vessels **(Figure 12).** When this has been done, the sac is treated as in the ordinary indirect inguinal hernia (Plate CLXII).

PLATE CLXVI   REPAIR OF DIRECT INGUINAL HERNIA

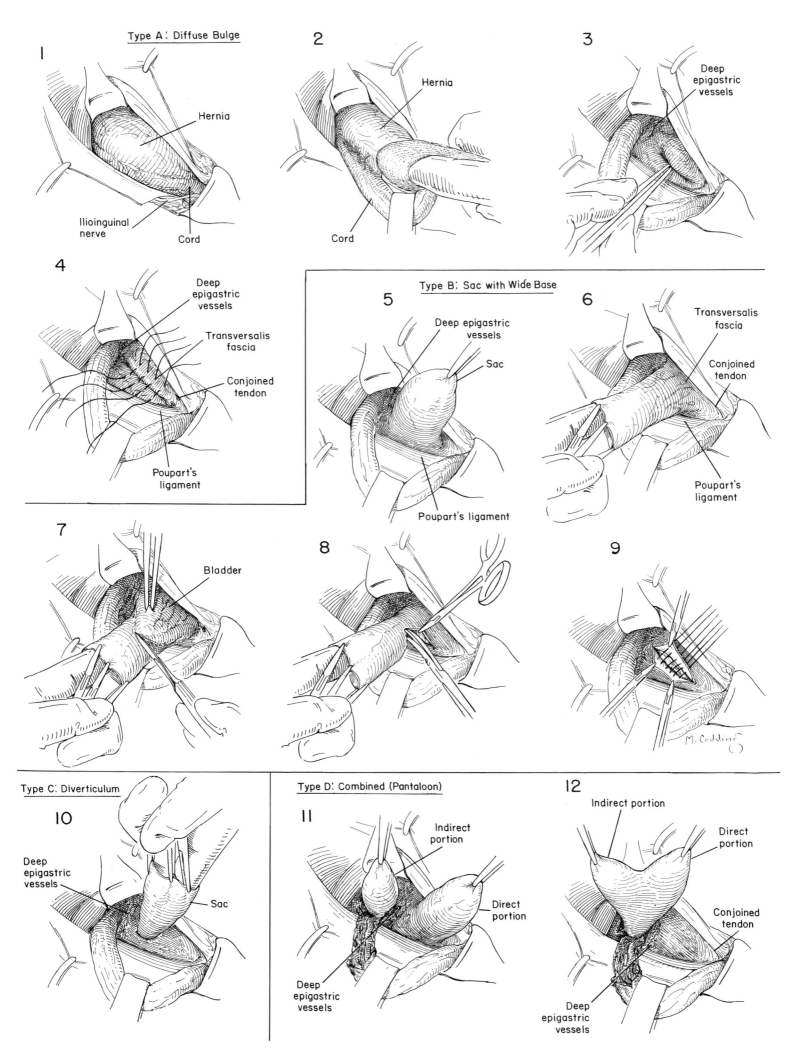

Type A: Diffuse Bulge

1 Hernia
Ilioinguinal nerve
Cord

2 Hernia
Cord

3 Deep epigastric vessels

4 Deep epigastric vessels
Transversalis fascia
Conjoined tendon
Poupart's ligament

Type B: Sac with Wide Base

5 Deep epigastric vessels
Sac
Poupart's ligament

6 Transversalis fascia
Conjoined tendon
Poupart's ligament

7 Bladder

8

9 M. Codding

Type C: Diverticulum

10 Deep epigastric vessels
Sac

Type D: Combined (Pantaloon)

11 Indirect portion
Direct portion
Deep epigastric vessels

12 Indirect portion
Direct portion
Conjoined tendon
Deep epigastric vessels

PLATE CLXVII · REPAIR OF DIRECT INGUINAL HERNIA (McVAY)

CLOSURE. After the hernial sac has been reduced and the rent in the transversalis fascia repaired, or the neck of the sac amputated, additional support may be obtained by approximating the transversalis fascia and the aponeurosis of the transverse abdominal muscle to either Poupart's or Cooper's ligament **(Figure 13).** The conjoined tendon is drawn upward with a small retractor, and the cord is retracted downward. Underneath the conjoined tendon the transversalis fascia can usually be identified as a strong but thin fibrous membrane. Sutures are taken in this structure above the level of closure of the hernial sac and in the iliopubic tract. The first suture includes a bite in the periosteum of the pubic spine as well as the above-mentioned structures **(Figure 13).** These interrupted 00 silk sutures are continued upward to the region of the deep epigastric vessels. Great care must be exercised to identify the deep epigastric vessels, or they may be injured accidentally. After the interrupted sutures have been tied to approximate the transversalis fascia and the inferior margin of the aponeurosis of the transverse abdominal muscle to the iliopubic tract, the region of the exit of the cord should be explored, and additional sutures should be placed to ensure that the cord is angulated outward.

As the cord is retracted downward, a second layer of sutures is placed to unite the conjoined tendon to Poupart's ligament. These sutures are carried outward to approximate the internal oblique muscle to Poupart's ligament in a similar fashion. Unequal bites are used throughout all structures, and the first sutures should likewise incorporate the periosteum of the pubic spine **(Figure 14).** If the tension is too great, multiple incisions are made in the anterior sheath of the rectus (Plate CLXV, **Figures 31** and **32**). Some prefer to reflect a curved flap of the rectus sheath downward and attach it to Poupart's ligament **(Figure 15).**

Instead of approximating the transversalis fascia and the aponeurotic margin of the transverse abdominal muscle to the iliopubic tract and to Poupart's ligament to repair either a direct or indirect hernia, a stronger repair results from their approximation to Cooper's ligament. To accomplish this it is necessary to retract the conjoined tendon upward and the cord downward, while the transversalis fascia adjacent to the pubic spine is freed from Cooper's ligament **(Figure 16).**

By blunt dissection and the use of a curved retractor **(Figure 17),** the region of Cooper's ligament can be visualized, and the external iliac vessels can be identified. As the conjoined tendon or internal oblique muscle is held upward, a firm aponeurotic margin of transverse abdominal muscle is exposed in order to facilitate the placement of interrupted sutures. As the bulge in this region is retracted upward and medially by an appropriate retractor, Cooper's ligament is clearly visualized as a white, fibrous ridge, deep in the wound at the innermost portion of the concavity and closely applied to the horizontal ramus of the pubis **(Figure 17).** Interrupted 00 silk sutures on small Mayo needles approximate the aponeurotic margin of the transverse abdominal muscle and the transversalis fascia to Cooper's ligament. The iliac vessels may be protected by the surgeon's left index finger or a narrow S retractor as the innermost suture is placed. The sutures are continued downward until the region of the pubic spine is included in the last one **(Figure 18).** Three to five interrupted sutures are usually required. In obese individuals it may be difficult to obtain an easy exposure in this location, and constant care must be exercised to avoid injury to the iliac vessels and to effect a complete and solid repair **(Figure 19).** Some operators prefer to make an incision in Cooper's ligament before placing the sutures in order to ensure a better fascial approximation. After the aponeurotic margin of the transverse abdominal muscle has been anchored as far medially to Cooper's ligament as can be safely done, more superficial sutures may be taken to approximate it to the iliopubic tract **(Figures 19** and **20).** Some surgeons prefer to reinforce the repair to Cooper's ligament by another row of sutures approximating Poupart's ligament to the aponeurosis of the transverse abdominal muscle **(Figure 21).** The suturing of the internal oblique muscle to Poupart's ligament is not considered worth while. The type of repair should be varied to suit the anatomic conditions encountered. A combination of the technics described may be advantageous to ensure a solid repair without tension upon the suture lines and an accurate approximation of fascia to fascia.

POSTOPERATIVE CARE. Care is routine. See Plate CLXIII.

PLATE CLXVII   REPAIR OF DIRECT INGUINAL HERNIA (McVAY)

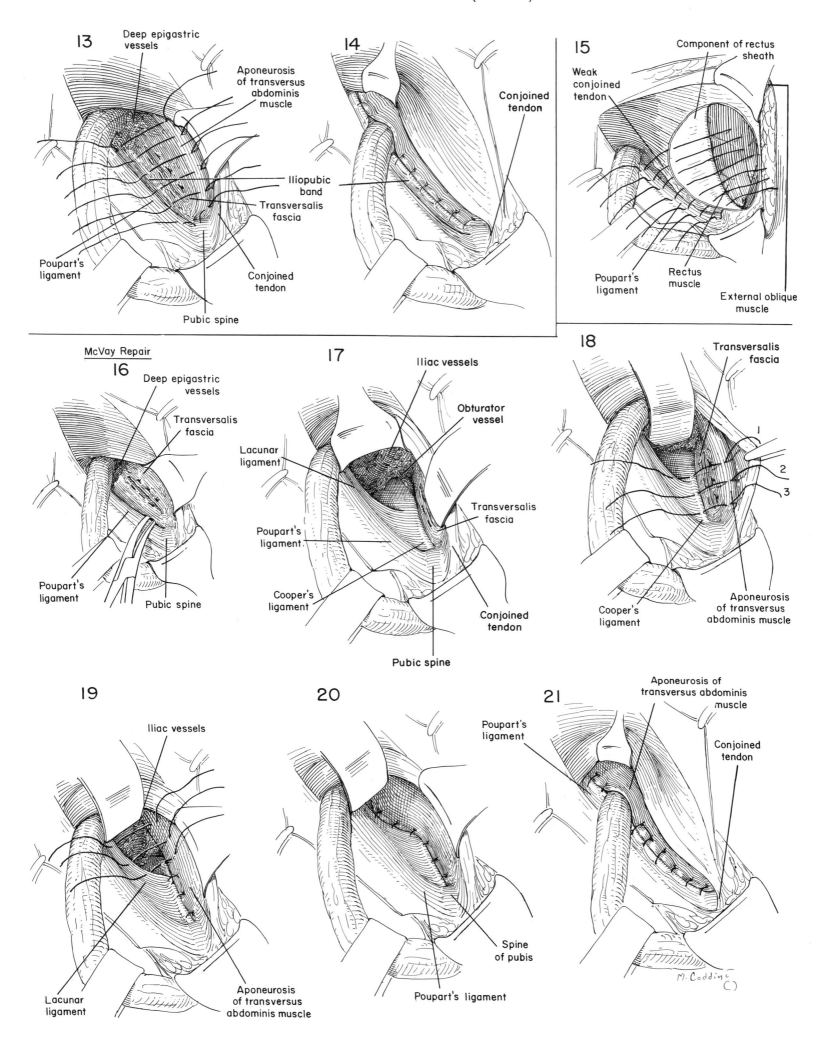

PLATE CLXVIII · REPAIR OF FEMORAL HERNIA

INDICATIONS. All femoral hernias should be repaired unless the patient's condition is unsatisfactory.

PREOPERATIVE PREPARATION. The preoperative preparation is directed by the patient's general condition. When the contents of the hernial sac are strangulated, the fluid and electrolyte balance is restored by 5 per cent dextrose in a balanced electrolyte solution administered intravenously. Antibiotics are instituted if the examination indicates the possibility of nonviability of the bowel and consequent necessity for resection of intestine. Sufficient time is taken to give the required amount of whole blood and plasma, depending upon the clinical and laboratory evaluation of the patient. Constant gastric suction is instituted. A slowing of the pulse and a good output of urine are signs favorable to early surgical intervention.

ANESTHESIA. See Plate CLXII.

POSITION. The patient is placed in a supine position with the knees slightly flexed to lessen the tension in the groin. The entire table is tilted slightly with the patient's head down.

OPERATIVE PREPARATION. The skin is prepared in the routine manner. A sterile transparent plastic drape may be used to cover the operative area.

INCISION AND EXPOSURE. The surgeon should have in mind the relationship of the hernial sac to the deep femoral vessels and Poupart's ligament **(Figure 1)**. The usual incision for inguinal hernia is made just above Poupart's ligament in the line of skin cleavage **(Figure 2)**. The incision above Poupart's ligament is preferred because it gives the best exposure of the neck of the sac and provides better exposure if bowel resection and anastomosis are necessary. The incision is made and carried down to the external oblique fascia. After the fascia has been dissected free of the subcutaneous fat, retractors are inserted in the wound. The external oblique fascia is divided in the direction of its fibers, as in the incision for inguinal hernia (Plate CLXII). The round ligament or spermatic cord is retracted upward along with the margin of the conjoined tendon **(Figure 3)**. The peritoneum, covered by transversalis fascia, now bulges in the wound. The neck of the hernial sac is freed from the surrounding tissues.

DETAILS OF PROCEDURE. The operator must now choose one of two procedures. If he can pull the sac upward through the femoral canal to the surface, it may be unnecessary to open the abdominal cavity until the sac itself is opened. This is facilitated by retracting the neck of the sac upward with forceps, while the operator applies counterpressure below Poupart's ligament through the hernial mass **(Figure 4)**. If the sac cannot be reduced from beneath Poupart's ligament by this maneuver, it becomes necessary to dissect the subcutaneous tissue from the lower leaf of the external oblique until the hernial sac is exposed as it appears in the femoral canal beneath Poupart's ligament **(Figure 5)**. Following this procedure it is frequently possible to withdraw the hernial sac from the femoral canal, converting the femoral hernia to a diverticular type of direct hernia **(Figure 6)**.

If the contents of the hernial sac appear to be reduced so that it can be opened without possible injury to incarcerated bowel, the sac is opened **(Figure 7)**. A purse-string suture, which should include transversalis fascia as well as peritoneum, is placed at the junction of the sac and the peritoneal cavity so that when it is tied, no residual peritoneal pouch remains **(Figures 8** and **9)**. Great care is taken that the suture closing the neck of the sac does not include intestine or omentum.

When operating for strangulated femoral hernia, the surgeon should open the peritoneal cavity before attempting to reduce the sac; otherwise gross contamination may occur **(Figure 10)**. An incision is made into the peritoneal cavity just above the neck of the hernial sac in order to visualize and evaluate its contents. If the omentum is incarcerated, traction is applied with forceps in an effort to reduce it within the abdominal cavity **(Figure 10)**. If the omentum is gangrenous, it is excised, and all bleeding points are controlled with fine silk. After its contents have been reduced, the hernial sac is completely everted into the peritoneal cavity **(Figure 11)**. The sac is amputated flush with the peritoneum, and the opening in the peritoneum is carefully closed with interrupted 00 silk mattress sutures **(Figure 12)**.

PLATE CLXVIII   REPAIR OF FEMORAL HERNIA

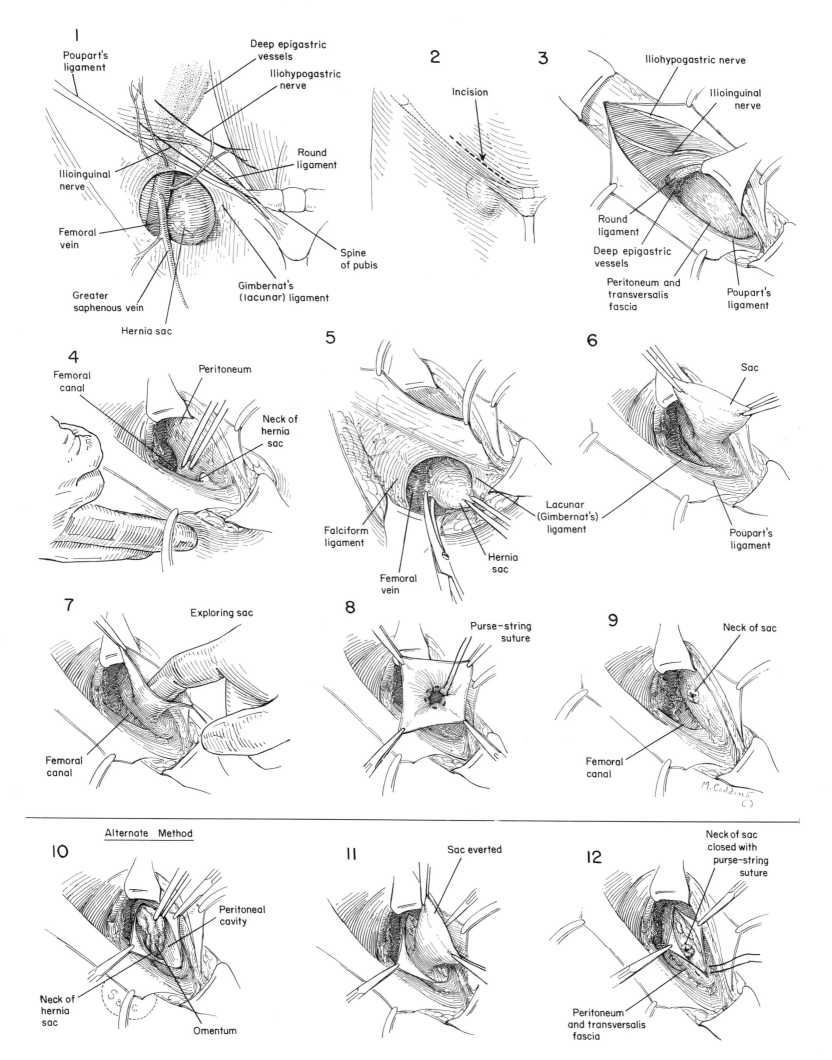

1

Poupart's ligament

Deep epigastric vessels

Iliohypogastric nerve

Round ligament

Ilioinguinal nerve

Femoral vein

Spine of pubis

Greater saphenous vein

Gimbernat's (lacunar) ligament

Hernia sac

2

Incision

3

Iliohypogastric nerve

Ilioinguinal nerve

Round ligament

Deep epigastric vessels

Peritoneum and transversalis fascia

Poupart's ligament

4

Femoral canal

Peritoneum

Neck of hernia sac

5

Falciform ligament

Femoral vein

Hernia sac

Lacunar (Gimbernat's) ligament

6

Sac

Poupart's ligament

7

Exploring sac

Femoral canal

8

Purse-string suture

9

Neck of sac

Femoral canal

M. Codding

Alternate Method

10

Neck of hernia sac

Peritoneal cavity

Omentum

11

Sac everted

12

Neck of sac closed with purse-string suture

Peritoneum and transversalis fascia

PLATE CLXIX · REPAIR OF FEMORAL HERNIA

DETAILS OF PROCEDURE (Dennis Technic). When operating for a strangulated femoral hernia, especially if nonviable bowel is practically a certainty, it is important that the contents of the sac be undisturbed to avoid gross contamination. Under such circumstances, after the external oblique has been divided, the sac is dissected from the surrounding tissues and Poupart's ligament divided down to the neck of the sac. It is advisable to divide the ligament in a Z-like fashion to facilitate its subsequent repair **(Figure 13).** The constricting band about the neck of the sac is retained to avoid contamination from the contents of the sac. After the hernial sac, including the constricting neck, has been isolated, the peritoneal cavity is opened in order to evaluate the contents of the sac more accurately **(Figure 14).** If abdominal exploration demonstrates the probability of strangulated bowel within the sac, the decision must be made whether to open the sac to determine the viability of the bowel or to divide the bowel proximal to the neck of the sac **(Figure 15).** If the duration of the acute strangulation combined with clinical and laboratory examination makes gangrenous bowel almost a certainty, it is desirable to divide the viable bowel as it enters the sac. The sac is then resected *en masse* proximal to the neck to avoid releasing any material from the contaminated sac **(Figure 16).** A direct end-to-end or lateral anastomosis of the bowel is carried out, followed by subsequent repair of the hernia.

In cases of strangulation of short duration the viability of the reduced bowel may be questionable, making it better judgment to divide the neck of the hernial sac after the field has been thoroughly walled off by warm, moist gauze sponges. It is advisable, therefore, to observe the bowel for a time after it has been released from the constriction of the neck of the hernial sac **(Figure 17).** The involved bowel should be wrapped in warm, moist gauze sponges. When viability is questionable, a local anesthetic agent may be injected into the mesentery to overcome arterial spasm. The presence of bloody fluid in the hernial sac, gangrenous odor, gangrenous appearance of the bowel, lack of arterial pulsations, absence of glossy sheen, and the failure of peristaltic waves to pass over the discolored area when the intestine is stimulated are all concrete evidence that the involved area should be resected. In some instances a small knuckle (Richter's hernia) of the convex portion of the involved loop is constricted within the femoral ring, and localized gangrene develops **(Figure 18).** Small areas of this type must be repaired by inversion with a purse-string suture unless this results in obstruction of the bowel; then segmental resection is required.

The sac is completely excised, and the opening in the peritoneal cavity is closed with interrupted mattress sutures **(Figures 18** and **19).** The Z-division of Poupart's ligament is repaired with interrupted sutures of fine silk **(Figure 20).**

CLOSURE. There are several methods of preventing recurrence of the hernia. The transversalis fascia and the aponeurotic margin of the transverse abdominal muscle may be approximated from the spine of the pubis upward along Cooper's ligament, as in the repair of a direct inguinal hernia (Plate CLXVII). It is essential to have an adequate exposure of the iliac vessels so that they are not accidentally injured when these interrupted sutures **(Figures 21** and **22)** are placed. After this procedure has been completed, several sutures are taken in Cooper's ligament and to the inferior margin of Poupart's ligament in order to close the femoral canal **(Figure 23).** The iliac vessels should not be constricted. The round ligament in the female or the cord in the male is returned to normal position or transplanted as in other types of hernia repair. A second layer of sutures may be placed between the aponeurosis of the transverse abdominal muscle and Poupart's ligament **(Figure 24).** The external oblique is closed without constriction about the cord or round ligament, followed by the usual approximation of the subcutaneous tissue and skin.

POSTOPERATIVE CARE. It is wise to keep the thigh slightly flexed during the immediate postoperative period. The patient is permitted out of bed within 24 hours after operation. Constant gastric suction is maintained for several days if resection of the intestine was required. Antibiotics, electrolytes, plasma, and whole blood are essential in the more complicated cases associated with intestinal obstruction and frequently are of greater importance than the technical steps of the repair. Heavy manual labor, especially that which greatly increases the intra-abdominal tension, must be avoided for at least six to eight weeks.

PLATE CLXIX   REPAIR OF FEMORAL HERNIA

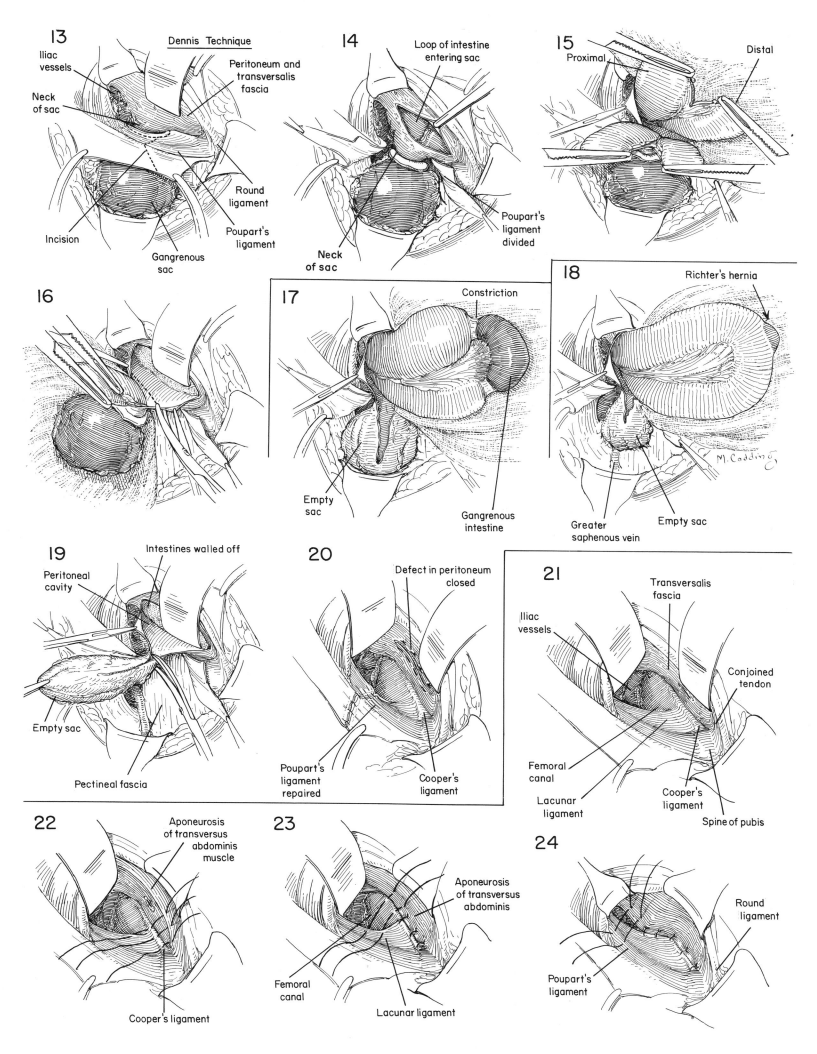

13 Dennis Technique
Iliac vessels
Neck of sac
Incision
Gangrenous sac
Peritoneum and transversalis fascia
Round ligament
Poupart's ligament

14 Loop of intestine entering sac
Neck of sac
Poupart's ligament divided

15 Proximal
Distal

16

17 Constriction
Empty sac
Gangrenous intestine

18 Richter's hernia
Greater saphenous vein
Empty sac
M. Codding

19 Intestines walled off
Peritoneal cavity
Empty sac
Pectineal fascia

20 Defect in peritoneum closed
Poupart's ligament repaired
Cooper's ligament

21 Transversalis fascia
Iliac vessels
Conjoined tendon
Femoral canal
Lacunar ligament
Cooper's ligament
Spine of pubis

22 Aponeurosis of transversus abdominis muscle
Cooper's ligament

23 Aponeurosis of transversus abdominis
Femoral canal
Lacunar ligament

24 Round ligament
Poupart's ligament

PLATE CLXX · HYDROCELE REPAIR

INDICATIONS. A hydrocele of the tunica vaginalis occurring within the first year of life seldom requires operation, since it will often disappear without treatment. Hydroceles that persist after the first year, or that appear later in life, usually require treatment, since they show little tendency toward spontaneous regression. All symptomatic hydroceles in adults or in children older than two years should be removed. Most hydroceles are painless, and symptoms arise only from the inconvenience caused by their size or weight. The long-continued presence of a hydrocele infrequently causes atrophy of the testicle. Open operation is the method of choice for removing the hydrocele. Aspiration of the hydrocele contents and injection with sclerosing agents are generally regarded as unsatisfactory treatment because of the high incidence of recurrences and the frequent necessity for repetition of the procedure. Occasionally, severe infection can be introduced by aspiration. Simple aspiration, however, may often be used as a temporary measure in those cases where surgery is contraindicated or must be postponed.

The accuracy of the diagnosis must be ascertained. Great care must be taken to differentiate a hydrocele from a scrotal hernia or tumor of the testicle. A hernia usually can be reduced, transmits a cough impulse, and is not translucent. A hydrocele cannot be reduced into the inguinal canal and gives no impulse on coughing unless a hernia is also present. In young children a hydrocele is often associated with a complete congenital type of hernial sac.

ANESTHESIA. Either spinal or general anesthesia is satisfactory in adults. General anesthesia is the choice in children. Local infiltration anesthesia is generally unsatisfactory because it fails to abolish abdominal pain produced by traction on the spermatic cord.

POSITION. The patient is placed on his back on a level table with his legs slightly separated. The surgeon stands on the side of the table nearest the operative site.

OPERATIVE PREPARATION. The skin is prepared routinely, with particular care given to scrubbing the scrotal area. Iodine should be avoided for preparation of the scrotal skin, since it will cause severe excoriation. The area is draped as for any other operation on the scrotum.

INCISION AND EXPOSURE. The relationship of the hydrocele of the tunica vaginalis testis to the testicle, epididymis, spermatic cord, and covering layers of the scrotum is shown in **Figure 1**. With the mass grasped firmly in one hand so as to stretch the scrotal skin and to fix the hydrocele, an incision 6 to 10 cm. long is made on the anterior surface of the scrotum, over the most prominent part of the hydrocele, well away from the testicle which lies inferiorly and posteriorly **(Figure 2)**. The skin, dartos muscle, and thin cremasteric fascia are incised and reflected back together as a single layer from the underlying parietal layer of the tunica vaginalis, which is the outer wall of the hydrocele **(Figures 3 and 4)**. If the hydrocele is associated with an inguinal hernia, the classic hernia incision should be made and extended downward to the scrotum if necessary. Usually, the hydrocele can be easily delivered up out of the scrotum into the wound.

DETAILS OF PROCEDURE. When the hydrocele is well separated laterally and medially from the overlying layers, its wall is grasped with two Allis forceps, and a trocar attached to a suction tube is thrust into it to evacuate the fluid **(Figure 5)**. With a finger in the opening of the sac acting as a guide and providing traction, the surgeon completely separates the wall of the hydrocele from the scrotum so that the spermatic cord and testicle with attached hydrocele sac lie entirely free in the operative field **(Figures 6, 7,** and **8)**. The hydrocele sac is then opened completely **(Figure 9)**. Some surgeons prefer to delay emptying the hydrocele until it has been dissected completely free from the surrounding tissues and delivered outside the scrotum.

In younger men particularly the testicle is carefully inspected and palpated, since hydrocele has been known to occur in the presence of testicular neoplasm.

The relationship of the testicle to the tunica vaginalis is shown in **Figure 10**. With the walls of the hydrocele sac completely freed and completely opened, the redundant sac wall is trimmed with scissors, leaving only a margin of about 2 cm. around the testicle, epididymis, and spermatic cord **(Figure 10, A and B)**. Great care must be taken to obtain absolute hemostasis, since the smallest bleeding point left uncontrolled is apt to ooze slowly into the loose scrotal tissues, producing a massive scrotal hematoma. Some of the largest, most painful, and most slowly absorbed postoperative hematomata have occurred following this procedure because of lack of complete hemostasis.

When the redundant portions of the sac have been excised, the edges are sewed behind the testicle and spermatic cord with interrupted fine silk or fine catgut, thus everting the retained portion of the old hydrocele sac **(Figures 11 and 12)**. Some surgeons prefer not to evert the sac but to place either interrupted or continuous fine catgut hemostatic sutures along its margin. In children, especially, the contents of the upper portion of the cord should be inspected for a possible hernial sac.

CLOSURE. The testicle and spermatic cord are carefully replaced in the scrotum, care being taken that no abnormal rotation of the cord has occurred. The testicle is anchored to the bottom of the wall of the scrotum with one or two chromic catgut or silk sutures to prevent torsion of the cord **(Figure 13)**. The dartos fascia is closed with interrupted fine silk or plain catgut sutures **(Figure 14)**. A small Penrose drain is always brought out through a small stab wound at the most dependent portion of the scrotum. This allows escape of blood and prevents hematomata. The skin is closed with interrupted fine silk or plain catgut sutures.

POSTOPERATIVE CARE. The scrotum should be supported by a suspensory for one to two weeks postoperatively. Ice bags should be placed under the scrotum for the first 24 hours. The dressing should be changed daily. The drain is removed in 24 to 48 hours, depending on the amount of drainage. Silk skin sutures should be removed on the seventh postoperative day. Plain catgut skin sutures will fall out as they disintegrate. The patient may be out of bed on the day of the operation. Fluid and electrolyte balance is carefully maintained.

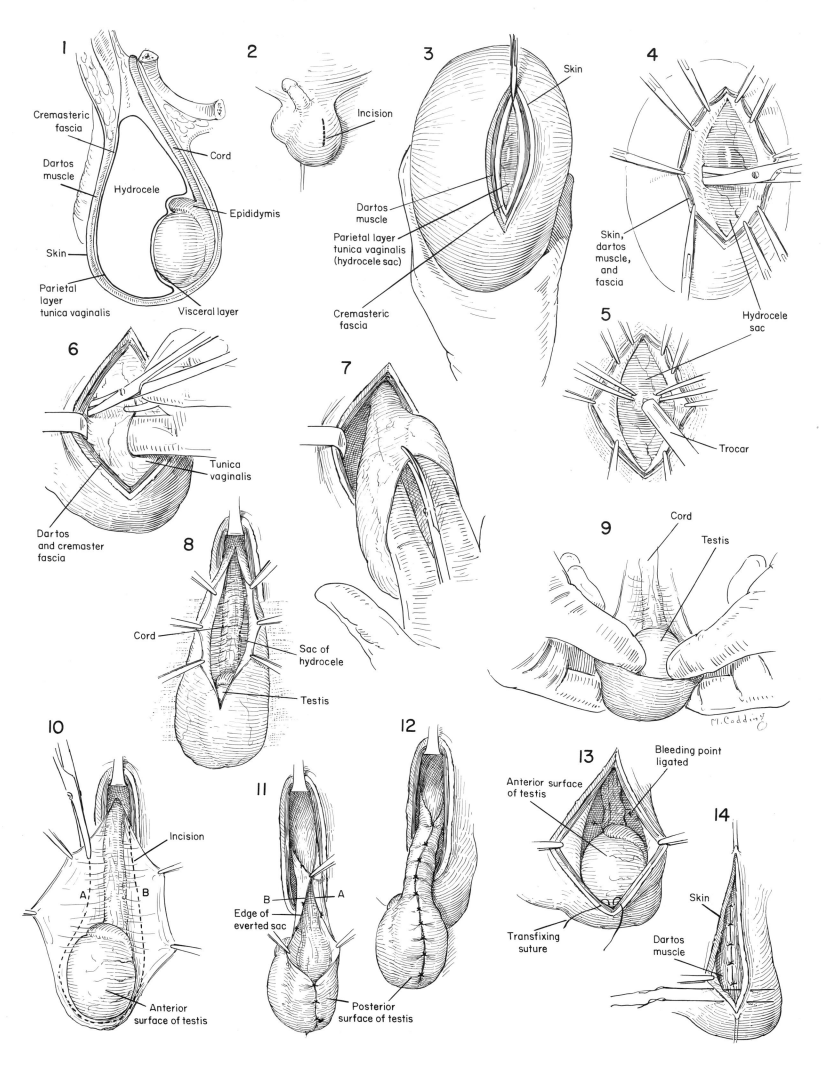

1
Cremasteric fascia
Dartos muscle
Hydrocele
Skin
Parietal layer tunica vaginalis
Cord
Epididymis
Visceral layer

2
Incision

3
Skin
Dartos muscle
Parietal layer tunica vaginalis (hydrocele sac)
Cremasteric fascia

4
Skin, dartos muscle, and fascia
Hydrocele sac

5
Trocar

6
Tunica vaginalis
Dartos and cremaster fascia

7

8
Cord
Sac of hydrocele
Testis

9
Cord
Testis

M. Codding

10
Incision
A   B
Anterior surface of testis

11
B   A
Edge of everted sac
Posterior surface of testis

12

13
Bleeding point ligated
Anterior surface of testis
Transfixing suture

14
Skin
Dartos muscle

PLATE CLXXI · RECTAL PROLAPSE, PERINEAL REPAIR

INDICATIONS. Operative correction of complete rectal prolapse in children is rarely indicated. However, in adults (especially in older groups) effective operative repair is worth while. Rectal prolapse is relatively commonly found to be associated with or related to neurologic and psychiatric disorders as well as degenerative arteriosclerotic diseases. True prolapse of the rectum involves a herniation of the pouch of Douglas through the dilated and incompetent sphincter muscles. To correct this defect, the hernial pouch must be eliminated and the weakened pelvic floor strengthened. Obliteration of the pouch of Douglas and fixation of the rectum can be accomplished by either the perineal, abdominal, or combined approach.

PREOPERATIVE PREPARATION. The patient is hospitalized five to seven days before operation. A barium enema and sigmoidoscopic examination are essential. The use of a low-residue diet, cathartics, and enemas is necessary to obtain a clean and empty large bowel. The prolapse is reduced and reduction sustained by the application of a T-binder to minimize the associated edema and encourage the healing of any superficial ulcerations. Systemic antibiotic therapy is started shortly before the operation and continued three or more days.

ANESTHESIA. General or spinal anesthesia is satisfactory.

POSITION. The patient is placed in a lithotomy position with the legs widely separated. The table is in a slight Trendelenburg position to decrease the venous ooze and enhance the anatomic dissection.

OPERATIVE PREPARATION. The prolapse is reduced and the rectum irrigated with sterile saline. The skin about the perineum is cleansed in a routine manner. The area may be dried and a plastic drape used if desired. The bladder is catheterized, and the catheter left in place.

INCISION AND EXPOSURE. The prolapse tends to present without difficulty **(Figure 1)**, and Babcock or Allis forceps are applied for traction purposes to determine the extent of the prolapse. The relationship of the prolapse to the pouch of Douglas and the sphincter muscles of the anus is shown in **Figure 2.** The protruding mass is palpated to make certain the small intestine is not entrapped in the hernia sac anteriorly. Sutures of 000 chromic catgut are placed in the midline **(Figure 3, A)** anteriorly, posteriorly, and at the halfway point on either side **(Figure 3, B and B₁)** near the anal margin, not only to serve as a retractor but for subsequent landmarks at the completion of the procedure. The identification of the pectinate line is important, since the incision through the presenting rectal mucosa will be made 3 mm. proximal to this anatomic landmark. This minimal amount of mucosa is adequate for the final anastomosis and is short enough to prevent postoperative protrusion. A sharp knife or an electric knife can be used **(Figure 3)**. This area tends to be quite vascular, and meticulous hemostasis by electrocoagulation or individual ligation is essential **(Figure 4)**. The incision through the outer sleeve should divide the full thickness of bowel wall, including mucosa as well as the muscularis. The pouch of Douglas is not entered. The dissection is facilitated if the surgeon inserts his index finger in a developed cleavage plane between the two layers of prolapsed bowel wall **(Figure 5)**.

PLATE CLXXI   RECTAL PROLAPSE, PERINEAL REPAIR

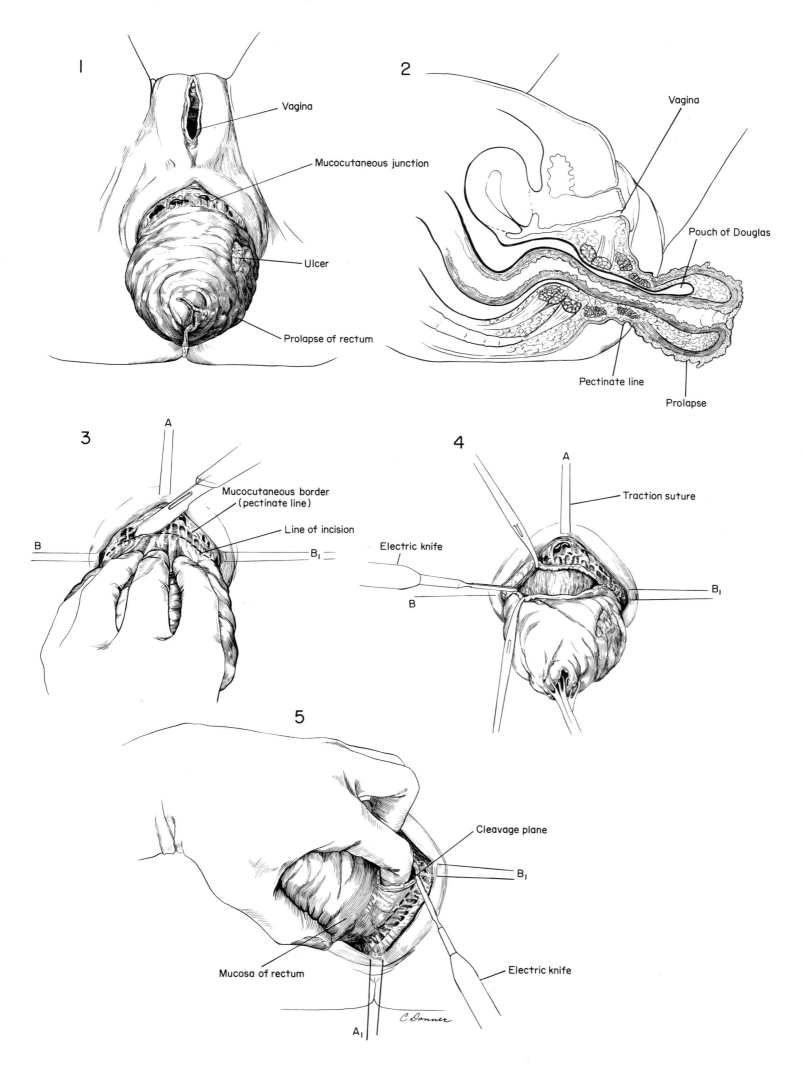

1

Vagina

Mucocutaneous junction

Ulcer

Prolapse of rectum

2

Vagina

Pouch of Douglas

Pectinate line

Prolapse

3

A

Mucocutaneous border
(pectinate line)

Line of incision

B

B₁

4

A

Traction suture

Electric knife

B

B₁

5

Cleavage plane

B₁

Mucosa of rectum

Electric knife

A₁

C Donner

PLATE CLXXII · RECTAL PROLAPSE, PERINEAL REPAIR

DETAILS OF PROCEDURE. After the mucosa and muscularis of the protruding segment have been completely divided, traction is maintained downward on the cuff of incised mucosa and muscularis **(Figure 6).** Any attachments between the bowel wall and the underlying segment are divided with the electrocoagulant unit or sharp knife, and all bleeding points are controlled. This cuff is easily pulled off and results in a segment twice as long as the original protrusion **(Figure 7).** The bowel wall is not amputated at this time, but downward traction is maintained as an attempt is made to identify the prolapsed pouch of Douglas **(Figure 7).** The resection may be started in the midline anteriorly and continued upward through the fat until the glistening wall of the peritoneum is identified. The peritoneum is gently opened **(Figure 8),** and the pouch of Douglas is explored with the examining finger. Any attachments between the small bowel or adnexa in the female should be separated to ensure freeing of as much of the pouch of Douglas as possible and to permit mobilization of the redundant rectosigmoid into the wound.

After the peritoneum is opened, the presenting intestine lying on the posterior side of the sliding hernia is grasped with forceps to determine how much mobile large intestine will require amputation to correct the tendency toward recurrent prolapse. The peritoneal opening should be extended laterally to either side. The blood supply, surrounded by a thick layer of fatty tissue, is usually identified posteriorly and on the right side of the presenting intestines **(Figure 9).** Half-length forceps and the surgeon's index finger are used as blunt dissectors until the mesentery to this

segment of the bowel has been separated without injuring the bowel wall itself. At least three half-length clamps are applied to ensure a safe double ligation with 0 chromic catgut **(Figure 10).** The most proximal one of these sutures should be of the transfixing type, since the tissues are under some tension, and bleeding may develop unless the contents of these clamps are securely tied. No effort should be made to strip the bowel from the mesentery; however, it may be necessary to reapply clamps from either side, as well as in the midline posteriorly, until all the redundant large intestine has been pulled freely into the wound.

After the blood supply has been ligated and as much of the intestines as necessary mobilized into the wound, the pouch of Douglas can be closed in several ways. If the opening is rather large and the prolapse has included a segment of the large intestine well above the base of the pouch of Douglas, an inverted T-type closure of the peritoneum can be carried out **(Figure 11).** The peritoneum is closed in the midline anteriorly with interrupted or continuous 00 chromic surgical catgut.

The closure approximates the peritoneum around the bowel wall, and the continuous suture is tied. A suture starting at this point, including a bite of the peritoneum as well as of the bowel wall, continues around to the right side until it is anchored in the region of the ligated mesentery blood supply **(Figure 11).** The attachment of the peritoneum is made secure in a similar manner on the left side. This accounts for the so-called inverted T closure of the peritoneum.

PLATE CLXXII   RECTAL PROLAPSE, PERINEAL REPAIR

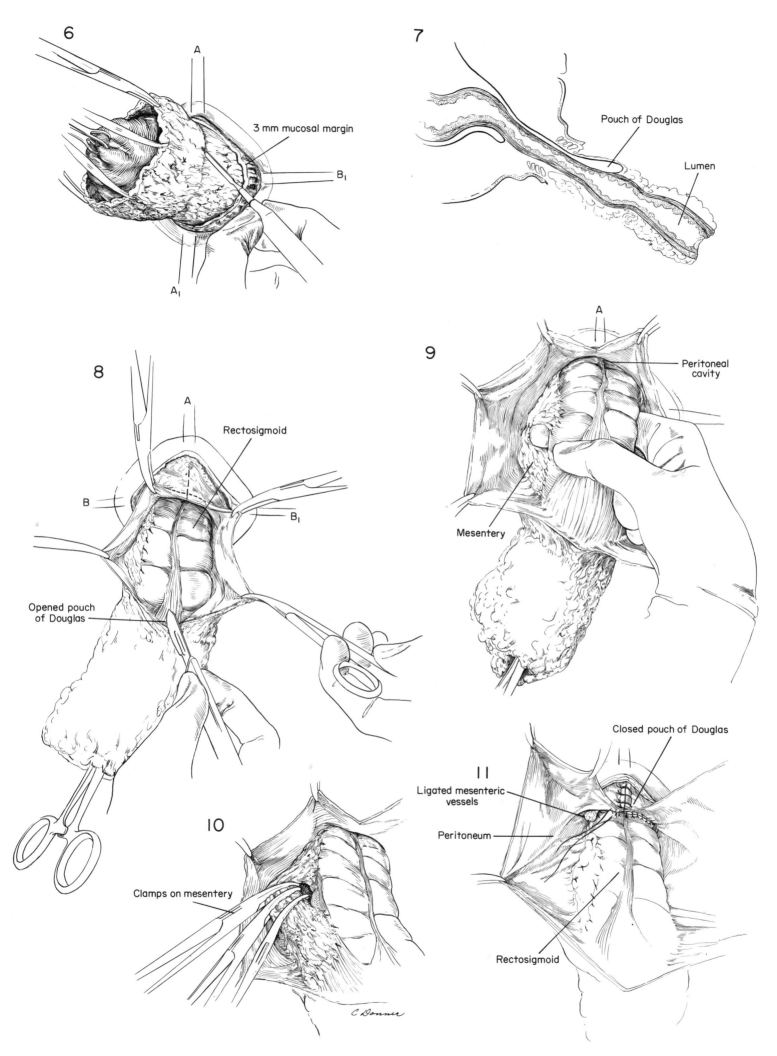

6

A

3 mm mucosal margin

B₁

A₁

7

Pouch of Douglas

Lumen

8

A

Rectosigmoid

B

B₁

Opened pouch
of Douglas

9

A

Peritoneal
cavity

Mesentery

10

Clamps on mesentery

11

Closed pouch of Douglas

Ligated mesenteric
vessels

Peritoneum

Rectosigmoid

C. Donner

PLATE CLXXIII · RECTAL PROLAPSE, PERINEAL REPAIR

DETAILS OF PROCEDURE (*Continued*). In some instances, especially when the prolapse is not particularly marked, the pouch of Douglas may be developed from the anterior rectal wall similar to a direct hernial sac **(Figure 12).** The peritoneum is then carefully incised and the margins held apart by traction with two or three forceps **(Figure 13).** The surgeon's index finger should be inserted to ascertain that the pouch of Douglas is free from attachments to either the small bowel or the adnexa in the female. It may be necessary to enlarge such an opening and insert a small retractor to accomplish this with good visualization. The pouch of Douglas should be closed as high as possible with a purse-string suture of 00 chromic catgut **(Figure 14).** Considerable time may be required to make certain that the pouch of Douglas has been obliterated as high as possible. If the obliteration cannot be done satisfactorily, it may be judicious to obliterate the pouch of Douglas by a transabdominal approach as part of a plan for a second-stage or a two-stage procedure. After the peritoneum has been closed, the redundant peritoneum is amputated, and additional sutures are taken to control bleeding and reinforce the pouch of Douglas **(Figure 15).**

The next step involves identification of the levator muscles, since the reinforcement of the pelvic floor is essential to prevent recurrence. The procedure to be followed is not unlike the approximation of the levator muscles in the performance of a posterior perineorrhaphy (Plates LIV and LV). A small narrow retractor can be inserted anteriorly as the surgeon inserts the index and middle fingers of his left hand to better define the levator ani muscles on the left side. An Allis or Babcock clamp grasps the levator muscles to better define their margins, and a deep suture of 00 chromic catgut is inserted **(Figure 16).** The first suture can be applied at either the top or the bottom of the proposed closure, depending on which is easier. In **Figure 17** the first suture shown is placed in the bottom of the approximation, and a right-angle clamp depresses the bowel wall to provide a snug approximation by the levators. An additional three or four sutures are required to approximate the levators further up in the midline **(Figure 18).**

Only after the levators are approximated should the prolapsed bowel be prepared for amputation. It is essential that the normal anatomic position of the bowel be retained. For this reason it has been found judicious to split the anterior as well as the posterior wall of the prolapsed large

intestine almost up to the region where the bowel will be divided. This should be done carefully so that sufficient bowel is available for approximation to the pectinate line, yet a sufficient amount is removed to prevent recurrence **(Figure 18).** After the bowel has been divided, the surgeon should insert his finger into the lumen of the bowel to again check snugness of the approximation of the levator muscles. Enough room should be available to admit the index and middle fingers easily. If the approximation of the levators seems to be too snug and the blood supply to the bowel compromised, one of the sutures may be removed; or if too large, an additional approximation of the levators should be considered.

Before the bowel wall is divided up as high as eventually required, the midline anteriorly should be tested for length. The bowel wall is divided up to a point where a retraction suture can be placed in the midline approximating the mucosa with the pectinate line without tension **(Figure 19).** A quadrant of the mucosa is then divided, and the mucosa is approximated to the pectinate line with either the continuous lock suture of 00 chromic catgut or interrupted 00 chromic sutures. The mucosa can be more accurately approximated if a planned quadrant anatomic fixation is carried out as shown in **Figures 19** and **20.** The importance of the traction sutures in the midline and at the halfway point on either side readily becomes apparent as the satisfactory approximation of the mucosa to the pectinate line is finally accomplished **(Figure 20).** There should be an easy approximation of the mucosa to the pectinate line, and it should have a nice pink color. The sutures should not be tied so tight as to produce bleaching of the mucosa. After completion of the procedure the surgeon should introduce his well-lubricated finger carefully through the anastomosis to make certain of its patency as well as its adequacy **(Figure 21).** No drainage is indicated.

POSTOPERATIVE CARE. Antibiotic therapy should be considered for at least three or more days. Fluid balance is maintained by intravenous administration of water, glucose, and electrolytes. A liquid diet is gradually progressed to a low-residue diet. Mineral oil in doses of one ounce two times per day is given. Digital examination is delayed unless undue distress develops about the site of operation. The possibility of development of a perirectal abscess, which may require incision and drainage, is an ever-present threat.

PLATE CLXXIII   RECTAL PROLAPSE, PERINEAL REPAIR

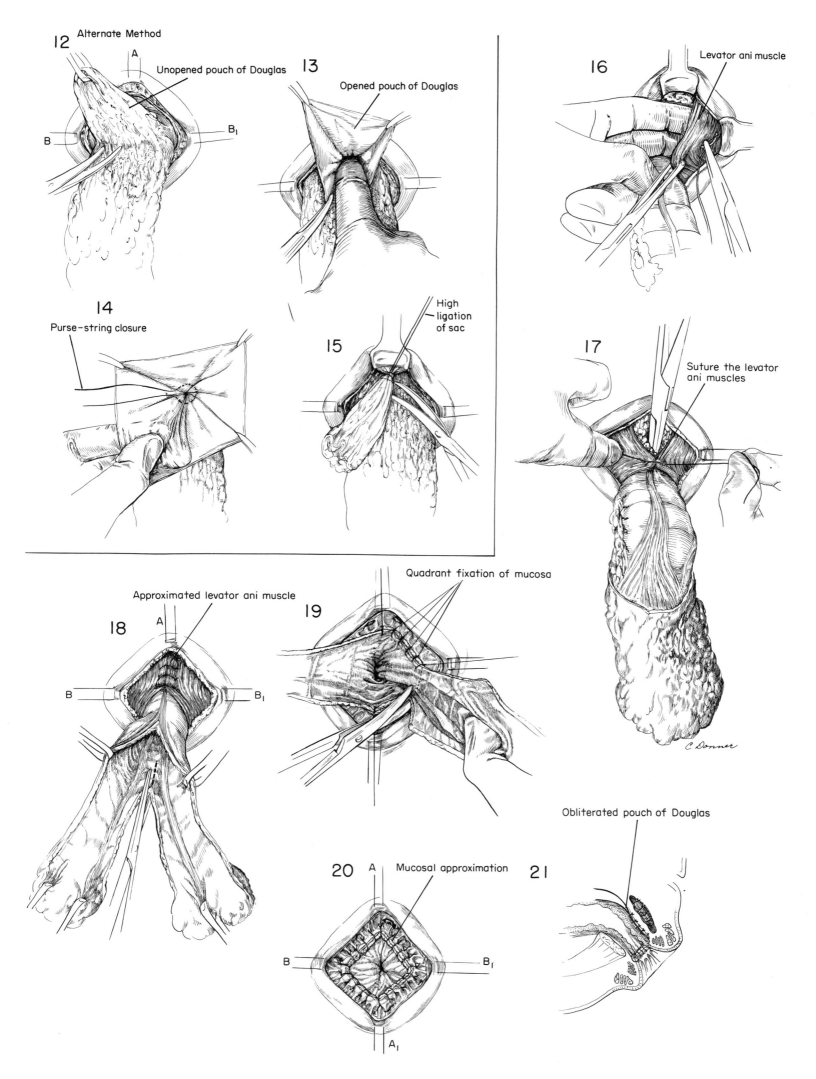

12 Alternate Method

A

Unopened pouch of Douglas

B

B₁

13 Opened pouch of Douglas

14 Purse-string closure

15 High ligation of sac

16 Levator ani muscle

17 Suture the levator ani muscles

C Donner

18 Approximated levator ani muscle

A

B

B₁

19 Quadrant fixation of mucosa

20 A

Mucosal approximation

B

B₁

A₁

21 Obliterated pouch of Douglas

PLATE CLXXIV · INJECTION AND EXCISION OF HEMORRHOIDS

A. Injection of Hemorrhoids

INDICATIONS. The injection of hemorrhoids is a palliative procedure. The patient is ambulatory. It may be used for the bleeding internal hemorrhoid that does not prolapse. It is not applicable to external hemorrhoids. Contraindications to the injection of the internal hemorrhoid are reactive inflammation or thrombosis, acute fissure, fistula or perianal abscess, severe cryptitis or papillitis, and an advanced degree of prolapse. The anatomy of internal and external hemorrhoids is shown in **Figure 1**. A sigmoidoscopic examination to rule out polyps and malignancy is mandatory before injection. A barium enema is also advisable.

PREOPERATIVE PREPARATION. No preoperative preparation is necessary other than a disposable commercial enema self-administered by the patient.

ANESTHESIA. No anesthesia is necessary. The procedure should be entirely painless. If pain is experienced, it indicates that the injection has been made too superficially or too close to the pectinate line. The injection is promptly discontinued.

POSITION. The patient is placed on the left side with the hips flexed and the right leg drawn up more than the left, or in a knee-chest position.

DETAILS OF PROCEDURE. An anoscope is inserted. The sclerosing solution is injected above the hemorrhoid about 3 mm. below the mucosa **(Figure 2)**. Slight distention of the mucosa will result, but it should not blanch. One to 2 ml. of solution are usually sufficient for one hemorrhoid. No more than three sites are injected at a single operation.

POSTOPERATIVE CARE. No postoperative care is necessary. If the patient complains of pain or discomfort, he is told to return promptly. Injections are usually repeated at intervals of about one week until all sites are injected. Keeping a chart of the exact site of each injection ensures that all quadrants receive one injection.

B. Excision of Hemorrhoids

INDICATIONS. Hemorrhoidectomy is usually an elective procedure performed in good-risk patients with persistent symptoms referable to proven hemorrhoids. Bleeding, protrusion, pain, pruritis, and infection are the more common indications when palliative medical measures have failed. Large external skin tags may require removal because of local pruritis. In the female a pelvic examination is made to eliminate tumor or pregnancy as the etiology. In the male the status of the prostate gland must be thoroughly evaluated. In all patients a thorough sigmoidoscopy and a barium enema are mandatory. The presence of a serious systemic disease, such as cirrhosis of the liver, or a probable short life expectancy from advanced age or any other cause should be a general contraindication to operation unless anal symptoms are marked.

PREOPERATIVE PREPARATION. No cathartic is given before operation. A thorough cleansing enema is given the night before or early the morning of operation, preferably several hours before operation, since residual enema fluid is more disturbing than the presence of a small amount of dry fecal material.

ANESTHESIA. Spinal, sacral, or local anesthesia is satisfactory. If an inhalation anesthesia is given, it should be remembered that dilatation of the anus stimulates the respiratory centers. Spinal anesthesia must be used with caution, because it may so completely relax the anal sphincter that it cannot be properly identified by palpation.

POSITION. The positioning of the patient depends on the type of anesthesia used. With spinal anesthesia the prone jack-knife position affords the surgeon the best exposure. If general anesthesia is used, an exaggerated dorsal lithotomy position is preferred with the buttocks extending beyond the edge of the table and the legs held in stirrups.

OPERATIVE PREPARATION. Dilatation of the anus before hemorrhoidectomy is undesirable because it distorts the anatomy, making it impossible to remove all hemorrhoids at one operation without fear of

stenosis. Gentle dilatation may be used if no more than three hemorrhoids are removed at one time.

DETAILS OF PROCEDURE. Anoscopy is done, and any associated pathology is identified so that hypertrophied papillae or deep crypts may be removed.

The anal canal may be gently dilated to about two fingers' width to permit adequate exposure. A suitable self-retaining retractor is inserted into the canal, and further inspection is made. A gauze sponge is introduced into the rectum, and the retractor is withdrawn **(Figure 3)**. The surgeon makes gentle traction on the sponge, reproducing, in effect, the passage of a bolus through the canal. As the sponge is withdrawn, the prolapsing hemorrhoids may be identified and are picked up with hemorrhoid clamps **(Figure 4)**. Clamps are placed on all the prolapsing hemorrhoids and left in place as markers during the operation. Opposite the hemorrhoid a straight hemostatic forceps is placed on the anal verge, which is the external boundary of the anal canal. The hemorrhoid is placed under tension by simultaneous traction on the forceps and the hemorrhoid clamp **(Figure 5)**. A triangular incision is made from the anal verge to the pectinate line **(Figure 6)**. By traction on the two clamps and careful blunt and sharp dissection with the scalpel, it is possible to dissect off the triangular area of skin and the hemorrhoidal tissue from the outer edge of the external sphincter muscle. Many small, fibrous bands will be found running upward into the hemorrhoidal mass. These represent the continuation downward of the longitudinal muscle and may be divided with impunity **(Figure 7)**. Dissection is carried to the outer edge of the external sphincter. The anal skin must be divided to and slightly beyond the pectinate line. There now remain mucosa and the deep veins entering the hemorrhoidal mass. The tissue is secured with a straight clamp and a transfixing suture placed at the apex of the hemorrhoidal mass **(Figure 8)**. The hemorrhoidal tissue is removed with a knife, and an over-and-over continuous suture is made in the mucosa **(Figure 9)**. The clamp is removed, and a continuous suture approximates the mucosa, including the two edges of the pectinate line. As the suture is continued externally, small bites are taken in the external sphincter muscle **(Figure 10)**. The deep portion of the skin is closed by a subcutaneous approximation **(Figure 11)**, and the skin edges are left open to provide for better drainage and to prevent postoperative edema **(Figure 12)**.

Each hemorrhoidal mass is similarly removed. All possible mucosal tissue must be preserved to prevent stenosis. However, relatively large areas of skin may be safely removed in the triangular incision.

With extensive hemorrhoids it may be necessary to excise one-half of the mucosa of the entire canal in this fashion. The triangular incision may extend from the anal verge and reach the pectinate anteriorly and posteriorly. The mucosa is divided horizontally, taking small bites of tissue in a series of hemostats **(Figure 13)**. This mucosal flap is sutured into the external sphincter horizontally to prevent stenosis **(Figure 14)**. All redundant incisional skin margins should be excised to minimize the subsequent development of potentially damaging perianal skin tabs.

POSTOPERATIVE CARE. A sterile protective dressing is applied to the anus. Petrolatum may be applied locally. The diet is restricted for the first two or three days, but by the third day the patient may be allowed a full diet. Mineral oil (30 ml.) is given nightly as soon as postoperative nausea has ceased. The patient is encouraged to have a bowel movement, and usually he will do so by the third day. Local application of heat is useful in alleviating discomfort. The patient may take sitz baths as desired. A daily rectal examination is performed. An anesthetic ointment is applied preliminary to the examination. Weekly anal dilatation is continued postoperatively until healing is complete.

C. Treatment of Thrombosed Hemorrhoids

Thrombosed external hemorrhoids may be removed in the patient who is ambulatory. The anus is cleansed, and anesthesia is administered by injection of 2 or 3 ml. procaine hydrochloride over the surface and just beneath the thrombosed hemorrhoids. An elliptical incision is made over the thrombosed area, and the clot is removed by finger compression or by introduction of a small curette **(Figures 15 and 16)**. This excision leaves no redundant scar tissue, and final healing occurs without tab formation. Gentle dissection of the clot causes no bleeding, and it should not be necessary to suture the wound. Rarely, a suture of fine catgut may be necessary. The patient may return home immediately.

PLATE CLXXIV   INJECTION AND EXCISION OF HEMORRHOIDS

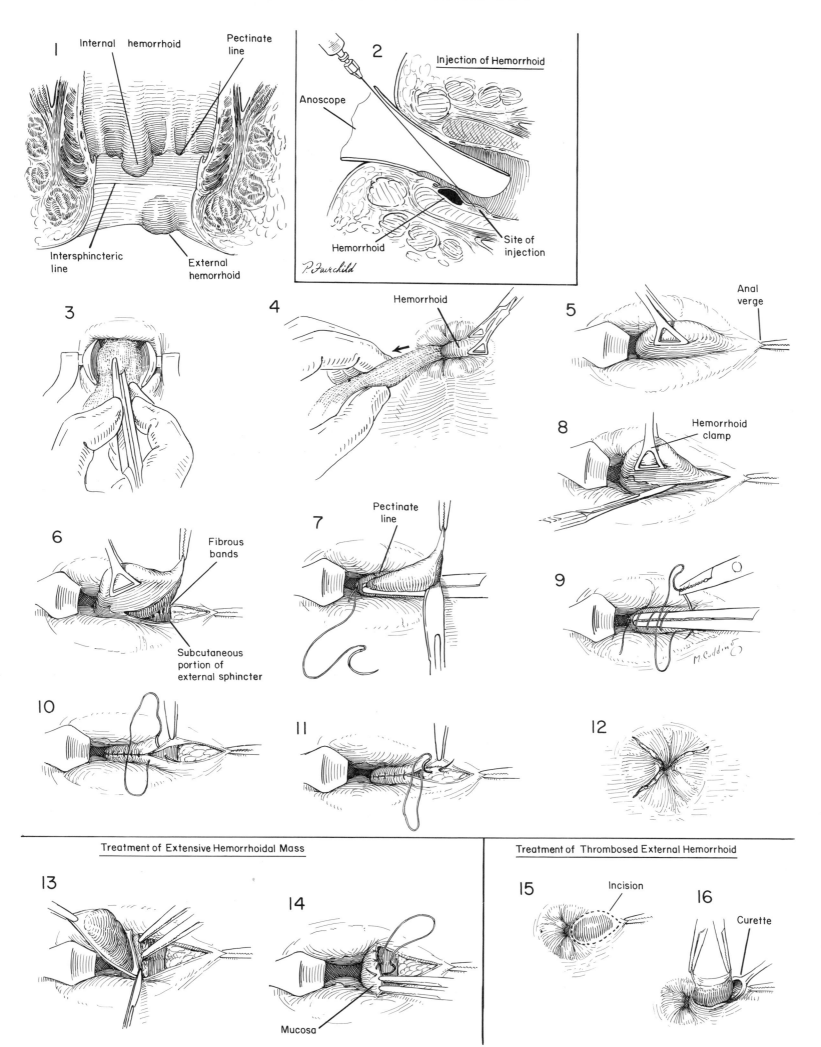

1 Internal hemorrhoid · Pectinate line · Intersphincteric line · External hemorrhoid

2 Injection of Hemorrhoid · Anoscope · Hemorrhoid · Site of injection · P. Fairchild

4 Hemorrhoid

5 Anal verge

6 Fibrous bands · Subcutaneous portion of external sphincter

7 Pectinate line

8 Hemorrhoid clamp

9 M. Codding

Treatment of Extensive Hemorrhoidal Mass

13

14 Mucosa

Treatment of Thrombosed External Hemorrhoid

15 Incision

16 Curette

PLATE CLXXV · DRAINAGE OF ISCHIORECTAL ABSCESS—EXCISION OF FISTULA IN ANO

A. Drainage of Ischiorectal Abscess

INDICATIONS. Ischiorectal abscesses are drained immediately. Careful palpation often shows evidence of fluctuation not seen in the perianal tissue. Operation is not delayed until fluctuation is obvious, because a perirectal abscess may rupture through the levator muscle into the retroperitoneal tissue.

PREOPERATIVE PREPARATION. No special preoperative preparation is required. Antibiotic therapy may be given.

ANESTHESIA. General anesthesia with endotracheal intubation may be used; however, regional anesthesia, either spinal or caudal, is satisfactory.

POSITION. The lithotomy position is preferred for drainage.

INCISION AND EXPOSURE. The common locations of ischiorectal abscesses are shown in **Figure 1.** Abscesses may be located extraperitoneally above the levator ani muscle. Careful rectal and sigmoidoscopic examination should be performed to detect associated pathologic processes after the patient has been anesthetized. An incision is made at the maximum point of tenderness **(Figure 1)** and placed either parallel or radial to the anus. If the abscess lies above the levator, the incision is deepened radially to avoid nerves and blood vessels.

DETAILS OF PROCEDURE. After incision and drainage, the cavity is explored with the index finger to ensure complete drainage and to ascertain that no foreign body is in the ischiorectal space. A specimen of the draining material is obtained for bacteriologic studies. Usually, there is no communication with the rectum. If the abscess is small, and a clear communication with the rectum is identified, the tract may be excised. The outer opening must be sufficiently large, for the common error is to drain a large cavity through a comparatively small incision, resulting in the development of a chronic abscess.

CLOSURE. The cavity is lightly packed with gauze in petrolatum.

POSTOPERATIVE CARE. Moist compresses and sitz baths reduce inflammation and promote rapid healing. Postoperative dressings to assure healing from the bottom are as important as the operation. An ischiorectal abscess is prone to result in an anal fistula; however, in about half of the cases, there will be primary healing with proper postoperative care.

B. Excision of Fistula in Ano

INDICATIONS. The majority of anal fistulae result from infection arising in a crypt, extending into the perianal musculature, and then rupturing either into the ischiorectal fossa or superficial perirectal tissues. Operative obliteration of the fistula is always indicated if the patient's general condition is good.

ANATOMIC CONSIDERATIONS. Treatment of anal fistulae presupposes a knowledge of anal anatomy, particularly of the sphincter muscles and their relation to the anal crypts. A study of **Figures 2, 3, 4,** and **5** will clarify several important points. As shown in **Figure 2,** the external sphincter muscle can be divided into three portions—the subcutaneous, superficial, and deep portions. The subcutaneous portion lies just beneath the skin and below the lower edge of the internal sphincter **(Figure 2, 1).** The superficial and deep portions surround the deeper part of the internal sphincter and continue upward to join with the levator muscle **(Figure 2, 2 and 3).** The levator ani surrounds the anal canal laterally and posteriorly, but it is absent anteriorly **(Figure 2, 5).** The longitudinal muscle of the anus is the continuation downward of the longitudinal muscle of the large bowel **(Figure 2, 6).** The internal sphincter muscle is a bulbous thickening of the circular muscle coat of the large bowel. The superficial external sphincter is palpated as a band surrounding the anal canal just beneath the skin **(Figure 2, 2).** Just above it is felt a slight depression, the intersphincteric line, and the slight swelling above this point is the lower edge of the internal sphincter **(Figure 2, 4).** If the finger is introduced into the canal and hooked around the entire anorectal ring anteriorly, it contacts the deep portion of the external sphincter, the levator being absent in this location **(Figure 2, 3).** As the finger is rotated posteriorly, in contact with the midline of the canal laterally, a distinct thickening is felt as the levator ani **(Figure 2, 5)** joins the canal, and posteriorly the anal canal feels thicker

than it does anteriorly. Incontinence will not occur if any portion of the external sphincter or levator muscle remains intact.

An anterior fistula involving only the subcutaneous and superficial portions of the external sphincter may be excised in one operation **(Figure 3, A, B, C, and D).** An anterior fistula involving the entire external sphincter **(Figure 3, E)** cannot be excised in one operation without producing total incontinence. Posteriorly, if the levator ani muscle is left intact, a fistula involving the entire external sphincter can be completely excised with far less danger of total incontinence.

Most fistulae arise in the anal glands at the base of the crypts of Morgagni; therefore, the abscess usually lies within the substance of the internal sphincter **(Figure 4).** It extravasates through the muscle, tending to follow the tissue planes created by the fibromuscular septa of the longitudinal muscle. Fistulae rarely arise from perforations of the anal canal associated with foreign bodies or abscesses, as in tuberculosis or ulcerative colitis. The internal opening may be above the pectinate line and may traverse the entire sphincter or portions of the levator **(Figure 3, F).** It may be necessary to operate in two stages to avoid incontinence.

Simple anal fistulae **(Figure 5, a)** follow a direct route into the anus. Complicated fistulae **(Figure 5, b and c)** follow a more devious route, often horseshoe in shape and with numerous openings. Most complicated fistulous tracts open into the posterior half of the anus. Should the fistula have multiple sinuses, the main exit will usually be posterior, even though one opening is anterior to the line **(Figure 5, x-x)**; a single fistulous opening anterior to x-x usually extends directly into the anterior half of the anus **(Figure 5, a)** (Goodsall's rule).

PREOPERATIVE PREPARATION. Local abscesses are drained if there is pocketing or cellulitis. If there is no severe local inflammation, a cleansing enema is given the night before operation. No cathartic is necessary.

ANESTHESIA. Inhalation anesthesia is the procedure of choice when dealing with a complicated fistula. Spinal anesthesia is satisfactory for simple fistulae and may be used for more complicated fistulae; however, it provides such complete relaxation of the musculature that palpation and recognition of the divisions of the external sphincter and levator are sometimes impossible.

POSITION. See Plate CLXXIV.

1. TREATMENT OF SIMPLE FISTULAE

DETAILS OF PROCEDURE. The anal canal may be dilated just enough to permit introduction of a self-retaining retractor. The pectinate line is directly visualized, and anal crypts that may reveal the internal opening are inspected. Gentle probing of suspected crypts may reveal an unusually deep crypt which, from the position of its external opening, can be recognized as the source of the fistula **(Figure 6).** If a normal pectinate line is found, with shallow crypts or no crypts at all, it is likely to be a local perianal abscess with no direct communication with the anal canal.

Some surgeons prefer to inject a dye into the external opening to trace the fistulous tract.

After the internal opening of a simple fistula has been identified, a probe is introduced into the external opening and gently passed down the tract into the external opening **(Figure 7).** The incision is made on the probe, and the tract is laid open. The edges of the tract are excised, taking care to saucerize the incision **(Figure 8).** The anal glands cause most fistulae, and particular care should be taken to excise the tissue around the internal opening **(Figure 9).** The tract should lie open as shown in **Figure 10.** In simple fistulae the entire tract may be stabilized with a probe as it is excised with scissors **(Figure 11).**

2. TREATMENT OF COMPLICATED FISTULAE

DETAILS OF PROCEDURE. The procedure is followed as outlined for simple fistulae. The internal opening is identified with a probe. One of the external openings is explored with a probe and opened as far as the tract can be readily identified. The probe usually enters the fistulous tract a short distance **(Figure 12).** The tract is incised down to this point **(Figure 13).** The direction of the tract may no longer be apparent. Traction is placed upon the inside edges of the wound, and the base of the tract is vigorously wiped with dry gauze **(Figure 14).** The granulations wipe off, leaving firm scar tissue. One point is found at which the granulations remain. This point marks the continuation of the tract **(Figure 15).** The probe is gently reinserted, the exact direction is appraised, and then the probe is carefully passed as far as possible. It may pass down into the internal opening; otherwise, the tract is again incised, and the wiping procedure is followed until the opening is rediscovered.

PLATE CLXXV   DRAINAGE OF ISCHIORECTAL ABSCESS—EXCISION OF FISTULA IN ANO

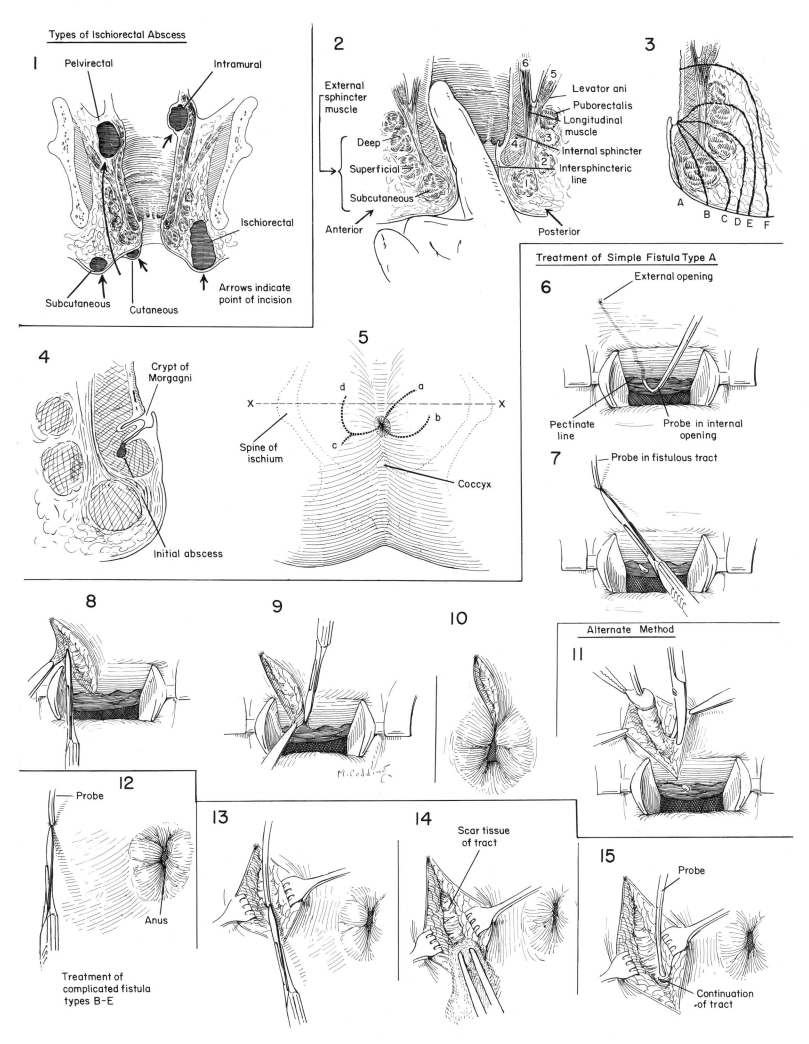

Types of Ischiorectal Abscess

1
Pelvirectal
Intramural
Ischiorectal
Subcutaneous
Cutaneous
Arrows indicate point of incision

2
External sphincter muscle
Deep
Superficial
Subcutaneous
Anterior
Levator ani
Puborectalis
Longitudinal muscle
Internal sphincter
Intersphincteric line
Posterior

3
A B C D E F

4
Crypt of Morgagni
Initial abscess

5
d   a
X — — — — — — X
c   b
Spine of ischium
Coccyx

Treatment of Simple Fistula Type A

6
External opening
Pectinate line
Probe in internal opening

7
Probe in fistulous tract

8

9
M. Codding

10

Alternate Method

11

12
Probe
Anus
Treatment of complicated fistula types B-E

13

14
Scar tissue of tract

15
Probe
Continuation of tract

PLATE CLXXVI · EXCISION OF FISTULA IN ANO—EXCISION OF FISSURE IN ANO

DETAILS OF PROCEDURE (*Continued*). All of the superficial tracts are outlined, defined, excised, and saucerized before carrying the dissection into the sphincter (**Figures 16** and **17**). Usually, only one internal opening is found. Again, as in a direct fistula, the tissues around the internal opening must be carefully excised in order to obliterate the anal glands. The sphincter muscle may be divided laterally or posteriorly, providing it is cut cleanly at the point where the tract traverses the muscle (**Figure 18**). The decision to complete the operation in one or two stages depends solely upon the depth of the tract traversing the sphincter. No matter how complicated the tract has been or how many superficial openings have been saucerized and laid open, if the internal opening can be reached without dividing the entire anorectal ring, and there is only one internal opening, a one-stage operation is done.

When the fistula has arisen above the pectinate line, usually because of the presence of a foreign body or some ulcerative process, a two-stage operation is done. The dissection is carried down to the external sphincter, but most of this is left intact. A small piece of braided silk is pulled through the fistulous tract and loosely tied to act as a seton (**Figure 19**). This allows the granulations to begin to form and the edges of the wound to become somewhat firm before the sphincter is completely divided.

It is not division of the sphincter that produces incontinence, but division of the sphincter and then its being allowed to retract widely and fill up with scar tissue. At the second stage, several weeks later, a probe is passed along the seton (**Figure 20**), and the sphincter is divided (**Figure 21**). The granulations will be firm enough around the wound so that the divided muscle will not retract widely. Rarely, a tract is found that appears to be a simple fistula, in the sense that there is only one external opening and only one internal opening with a direct tract between the two; yet this may pass at a level above the deep external sphincter anteriorly, or the levator posteriorly, and the operation must be performed in two stages.

CLOSURE. At the completion of the operation the tract is gently packed with gauze in petrolatum, and a sterile dressing is applied.

POSTOPERATIVE CARE. The patient may be out of bed as soon as the anesthesia has worn off. In most instances it is not necessary to disturb the pack for the first 48 hours. The patient is allowed a light diet, and there is no attempt to restrain bowel movements. Hot sitz baths are started on the second day following operation, and daily rectal examination is then performed. The area of the internal opening is gently massaged to prevent the formation of excessive granulations that protrude into the anal canal. Careful postoperative dressings and the removal of detritus or slough from the wound surface will ensure the development of healthy granulations. Once they begin to form, they are gently pressed down at each dressing in order to prevent pocketing. The care with which postoperative dressings are performed is as important in the prevention of a local recurrence as is the operation. Many so-called "recurrences" are the result of careless postoperative care. Patients may be discharged from the hospital in four or five days, but biweekly postoperative examinations are continued until healing is complete.

C. Treatment of Fibrotic External Sphincter Ani

INDICATIONS. As a result of low-grade chronic cryptitis or papillitis, combined with the prolonged use of saline or mineral oil cathartics which make the stools liquid, the subcutaneous and superficial portions of the external sphincter undergo a progressive contraction and fibrosis (**Figure 22,** A and B). The fibrotic sphincter may be differentiated from a spastic sphincter by the introduction of a local anesthetic into the muscle. The sphincter in spasm will relax, whereas the fibrosed sphincter will not permit the introduction of more than one finger into the anal canal. Rectal examination or anoscopy may be so painful as to require postponement until complete anesthesia is induced. The operation for correcting this condition is sometimes referred to as pectinotomy, under the mistaken assumption that the fibrotic area lies at the pectinate line; however, the fibrotic ring is a portion of the fibrosed internal sphincter (**Figure 22,** A and B).

PREOPERATIVE PREPARATION. No special preoperative preparation is necessary, other than ascertaining that the patient's general condition is good. It is desirable to give a cleansing enema the night before operation. If there are associated spasm and pain, this may be omitted.

ANESTHESIA. Local, general, or spinal anesthesia, as acceptable to the patient, is satisfactory.

POSITION. See Plate CLXXIV.

OPERATIVE PREPARATION. The field is prepared as described previously.

DETAILS OF PROCEDURE. A self-retaining retractor is introduced into the anal canal. It will not open widely because of the marked stenosis in the canal. Attempting to stretch or dilate the canal is very unwise, as it produces trauma and hemorrhage and may result in recurrent fibrosis. After introduction of the retractor the fibrotic subcutaneous portion of the internal sphincter is identified by palpation as a firm, ringlike contracture of the canal (**Figure 23**). An incision is made directly over the ring and deepened down to the outer edge of the muscle (**Figure 24**). The incision is placed to the side of the midline to avoid dividing the fibrous attachments of the sphincter to the coccyx posteriorly. A small pair of dissecting scissors may be inserted beneath the fibrotic muscle, and the muscle may be divided with a knife on top of the scissors (**Figure 25**). The canal then completely relaxes. The retractor is spread, and the entire canal is thoroughly inspected. If complete relaxation does not occur, it is because the superficial portion of the sphincter is also involved in the inflammation, and dissection must be made further into the muscle. The process, however, is usually localized to the subcutaneous or at most the subcutaneous and superficial portions of the sphincter, so the fibrotic area can be divided with impunity.

After the sclerotic portion has been divided, the remainder of the canal is thoroughly inspected, and any associated pathology, such as cryptitis or papillitis, is corrected.

D. Excision of Fissure in Ano

INDICATIONS. Fissures are acute or chronic. Acute fissures are superficial breaks in the anal mucosa. A chronic fissure results from recurrent acute fissures and is accompanied by persistent pain. It is ordinarily associated with pathology such as markedly hypertrophied papillae at the upper edge of the fissure and/or a sentinel pile externally. Palpation reveals induration and ulceration of the base of the fissure. The treatment is total excision, including division of the scarred subcutaneous portion of the external sphincter muscle.

PREOPERATIVE PREPARATION. No preoperative preparation is necessary. The cleansing enema, which is such an excruciating procedure to this patient, is omitted.

ANESTHESIA. Spinal, sacral, or local anesthesia is satisfactory.

OPERATIVE PREPARATION. The field is prepared with local antiseptic solution. No attempt is made to dilate the canal and irrigate the rectum.

DETAILS OF PROCEDURE. The self-retaining retractor is inserted into the canal to permit adequate exposure of the fissure. A triangular incision is made from the outer edge of the fissure down to and including the edge of the pectinate line (**Figure 26**). The incision is deepened to include all the indurated and inflamed scar tissue (**Figure 27**). The anal skin, the fissure, and a small portion of the rectal mucosa are then excised as a large triangular flap (**Figure 28**). The scarred portion of the internal sphincter will be seen crossing the base of the wound (**Figure 29**). If there are local scarring and contracture, the scars should be divided, and the fibrotic edges should be excised (**Figure 30**). A new pectinate line is reconstructed by sewing the edge of the rectal mucosa into the lower edge of the internal sphincter (**Figure 31**). It is important to place the sutures so that the line of closure is continuous with the adjacent pectinate line.

POSTOPERATIVE CARE. Patients are allowed out of bed and encouraged to move their bowels as soon as possible after operation. Daily sitz baths and daily rectal examinations are indicated to ensure that granulations do not build up and protrude into the anal canal. A daily rectal examination keeps the healing surface firm and encourages epithelization. The patient should be kept under weekly observation after discharge until healing is complete.

PLATE CLXXVI   EXCISION OF FISTULA IN ANO—EXCISION OF FISSURE IN ANO

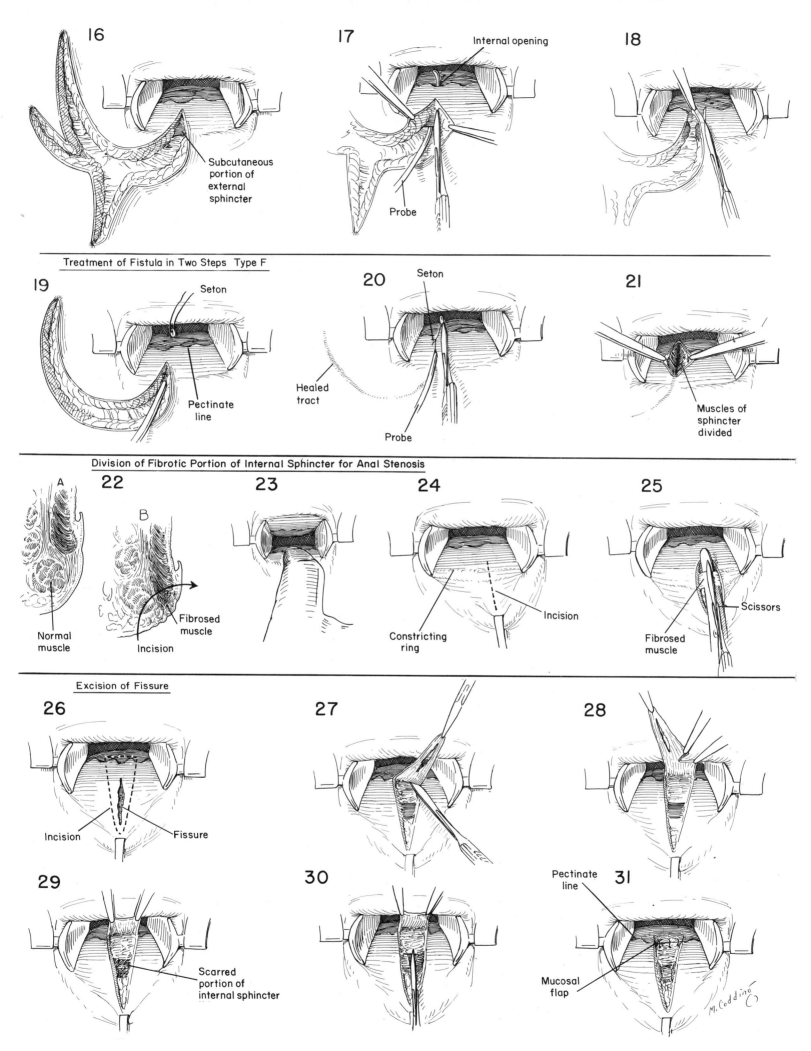

16

Subcutaneous portion of external sphincter

17

Internal opening

Probe

18

Treatment of Fistula in Two Steps Type F

19

Seton

Pectinate line

20

Seton

Healed tract

Probe

21

Muscles of sphincter divided

Division of Fibrotic Portion of Internal Sphincter for Anal Stenosis

22

A

B

Normal muscle

Incision

Fibrosed muscle

23

24

Constricting ring

Incision

25

Fibrosed muscle

Scissors

Excision of Fissure

26

Incision

Fissure

27

28

29

Scarred portion of internal sphincter

30

31

Pectinate line

Mucosal flap

M. Coddino

PLATE CLXXVII · EXCISION OF PILONIDAL SINUS

INDICATIONS. Pilonidal cysts and sinuses should be completely excised or exteriorized **(Figure 3, A and B)**. Acutely infected sinuses should be incised and drained, followed later by complete excision after the acute infection subsides. The more limited procedure of exteriorization is effective when the sinus tract is well defined **(Figure 3, B)**. Regardless of the various surgical approaches, a definite incidence of recurrence should be anticipated.

PREOPERATIVE PREPARATION. In complicated sinuses with several tracts present, a dye such as methylene blue may be injected for better identification, although if a careful dissection is carried out in a bloodless field, the surgeon can recognize and avoid the sinus tracts. It is important that this be done several days before operation to avoid excessive staining of the operative area, which may occur if the injection is done at the time of operation.

ANESTHESIA. Light general or intravenous anesthesia is satisfactory. The patient's position requires that special care be taken to maintain an unobstructed airway. Spinal anesthesia should not be used in the presence of infection near the site of lumbar puncture.

POSITION. The patient is placed on his abdomen with the hips elevated and the table broken in the middle **(Figure 1)**.

OPERATIVE PREPARATION. Two strips of adhesive tape are anchored snugly and symmetrically about 10 cm. from the midline at the level of the sinus and pulled down and fastened beneath the table **(Figure 2)**. This spreads the intergluteal fold for better visualization of the operative area. A routine skin preparation follows.

DETAILS OF PROCEDURE. An ovoid incision is made around the opening of the sinus tract about 1 cm. away from either side. Firm pressure and outward pull make the skin taut and control bleeding.

An Allis forceps is placed at the upper angle of the skin to be removed, and the sinus is cut out *en bloc* **(Figure 5)**. The subcutaneous tissue is excised downward and laterally to the fascia underneath. Great care is exercised to protect this fascia from the incision, as it offers the only defense against deeper spread of infection **(Figure 6)**. Small, pointed hemostats should be used to clamp the bleeding vessels in order that the smallest amount of tissue reaction be incurred. Electrocoagulation may be used to control bleeding and to keep the amount of buried suture material to a minimum. Some prefer to avoid burying any suture material by using compression or electrocoagulation to control all the bleeding points. Extreme care should be taken in the dissection of the lower end of the incision, as many small, troublesome vessels are frequently encountered which tend to retract when divided. After careful inspection of the wound to make sure that all sinus tracts have been removed, the subcutaneous fat is undercut at its junction with the underlying fascia **(Figure 7)**. This under-

cutting should extend only far enough to allow approximation of the edges without tension **(Figure 8)**.

CLOSURE. After all bleeding points are controlled, the wound should be thoroughly washed with saline. The chances for primary healing are greatly enhanced if the field is absolutely dry. If unexpected infection has been encountered, the wound should be packed open. In uncomplicated sinuses the wound is closed after all bleeding is controlled. Rather than bury sutures, the skin can be closed and the dead space eliminated by a series of interrupted vertical mattress sutures **(Figure 9)**. The suture is introduced a centimeter or a little more from the margins of the wound to include the full thickness of the mobilized flap of skin and subcutaneous tissue. A second bite includes the fascia in the bottom of the wound **(Figure 9)**. The suture is then continued deep into the opposite flap. The suture is directed back to the original side as it passes back through the skin margins **(Figure 10)**. When tied, this obliterates the dead space and accurately approximates the skin margins **(Figure 11)**. The sutures should be placed at intervals of not more than 1 cm. Skin approximation must be very accurate, since even a small overlap may be surprisingly slow to heal in this area. A pressure dressing is applied with great care, and the sutures are allowed to remain in place for 10 to 14 days.

When the sinus appears small and in the presence of recurrence, a probe may be inserted into the sinus, and the skin and subcutaneous tissue divided **(Figure 3, A)**. The entire sinus, including any tributaries, must be laid wide open and all granulation tissue wiped away repeatedly with sterile gauze. The thick lining of the sinus forms the bottom of the wound. A wedge of subcutaneous tissue is excised to facilitate the sewing of the mobilized skin margins to the thick wall of the retained sinus. This ensures a cavity that can be easily dressed with a minimum of drainage as well as discomfort to the patient. The raw margins of the wound are held apart by a gauze pack until healing is complete **(Figure 3, B)**. This method has the advantage of being a procedure of less magnitude than complete excision. The period of hospitalization and rehabilitation is shortened and insurance against recurrence enhanced.

POSTOPERATIVE CARE. Complete immobilization of the area and protection against contamination are essential. Early ambulation is not advisable. The patient is kept on his abdomen or flat on his back with the head resting near the foot of the bed. This reversal of the usual position permits eating, etc., from trays placed near the foot of the bed with a minimum of physical effort. The diet is restricted to clear liquids for several days, followed by a low-residue diet to decrease the chances of contamination from a bowel movement. When the sinus is packed open or exteriorized, the patient is not immobilized. Regardless of the method used, frequent and repeated dressings are indicated to avoid possible early bridging of the skin with recurrence and prolonged discomfort and disability. The importance of keeping all hair removed from the intergluteal fold until healing is complete cannot be overemphasized. Depilatory agents may be used several times per month, providing pretesting for sensitivity to the agent has been negative.

PLATE CLXXVII   EXCISION OF PILONIDAL SINUS

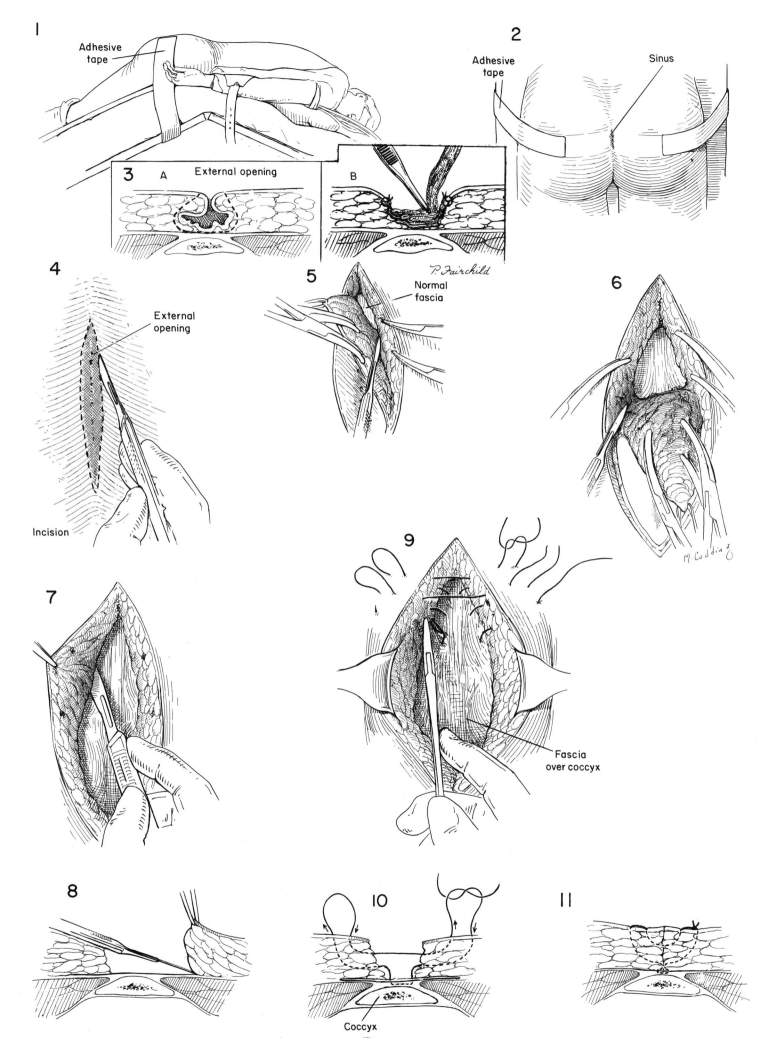

1

Adhesive
tape

2

Adhesive
tape   Sinus

3   A   External opening   B

P. Fairchild

4

External
opening

Incision

5

Normal
fascia

6

M. Coddin Jr.

7

9

Fascia
over coccyx

8

10

Coccyx

11

PLATE CLXXVIII · PRINCIPLES OF AMPUTATION

INDICATIONS. The common factors indicating amputation of a part of the body are trauma, interference with the vascular supply, malignant neoplasm, chronic osteomyelitis, life-threatening infections, congenital limb deformity in children, the need to increase function, and, occasionally, the cosmetic effect.

PREOPERATIVE PREPARATION. In the presence of trauma it is first necessary to evaluate carefully the extent of tissue and vascular damage in terms of possibly salvaging the extremity. With the recent advances in peripheral vascular repair and grafting, reestablishment of distal blood flow following arterial injury, blockage by arteriosclerosis, or embolus is often possible. It is essential to combat shock with whole blood transfusions and with intravenous administration of fluids until the patient's general condition is improved sufficiently to withstand the operation. With diabetes or advanced vascular disease the usual strict medical measures are taken to regulate these associated diseases. If there is localized skin infection at the proposed level for amputation, the procedure is delayed whenever possible. In the presence of wet gangrene, packing the leg in ice or dry ice, combined with the application of a tourniquet just below the site of proposed amputation, not only may lessen toxicity but also may decrease the incidence of wound infection, since the lymphatics may be cleared before amputation. The threat of gas gangrene may be a real one when the arterial supply to the extremity has been severely compromised, either by intra-arterial occlusion or trauma with inadequate debridement and a closed space infection.

ANESTHESIA. Spinal anesthesia is commonly used for major amputation of the lower extremities, inhalation anesthesia for major amputations of the upper extremities, and plexus block or local infiltration anesthesia for amputation of the fingers and toes.

POSITION. See Plate CLXXIX. In amputations of the upper extremity, the patient is placed near the edge of the table with the arm extended and abducted to the desired position. For amputations of the lower extremity, the leg may be elevated with several sterile towels under the calf.

OPERATIVE PREPARATION. In the absence of infection, the extremity is elevated to encourage venous drainage before a tourniquet is applied. The tourniquet is placed above the knee for amputations of the lower leg and foot, high in the thigh for amputations of the knee and lower thigh, and above the elbow to control the brachial artery for major amputations of the forearm. In cases of arteriosclerosis, the tourniquet should not be used, because of the possibility of damaging the blood supply to the stump. Sterile elastic bands may be applied to the base of the digit for minor amputations. The skin is prepared with the usual antiseptic solutions well above and below the proposed site of amputation. In major amputations the entire extremity may be wrapped in sterile adherent plastic drapes to enable the assistant to hold it and change its position as desired.

SITES FOR AMPUTATION. The efficiency of modern prostheses has eliminated the time-honored "sites of election." Generally, the pathology and age, as well as occupation, of the patient dictate the site of amputation, with the goal of preserving all possible length. This is particularly true of the upper extremity.

The rule of saving all possible length does not necessarily apply to the lower extremity. However, whenever possible, the knee should be saved since it provides major functional advantages. While the blood supply to the upper extremity is usually adequate, the reverse is often true for the lower extremity. Furthermore, the problems of weight-bearing and retaining adequate soft tissue to cover the stump affect the site of election in the lower extremity, since an inadequate blood supply, often after failure of a vascular bypass graft, is the most common indication for amputating the lower extremity.

Since the profunda femoral artery tends to be the main channel after occlusion of the superficial femoral vessels or a femoral-popliteal bypass graft, the site of amputation must be selected well within the zone adequately supplied by this vessel. Accordingly, the amputation is usually above the knee. For this reason the supracondylar amputation **(Figure 1, A)** continues to be the most frequent site for amputation in the presence of arterial insufficiency, although a below-knee one is preferred if possible.

It can be technically performed in a short time with the best assurance of primary healing of the flaps. Knee disarticulation (C) and transcondylar amputation (B) yield an enlarged, rounded end that is cumbersome and difficult to fit with a prosthesis.

The rule of saving all possible length does not apply to below-knee amputation. Long leg stumps are not recommended because of their poor tolerance of prosthesis. Since the anterior margin of the tibia is usually beveled, there must be enough solid tissue with good blood supply to cover it as provided by a longer posterior flap. The optimum length of the stump is between 12 and 18 cm. A short below-knee stump is preferable to knee disarticulation, for it is possible to utilize the short stump for fitting a prosthesis with use of the patient's own knee joint. It should be emphasized that the fibula does not bear the pressure of a prosthetic appliance well and will become tender and painful. It should be amputated 3 to 5 cm. higher than the tibia, and with a short below-knee stump it is wise to remove the fibula completely.

Although ankle amputations have few indications, chiefly trauma, the Syme amputation lends itself to a very serviceable end-weight-bearing prosthesis but has cosmetic disadvantages in females **(Figure 1, D)**. There is general agreement that a most satisfactory foot amputation is the transmetatarsal. In the presence of vascular insufficiency to the lower extremity, amputations about the ankle or foot should be performed cautiously for secure indications, especially in the presence of infection, as they frequently heal poorly, necessitating secondary procedures.

Formerly, the junction of lower and middle thirds of the forearm was considered the optimum site for amputations; however, newer artificial limbs which include pronation and supination movements make it desirable to save all possible length. Length is again important in the hand, where a partial amputation of the fingers or of all fingers, leaving an opposing surface at the thumb for gripping, allows better function than can be provided by any prosthesis. A stump of any length in the forearm will give better function than an amputation above the elbow, and it eliminates a turntable included in a prosthesis.

TYPES OF FLAPS. As a general rule it is desirable to have the scar at the end of the stump in the upper extremity, since the prosthesis bears largely on the lateral surfaces of the stump. The scar for end-bearing stumps of the lower extremity should preferably be anterior or posterior to the end of the stump. In minor amputations of the fingers and toes, long palmar and plantar flaps are made to cover the stump with a thick, protective pad of tissue **(Figures 2 and 5)**. Racket incisions are advisable for amputations of the toes, since they may be extended upward to permit exposure of the metatarsals **(Figure 3)**, or they may be used for amputations of digits where all possible length must be preserved. This is especially true for injuries of the thumb (Incisions B, C, and D, **Figure 6**). Racket incisions with removal of the head of the metacarpal or metatarsal give a good appearance to the extremity but considerably diminish the breadth of the foot or palm.

DETAILS OF PROCEDURE. Sufficient soft tissue must be present to approximate easily over the end of the bone, but excessive amounts are avoided, since bulky soft tissue hinders the fitting of a prosthesis. Arteries and veins should be individually tied. Nerves are divided at as high a level as possible. Two Kocher clamps are placed on large nerves 0.5 cm. apart before division of the nerve. The nerve is then sharply severed just beyond the distal clamp, and the nerve is doubly ligated with 00 silk just distal to the clamps. This aids in the prevention of symptomatic neuromas.

The bone should be divided at a sufficiently high level to permit the soft parts to approximate, producing a thick covering for its end. The sharp margins of bone are beveled either with a rongeur or rasp.

CLOSURE. All bleeding points are tied carefully so that, in the ordinary case, drainage is unnecessary. The investing fascia rather than the deep muscles is loosely approximated with interrupted silk sutures. When there has been considerable oozing or a moderate amount of infection distal to the site of amputation, through-and-through drainage may be instituted. If a guillotine type of amputation was carried out in the presence of a progressing infection, the wound is left open to be closed secondarily later, or the extremity is reamputated later at a higher level to permit primary closure.

POSTOPERATIVE CARE. See Plate CLXXX.

PLATE CLXXVIII   PRINCIPLES OF AMPUTATION

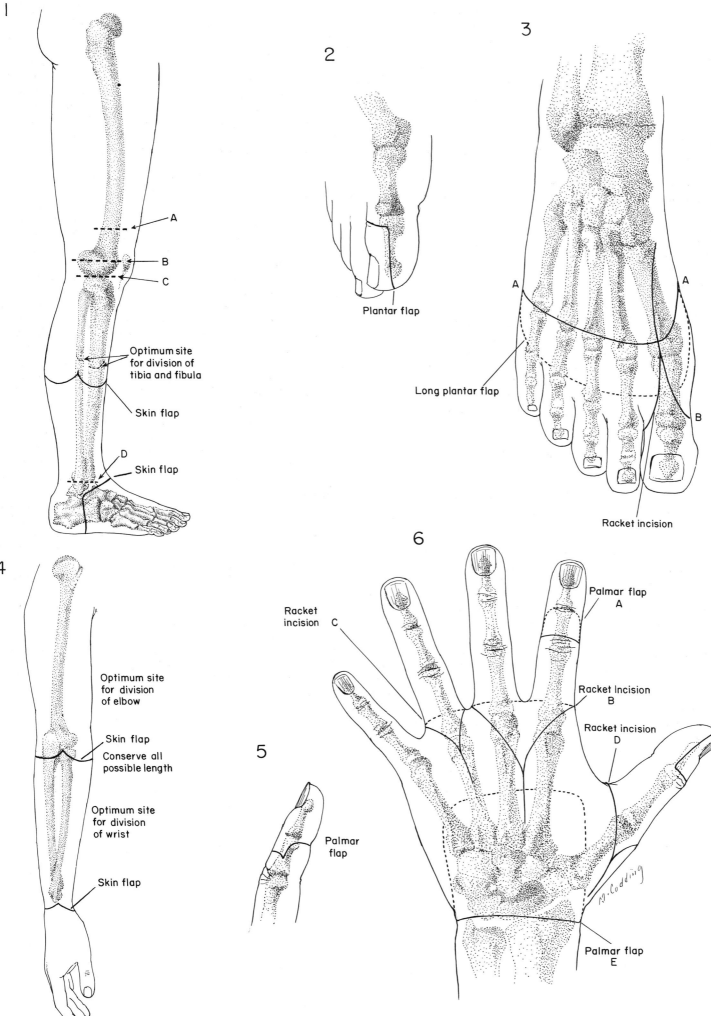

1

A

B

C

Optimum site
for division of
tibia and fibula

Skin flap

D

Skin flap

2

Plantar flap

3

A

A

B

Long plantar flap

Racket incision

4

Optimum site
for division
of elbow

Skin flap

Conserve all
possible length

Optimum site
for division
of wrist

Skin flap

5

Palmar
flap

6

Racket
incision   C

Palmar flap
A

Racket Incision
B

Racket incision
D

Palmar flap
E

M. Codding

PLATE CLXXIX · AMPUTATION, SUPRACONDYLAR

INDICATIONS. Common indications for supracondylar amputation are trauma, interference with the blood supply, tumor, infections that are dangerous to life, the need for increased function, etc. Amputation should not be performed unless all conservative measures have failed.

The amputation at the thigh is described in detail. This is a frequent site following failure of reconstructive or bypass arterial procedures or in the presence of unreconstructable circumstance as documented with proximal and distal arteriography.

PREOPERATIVE PREPARATION. The preoperative preparation must of necessity vary with the indications for amputation as outlined in the preceding section. Medical management may be supplemented by sympathectomy in those instances where the decreased blood supply can be demonstrated to be the result of vascular spasm or where a transient small increase in local blood flow will tip the balance to successful healing. Careful evaluation must be made to determine whether there is a localized arterial obstruction, and arteriography is essential. If localized obstruction is present, a proximal (for example, aortofemoral) reconstructive procedure may restore an adequate blood inflow, or a distal (for example, femoral-popliteal) bypass arterial graft may eliminate the need for amputation.

When infection is present, vigorous therapeutic measures are needed. After bacterial cultures with drug sensitivities are obtained, the appropriate chemotherapy or antibiotic is administered. Should there be a localized skin infection at the proposed level for amputation, the procedure is delayed if improvement is possible. In the presence of an advancing infection a guillotine or open amputation is done above the level of the infection, with a subsequent definitive amputation at a higher point of election.

The night before operation, the thigh from the groin to well below the knee is shaved carefully, although some prefer depilatories or preparation within the operating room. In addition, the area should be scrubbed either with green soap or a soap containing hexachlorophene, and the extremity should be wrapped.

ANESTHESIA. Low spinal anesthesia is used most frequently, although inhalation anesthesia may be administered unless the patient's condition contraindicates it.

POSITION. The patient is placed with the hip on the affected side out to the margin of the table to allow full abduction of the thigh by an assistant, and the calf or ankle may be elevated with several sterile towels.

OPERATIVE PREPARATION. The foot is held in abduction while the leg from below the knee to high in the groin is cleaned with appropriate antiseptics. A sterile sheet is placed beneath the thigh. The foot and lower leg up to the knee are covered with a sterile sheet or plastic drape **(Figure 1)**. Unless there is evidence of progressive infection, the extremity is elevated by the assistant to encourage venous drainage.

INCISION AND EXPOSURE. The type of flap that is used varies. With progressive infection of the lower leg a circular incision is made for a guillotine amputation. However, when possible, anterior and posterior flaps are outlined with a sterile marking pen, assuring an appropriate stump length **(Figure 1)**. Either equal anterior and posterior flaps are used or, more commonly, a larger anterior flap with a length one and one-half times the diameter of the thigh at the level of the division of the femur.

The surgeon stands on the inner side of the thigh, to visualize better the main arterial and nerve supply, and outlines the selected incision. Since the soft parts retract considerably, the skin incision must extend at least 15 cm. below the point where the bone is to be divided. The incision is carried through the skin and subcutaneous tissue down to the fascia over the underlying muscles. All bleeding points are clamped and tied.

DETAILS OF PROCEDURE. The surgeon must be familiar with the location of the major nerves and vessels **(Figure 2)**. The first blood vessel of any size to be clamped and tied is the great saphenous vein, located on the medial or posteromedial aspect of the thigh, depending on the level of amputation **(Figures 2 and 4)**. The muscles, which should be divided at a slightly higher level than the skin and fascia, retract upward so that the flaps will consist chiefly of skin and fascia **(Figure 3)**. Those on the lateral and anterior aspects of the thigh are first divided, and the few bleeding points found are clamped and tied.

The median incision into the muscle layer is made carefully until the femoral vessels are exposed deep on the posteromedial aspect of the thigh **(Figure 5)**. If a tourniquet has not been applied, the surgeon should locate the major vessel by palpation or by its visible pulsation. If a tourniquet has been used, the dissection is carried out directly until the femoral vein is exposed. This is divided between half-length clamps. Both artery and vein are tied separately **(Figure 6)**, and, if desired, a transfixing tie may be added distal to the original ligature on the femoral artery.

The sciatic nerve is next located posterior to the femoral vessels and is isolated from the surrounding tissues by a blunt-nosed, curved, half-length clamp passed beneath the nerve or the common peroneal and posterior tibial branches, in the event of a high bifurcation of the sciatic nerve. In an effort to minimize the formation of an amputation neuroma, the nerve is pulled down as far as possible, and a strong straight Ochsner clamp is applied. A second similar crushing clamp is applied about 5 mm. distal to the untied clamp and the nerve divided immediately below the second clamp. The proximal clamp is removed, and the crushed area is ligated with a heavy 0 ligature of silk. Fine ligatures are avoided lest the epineural sheath be cut through, permitting the formation of a neuroma. Catgut ligatures are avoided since they may be absorbed before the epineural sheath has united, causing the sheath to reopen with the formation of a neuroma. The distal clamp is then removed, leaving a crushed and flattened short segment of nerve that tends to prevent the ligature from slipping off. The nerve is allowed to retract well upward into the muscle layers. It should never be anchored to adjacent structures. When the sciatic nerve has retracted upward, the tissues are further freed from the posterior surface of the femur. The profunda femoris artery and vein must be secured and ligated in the posterior group of muscles **(Figure 2)**.

PLATE CLXXIX   AMPUTATION, SUPRACONDYLAR

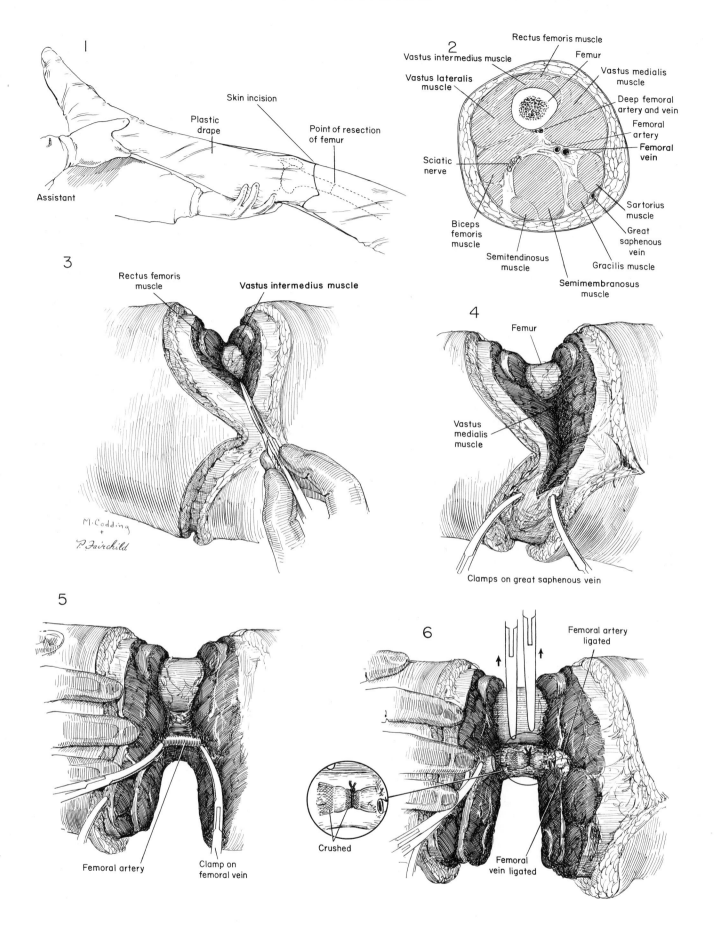

1

Assistant

Plastic drape

Skin incision

Point of resection of femur

2

Vastus intermedius muscle

Rectus femoris muscle

Femur

Vastus medialis muscle

Vastus lateralis muscle

Deep femoral artery and vein

Femoral artery

Femoral vein

Sciatic nerve

Sartorius muscle

Great saphenous vein

Biceps femoris muscle

Gracilis muscle

Semitendinosus muscle

Semimembranosus muscle

3

Rectus femoris muscle

Vastus intermedius muscle

M. Codding + P. Fairchild

4

Femur

Vastus medialis muscle

Clamps on great saphenous vein

5

Femoral artery

Clamp on femoral vein

6

Femoral artery ligated

Crushed

Femoral vein ligated

PLATE CLXXX · AMPUTATION, SUPRACONDYLAR

DETAILS OF PROCEDURE (*Continued*). The gauze sponges are removed, and all bleeding points are clamped. Only those on the proximal side are tied, while the clamps on the distal side, which are to be removed, may be left in place. A circular incision is made through the periosteum of the femur **(Figure 7),** and the periosteum is pushed downward *only* for several centimeters with a periosteum elevator **(Figure 8).** During this procedure the muscle of the upper flap may be retracted upward by means of a sterile towel or bandage placed over the muscle surface. Retraction and covering of the muscle are maintained while the femur is divided with a saw at the desired level **(Figure 9).** The amputated part is removed from the surgical field.

The sharp margins of the bone at the site of amputation are beveled off with a rougeur or rasp **(Figure 10).** If a tourniquet has been used, it is now removed, and any additional bleeding points are clamped and tied. The muscle surface is washed with warm isotonic saline until the surgeon is assured that there is good hemostasis and all bone fragments are washed away. The thigh is held moderately flexed by an assistant to permit a full exposure of the entire field, although sterile towels beneath the proximal thigh may perform the same function.

CLOSURE. The deep investing fascia to the muscles in the anterior and posterior flaps is approximated with interrupted sutures over the end of the femur **(Figure 11).** After all dead space has been obliterated by the careful approximation of the muscle layers, the fascia over the muscles in the anterior and posterior flaps is approximated with interrupted silk sutures **(Figure 11).** With adequate hemostasis drainage should be unnecessary, but if serious infection existed distal to the site of amputation, it may be advisable to institute drainage. A through-and-through rubber tissue drain may be placed at the base of the flaps, and the muscles may be closed over it. If a guillotine type of amputation was carried out, the wound is left open, to be closed later in a delayed manner or reamputated at a higher level to permit primary closure.

Any excess or irregular tissue about the skin flaps is excised, and the subcutaneous tissue is approximated with interrupted silk sutures. The skin flaps are brought together by the two hands of the assistant, who holds the stump at a convenient level for the surgeon, while the subcutaneous and skin sutures are inserted **(Figures 11** and **12).** The skin is closed with interrupted silk sutures except while infection is present, and the use of forceps on the skin edges should be avoided.

POSTOPERATIVE CARE. The stump is covered with a nonadherent dressing and fluffs of sterile gauze and is encased in a dressing that is snug but not too tight. This dressing may have to be changed in 24 hours, since the stump may swell, resulting in pain as well as interference with the blood supply. The immediate postoperative care includes continued insulin regulation in the diabetic and elevation of the stump on several pillows to combat the swelling. After 24 to 48 hours the stump should be kept flat on the bed, as continued elevation leads to a flexion contracture. Splints may be applied at the time of surgery to maintain extension and prevent flexion contractures, but these must be removed early so that exercises can be started on the fourth or fifth day.

Guillotine amputations require special care. The raw surface is covered with sterile gauze. Circumferential traction is usually applied to the proximal skin soon after surgery to prevent skin edge retraction. In some cases this will be sufficient to cover the bone ends, and healing will take place; however, when the skin cannot be brought together in this way, skin grafts may have to be applied at a later date to cover persistent areas of granulation tissue.

The earlier the rehabilitation of the patient is started, the shorter the period of the postamputation depression. It has been found desirable to fit a temporary well-fitted limb as soon as the sutures are removed or within two or three weeks in below-the-knee amputations. The immediate postsurgical fitting of a prosthesis has many advantages. These include accelerated healing and less postsurgical pain, prevention of contractures, fewer psychological problems, and the return of the patient to work or home much earlier. Some prefer the immediate application of a rigid plaster dressing snugly over the sterile dressings of the below-the-knee amputation before the patient leaves the operating room. A socket is secured into its base, and an adjustable pylon can be immediately fitted for ambulation within a few days after surgery. After the sutures have been removed and wound healing evaluated, a new cast-socket is reapplied. The original prosthetic unit is replaced and realigned. After the second cast-socket has been worn for ten days, a new cast can be taken for the permanent prosthesis. Regular instructions by a physiotherapist are essential to ensure exercises designed to strengthen the hip extensors and stretch the hip abductors and flexors.

When immediate postsurgical fitting is not carried out, it is most important that exercises administered by a therapist or a nurse be followed. In order to aid shrinkage of the stump, cotton-elastic bandages are wrapped around the stump and worn continuously. The bandage is removed and properly reapplied every four hours and at bedtime. A clean bandage should be available each day. The amputee as well as members of the family should be taught to apply the bandage. Lower extremity stumps should not be propped up on pillows lest contractures develop, and lying prone on a flat bed will demonstrate hip or knee contractures. Crutch walking is preferred to use of wheelchairs for the same reason. It takes less energy for the patient to walk with a prosthesis than with crutches. However, many factors must be considered, including whether the patient walked before amputation, the presence of other serious illnesses, poor vision, condition of the other leg, degree of cooperation and alertness, as well as balance and degree of coordination. A planned program of rehabilitation is very important regardless of the type and extent of the amputation, and a coordinated follow-up involving the surgeon, physiotherapist, and prosthetist is desirable.

PLATE CLXXX   AMPUTATION, SUPRACONDYLAR

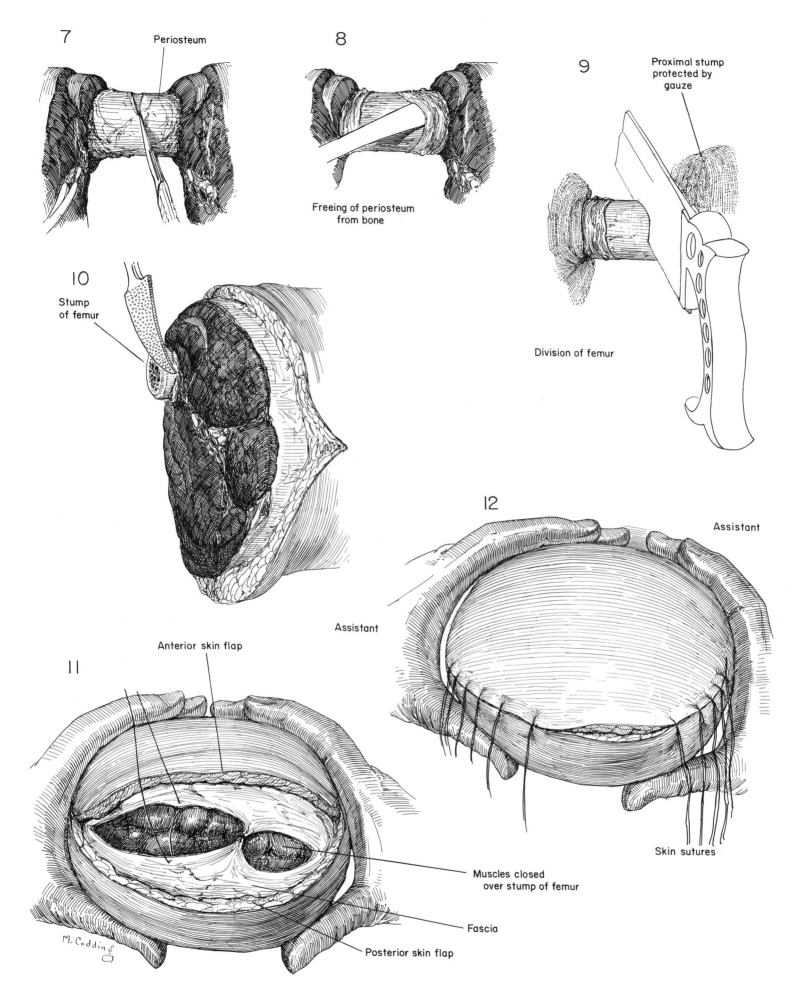

7

Periosteum

8

Freeing of periosteum
from bone

9

Proximal stump
protected by
gauze

Division of femur

10

Stump
of femur

12

Assistant

Assistant

Skin sutures

11

Anterior skin flap

Muscles closed
over stump of femur

Fascia

Posterior skin flap

M. Codding

PLATE CLXXXI · INCISION AND DRAINAGE OF INFECTIONS OF THE HAND

INDICATIONS. The indications for incision and drainage of infections of the hand vary with the location, duration, extent, and severity of the infection. For localized infections, other than cellulitis or lymphangitis of streptococcal origin, incision and drainage are carried out. It should be remembered that most infections arising on the volar surface of the hand produce maximal swelling on the dorsum; however, dorsal drainage is used only when suppuration presents on the dorsum. As a rule, surgery is contraindicated in the presence of a spreading streptococcal infection.

PREOPERATIVE PREPARATION. Immobilization, rest, and elevation in combination with antibiotic therapy are used to treat insufficiently localized infections. Once the diagnosis of abscess is made, incision and drainage are performed. Soiled hands are cleansed with soft soap and water; hands that have been in contact with grease should first be washed with ether or some other solvent. Regardless of how minor the infection that involves the extremity, the possibility of diabetes should be considered. The successful treatment of the infection may depend upon adequate control of diabetes if it is present.

ANESTHESIA. Axillary or brachial nerve plexus block may be used. Digital nerve block or regional block of the ulnar, radial, or median nerves provides satisfactory anesthesia for minor incision of the digits in the absence of lymphangitis. Digital blocks should be carried out either in the palm or in the loose tissue of the web spaces of the fingers. Blocks at the base of the fingers can cause serious interference with circulation because of the lack of room for expansion and the increased pressure within the sheath. Epinephrine should never be employed with the local anesthetic because of the danger of subsequent gangrene of the digit. General anesthesia is used for infections proximal to the middle phalanx or in those cases in which incision is required but cellulitis is still present. It may also be used in more extensive and neglected infections.

POSITION. The patient is placed in a supine position with the involved hand on an arm table.

OPERATIVE PREPARATION. Routine skin preparation of the hand is performed. In all but minor procedures a bloodless field is essential. Usually, in the adult this is obtained by inflating a blood pressure cuff to 250 mm. of mercury after venous drainage of the arm by elevation without the use of an elastic bandage.

A. Felon

DETAILS OF PROCEDURE. When infection is limited to the pulp of the terminal phalanx, immediate drainage is imperative to relieve the increased tension, which may compromise the blood supply and lead to loss of the terminal segment of bone. Superficial infections may be drained through incisions directly overlying the site of infection. For a deeply situated abscess the incision should be made to one side of the fingernail, across under the free edge of the nail, and extended well down into the pulp of the finger anterior to the terminal phalanx until all compartments have been opened and the abscess cavity completely drained **(Figures 1 and 2).** Care must be taken not to enter the tendon sheath. Bilateral incisions are avoided.

B. Paronychia

DETAILS OF PROCEDURE. Treatment depends upon the stage of development of the infection. Acute unilateral paronychia requires elevation of the cuticle from the nail at the site of infection **(Figure 3).** If the infection is advanced or with subungual abscess, removal of the proximal portion of the nail is preferred **(Figures 4 and 5).** If necessary to ensure adequate drainage, an incision may be made in the skin below the corner of the nail, placed laterally to avoid damage to the nail bed **(Figure 3),** since a permanent ridge with deformity may result from disruption of the nail bed. Similar treatment plus removal of infected granulations is usually necessary for chronic paronychia. Underlying fungus infection should be considered in recurrent paronychia.

C. Infections of Tendon Sheaths and Palmar Spaces

DETAILS OF PROCEDURE. While a felon is limited to the closed space of the terminal phalanx, infections proximal to this region may extend into the tendon sheaths. The flexor tendon sheaths of the index, middle, and ring fingers extend approximately one fingerbreadth proximal to the base of the finger. The sheath of the flexor pollicis longus is continued into the wrist as the radial bursa, that of the flexor tendons of the little finger is confluent with the ulnar bursa **(Figure 6).**

If early treatment with immobilization, elevation, and antibiotics has not been successful, surgical drainage will be necessary. If a wound is present, this should be opened and exudate sent to the laboratory for smear, culture, and sensitivities. If extensive infection is present, drainage is carried out through transverse incisions, as indicated by the dotted lines in **Figure 6,** opening the sheath distally and proximally. The distal incision should be placed just proximal to the interphalangeal crease and the proximal incision about a fingerbreadth below the metacarpophalangeal crease for the index, middle, ring, and little fingers. The proximal transverse incision for the thumb must be placed just proximal to the wrist, at the base of the radial bursa, and a similar incision may be required in the ulnar bursa for drainage of infection in the flexor tendon sheath of the little finger if it has spread into the palm. A small catheter may be introduced into the sheath for irrigation with saline or the appropriate antibiotic solution. In neglected cases more classic midlateral digital incisions may be required, as illustrated in **Figures 7 and 8.**

Abscesses of the interdigital spaces may be drained through incisions placed directly over the site of abscess, with care taken not to spread the infection to the tendon sheaths. Such incisions should be curved and transverse on the palmar surface, avoiding the motor branch of the median nerve **(Figures 6 and 7).** Double abscesses ("collar button" type), with pockets of pus on both dorsal and palmar aspects of the hand connected by a narrow tract, will require both a transverse palmar incision and a longitudinal dorsal incision.

POSTOPERATIVE CARE. Dry dressings and early return of motion, usually on the following day, with gradual increase in range of motion, are indicated in uncomplicated felon and paronychia. In tendon sheath infections antibiotics are continued for a week. Gentle movements are encouraged and increased as tolerated. Elevation of the extremity to heart level will lessen discomfort during the period of immobilization and until swelling has cleared. The rehabilitation of the infected hand requires careful supervision.

PLATE CLXXXI   INCISION AND DRAINAGE OF INFECTIONS OF THE HAND

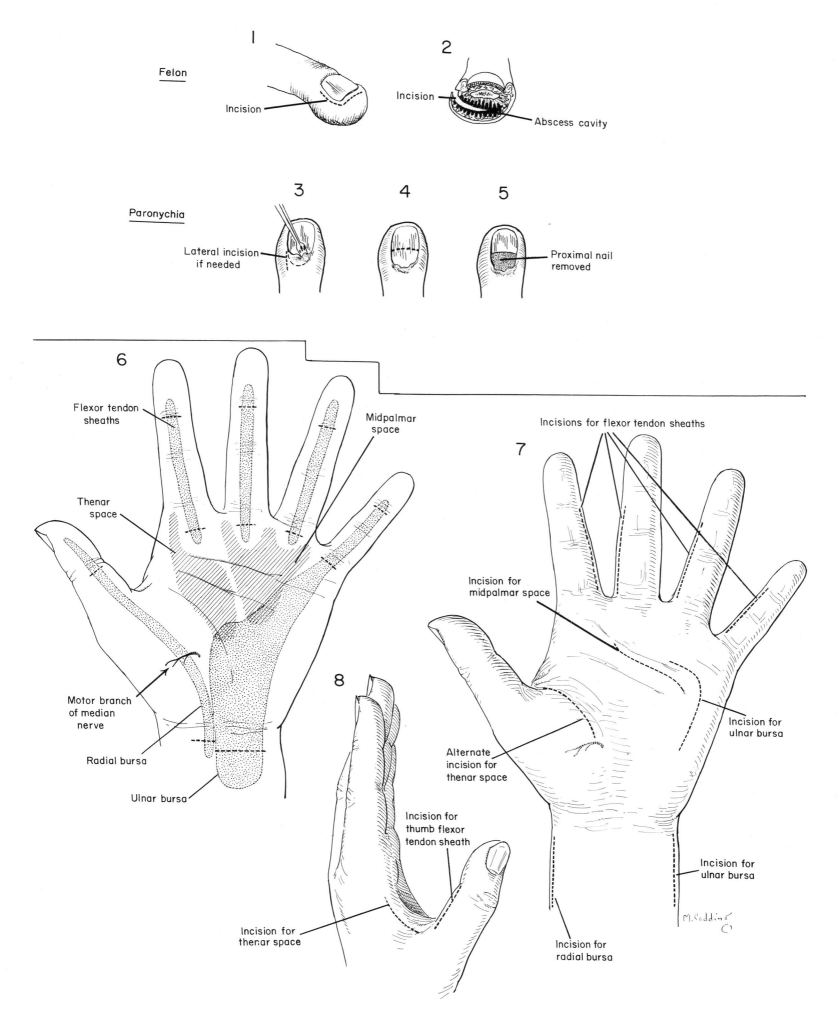

PLATE CLXXXII · SUTURE OF NERVE

INDICATIONS. Following traumatic division of a nerve **(Figure 1),** either primary or delayed (secondary) repair is required. Primary nerve repair should be performed except in the presence of other extensive injuries precluding additional surgery, or severe contamination. With magnification and technical improvements few nerves are too small to be repaired in hand injuries. Involved digital nerves or severed median and ulnar motor branches should be identified and repaired if they are divided.

In a wound in which primary repair would be jeopardized, severed nerve ends may be identified and loosely approximated to prevent retraction and loss of proper anatomic rotation. This will facilitate secondary repair.

ANESTHESIA. General or axillary block anesthesia is used, depending on the anticipated duration and the site of the operation.

OPERATIVE PREPARATION. With the wound protected with sterile gauze to avoid further contamination, the surrounding skin is shaved and carefully prepared. The wound is then uncovered and thoroughly irrigated with several liters of warm saline.

A smooth sheet wadding is applied and a pneumatic tourniquet placed halfway between axilla and elbow. The extremity is first elevated above the level of the heart to permit venous drainage, after which an elastic bandage is applied from the tip of the extremity upward. In the normal adult a blood pressure cuff is inflated to 250 mm. mercury, or at least 80 mm. above the systolic blood pressure, and finally the elastic bandage is removed. This tourniquet may be left inflated with safety for one and one-half hours. It may be reinflated for a second hour after a 15-minute period of normal circulation.

INCISION AND EXPOSURE. For thorough debridement and to provide adequate exposure for exploration of the nerve segments, the limits of a laceration usually must be extended to the full depths of the wound. The surgeon should not hesitate to do this, but at the same time he should take care that the extended incisions do not cross flexion creases at right angles **(Figure 1).**

Local skin flaps are raised and retracted, and normal nerve above and below the lacerated portions is isolated. Dissection is carried out along the axis of the nerve toward the laceration, care being taken to preserve the small nerve branches and adjacent structures **(Figure 2).**

For the excision of a scar or neuroma a liberal incision is made to one side of and parallel with the nerve. The dissection is carried down through muscle and tissue planes along the same axis. Before the lesion is isolated, normal nerve is exposed 1 to 2 cm. above and below the lesion. Retraction of the nerve trunks, if necessary, is accomplished by moist cotton tapes **(Figure 5).** All sponging is done with moist gauze, and tissues must be moistened with saline at frequent intervals.

DETAILS OF PROCEDURE. As soon as the severed nerve ends have been identified, guide sutures of fine suture material swaged on small, curved cutting needles (atraumatic) may be placed in the epineurium of the proximal and distal segments to aid later in funicular alignment **(Figure 3).** A small ribbon retractor or tongue blade, covered with moist gauze and placed beneath the line of resection, provides a support for cutting the nerve **(Figure 3).** The nerve ends are then freed, and the frayed or damaged portions are resected in thin serial sections with a sharp knife or razor blade held perpendicular to the long axis of the nerve, until normal funiculi are observed **(Figures 3 and 4).**

A neuroma, or combination of proximal neuroma and distal glioma as is found at the time of secondary nerve repair, is similarly excised **(Figures 5, 6,** and **7).** It is helpful in making serial cuts to leave a small bridge of tissue that can serve as a handle for manipulation of the nerve **(Figure 7).** This is divided when the nerve suture is started. It is essential that all abnormal tissue be removed and that the cut surface present the appearance of normal nerve. In the course of this procedure 1 cm. or more of nerve length may be lost. This is usually of no consequence in repair, since moderate flexion of the wrist will make up the loss. During the postoperative healing period enough relaxation must be maintained to prevent tension on the anastomosis. Additional length may be obtained by carefully mobilizing the nerve trunks for several centimeters away from the cut end. If still more relaxation is needed, the proximal course of the nerve may be shortened by transplantation, as, for example, in rerouting the ulnar nerve. Nerve graft is indicated where the gap cannot be overcome without tension. The free nerve ends are then approximated and their funiculi matched as accurately as possible to restore continuity of normal pathways **(Figure 9).** The success of the repair depends largely on the precision of this maneuver. Other aids to alignment of cut ends, particularly of larger nerves, are their typical cross-sectional shape and longitudinal vessels visible on the epineurium. The previously placed guide sutures also give some idea as to the amount of rotation of a segment.

With the nerve ends properly aligned, a fine (000000) suture with swaged needle is placed across the defect, the suture picking up 1 to 2 mm. of the epineurium of each nerve end **(Figure 10).** A second suture is placed and tied on the opposite side of the nerve, approximately 120 degrees from the first. These two sutures are now used to rotate the nerve, while the edges of epineurium are approximated with 0000000000 interrupted sutures around the line of anastomosis **(Figure 12).** These sutures can be more accurately placed with the use of a loupe or other type of magnification. The sutures should include the epineurium only. Sufficient sutures are used to secure firm and accurate apposition of the cut surfaces; these are cut on the knot to reduce foreign body irritation **(Figure 13).**

The tourniquet is deflated, bleeders are clamped and ligated, and oozing is controlled by moderate local pressure. An absolutely dry field is obtained, and the wound is irrigated with warm saline to remove all clots and debris. Guide sutures are removed before closure.

CLOSURE. The wound is closed in layers, interrupted 00000 sutures being used throughout. Gauze dressing is applied, mild pressure being maintained by elastic bandage over mechanics' waste or fluffed gauze sponges to prevent oozing and hematoma formation. A plaster slab included in the dressing maintains immobilization and any relaxation of a nerve previously obtained by joint flexion.

POSTOPERATIVE CARE. An extremity with a nerve repair is kept elevated postoperatively, careful watch being maintained for signs of ischemia or hematoma formation. After four weeks, healing of the repair is such that relaxation splinting may be gradually diminished over the next three to four weeks. However, if motor paralysis and concomitant deformity such as wrist drop should follow division of the radial nerve, the deformity is corrected by proper splinting until the motor function returns. No splint should remain in place all the time, lest stiffness of joints result. Physiotherapy is used to preserve good muscle tone and to prevent ankylosis of the joints.

Protection of anesthetic areas from injury is vital. Early determination of muscle and sensory deficits is useful as a base line in evaluating subsequent rate of return of function. Electrical stimulation of denervated muscle may be used to prevent atrophy.

PLATE CLXXXII   SUTURE OF NERVE

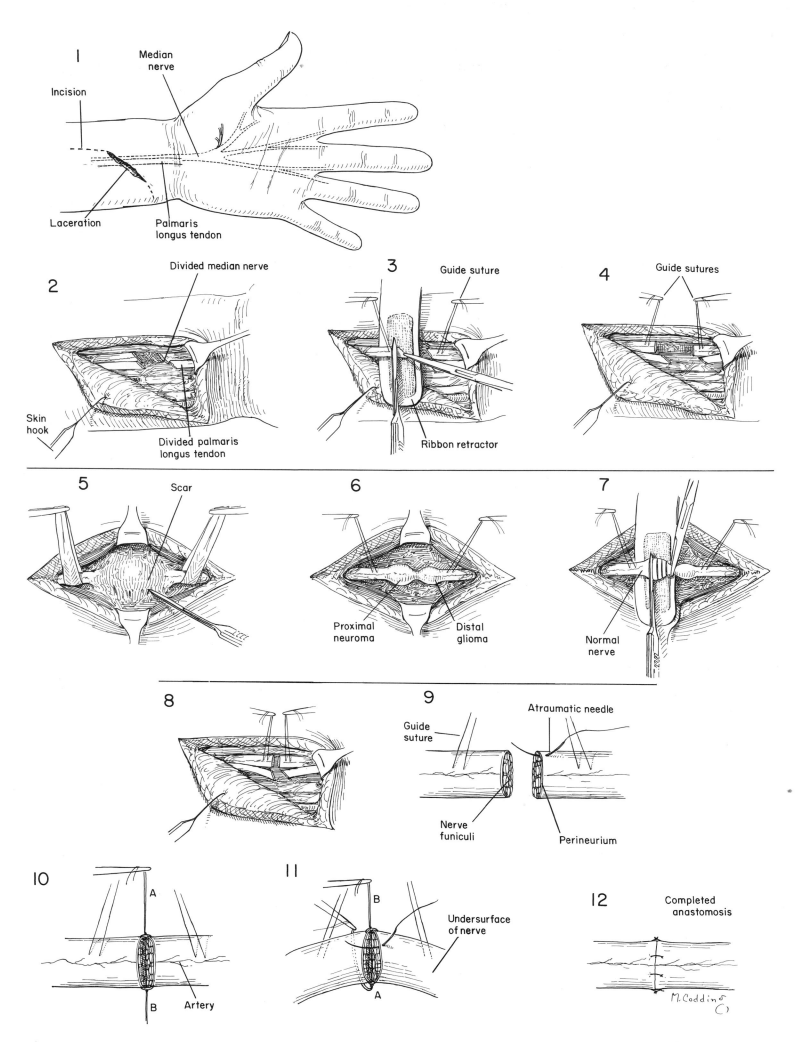

I

Incision

Median nerve

Laceration

Palmaris longus tendon

2

Divided median nerve

Skin hook

Divided palmaris longus tendon

3

Guide suture

Ribbon retractor

4

Guide sutures

5

Scar

6

Proximal neuroma

Distal glioma

7

Normal nerve

8

9

Guide suture

Atraumatic needle

Nerve funiculi

Perineurium

10

A

B

Artery

11

B

A

Undersurface of nerve

12

Completed anastomosis

M. Codding

PLATE CLXXXIII · SUTURE OF TENDON

INDICATIONS. Following trauma, primary repair of tendons is indicated, except in the presence of severe contamination or massive tissue destruction. In addition, controversy continues over the management of tendon lacerations in "no man's land" **(Figure 1),** which also includes an area at the base of the thumb over the metacarpophalangeal joint. Although flexor tendon repair in these areas is successful in children under eight years of age, a satisfactory result in an adult is difficult to attain, and a primary repair in this area should be carried out by a surgeon experienced in tendon surgery.

Repair of tendon injuries is usually undertaken no later than six hours after injury. The absence of contamination and proper local and general care of the patient may extend this period to as much as 24 hours on rare occasions. It must be remembered that tendon surgery demands precision and delicate handling of tissue and should be performed only by one thoroughly familiar with the principles involved. In this instance a poor repair is worse than none, since excess scarring inevitably produces failure. Tendon repair is contraindicated in the presence of infection.

ANESTHESIA. General or axillary block anesthesia may be used.

OPERATIVE PREPARATION. With the laceration protected by moist, sterile gauze to prevent further contamination, the surrounding skin is shaved and thoroughly cleansed with soft soap and water. Grease and other water-insoluble contaminants are removed with a suitable solvent, and the skin is prepared.

The wound is then uncovered and thoroughly irrigated with several liters of warm saline. A bloodless field is essential. A smooth sheet wadding is applied and a tourniquet placed halfway between axilla and elbow. The extremity is first elevated above the level of the heart to permit venous drainage, after which an elastic bandage is applied from the tip of the extremity upward. In the normal adult a blood pressure cuff is inflated to 250 mm. mercury, or at least 80 mm. above systolic blood pressure, and finally the elastic bandage is removed. This tourniquet may be left inflated with safety for one and one-half hours. It may be reinflated for a second hour after a 15-minute period of normal circulation.

INCISION AND EXPOSURE. Exposure must be adequate. It is usually necessary to extend the original limits of the wound **(Figure 2).** However, care must be taken that the extending incisions are anatomic, that they are on the lateral aspects of digits, that they parallel flexion creases in the palm, and that they do not cut across flexion creases in the wrist. Poorly made incisions may result in deformity.

DETAILS OF PROCEDURE. Debridement and exploration of the involved area are carried out. Adjacent nerves and vessels are identified and retracted. If possible, the tendon ends are located in the wound and grasped with forceps **(Figure 3).**

In some cases, such as lacerations of the flexor pollicis tendon, the proximal tendon stump may retract into the wrist. It is then found through a small transverse wrist incision and is threaded back through its canal by means of a metal probe and wire suture **(Figure 4).** The incision in the wrist is closed. The distal ends of most flexor tendons cut in the palm will appear in the wound on flexion of the phalanges. The proximal ends may often be forced into the wound by pressure on the corresponding muscle belly in the forearm. Blind searching for a missing tendon end should be avoided. A second incision along the course of the tendon is always preferable.

The tendon ends are manipulated by means of small, straight hemostats placed close to the cut surface. A single nonabsorbable suture with two straight needles is used for the repair. The first needle is passed through the tendon 1.5 cm. from the cut end **(Figure 5, A).** The length of the suture is made equal, and then the second needle (B) is passed obliquely about one-third of the distance to the cut end. To avoid cutting the suture with the needle, the second needle is passed obliquely through the tendon before the first is pulled through. The damaged portion of the tendon is partially cut through **(Figure 7),** and the first needle is passed obliquely through the cut end. The second suture is then placed. The opposite tendon end is opened **(Figure 8)** and the needles are passed through to the side of the tendon, then completed as illustrated **(Figures 9 and 10).** The suture ends are tightened, one at a time, by holding the tendon atraumatically just distal to the site of exit of suture **(Figure 11).** The suture is then tied. A few 000000 mattress sutures may be used at the site of anastomosis to smooth out the irregular or frayed areas.

When the anastomosis has been completed, the tourniquet is released. Hemostasis is established by pressure to control oozing and fine ties on larger vessels. The field must be dry before closure is attempted.

CLOSURE. Deep soft tissues are approximated to eliminate dead space; subcutaneous tissue and skin are closed in the usual manner with fine sutures.

Nonadherent gauze is placed over the wound, and a bulky dressing of fluffed gauze is formed. Elastic bandage should be used to maintain moderate pressure. The elastic bandage is rolled on the arm without stretching to avoid pain from excessive pressure. A dorsal or volar plaster slab incorporated in the outer layers of the dressing is used to maintain immobilization following flexor tendon repair **(Figure 13).** The wrist is held in slight flexion.

POSTOPERATIVE CARE. The extremity is kept elevated for several days at shoulder level or above with frequent exercises of the shoulder and elbow. If the patient complains of severe pain or throbbing at any time, the wound should be examined. Complete immobilization is maintained for four weeks; then the splint is removed and motion gently commenced. A week later more vigorous exercises are started and continued for three more weeks.

PLATE CLXXXIII   SUTURE OF TENDON

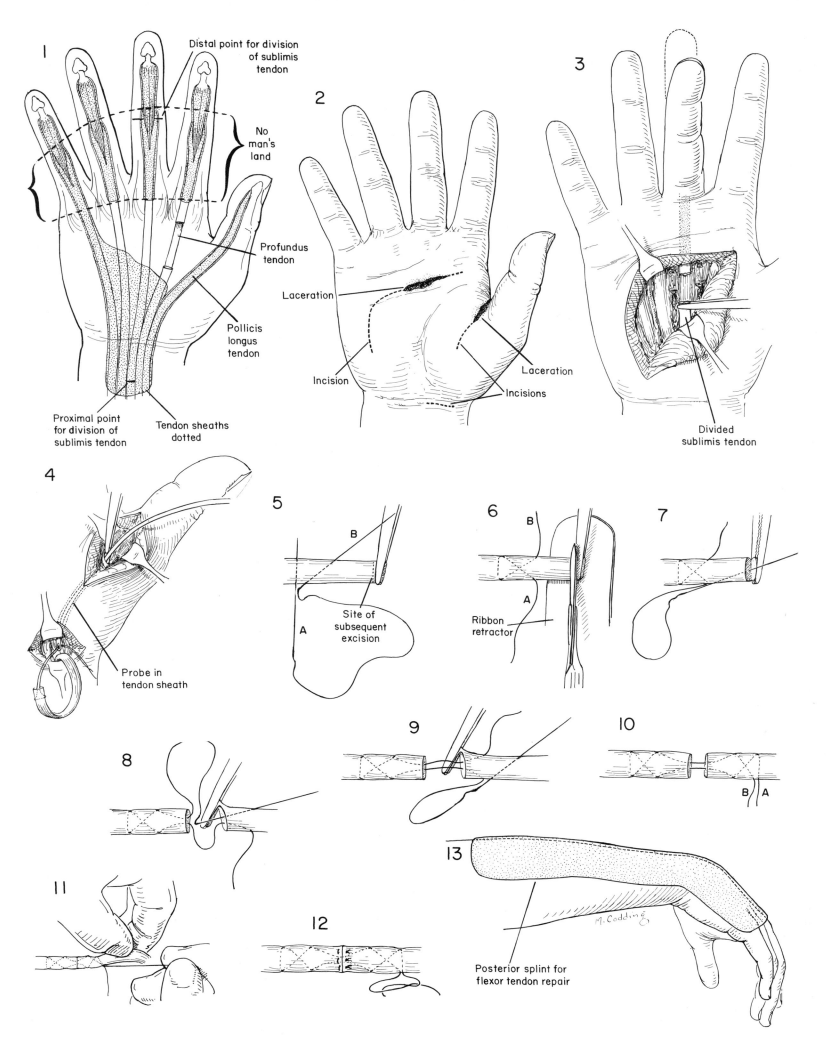

1

Distal point for division of sublimis tendon

No man's land

Profundus tendon

Pollicis longus tendon

Proximal point for division of sublimis tendon

Tendon sheaths dotted

2

Laceration

Incision

Laceration

Incisions

3

Divided sublimis tendon

4

Probe in tendon sheath

5

B

A

Site of subsequent excision

6

B

A

Ribbon retractor

7

8

9

10

B A

11

12

13

M. Codding

Posterior splint for flexor tendon repair

PLATE CLXXXIV · SKIN GRAFT

INDICATIONS. Skin defects resulting from full-thickness skin loss can be repaired by transplanting skin. The transplant may be a split-thickness free graft, a full-thickness free graft, or a pedicle flap.

Free skin grafts should be considered when the recipient site is of sufficient quality to sustain the viability of the graft during the 48 hours preceding revascularization. They are also useful when good bearing surfaces are not required, and no surgery is contemplated through the grafted area in the future. These grafts do not prevent wound contracture completely and give a less than optimum cosmetic appearance.

The thin (20- to 30-micron) grafts **(Figure 1)** are most applicable in covering granulating areas, particularly those resulting from burns. Rapid reepithelization of the donor site occurs, and this may allow additional grafts to be taken from the same area. The thin graft should not be used as a permanent cover in areas where contractures will result in functional difficulty or cosmetic deformity.

The intermediate (30- to 45-micron) and thick (56- to 66-micron) grafts **(Figure 1)** are widely applicable when the recipient site is of good quality to sustain its viability. This is most commonly found in a freshly created surgical defect. There is better resistance to contracture, and these grafts will simulate normal skin more closely than the thin graft.

Full-thickness skin graft gives the closest approximation to normal skin in appearance and is usually reserved for certain areas about the face and palmar surface of the hands and fingers. On many body surfaces, particularly areas of motion such as the axilla, elbow, and knee, a thin graft will not serve the local functional requirements and may allow contracture, fissure formation, and ulceration.

The buttocks and lateral hip areas will supply large quantities of skin as split-thickness skin graft when needed. The surgeon should be reluctant to use a donor site that will be exposed with normal dress patterns. Skin grafts taken from below the nipple line and out of the blush area will tend to develop a yellow-brown discoloration when placed on the face and neck. For this reason other donor sites in the supraclavicular area, neck, and scalp may be used for better color match for defects on the face. Hair-bearing skin should not be transplanted to a normally hairless area such as the forehead.

PREOPERATIVE PREPARATION. In the case of the burned patient, where primary excision is not to be carried out, a firm, red granulating bed is the ideal recipient site. The use of chemotherapeutic agents, wet and dry dressings, and frequent changing of dressings will aid in reducing bacterial activity. Debridement of devitalized tissue is carried out at each dressing change. The hypoproteinemia and anemia of the chronically ill, severely burned patient are barriers to successful grafting, and any such deficiencies should be corrected. Blood volume should be restored to normal. Supplementation of the oral intake by means of hyperalimentation may be required. The patient is weighed daily and his weight trend carefully observed.

ANESTHESIA. Generally, local anesthesia can be used for small excisions and skin graft. Where extensive skin grafting must be carried out, general anesthesia is usually indicated.

POSITION. The patient's position is determined by the field of operation. Not uncommonly, the patient will be on his abdomen while the graft is obtained from the back and, following dressing of the donor site, will be turned for placement of the graft on the recipient site. If a donor area is available on the same side as the recipient site, the patient's postoperative position will be one of greater comfort.

DETAILS OF PROCEDURE. A variety of instruments are available for use in obtaining split-thickness skin grafts. The choice will depend upon the individual case and the surgeon's experience. Since the invention of the dermatome the use of skin knives for free-hand cutting of a skin graft has been limited more to the rapid acquisition of small skin grafts.

Padgett Dermatome

The Padgett dermatome is the prototype for the drum dermatomes of various other designs. They may be obtained with throw-away blades and an adaptor or with a resharpenable blade. The drum and knife blade are carefully adjusted and checked, and the thickness gauge is set **(Figures 2 and 2A)**. The drum and donor site are cleansed with ether or acetone to remove grease. With either a folded sponge or a fine-bristle brush, the drum and donor site are painted with dermatome glue **(Figures 3 and 4)**. The glue must run easily. The addition of solvent will aid in obtaining the proper viscosity if the glue is too thick. Sufficient time is allowed for the glue to dry. The leading edge of the drum is placed in contact with the cemented skin and pressed firmly **(Figure 5)**. The leading drum margin is slightly raised before cutting is initiated. Constant drum pressure and rhythmical blade motion are obtained with gradual rolling of the drum upward as the cutting progresses. Care is taken that the blade does not make full-thickness cuts at the drum periphery. The attached margin of the elevated graft is severed with a sharp scalpel against the drum surface **(Figure 6)**. The graft is removed from the drum by gentle traction and rolled gently into a sponge moistened with saline until it is needed. Application of a moist compress will control bleeding from the donor area while the operation continues.

Electric and Air-Powered Dermatomes

The donor site must be a flat firm surface, the back and thighs being commonly used donor sites. The blade is checked carefully, inserted into the dermatome, and secured. When the desired width and thickness calibrations are determined and settings made, a thin layer of mineral oil is spread over the donor site, and the dermatome is placed flat on the surface. The dermatome is advanced until the desired length of skin is obtained. If a long segment of skin is to be obtained, the assistant may grasp the skin and hold it taut as the dermatome advances **(Figure 7)**. Too great a pressure may produce a greater thickness of skin than is desired; therefore, in using these dermatomes, the amount of pressure exerted becomes important. If large areas need grafting, as in extensive burns, meshing techniques may be used for greater coverage.

It is imperative that hemostasis be complete before application of the graft. If the area to be grafted is one that would be difficult to dress with a simple external pressure dressing, then a tie-over-bolus dressing may be utilized. The graft is placed into the defect. Excessive skin is trimmed from the edges, and the graft is carefully sutured to the adjacent skin with an equal number of interrupted sutures of fine silk on each side of the defect. These are tied but left uncut **(Figure 8)**. More accurate approximation of the remaining skin edges can be accomplished by further interrupted or continuous sutures as the case requires. One layer of nonadherent gauze is placed over the graft, and the area is then covered with fluffed gauze. The long sutures are then tied securely over the mound of fluffed gauze. The **(Figure 9)**. Immobilization of the area is extremely important. If the recipient site is a granulating surface, the graft is sutured to the edge of the defect with fewer sutures or held in place with adhesive strips or tissue adhesive. Before application of the dressing, the wound is checked for the presence of any blood clots under the graft. The external dressing is then applied with nonadherent gauze adjacent to the graft, supported by a firm compression dressing, carefully applied and immobilized.

Management of the Donor Area

Nonadherent gauze is applied as a single layer over the donor area. This is supported by a bulky nonocclusive gauze dressing. On the following day the outer dressing should be removed from the donor site, leaving the inner gauze adjacent to the wound. This can be left in place until it falls off as the donor site reepithelizes. If there is a large accumulation of dried serum included in this dressing, it may be advantageous to allow the patient to soak this off in the bathtub.

POSTOPERATIVE CARE. The frequency with which the dressing is changed will vary with the case. If it is elected to use no dressing over a graft, it should be protected from being rubbed or damaged by a wire cage or other protective structure. This type of dressing will allow the surgeon to evacuate seromas and hematomas as they collect beneath the graft and is used when the recipient site is less than optimal. When a tie-over dressing is used, it may be left in place for five to seven days. Inspection around the periphery of the bolus dressing from time to time will give an indication of the accumulation of fluid. When the dressing is changed, the presence of a seroma beneath the graft does not necessarily indicate a loss of the graft. The graft should be incised over the seroma and the seroma evacuated, and a firm dressing reapplied for 24 to 48 hours. However, if a hematoma is present beneath the graft and is evacuated in a similar fashion, one can expect to lose a large portion of the graft. Nevertheless, the hematoma should be evacuated and the graft redressed. Function should be resumed gradually. Grafts on the lower extremities should not be allowed to become dependent without guarded ambulation, particularly in those individuals with venous insufficiency. Increased venous pressure can cause an accumulation of edema fluid beneath the graft and cause loss of the graft as late as 14 to 21 days after grafting. After the graft has healed fully, the daily application of cold cream, lanolin, or other hydrophilic salve in small amounts will help keep it from scaling and keep it pliable. The donor area should be healed in 8 to 14 days.

PLATE CLXXXIV   SKIN GRAFT

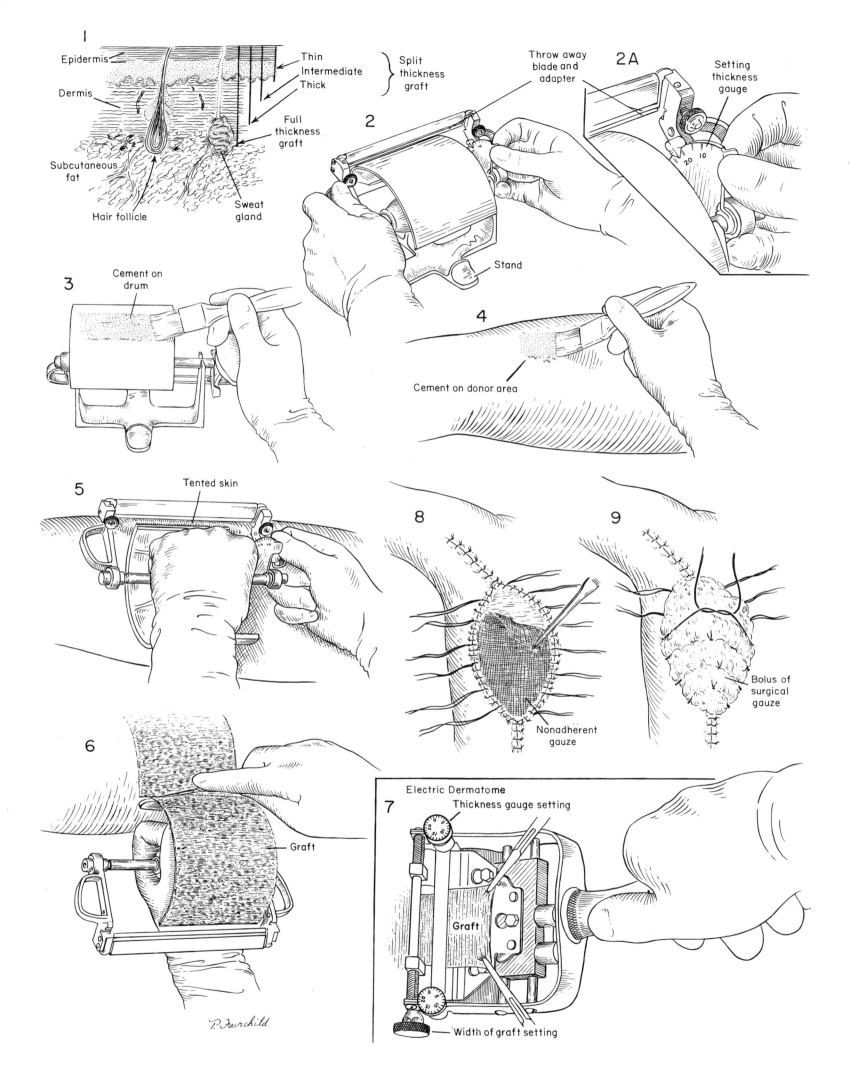

1
Epidermis
Dermis
Subcutaneous fat
Hair follicle
Sweat gland
Thin / Intermediate / Thick — Split thickness graft
Full thickness graft

2
Throw away blade and adapter
Stand

2A
Setting thickness gauge
20 10

3
Cement on drum

4
Cement on donor area

5
Tented skin

6
Graft

7
Electric Dermatome
Thickness gauge setting
Graft
Width of graft setting

8
Nonadherent gauze

9
Bolus of surgical gauze

P. Fairchild